Trace Elements in Human Health and Disease

Volume II
Essential and Toxic Elements

THE NUTRITION FOUNDATION

A Monograph Series

HORACE L. SIPPLE AND KRISTEN W. MCNUTT, EDS.: *Sugars in Nutrition*, 1974

ROBERT E. OLSON, ED.: *Protein-Calorie Malnutrition*, 1975

ANANDA S. PRASAD, ED.: *Trace Elements in Human Health and Disease, Volume I, Zinc and Copper, 1976; Volume II, Essential and Toxic Elements,* 1976

MORLEY R. KARE AND OWEN MALLER, EDS.: *The Chemical Senses and Nutrition,* 1977

JOHN N. HATHCOCK AND JULIUS COON, EDS.: *Nutrition and Drug Interrelations,* 1978

Trace Elements in Human Health and Disease

Volume II
Essential and Toxic Elements

EDITOR

Ananda S. Prasad

Division of Hematology
Department of Medicine
Wayne State University School of Medicine
Detroit, Michigan
and
Veterans Administration Hospital
Allen Park, Michigan

ASSOCIATE EDITOR

Donald Oberleas

Department of Medicine
Wayne State University School of Medicine
Detroit, Michigan
and
Research Service
Veterans Administration Hospital
Allen Park, Michigan

ACADEMIC PRESS   New York San Francisco London   1976

A Subsidiary of Harcourt Brace Jovanovich, Publishers

ACADEMIC PRESS, INC.
111 Fifth Avenue, New York, New York 10003

United Kingdom Edition published by
ACADEMIC PRESS, INC. (LONDON) LTD.
24/28 Oval Road, London NW1

Library of Congress Cataloging in Publication Data

Main entry under title:

Trace elements in human health and disease.

    (Nutrition Foundation monograph series)
    Based on the papers presented at an international
symposium on trace elements held in Detroit on
July 10–12, 1974.
    Includes bibliographies.
    CONTENTS: v. 1.   Zinc and copper.–v.2.
Essential and toxic elements.
    1.   Deficiency diseases–Congresses.   2.   Trace
element metabolism–Congresses.   3.   Trace elements
–Toxicology–Congresses.   I.   Prasad, Ananda
Shiva.   II.   Oberleas, Donald.   III.   Series:
Nutrition Foundation, New York.   Nutrition
Foundation monograph series,   [DNLM: 1.   Trace
elements–Congresses. QU130 I636t 1974]
RC623.5.T7   616.3'99   75-30471
ISBN 0–12–564202–4

Contents

26 Magnesium Deficiency and Magnesium Toxicity in Man
Edmund B. Flink

27 Magnesium Deficiency and Calcium and Parathyroid Hormone Interrelations
Maurice E. Shils

28 Biochemistry and Physiology of Magnesium
Jerry K. Aikawa

33 Metabolism and Function of Manganese
R. M. Leach, Jr.

34 Fluoride Metabolism—Effect of Preeruptive or Posteruptive Fluoride Administration on Rat Caries Susceptibility
J. M. Navia, C. E. Hunt, F. B. First, and
A. J. Narkates

35 Methodology of Trace Element Research
E. J. Underwood

36 Mineral Interrelationships
C. H. Hill

37 Perinatal Effects of Trace Element Deficiencies
Lucille S. Hurley

List of Contributors

Numbers in parentheses indicate the pages on which the authors' contributions begin.

Jerry K. Aikawa (47), Department of Medicine, School of Medicine, University of Colorado, Denver, Colorado

Ellen D. Brown (315), Department of Biochemistry, School of Medicine, George Washington University, Washington, D.C.

Raymond F. Burk (105), Department of Internal Medicine, Medical School at Dallas, University of Texas Southwestern, Dallas, Texas

Thomas W. Clarkson (453), The Medical College, Baghdad, Iraq

R. J. Doisy (79), Department of Biochemistry, State University of New York, Upstate Medical Center, Syracuse, New York

F. B. First (249), Institute of Dental Research, Department of Comparative Medicine, School of Dentistry, The University of Alabama in Birmingham, Birmingham, Alabama

Edmund B. Flink (1), Department of Medicine, West Virginia University, Morgantown, West Virginia

J. M. Freiberg (79), Departments of Biochemistry, Medicine, and Pediatrics, State University of New York, Upstate Medical Center, Syracuse, New York

H. E. Ganther (165), Department of Nutritional Sciences, University of Wisconsin, Madison, Wisconsin

D. G. Hafeman (165), Departments of Nutritional Sciences and Biochemistry, University of Wisconsin, Madison, Wisconsin

A. E. Harper (371), Departments of Nutritional Sciences and Biochemistry, University of Wisconsin, Madison, Wisconsin

C. H. Hill (281), Department of Poultry Science, North Carolina State University, Raleigh, North Carolina

W. G. Hoekstra (165), Departments of Nutritional Sciences and Biochemistry, University of Wisconsin, Madison, Wisconsin

C. E. Hunt (249), Institute of Dental Research, Department of Comparative Medicine, School of Dentistry, The University of Alabama in Birmingham, Birmingham, Alabama

Lucille S. Hurley (301), Department of Nutrition, University of California, Davis, California

R. A. Lawrence (165),* Department of Biochemistry, University of Wisconsin, Madison, Wisconsin

R. M. Leach, Jr. (235), Department of Poultry Science, The Pennsylvania State University, University Park, Pennsylvania

Orville A. Levander (135), Nutrition Institute, Agricultural Research Service, U.S. Department of Agriculture, Beltsville, Maryland

A. J. Narkates (249), Institute of Dental Research, Department of Comparative Medicine, School of Dentistry, The University of Alabama in Birmingham, Birmingham, Alabama

J. M. Navia (249), Institute of Dental Research, Department of Comparative Medicine, School of Dentistry, The University of Alabama in Birmingham, Birmingham, Alabama

F. H. Nielsen (379), Human Nutrition Laboratory, Agricultural Research Service, U.S. Department of Agriculture, Grand Forks, North Dakota

H. Mitchell Perry, Jr. (417), Medical Service, Veterans Administration Hospital, and the Hypertension Division, Department of Internal Medicine, Washington University School of Medicine, St. Louis, Missouri

Magnus Piscator (431), Department of Environmental Hygiene, Karolinska Institute, Stockholm, Sweden

A. J. Schneider (79), Departments of Biochemistry, Medicine, and Pediatrics, State University of New York, Upstate Medical Center, Syracuse, New York

R. E. Serfass (165), Department of Food and Nutrition, School of Home Economics, Winthrop College, Rock Hill, South Carolina

Maurice E. Shils (23), Department of Medicine, Memorial Hospital for Cancer and Allied Diseases, New York, New York

J. Cecil Smith, Jr. (315), Trace Element Research Laboratory, Veterans Administration Hospital, Washington, D.C.

Jack L. Smith (443), Department of Biochemistry, University of Nebraska Medical Center, and Swanson Center for Nutrition, Inc., Omaha, Nebraska

M. R. Spivey Fox (401), Division of Nutrition, Bureau of Foods, Food and Drug Administration, Department of Health, Education and Welfare, Washington, D.C.

D. H. P. Streeten (79), Departments of Biochemistry, Medicine, and

* Present address: Department of Internal Medicine, Health Science Center at Dallas, University of Texas, Dallas, Texas.

Pediatrics, State University of New York, Upstate Medical Center, Syracuse, New York

E. J. Underwood (269), Commonwealth Scientific and Industrial Research Organization, Wembley, Western Australia

Carol I. Waslien (347),* Vanderbilt University, Nashville, Tennessee, and U.S. Naval and Medical Research, Cairo, Egypt

* Present address: Department of Nutrition and Foods, Auburn University, Auburn, Alabama.

Preface

During the past decade, we have witnessed remarkable advances in the field of trace element research. Although iron and iodine have been known to be essential to man for a long period of time, it is only within the past ten years that the important role of zinc in growth and gonadal function has been recognized. The recent discovery that chromium may play an important role in late onset diabetes as an integral part of the glucose tolerance factor provides exciting possibilities for future research in clinical medicine. Basic research demonstrating the essential role of zinc in nucleic acid metabolism, the role of copper in collagen, and that of manganese in the metabolism of cartilage has been accomplished only during the past decade. Recently it has been shown that selenium is an integral part of the human red cell enzyme glutathione peroxidase, thus establishing its essential role in man. Deficiency of copper occurring in infants has been reputed, but so far manganese deficiency in man has not been recognized. A greater awareness of the basic biochemical roles of these elements is likely to uncover diseased states in man that may be influenced by use of such elements. Recent advances in analytical techniques now make it possible to measure trace elements more rapidly and with greater accuracy in biological fluids, thus allowing use of this parameter for management of certain diseased conditions in man.

Nutritionally speaking, it has become obvious that the availability of trace elements in the human diet is a complex problem which needs considerably more research. For example, the requirement of zinc may vary widely depending upon the phytate and fiber content of the diet. This presents great problems in defining requirements of zinc for different human populations.

At present, iron, iodine, copper, zinc, manganese, cobalt, molybdenum, selenium, chromium, and tin are recognized to be essential for animals. In man, deficiencies of iron, iodine, copper, and zinc have been recognized. With respect to iron and zinc, nutritional availability poses serious problems in certain segments of the human population. Cobalt is an essential part of the B_{12} molecule, and xanthine oxidase requires molybdenum for its activity. Although cobalt and molybdenum are regarded as essential elements, at least from the biochemical point of view, there is little evidence that these elements play significant roles in any aspect of human health or disease.

In this two-volume work, zinc, copper, manganese, chromium, and selenium have been included; iron and iodine have not since many reviews are available on these elements. Cobalt, molybdenum, and tin were excluded inasmuch as their specific roles in human health and disease have not been established at present, and very little is known with respect to their metabolism in man. Although classically magnesium is not considered to be a trace element it has been included because its biochemical role is similar to that of a trace element and its importance in human metabolism is unquestioned. Fluoride, although not essential, is considered to be a beneficial element for dental health, and therefore it has also been included. During the past decade, increasing interest has been aroused regarding the possible chronic deleterious effects of trace element burdens arising from the growing industrialization, motorization, and urbanization of large sections of the human race. Mercury, cadmium, and lead fall into this category, and, therefore, have also been included.

The importance of interaction between various elements is exemplified by the adverse effect of cadmium (a toxic element) on the metabolism of zinc (an essential element) in man. Such studies provide further insight into the mechanisms of toxic effects of trace elements and their correction by proper management. These aspects of trace elements provide exciting possibilities for future research in many areas of human health and disease.

I hope that this two-volume work will be useful to physicians, researchers, nutritionists, and toxicologists alike. It is based on papers presented at an International Symposium on Trace Elements and Human Disease held at Wayne State University School of Medicine, Detroit, Michigan, July 10–12, 1974. I wish to thank the contributors and reviewers of the manuscripts for their excellent cooperation. This work would not have been possible without the excellent support of The Nutrition Foundation, Dr. W. J. Darby, Dr. C. O. Chichester, Mr. Richard M. Stalvey, and Miss Kathy Hart. I wish to express my gratitude for their help. I owe thanks to my secretary Ms. Karen Harrington and to many others in my division who helped me throughout its preparation. Finally I wish to express my sincere appreciation of the understanding and unselfish support of my wife, Dr. Aryabala Prasad.

Ananda S. Prasad

Contents of Volume I: Zinc and Copper

26

Magnesium Deficiency and Magnesium Toxicity in Man

Edmund B. Flink

I. INTRODUCTION

Magnesium deficiency is fairly common in man. The principle causes are interruption of intake for prolonged periods; failure of absorptive processes for various reasons; renal wastage due to drugs, chemicals, or renal pathology; or neonatal factors, including renal wastage or intestinal malabsorption of magnesium. There may be a combination of these pathogenic factors. Magnesium deficiency is often missed or ignored. Knowledge of specific causes of magnesium depletion and of some often subtle signs and symptoms is obviously important to its recognition.

II. MAGNESIUM DEFICIENCY

A. Nutritional Aspects

Magnesium is absorbed from the entire small bowel and to a small extent from the colon, particularly in infants. Fatal intoxication has occurred in infants given magnesium sulfate enemas. The ileum is the main site for absorption (MacIntyre and Robinson, 1969). The kidneys normally conserve magnesium avidly (Barnes, 1969). The normal mean

1

serum or plasma magnesium in our laboratory is 1.77 ± 0.13 meq/liter. This value is also approximately the median value for many published reports. Jackson and Meier (1968) studied 5100 unselected consecutive patients and found a mean of 1.78 ± 0.15 meq/liter. Much has been written about methods for magnesium determinations. The most precise method is atomic absorption spectrophotometry, but similar means and ranges of values have been obtained by flame emission spectrophotometry, EDTA titration and colorimetric and fluorometric methods in our and many other laboratories. The adult human body contains from 21 to 28 gm of magnesium, or approximately 2000 meq in a 70 kg man (Whang et al., 1967). Since the skeleton has 55–60% of the magnesium, it is clear that the size of the skeleton makes a difference in the total amount in the body. Soft tissues have 40–45% of the magnesium, and extracellular fluid has less than 1%.

Magnesium is the fourth cation in terms of abundance in the human and animal body. Its high concentration in cells is like that of potassium. There are many similarities between potassium and magnesium metabolism, although magnesium is much harder to displace from the cell than potassium. In 1951, Cotlove et al. found that the concentration of potassium in cells was reduced by magnesium deficiency and that the potassium concentration in cells did not return to normal until magnesium deficiency was corrected. This has been confirmed by others (Whang et al., 1967), and the same phenomenon has been found in man by our group. Certain parallels between potassium and magnesium deficiency need to be kept in mind, since many of the causes of magnesium deficiency also cause potassium deficiency.

According to Jones et al. (1967) optimal daily intake of magnesium is 0.33–0.35 meq/kg/day in adults, but Seelig (1971) recommends 0.5 meq/kg/day. During pregnancy, the need increases to 0.5 meq/kg/day. The requirement for infants is 0.8–1.6 meq/kg/day, and for young children about 1.0 meq/kg/day. Patients have been maintained in balance with much less magnesium than cited above, but it is wise to provide what is considered optimum as indicated by these figures. Magnesium is found in abundance in both plant and animal foods. Highly purified foods such as sugars and starches and beverages such as soft drinks and alcohol have no magnesium. Cow's milk has magnesium in reasonable amount, but the high phosphate and calcium content adversely affect the magnesium utilization. This is important in infancy and early childhood. Experimental and biochemical aspects of magnesium metabolism will be discussed by Aikawa in this monograph. The reader may also be interested in comprehensive reviews by Walser (1967) and Wacker and Parisi (1968).

B. Etiology

There are many causes of clinical magnesium deficiency. Grouping the causes according to broad categories simplifies understanding of pathogenesis. An outline of causes is found in Table I. Symptomatic magnesium deficiency, of course, usually depends on severity and duration. The causes listed in Table I will be discussed in enough detail to permit a better understanding of the processes involved. In 1951, we reported an instance of prolonged parenteral magnesium-free fluid administration that resulted in hypomagnesemia and clinical manifestations that are now considered by many to be characteristic of magnesium deficiency (Fraser and Flink, 1951). This cause has been reported frequently since then. High calorie amino acid hyperalimentation fluid without adequate magnesium enhances the rate of development of deficiency. In a previously well-nourished individual, magnesium-free fluid administration of 3 weeks or longer is necessary to produce depletion. Experimental magnesium depletion in animals is enhanced by high protein and high calcium intake (Bunce et al., 1963; Colby and Frye, 1951). Large volume losses of gastrointestinal fluids simultaneously enhance deficiency, partly because of the associated interruption of food intake, but also because of significant loss of magnesium in the fluid when the volume is large (Barnes, 1969; Thoren, 1963). Burn patients are particularly vulnerable to depletion because of large volumes of exudate formed and also because of the prolonged parenteral therapy needed (Broughton et al., 1968). Complicated surgical problems resulting from trauma or mishap and requiring long maintenance on parenteral nutrition predispose the patient to magnesium depletion unless adequate magnesium supplements are used as a preventive measure during the entire illness (Baron, 1960; Broughton et al., 1968; Flink et al., 1954, 1957; Fletcher et al., 1960; Kallas, 1970; Randall et al., 1959; Smith, 1963; Thoren, 1963).

Prolonged severe diarrhea from any cause can result in magnesium depletion. Therefore, chronic ulcerative colitis and regional enteritis in an active phase, amebic colitis, or chronic laxative abuse can result in magnesium depletion. Some of these have been studied in detail by Thoren (1963), but there have been many reports of series of patients with magnesium depletion resulting from severe chronic diarrhea (Gerlach et al., 1970; Hammarsten and Smith, 1957; Thoren, 1963). In a recently studied patient, we underestimated the ongoing need for replacement, resulting in critical relapses of symptoms. Although the subject will be discussed under therapy, it is helpful to emphasize here that complete repletion is a slow process in at least some illnesses, par-

TABLE I   Causes of Magnesium Deficiency and Hypomagnesemia

A. Gastrointestinal and nutritional causes
　　1. Prolonged parenteral fluid administration without magnesium (beginning after 3 weeks)
　　2. Prolonged severe diarrhea, e.g., ulcerative colitis, regional enteritis, and chronic laxative abuse
　　3. Intestinal malabsorption
　　　　a. Idiopathic steatorrhea
　　　　b. Tropical sprue
　　　　c. Short bowel syndrome from any cause, resection for enteritis or vascular lesion, jejunocolic fistula for weight reduction, gastrojejunocolic fistula
　　4. Alcoholism
　　5. Acute and recurrent pancreatitis
　　6. Starvation with attendant metabolic acidosis
　　7. Diabetic ketoacidosis
　　8. Protein calorie malnutrition including kwashiorkor
B. Renal causes
　　1. Prolonged use of the diuretics (especially furosemide and ethacrynic acid)
　　2. Renal diseases
　　　　a. Renal tubular acidosis
　　　　b. Recovery from acute tubular necrosis (diuretic phase)
　　　　c. Chronic glomerulonephritis and pyelonephritis (rarely)
　　　　d. Familial renal magnesium wastage
　　　　e. Gentamycin induced renal injury
C. Endocrine and metabolic causes
　　1. Hyperthyroidism
　　2. Hyperparathyroidism with osteitis fibrosa cystica
　　3. Malacic bone disease with hypercalcemia
　　4. Primary and secondary aldosteronism (mineralocorticoid excess)
　　5. Excessive lactation
　　6. Congenital hypoparathyroidism
　　7. Infant born of mother with hyperparathyroidism
D. Neonatal and childhood causes
　　1. Infantile convulsions with hypomagnesemia and hypocalcemia
　　2. Newborns of diabetic mothers
　　3. Genetic (male) hypomagnesemia
　　4. Exchange transfusions

---

ticularly ongoing illnesses. Obviously, effective therapy of the primary illness is required.

Intestinal malabsorption for a number of reasons is a common factor in magnesium deficiency (Balint and Hirschowitz, 1961; Booth et al., 1963; Fletcher et al., 1960; Gerlach et al., 1970; Goldman et al., 1962; Heaton and Fourman, 1965; McIntyre et al., 1961; Muldowney et al., 1970; Nielsen and Thaysen, 1971; Opie et al., 1964). The simplest form is extensive resection of the small bowel, particularly when the ileum is resected for any reason. Malabsorption of many nutrients results. Spontaneous enterocolonic fistulae or surgically induced fistulae are also obvious causes of malabsorption. One of the complications of enterocolonic fistulae for treatment of obesity is magnesium deficiency. Steatorrhea from any cause, e.g., nontropical sprue (celiac disease), tropical sprue, or chronic pancreatic insufficiency, may result in magnesium deficiency. Steatorrhea could have an enhancing effect in addition to large intestinal fluid loss because of the loss of fats and fatty acids. Magnesium and calcium have the chemical property of combining with fatty acids to make soaps. Steatorrhea therefore can enhance magnesium and calcium loss. Some striking examples of hypocalcemia have been reported in patients with steatorrhea. The implications of low calcium due to magnesium depletion will be discussed in detail by Shils in Chapter 27. Suffice it to say that correction of magnesium depletion is necessary to correct hypocalcemia (Estep et al., 1969; Heaton and Fourman, 1965; Muldowney et al., 1970).

Alcoholism was recognized as a cause of magnesium deficiency by Flink et al. in 1954. Evidence to support this concept includes the following: hypomagnesemia occurs often (Flink et al., 1954; Heaton et al., 1962; Martin et al., 1959; Mendelson et al., 1959; Milner and Johnson, 1965; Nielsen, 1963; Smith and Hammarsten, 1959; Stutzman and Amatuzio, 1953; Sullivan et al., 1968; Sutter and Klingman, 1955); alcohol induces magnesium diuresis (Heaton et al., 1962; Kalbfleisch et al., 1963; McCollister et al., 1958, 1963); a positive external balance of magnesium amounting to a mean of 1.0 meq/kg during recovery has been demonstrated (Flink et al., 1957; Jones et al., 1969; Lim and Jacob, 1972a; McCollister et al., 1960). Low exchangeable magnesium (^{28}Mg) has been found by three groups with similar results (Jones et al., 1969; Martin and Bauer, 1962; Mendelson et al., 1965). Low magnesium concentration in muscles of patients with alcoholism at the beginning of withdrawal has been demonstrated by several investigators (Jones et al., 1969; Lim and Jacob, 1972a) to be similar to decreases observed in celiac disease and kwashiorkor (MacIntyre et al., 1961; Metcoff et al., 1960; Montgomery, 1960). Favorable response to magnesium therapy has been observed often, but not always, and low serum magnesium levels have been reported many times. Instances of severe hypomagnesemia associated with cardiac irregularity (Chadda et al., 1973; Kim et al., 1961; Loeb et al., 1968; Ricketts et al., 1969) and hypocalcemia responsive only to magnesium repletion (Estep et al., 1969) have been found in the withdrawal period. The pathogenesis of magnesium depletion in chronic alcoholism is related to magnesium loss in the urine as a result of alcohol ingestion and to the malnutrition resulting from ingestion mainly of magnesium-free calories. The malnutrition is probably the more important. Because of the high incidence of serious alcoholism world wide, alcohol is the most important cause of magnesium deficiency in adults.

Although cerebrospinal fluid has not been extensively studied, Glickman et al. (1962) found lower mean values of cerebrospinal fluid magnesium in alcoholic patients with delirium tremens than normal. The means were not significantly lower by statistical analysis, but some of the values were beyond 3 standard deviations of the mean. Chutkow and Myers (1968) has found low cerebrospinal fluid magnesium in non-alcoholic patients with magnesium deficiency and in experimental magnesium deficiency.

One of the first diseases to be identified as accompanied by hypomagnesemia are acute pancreatitis and recurrent acute pancreatitis (Edmondson et al., 1952). The more severe the episode, the more severe is the hypomagnesemia and hypocalcemia. Prolonged illness due to pancreatitis necessitating total parenteral nutrition can accentuate magnesium depletion. When alcoholism is the cause of the pancreatitis it can be an important contributing factor to magnesium depletion.

Starvation during World War II was the first recognized nutritional cause of magnesium depletion (Mellinghoff, 1949). Symptoms were not noted. The mechanism of magnesium deficiency during starvation was elucidated in the study of patients undergoing voluntary starvation for obesity (Jones et al., 1966a). An average loss of 10 meq of magnesium per day was found during total starvation. Ketoacidosis appears to be the principle pathogenic mechanism. Symptomatic magnesium deficiency has been reported after prolonged starvation for obesity. Butler et al. (1947) and Nabarro et al. (1952) demonstrated significant magnesium depletion during diabetic ketoacidosis, but no symptoms related to this were reported. Martin and Wertman (1947) reported a high incidence of hypomagnesemia in diabetic ketoacidosis. Occasionally, symptoms do occur from this cause, especially if there has been a prolonged period of acidosis.

Protein–calorie malnutrition and kwashiorkor have been recognized as causes of serious magnesium depletion since 1960 (Caddell, 1969; Metcoff et al., 1960; Muldowney et al., 1970). Evidence of this are low muscle magnesium concentration, retention of a large amount of infused magnesium, and favorable response to magnesium therapy (Caddell, 1969; Caddell et al., 1973; Montgomery, 1960, 1961). However, there is not universal agreement about the therapeutic benefits of magnesium (Rosen et al., 1970). Early serial studies (Caddell, 1969) as well as recent serial studies (Caddell et al., 1973) have demonstrated slow repletion of magnesium in muscle in this group of patients. By means of a magnesium infusion test, Caddell *et al.* (1973) has been able to demonstrate a prolonged period before there is return to a normal response, suggesting prolonged period of recovery until magnesium homeostasis is reestablished.

Diuretics have been studied intensively with respect to magnesium and calcium as well as to all electrolytes. The diuretic agents furosemide and ethacrynic acid cause a twofold or more increase in magnesium excretion (Hänze and Seyberth, 1967). Thiazide diuretics increase magnesium excretion less than furosemide and ethacrynic acid (McCollister *et al.*, 1958). Ammonium chloride and mercury diuretics also cause increased magnesium excretion in some patients. Magnesium and potassium depletion can occur simultaneously and cause serious cardiac arrhythmia or enhanced digitalis toxicity. Prescription of potassium supplementation is common, so diuretics can result in magnesium depletion, which goes undetected (Lim and Jacob, 1972b).

Renal causes of hypomagnesemia include renal tubular acidosis, recovery from acute tubular necrosis, chronic glomerulonephritis and pyelonephritis, gentamycin-induced renal injury (Holmes *et al.*, 1969), and familial renal magnesium wastage (Glickman *et al.*, 1962). Clinical symptoms of hypomagnesemia were first reported by Hirschfelder and Haury (1934) in patients with chronic renal diseases. Severe chronic renal failure as defined by a glomerular clearance rate of less than 10 ml/min is often associated with hypermagnesemia, but above this, clearance hypomagnesemia also may occur. Randall (1969) was able to produce a sharp decrease in magnesium level from high values to normal or low levels by correction of acidosis with sodium bicarbonate in patients with serious renal failure. This study illustrates the importance of knowing the condition of patients at time of blood sampling. Familial magnesium wastage is often but not always associated with hypokalemic metabolic alkalosis (Gitelman *et al.*, 1969). The critical evidence to support this diagnosis is lack of renal conservation of magnesium in spite of hypomagnesemia. The syndrome may be asymptomatic but usually has one or more of the manifestations discussed below. This is particularly true in young children. No other renal lesion is demonstrable other than renal wastage of magnesium and also potassium.

There are several endocrine disturbances associated with hypomagnesemia. Hyperthyroidism is associated with hypomagnesemia, while hypothyroidism is associated with hypermagnesemia (Jones *et al.*, 1966b; Tapley, 1955). By means of balance studies, it has been possible to demonstrate retention of magnesium during therapy of hyperthyroidism and a negative balance during thyroid replacement. It is possible that some of the manifestations of thyroid crises are due to magnesium deficiency, but this is not clearly established. When ^{28}Mg is used as a tracer, exchangeable magnesium actually is diminished in hypothyroidism (Dimich et al., 1966). The paradoxically diminished exchangeable magnesium in the face of demonstrated increase of body magnesium makes interpretation of ^{28}Mg studies more difficult.

Hyperparathyroidism has resulted in symptomatic magnesium deficiency in isolated instances (Agna and Goldsmith, 1958; Harman, 1956; Heaton and Pyrah, 1963; Potts and Roberts, 1958). It appears that the patients who develop hypomagnesemia with or without symptoms postoperatively are primarily those with osteitis fibrosa cystica or marked hypercalcemia. Hypercalcemia from other causes also may be associated with hypomagnesemia, with or without symptoms (Eliel et al., 1969), probably because hypercalcemia promotes magnesium excretion. Parathyroid extract administration to hypoparathyroid patients produces increased renal conservation initially, followed by increased magnesium excretion, but many variations in response to parathyroid extract occur. Hypomagnesemia may be associated with congenital hypoparathyroidism and is either transient due to maternal hyperparathyroidism, or permanent due to a rare instance of familial hypoparathyroidism. Of course, hypocalcemia is a prominent or dominant feature of such instances.

Primary and secondary aldosteronism causes magnesium loss (Cohen et al., 1970; Gitelman et al., 1969; Mader and Iseri, 1955). A patient with mineralocorticoid excess due to tumor of the adrenal cortex had quite low magnesium levels and had intermittent tetany. A number of patients with aldosteronism have had tetany. Secondary aldosteronism in cirrhosis accounts for the hypomagnesemia found in children and adults with cirrhosis and ascites and edema. The hypomagnesemia responds to an aldosterone antagonist. Deoxycorticosterone also causes magnesium loss. Lactation has resulted in hypomagnesemia and tetany in a "wet nurse" producing a very large volume of milk (Greenwald et al., 1963).

There are many instances of infantile hypomagnesemia, which often is associated with hypocalcemia (Black et al., 1962; Friedman et al., 1967; Haijamae and MacDowall, 1972; Keipert, 1969; Nordia et al., 1971; Paunier et al., 1965; Skyberg et al., 1967; Strømme et al., 1969; Tsang, 1972; Wong and Teh, 1968). The pathogenesis is varied and complex as outlined in an excellent summary by Tsang (1972). Among those cases most easily explained are infants born to diabetic mothers or mothers with sprue who have low serum magnesium levels (Clarke and Carré, 1967). Exchange transfusions to infants result in chelation of magnesium and calcium by citrate. Symptoms are usually transient but can be serious (Bajpai et al., 1967).

A syndrome in male infants is characterized by hypomagnesemia and hypocalcemia and is due to malabsorption of magnesium from the gut (Friedman *et al.*, 1967; Haijamae and MacDowall, 1972; Keipert, 1969; Nordia *et al.*, 1971; Paunier *et al.*, 1965, 1968; Skyberg *et al.*, 1967; Strømme *et al.*, 1969). Therapy with parenteral magnesium salts initially followed by oral magnesium supplements corrects the symptoms. In addition to this fairly specific syndrome dependent on intestinal malabsorption, there are many infants and young children of both sexes who develop hypomagnesemia and hypocalcemia with symptoms responding only to magnesium therapy. These patients usually recover completely without need for continued therapy. These patients include those with protracted diarrhea and those who fail to thrive and feed properly. The feeding of cow's milk formula (high phosphate) appears to be important in many patients with transient symptoms (Tsang, 1972). Recognition of the high probability of hypomagnesemia as a cause of neonatal or early childhood convulsions is important, since therapy is specific and may be lifesaving and prevent brain damage.

In a patient with any of the above causes, establishing a diagnosis of magnesium deficit is still difficult. Hypomagnesemia (more than 2 standard deviations below the mean) is not conclusive evidence per se, and a big deficit can occur without hypomagnesemia (Caddell and Olson, 1973; Caddell *et al.*, 1973; Jones *et al.*, 1969; Opie *et al.*, 1964). Erythrocyte magnesium concentration has been used by man, but red cells are not quickly responsive to a deficit (Smith and Hammarsten, 1959). Total external balance studies are the most convincing evidence, but such a study is often not feasible. Magnesium infusion tests afford fairly good evidence and often are feasible. The amount of magnesium in the urine in 24 hr or 48 hr, depending on test, is subtracted from the amount of magnesium given intravenously over a 6 hr period (Caddell *et al.*, 1973; Thoren, 1963). Unequivocal response of patients' symptoms that have not responded to other measures is also good evidence. Muscle biopsy and chemical analysis are good evidence, but are of no use in assessing immediate need and also are not generally available. A sum of clinical evidence and chemical evidence ultimately is needed to establish a diagnosis of magnesium-deficiency syndrome.

C. Manifestations

There is no doubt that even severe hypomagnesemia associated with a significant deficit may be totally asymptomatic and remain undetected clinically (Flink *et al.*, 1957; Hanna *et al.*, 1960; Martin *et al.*, 1952). There has been considerable controversy about characteristic manifestations, but many investigators during the past twenty years have supported the concept of a multifaceted and varied syndrome. There is no consensus on the matter.

It is quite clear that the word tetany is far too restrictive and not really descriptive. Hirschfelder and Haury (1934) reported seven patients who had low magnesium and had muscular twitching or convulsions and concluded that "there is a clinical syndrome of low magnesium (hypomagnesemia) accompanied by muscular twitching or by convulsions." Miller (1944) reported the occurrence of tremor and muscular twitching in a 6-year-old boy with magnesium as low as 0.5 meq/liter. In 1951, we reported a patient who had remarkable symptoms and signs following prolonged parenteral fluid administration (Fraser and Flink, 1951). The manifestations cleared in 24 hr after parenteral magnesium sulfate. These manifestations and further observations on many patients resulted in the following description (Flink et al., 1957): "A clinical syndrome characterized by muscle tremor, twitching and more bizarre movements, occasionally by convulsions and often by delirium, has been described and is considered to be characteristic of magnesium deficiency." Sudden onset of symptoms has been noted repeatedly, and Kellaway and Ewen (1962) described this very well: "It appeared remarkable that a gradual magnesium depletion which occurred over the course of some thirty days should blossom forth into such a florid 'syndrome' during an interval of a few hours." Hanna et al. (1960) emphasized the sudden occurrence of convulsions in a previously asymptomatic patient.

For sake of clarity a list of manifestations that have been reported many times is as follows (note that an individual may have one or many manifestations but not all at one time).

1. Muscular twitching and tremor of any or all muscles including the tongue
2. Athetoid and choreiform movements (rare)
3. Vertigo, ataxia and nystagmus (rare)
4. Muscle wasting muscle weakness
5. Positive Chvostek sign (fairly common)
6. Numbness and tingling (fairly common)
7. Positive Trousseau sign (rare)
8. Spontaneous carpopedal spasm or tetany (rare)
9. Convulsions
10. Sweating and tachycardia
11. Apathy, depression, and poor memory

12. Mild to severe delirium (confusion, disorientation, hallucinations, and paranoia)

13. Premature ventricular beats, ventricular tachycardia, and ventricular fibrillation

14. Coma

15. Death

Emphasis should be placed on neuromuscular and psychiatric aspects of the above list rather than on the more restrictive idea of tetany. When a patient has one of the causes and any of the manifestations listed above, the possibility of magnesium deficiency must be considered.

The frequent association of hypocalcemia with hypomagnesemia of infancy or in alcoholism, steatorrhea, and malabsorption from any cause has become apparent in the past decade but has been reported as an isolated finding in individual patients before this. The failure of intravenous calcium infusion to influence symptoms and signs, the failure to correct the hypocalcemia, and the correction of hypocalcemia symptoms and signs and hypomagnesemia by parenteral magnesium and later large oral doses is noteworthy. Magnesium and parathyroid interrelationships have been discussed in Chapter 27 by Shils.

Tetany in the sense of carpal and pedal spasm, muscle rigidity, and even opisthotonus occurs particularly in infants and young children but can also occur in adults, particularly in those with malabsorption. It usually is associated with hypocalcemia, as noted above, but may occur with normal or near normal calcium. I have seen only one adult patient with hypomagnesemia and normal calcium who had typical tetany with spontaneous carpal and pedal spasms and muscle rigidity.

Cardiac symptoms and signs deserve special mention. Cardiac arrhythmia, including frequent premature ventricular contractions, ventricular tachycardia, and ventricular fibrillation, have been reported (Chadda et al., 1973; Kim et al., 1961; Loeb et al., 1968; Ricketts et al., 1969; Seller et al., 1970). Digitalis toxicity is enhanced by magnesium deficiency in animals and man. Sudden death (Miller, 1944) in alcoholism, especially during withdrawal, could be related to tachyarrhythmia associated with hypomagnesemia. The danger is enhanced by hypokalemia, of course. The role of magnesium depletion in alcoholic cardiomyopathy is not clear at present (Alexander, 1966; Sullivan et al., 1968).

Magnesium depletion is important in the early manifestations of the alcohol withdrawal syndrome. Wolfe and Victor (1969) showed that there was a greatly exaggerated photic sensitivity as measured by photomyoclonus. The sensitivity was directly proportionate to the severity of hypomagnesemia. The sensitivity could be abolished by an intravenous infusion of magnesium sulfate. They also clearly documented the occurrence of hyperventilation alkalosis during the first 48 hr after withdrawal from alcohol.

Controversy still surrounds the role of magnesium deficiency in pathogenesis of the alcohol withdrawal syndrome. Delirium (confusion, hallucinations, delusions, violent behavior), tremor, and convulsions may occur in alcoholism as well as in nonalcohol-induced magnesium deficiency. Because of the dramatic improvement of neuromuscular symptoms in a number of patients treated with magnesium salts and symptomatology in common with magnesium deficiency from other causes, manifestations of alcohol withdrawal have been ascribed to magnesium depletion (Flink et al., 1954, 1957, 1973). The apparent complete failure to alter the course of some delirious patients with magnesium therapy is unexplained at present and is the principle reason for doubting the validity of the above hypothesis (Vallee et al., 1960). It is possible that the regular occurrence of an elevation of free fatty acids accounts for the seeming paradox (Flink et al., 1973). Chelation of Mg^{2+} by free fatty acids could produce significant lowering of Mg^{2+} in serum and also affect magnesium at the cell membrane. Magnesium at physiological concentration is precipitated by free fatty acids in concentrations that occur in alcohol withdrawal.

Durlach (1969) has been a strong proponent for the view that many patients with none of the usual causes listed above have magnesium deficiency and "spasmophilia." The diagnosis is based on decreased erythrocyte magnesium; abnormal and characteristic electroencephalogram, electronystagmogram, and electromyogram; and a positive Chvostek's sign. Oral magnesium supplements are used with success usually after many months. The inclusion of these patients as examples of magnesium deficiency is still not accepted generally.

D. Therapy

Therapy of patients with magnesium salts can be safely carried out by following the guidelines below. The program has been used with many hundreds of patients and is safe and effective (Flink, 1969). It is worth noting that this schedule of treatment calls for about one-fourth of the dose given in the treatment of eclampsia (Flowers et al., 1962). The following guidelines are suggested for treatment of magnesium deficiency regardless of etiology:

1. It is important to know that the kidneys are producing urine and the BUN (blood urea nitrogen) and/or creatinine are normal. Mag-

nesium may be needed and may be administered even in an instance of renal insufficiency, but the treatment must be monitored by serum or plasma levels frequently.

2. On the first day of therapy at least 1 meq Mg/kg/day should be given parenterally. Subsquently, at least 0.5 meq Mg/kg/day should be given for 3–5 days. If parenteral fluid therapy continues, at least 0.2 meq/kg/day should be given.

3. Give the above in intravenous infusions if such infusions are being given anyway; otherwise, intramuscular administration is satisfactory.

4. The following schedule for an average adult is safe and effective. (a) *Intramuscular route* (ampules with 1 gm $MgSO_4 \cdot 7H_2O$—50% solution = 8.13 meq Mg) Day 1: 2.0 gm (16.3 meq) every 4 hr for six doses. Day 2–5: 1.0 gm (8.1 meq) every 6 hr. (b) *Intravenous route* (same ampules) Day 1: 5 gm (41 meq) in each liter of fluid and at least 2 liters of 83 meq. Day 2–5: A total of 6 gm (49 meq) distributed equally in total fluids of the day.

If the patient's condition requires continued intravenous infusions, 2 gm of $MgSO_4$ should be given daily in the infusion as long as infusions are necessary. When a patient who has a reason to have magnesium deficiency *is* convulsing, 2.0 gm of $MgSO_4$ solution should be administered intravenously in a 10 min period. For infants and children, the dose should be 0.025 gm $MgSO_4$/kg in 10 min.

Magnesium repletion may be slow particularly in malnourished children (Caddell and Olson, 1973; Caddell *et al.*, 1973; Montgomery, 1961), in malabsorption syndromes (Goldman *et al.*, 1962; Heaton and Fourman, 1965; Opie *et al.*, 1964) and in alcoholism (Flink *et al.*, 1957; Jones *et al.*, 1969). Chutkow (1974) demonstrated a time lag or slow response to injected magnesium for the correction of sensitivity to audiogenic seizures in magnesium-deficient rats. This confirms clinical impressions. The response is quite different from the immediate response of hypocalcemic tetany to calcium injection. Magnesium therapy must be continued to 4 days intensively, as noted above, and at a lower dose, as noted above, if interference with normal oral feedings continues. Unless therapy is continued, relapses are apt to occur in the most severely depleted patients.

III. MAGNESIUM INTOXICATION

Magnesium intoxication and hypermagnesemia occur primarily in patients with serious renal insufficiency and in eclampsia when magnesium salts are administered in large doses. Excess magnesium appears to block neuromuscular transmission owing to diminution in endplate potential (Engbaek, 1952; Goodman and Gilman, 1970). As levels begin to exceed 4 meq/liter, the deep tendon reflexes are decreased and may be absent at levels approaching 10 meq/liter. At this point, respiratory paralysis is a hazard. Cardiac consequences may be seen in the form of heart block at levels below 10 meq/liter. As long as deep tendon reflexes are active, it is probable that the patient will not develop respiratory paralysis. The central depression and peripheral nerve transmission defects produced by the magnesium ion can be antagonized by a calcium injection. Calcium salt solution for intravenous use should be available immediately whenever large doses of magnesium salts are used in therapy for eclampsia, for instance.

Infants born to mothers who have had $MgSO_4$ treatment for eclampsia are at risk to develop magnesium intoxication manifested as depression and hypotonia. Lipsitz and English (1967) reported 16 infants of mothers treated with doses of 16–60 gm of $MgSO_4$ in 8–33 hours. Cord blood magnesium was 3.0–11.5 meq/liter in this group. Three exhibited severe depression and died. If $MgSO_4$ is going to be used in treatment of eclampsia, the dose should be determined by careful monitoring of blood levels and the avoidance of levels sufficient to abolish tendon reflexes. Marked hypermagnesemia in man and animals is associated with hypocalcemia (Monif and Savory, 1972).

Birth asphyxia can cause significant hypermagnesemia and hyperkalemia. Hypermagnesemia in infants induces hypothermia. Hypermagnesemia induced in infants of mothers with eclampsia also may develop meconium plug syndrome (Sokal et al., 1972).

An important cause of magnesium intoxication is the use of magnesium-containing antacids such as $Mg(OH)_2$ or magnesium trisilicate, as described by Randall (1969; Randall et al., 1964) in patients with renal failure. One interesting facet of these studies is the relatively low concentrations that contribute to intoxication. This phenomenon could be due to the observation by Fishman and Raskin (1967) that a high urea concentration results in transcellular transfer of cations. The warning about hazards of magnesium toxicity in patients with renal failure who use magnesium-containing antacids is important.

Magnesium has been used in anesthesia. Belsche et al. (1964) used various calcium and magnesium salts in dogs and rabbits and found that calcium gluconate and magnesium gluconate produced clinically satisfactory spinal anesthesia lasting 2 hr. There were no neurological sequelae. Aldrete et al. (1968) produced muscle relaxation with magnesium intravenously in dogs at about 12 meq/liter, but no real anesthesia at even higher levels. Muscle paralysis caused respiratory insufficiency with hypoxia and a sleeplike state. Somjen *et al.* (1960) also failed to produce anesthesia with magnesium infusions given to humans.

IV. SUMMARY

The magnesium deficiency syndrome can be caused by a large number of physiological disturbances, such as malabsorption, renal wastage, or inadequate food intake, and is characterized by a wide spectrum of manifestations, particularly neuromuscular disturbances and delirium. Knowledge of these causes and manifestations is necessary to detect and treat this often neglected syndrome.

Magnesium intoxication occurs primarily in three settings—treatment of eclampsia with attendant neonatal depression of vital functions; accidental or intentional poisoning; and moderately severe to severe renal failure. When magnesium-containing medications are taken by a patient with renal failure, intoxication often results.

REFERENCES

Agna, J. W., and Goldsmith, R. E. (1958). Primary hyperparathyroidism associated with hypomagnesemia. *N. Engl. J. Med.* **258,** 222–225.

Aldrete, J. A., Barnes, D. R., and Aikawa, J. K. (1968). Does magnesium produce anesthesia? *Anesth. Anal. (Cleveland)* **47,** 428–433.

Alexander, C. (1966). Idiopathic heart disease. Electron microscopic examination of myocardial biopsy in alcoholic heart disease. *Amer. J. Med.* **41,** 229–234.

Bajpai, P. C., Sugden, D., Stern, L., and Denton, R. L. (1967). Serum ionic magnesium in exchange transfusion. *J. Pediat.* **70,** 193–199.

Balint, J. A., and Hirschowitz, B. I. (1961). Hypomagnesemia with tetany in nontropical sprue. *N. Engl. J. Med.* **265,** 631–633.

Barnes, B. A. (1969). Magnesium conservation, a study of surgical patients. *Ann. N.Y. Acad. Sci.* **162,** 786–802.

Baron, D. N. (1960). Magnesium deficiency after gastrointestinal surgery and loss of excretions. *Brit. J. Surg.* **48,** 344–346.

Belsche, J. D., Buckley, J. J., and VanBergen, F. H. (1964). Use of calcium and magnesium cations as spinal anesthetics. *Univ. Minn. Med. Bull.* **35,** 369–370.

Black, E. H., Montgomery, R. D., and Ward, E. E. (1962). Neurological manifestations in infantile gastroenteritis and malnutrition. *Arch. Dis. Childhood* **37,** 106–109.

Booth, C. C., Babouris, N., Hanna, S., and MacIntyre, I. (1963). Incidence of hypomagnesemia in intestinal malabsorption. *Brit. Med. J.* **2,** 141–144.

Broughton, A., Anderson, I. R. M., and Bowden, C. H. (1968). Magnesium deficiency syndrome in burns. *Lancet* **2,** 1156–1158.

Bunce, G. E., Reeves, P. G., Oba, T. S., and Sauberlich, H. E. (1963). Influence of the dietary protein level on the magnesium requirement. *J. Nutr.* **79,** 220–226.

Butler, A. M., Talbot, N. B., Burnett, C. H., Stanbury, J. B., and MacLachlan, E. A. (1947). Metabolic studies in diabetic coma. *Trans. Ass. Amer. Physicians* **60,** 102–109.

Caddell, J. L. (1969). Magnesium deficiency in protein-calorie malnutrition: A follow-up study. *Ann. N.Y. Acad. Sci.* **162,** 874–890.

Caddell, J. L., and Olson, R. E. (1973). An evaluation of the electrolyte status of malnourished Thai children. *J. Pediat.* **83,** 124–128.

Caddell, J. L., Suskind, R., Sillup, H., and Olson, R. E. (1973). Parenteral magnesium load evaluation of malnourished Thai children. *J. Pediat.* **83,** 129–135.

Chadda, H. D., Lichstein, E., and Gupta, P. (1973). Hypomagnesemia and refractory cardiac arrhythmias in a nondigitalized patient. *Amer. J. Cardiol.* **31,** 98–100.

Chutkow, J. G. (1974). Clinical-chemicl correlations in the encephalopathy of magnesium deficiency. *Mayo Clin. Proc.* **49,** 244–247.

Chutkow, J. G., and Myers, S. B. (1968). Chemical changes in cerebrospinal fluid and brain in magnesium deficiency. *Neurology* **18,** 963–974.

Clarke, P. C. N., and Carré, I. J. (1967). Hypocalcemic, hypomagnesemic convulsions. *J. Pediat.* **70,** 806–809.

Cohen, M. I., McNamera, H., and Finberg, L. (1970). Serum magnesium in children with cirrhosis. *J. Pediat.* **76,** 453–455.

Colby, R. W., and Frye, C. M. (1951). Effect of feeding high levels of protein and calcium in rat rations on magnesium deficiency syndrome. *Amer. J. Physiol.* **166,** 408–412.

Cotlove, E., Holliday, M. A., Schwartz, R., and Wallace, W. M. (1951). Effect of electrolyte depletion and acid-base disturbance on muscle cations. *Amer. J. Physiol.* **167,** 665–675.

Dimich, A., Rizek, J. E., Wallach, S., and Silver, W. (1966). Magnesium transport in patients with thyroid disease. *J. Clin. Endocrinol. Metab.* **26,** 1081–1092.

Durlach, J. (1969). "Spasmophilia and Magnesium Deficit." Masson, Paris.

Edmonson, H. A., Berne, C. J., Homann, R. E., and Wertman, M. (1952). Calcium, potassium, magnesium and amylase disturbances in acute pancreatitis. *Amer. J. Med.* **12,** 34–42.

Eliel, L. P., Smith, W. O., Chanes, R., and Howrylko, J. (1969). Magnesium metabolism in hyperparathyroidism and osteolytic disease. *Ann. N.Y. Acad. Sci.* **162,** 810–830.

Engbaek, L. (1952). Pharmacological actions of magnesium ions with particular reference to neuromuscular and cardiovascular system. *Pharmacol. Rev.* **4,** 396–414.

Estep, H., Shaw, W. A., Waltington, C., Hobe, R., Holland, W., and Tucker, S. G. (1969). Hypocalcemia due to hypomagesemia and reversible parathyroid hormone unresponsiveness. *J. Clin. Endocrinol. Metab.* **29,** 842–848.

Fishman, R. A., and Raskin, N. H. (1967). Experimental uremic encephalopathy. Permeability and electrolyte metabolism of brain and other tissues. *Arch. Neurol. (Chicago)* **17,** 10–21.

Fletcher, R. F., Henly, A. A., Sammons, H. G., and Squire, J. R. (1960). A case of magnesium deficiency following massive intestinal resection. *Lancet* **1,** 522–525.

Flink, E. B. (1956). Magnesium deficiency syndrome in man. *J. Amer. Med. Ass.* **160,** 1406–1409.

Flink, E. B. (1969). Therapy of magnesium deficiency. *Ann. N.Y. Acad. Sci.* **162,** 901–905.

Flink, E. B., Stutzman, F. L., Anderson, A. R., Konig, T., and Fraser, R. (1954). Magnesium deficiency after prolonged parenteral fluid administration and after chronic alcoholism, complicated by delirium tremens. *J. Lab. Clin. Med.* **43,** 169–183; *J. Clin. Invest.* **32,** 568 (1953) (abst.).

Flink, E. B., McCollister, R., Prasad, A. S., Melby, J. D., and Doe, R. P. (1957). Evidences for clinical magnesium deficiency. *Ann. Intern. Med.* **47,** 956–968.

Flink, E. B., Flink, P. F., Shane, S. R., Jones, J. E., and Steffes, P. E. (1973). Magnesium and free fatty acids in alcoholism. *Clin. Res.* **21,** 884.

Flowers, C. E., Jr., Easterling, W. E., Jr., White, F. D., Jung, J. M., and Fox, J. T., Jr. (1962). Magnesium sulfate in toxemia of pregnancy. *Obstet. Gynecol.* **19,** 315–327.

Fraser, R., and Flink, E. B. (1951). Magnesium, potassium, phosphorus, chloride and vitamin deficiency as a result of prolonged use of parenteral fluids. *J. Lab. Clin. Med.* **38,** 809.

Friedman, M., Hatcher, G., and Watson, L. (1967). Primary hypomagnesemia with secondary hypocalcemia in an infant. *Lancet* **1,** 703–705.

Gerlach, K., Morowitz, D. A., and Kirsner, J. B. (1970). Symptomatic hypomagnesemia complicing regional enteritis. *Gastroenterology* **59,** 567–574.

Gerst, P. H., Porter, M. R., and Fishman, R. A. (1964). Symptomatic magnesium deficiency in surgical patients. *Ann. Surg.* **159,** 402–406.

Gitelman, H. J., Graham, J. B., and Welt, L. G. (1969). A familial disorder characterized by hypokalemia and hypomagnesemia. *Ann. N.Y. Acad. Sci.* **162,** 856–864.

Glickman, L. S., Schenker, V., Gronick, S., Green, A., and Schenker, A. (1962). Cerebrospinal fluid cation levels in delirium tremens with special reference to magnesium. *J. Nerv. Ment. Dis.* **134,** 410–414.

Goldman, L. A., Fossan, D. D. V., and Baird, E. E. (1962). Magnesium deficiency in celiac disease. *Pediatrics* **29,** 948–952.

Goodman, L. S., and Gilman, A., eds. (1970). "Pharmacological Basis of Therapeutics," 4th ed., pp. 811–814. Macmillan, New York.

Greenwald, J. H., Dubin, A., and Cardon, L. (1963). Hypomagnesemic tetany due to excessive lactation. *Amer. J. Med.* **35,** 854–860.

Haijamae, H., and MacDowall, I. G. (1972). Distribution of divalent cations at the cellular level during primary hypomagnesemia in infancy. *Acta Paediat. Scand.* **61,** 591–596.

Hammarsten, J. F., and Smith, W. O. (1957). Symptomatic magnesium deficiency in man. *N. Engl. J. Med.* **256,** 897–899.

Hanna, S., MacIntyre, I., Harrison, M., and Fraser, R. (1960). The syndrome of magnesium deficiency in man. *Lancet* **2,** 172–175.

Hänze, S., and Seyberth, H. (1967). Untersuchungen zur Wirkung der Diuretica Furosemide, Ethacrynsaure and Triamiteren auf die renale Magnesium und Calcium-ausscheidung. *Klin. Wochenschr.* **45,** 313–314.

Harman, M. (1956). Parathyroid adenoma in a child. *Amer. J. Dis. Child.* **91,** 313–325.

Heaton, F. W, and Fourman, P. (1965). Magnesium deficiency and hypocalcemia in intestinal malabsorption. *Lancet* **2,** 50–52.

Heaton, F. W., and Pyrah, L. N. (1963). Magnesium metabolism in patients with parathyroid disorders. *Clin. Sci.* **25,** 475–485.

Heaton, F. W., Pyrah, L. N., Beresford, C. C., Bryson, R. W., and Martin, D. F. (1962). Hypomagnesmia in chronic alcholism. *Lancet* **2**, 802–805.

Hirschfelder, A. D., and Haury, V. G. (1934). Clinical manifestations of high and low plasma magnesium. Dangers of Epsom salt purgation in nephritis. *J. Amer. Med. Ass.*, **102**, 1138–114.

Holmes, A. M., Hesling, C. M., and Wilson, T. M. (1969). Drug induced secondary aldosteronism in patients with pulmonary tuberculosis. *Quart. J. Med.* **39**, 299–315.

Jackson, C. E., and Meier, D. W. (1968). Routine serum magnesium analysis. *Ann. Intern. Med.* **69**, 743–748.

Jones, J. E., Albrink, M. J., Davidson, P. D., and Flink, E. B. (1966a). Fasting and refeeding of various suboptimal isocaloric diets. *Amer. J. Clin. Nutr.* **19**, 320–328.

Jones, J. E., Desper, P. C., Shane, S. R., and Flink, E. B. (1966b). Magnesium metabolism in hyperthyroidism and hypothyroidism. *J. Clin. Invest.* **45**, 891–900.

Jones, J. E., Manalo, R., and Flink, E. B. (1967). Magnesium requirements in adults. *Amer. J. Clin. Nutr.* **20**, 632–635.

Jones, J. E., Shane, S. R., Jacobs, W. H., and Flink, E. B. (1969). Magnesium balance studies in chronic alcoholism. *Ann. N.Y. Acad. Sci.* **162**, 934–946.

Kalbfleisch, J. M., Lindeman, R. D., Ginn, H. E., and Smith, W. O. (1963). Effects of ethanol administration on urinary excretion of magnesium and other electrolytes in alcoholic and normal subjects. *J. Clin. Invest.* **42**, 1471–1475.

Kallas, T. (1970). Symptomatic magnesium deficiency in urological patients. *J. Urol.* **104**, 325–327.

Keipert, J. A. (1969). Primary hypomagnesemia with secondary hypocalcemia in an infant. *Med. J. Aust.* **2**, 242–244.

Kellaway, G., and Ewen, K. (1962). Magnesium deficiency complicating prolonged gastric suction. *N. Z. Med. J.* **61**, 137–142.

Kim, Y. W., Andrews, C. E., and Ruth, W. E. (1961). Serum magnesium and cardiac arrhythmias with special reference to digitalis intoxication. *Amer. J. Med. Sci.* **242**, 87–92.

Lim, P., and Jacob, E. (1972a). Magnesium status of alcoholic patients. *Metab., Clin. Exp.* **21**, 1045–1051.

Lim, P., and Jacob, E. (1972b). Magnesium deficiency in patients on long-term diuretic therapy for heart failure. *Brit. Med. J.* **3**, 620–622.

Lipsitz, P. J., and English, I. C. (1967). Hypermagnesemia in the newborn infant. *Pediatrics* **40**, 856–862.

Loeb, H. S., Pietras, R. P., Gunnar, R. M., and Tobin, J. R. (1968). Paroxysmal ventricular fibrillation in two patients with hypomagnesemia. *Circulation* **37**, 210–215.

McCollister, R. J., Prasad, A. S., Doe, R. P., and Flink, E. B. (1958). Normal renal magnesium clearance and the effect of water loading, chlorthiazide and ethanol on magnesium excretion. *J. Lab. Clin. Med.* **52**, 928.

McCollister, R. J., Flink, E. B., and Doe, R. P. (1960). Magnesium balance studies in chronic alcoholism. *J. Lab. Clin. Med.* **55**, 98–104.

McCollister, R. J., Flink, E. B., and Lewis, M. (1963). Urinary excretion of magnesium in man following ingestion of ethanol. *Amer. J. Clin. Nutr.* **12**, 415–420.

MacIntyre, I., and Robinson, C. J. (1969). Magnesium and the gut. *Ann. N.Y. Acad. Sci.* **162**, 865–873.

MacIntyre, I., Hanna, S., Booth, C. C., and Read, A. E. (1961). Intracellular magnesium deficiency in man. *Clin. Sci.* **20**, 297–305.

Mader, I. J., and Iseri, L. T. (1955). Spontaneous hypopotassemia, hypomagnesemia, alkalosis and tetany due to hypersecretion of corticosterone-like mineralocorticoid. *Amer. J. Med.* **19**, 976–988.

Martin, H. E., and Bauer, F. K. (1962). Magnesium[28] studies in the cirrhotic and alcoholic. *Proc. Roy. Soc. Med.* **55** (11), 912–914.

Martin, H. E., and Wertman, M. (1947). Serum potassium, magnesium and calcium levels in diabetic acidosis. *J. Clin. Invest.* **26**, 217–228.

Martin, H. E., Mehl, J., and Wertman, M. (1952). Clinical studies of magnesium metabolism. *Med. Clin. N. Amer.* **36**, 1157–1171.

Martin, H. E., McCuskey, C., Jr., and Tupikova, N. (1959). Electrolyte disturbance in acute alcoholism with particular reference to magnesium. *Amer. J. Clin. Nutr.* **7**, 191–196.

Mellinghoff, K. (1949). Magnesium Stoffwechselstorungen bei Inanition, Deutches. *Arch. Klin. Med.* **195**, 475.

Mendelson, J., Wexler, D., Kubzansky, P. Leiderman, H., and Solomon, P. (1959). Serum magnesium in delirium tremens and alcoholic hallucinosis. *J. Nerv. Ment. Dis.* **128**, 352–357.

Mendelson, J. H., Barnes, B., Mayman, C., and Victor, M. (1965). The determination of exchangeable magnesium in alcoholic patients. *Metab., Clin. Exp.* **14**, 88–98.

Metcoff, J., Frenk, S., Antonowicz, I., Gordillo, G., and Lopez, E. (1960). Relations of intracellular ions to metabolite sequences in muscle in kwashiorkor. *Pediatrics* **26**, 960–972.

Miller, J. F. (1944). Tetany due to deficiency in magnesium. Its occurrence in a child of six years with associated osteochondrosis of capital epiphysis of femurs. *Amer. J. Dis. Child.* **67**, 117–119.

Milner, G., and Johnson, J. (1965). Hypomagnesemia and delirium tremens: Report of case with fatal outcome. *Amer. J. Psychiat.* **122**, 701–702.

Monif, G. R. G., and Savory, J. (1972). Iatrogenic maternal hypocalcemia following magnesium sulfate therapy. *J. Amer. Med. Ass.* **219**, 1469–1470.

Montgomery, R. D. (1960). Magnesium deficiency and tetany in kwashiokor. *Lancet* **2**, 264.

Montgomery, R. D. (1961). Magnesium balance studies in marasmic kwashiorkor. *J. Pediat.* **59**, 119–123.

Muldowney, F. P., McKenna, T. J., Kyle, L. H., Freaney, R., and Swan, M. (1970). Parathormone-like effect of magnesium replenishment in steatorrhea. *N. Engl. J. Med.* **281**, 61–68.

Nabarro, J. D. N., Spencer, A. G. D., and Stowers, J. M. (1952). Metabolic studies in severe diabetic ketosis. *Quart. J. Med.* **21**, 225–248.

Nielsen, J. (1963). Magnesium metabolism in an acute alcoholic. *Dan. Med. Bull.* **10**, 225–233.

Nielsen, J. A., and Thaysen, E. H. (1971). Acute and chronic magnesium deficiency following extensive small gut resection. *Scand. J. Gastroenterol.* **6**, 663–666.

Nordia, S., Donath, F., Macagno, R., and Gatti, T. (1971). Chronic hypomagnesemia with magnesium dependent hypocalcemia. *Acta Paediat. Scand.* **60**, 441–448.

Opie, L. H., Hurst, B. J., and Finlay, J. M. (1964). Massive small bowel resection with malabsorption and negative magnesium balance. *Gastroenterology* **47**, 415–420.

Paunier, L., Radde, I. C., Kooh, S. W., and Fraser, D. (1965). Primary hypomagnesemia with secondary hypocalcemia. *J. Pediat.* **67**, 945.

Paunier, L., Raddle, I. C., Kooh, S. W., Conen, P. E., and Fraser, D. (1968). Primary hypomagnesemia with secondary hypocalcemia in an infant. *Pediatrics* **41**, 385–402.

Potts, J. T., Jr., and Roberts, B. (1958). Clinical significance of magnesium deficiency and its relation to parathyroid disease. *Amer. J. Med. Sci.* **235**, 206–219.

Randall, R. E., Jr. (1969). Magnesium metabolism in chronic renal disease. *Ann. N.Y. Acad. Sci.* **162**, 831–842.

Randall, R. E., Jr., Rossmeisl, E. C., and Bleifer, K. H. (1959). Magnesium depletion in man. *Ann. Intern. Med.* **50**, 257–287.

Randall, R. E., Jr., Chen, M. D., Spray, C. C., and Rossmeisl, E. C. (1949). Hypermagnesemia in renal failure. *Ann. Intern. Med.* **61**, 73–88.

Ricketts, H. H., Denton, E. K., and Haywood, L. J. (1969). Unusual T-wave abnormality. Repolarization alternans associated with hypomagnesemia, acute alcoholism, and cardiomyopathy. *J. Amer. Med. Ass.* **207**, 365–366.

Rosen, E. A., Campbell, P. G., and Moosa, G. M. (1970). Hypomagnesemia and magnesium therapy in protein-calorie malnutrition. *J. Pediat.* **77**, 709–714.

Seelig, M. S. (1971). Human requirements of magnesium. Symposium Internationale sur le Déficit Magnésique in Pathologie Humaine, pp. 11–38. Vittel, France.

Seller, R. H., Cangiano, J., Kim, K. E., Mendelssohn, S., Brest, A. N., and Swartz, C. (1970). Digitalis toxicity and hypomagnesemia. *Amer. Heart J.* **79**, 57–68.

Skyberg, D., Stromme, J. H., Nesbakken, R., and Harnas, K. (1967). Congenital primary hypomagnesemia, an inborn error of metabolism. *Acta Paediat. Scand., Suppl.* **177**, 26–27.

Smith, W. O. (1963). Magnesium deficiency in the surgical patient. 1963. *Amer. J. Cardiol.* **13**, 667.

Smith, W. O., and Hammarsten, J. F. (1959). Intracellular magnesium in delirium tremens and uremia. *Amer. J. Med. Sci.* **237**, 413–417.

Sokal, M. M., Koenigsberger, M. R., Rose, J. S., Berdon, W. E., and Santulli, T. V. (1972). Neonatal hypermagnesemia and the meconium-plug syndrome. *N. Engl. J. Med.* **286**, 823–825.

Somjen, G. G., Hilmy, M., and Stephen, C. R. (1960). Failure to anesthesize human subjects by intravenous administration of magnesium sulfate. *J. Pharmacol. Exp. Ther.* **154**, 652–659.

Strømme, J. H., Nesbakken, R., Norman, T., Skjørten, F., Skyberg, D., and Johannessen, B. (1969). Familial hypomagnesemia, biochemical, histological and hereditary aspects studied in two brothers. *Acta Paediat. Scand.* **58**, 433–444.

Stutzman, F. L., and Amatuzio, D. S. (1953). Blood serum magnesium in portal cirrhosis and diabetes mellitus. *J. Lab. Clin. Med.* **41**, 215–219.

Sullivan, J. F., Lankford, H. G., Swartz, M. J., and Farrell, C. (1963). Magnesium depletion in alcoholism. *Amer. J. Clin. Nutr.* **13**, 297–303.

Sullivan, J. F., Parker, M., and Carsons, S. B. (1968). Tissue cobalt in beer drinkers myocardiopathy. *J. Lab. Clin. Med.* **71**, 893–911.

Suter, C., and Klingman, W. O. (1955). Neurological manifestations of magnesium depletion states. *Neurology* **5**, 691–699.

Tapley, D. F. (1955). Magnesium balance in myxedematous patients treated with triiodothyronine. *Bull. Johns Hopkins Hosp.* **96,** 274–278.

Thoren, L. (1963). Magnesium deficiency in gastrointestinal fluid loss. *Acta Chir. Scand., Suppl.* **306,** 1–65.

Tsang, R. C. (1972). Neonatal magnesium disturbances. *Amer. J. Dis. Child.* **124,** 282–293.

Vallee, B., Wacker, W. E., and Ulmer, D. D. (1960). The magnesium deficiency tetany syndrome in man. *N. Engl. J. Med.* **262,** 155–161.

Wacker, W. E., and Parisi, A. F. (1968). Magnesium metabolism. *N. Engl. J. Med.* **278,** 658–663, 712–717, and 772–776.

Walser, M. (1967). Magnesium metabolism. *Ergeb. Physiol., Biol. Chem. Exp. Pharmakol.* **59,** 185–296.

Whang, R., Morosi, H. J., Rogers, D., and Reyes, R. (1967). The influence of sustained magnesium deficiency on muscle potassium repletion. *J. Lab. Clin. Med.* **70,** 895–902.

Widdowson, E. M., McCance, R. A., and Spray, C. M. (1951). Chemical composition of human body. *Clin. Sci.* **10,** 113–125.

Wolfe, S., and Victor, N. (1969). The relationship of hypomagnesemia to alcohol withdrawal symptoms. *Ann. N.Y. Acad. Sci.* **162,** 973–984.

Wong, H. B., and Teh, Y. F. (1968). An association between serum magnesium and convulsions in infants and children. *Lancet* **2,** 18–21.

27

Magnesium Deficiency and Calcium and Parathyroid Hormone Interrelations

Maurice E. Shils

I. INTRODUCTION

Since the initial detailed observations of the effect of magnesium depletion in the rat in 1932, this deficiency has been associated in most species with neurologic manifestations (Kruse *et al.*, 1932).

The first observations concerning magnesium deficiency in man were those of Hirschfelder (1934). In a relatively small number of hypomagnesemic patients with renal insufficiency or hypoparathyroidism, he noted twitching and convulsions, some of which improved with magnesium. However, it was Flink and his associates (1954) who first brought magnesium deficiency solidly into clinical medicine with their studies of patients with acute alcoholism superimposed on chronic alcoholism, and in others who had been maintained on prolonged intravenous fluids without magnesium. They described personality changes, tremors, athetoid movements, and convulsions, and made certain observations relative to magnesium and potassium levels. Nevertheless, the symptomatology and biochemical abnormalities ascribable to deficiency of this ion were not adequately defined and were a matter of some disagreement despite

23

various individual case reports. This lack of clarity was ascribable to two major facts. (1) Despite various attempts, experimentally induced *symptomatic* human deficiency had not been induced. (2) The accounts of symptomatic clinical depletion always occurred in the setting of predisposing diseases and clinical situations that were usually very complex. These included severe malabsorption of various etiologies, chronic alcoholism with malnutrition, and illnesses requiring prolonged parenteral infusions that did not include magnesium, usually in association with serious losses of gastrointestinal secretions, renal disease, lactation losses, childhood malnutrition, and parathyroid disorders. In such circumstances, associated complex and uncontrollable variables such as multiple dietary inadequacies, metabolic abnormalities, manifestations of basic disease, severe infection, and treatments given in close proximity to the magnesium supplementation made it difficult and potentially misleading to ascribe certain clinical manifestations specifically to magnesium deficiency. Furthermore, at this time, the clinical literature was in disagreement concerning the relation of magnesium deficiency to serum calcium levels and to the occurrence of latent or overt tetany, defined here as a positive Trousseau sign or spontaneous carpopedal spasm. Some investigators expressed the opinion that tetany was not a manifestation of magnesium deficiency per se, and that a coexisting hypocalcemia was not related to the magnesium depletion. Others suggested that there was a relationship, since hypomagnesemia, hypocalcemia, and neurological symptoms improved in relation to magnesium therapy but not to calcium. Still another type of clinical picture was reported in which hyperirritability, tetany, and other neuromuscular abnormalities occurred in the setting of hypomagnesemia but where the serum calcium was normal; this syndrome was claimed to respond to magnesium but not to calcium salts.

II. EXPERIMENTAL SYMPTOMATIC MAGNESIUM DEFICIENCY IN MAN

In an attempt to develop a better understanding of the role of this ion, an effort was made to induce by dietary means magnesium depletion in adult human volunteers with normal absorption and renal function who were under close clinical supervision. These results have been published (Shils, 1964, 1969). In this study, individuals were maintained on a highly purified tube-fed diet supplemented with magnesium during a control period. The basal diet supplied 800 mg of calcium per day throughout the study and adequate amounts of vitamin D. Observations were made during the control period, in the depletion period when magnesium was omitted from the diet, and during the subsequent repletion period. Figure 1 summarizes some of the biochemical changes that were noted. All the seven subjects became markedly hypomagnesemic in the course of the depletion, as indicated by low serum and red cell magnesium. Six of the seven subjects became significantly hypocalcemic. The serum phosphorus was normal or slightly low in most of the patients but was elevated in one of the patients. Following repletion, three of the patients had a marked fall in phosphorus. Despite the adequacy of intake of calcium and vitamin D, all of the patients who became symptomatic had developed hypocalcemia. The time preceding neurological changes varied greatly, appearing anywhere from 25 to 110 days. Neurological changes included positive Chvostek and Trousseau signs, tremor and muscle fibrillations, and spasticity (Table I). An example

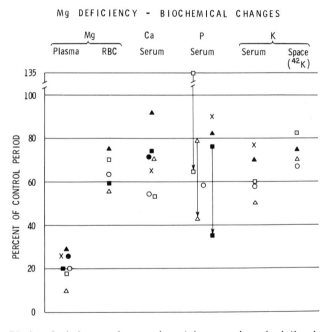

FIG. 1. Biochemical changes in experimental magnesium depletion in man. Each symbol represents one patient. The maximum change observed in the course of the depletion is indicated as a percentage of the average control levels for that individual. The transient decrease in plasma inorganic phosphate following magnesium repletion is indicated by a line connecting the values obtained late in the deficiency periods with those in the early repletion periods for three subjects. All values returned to normal following magnesium repletion. (From Shils, 1969.) (Permission granted by the copyright owner © (1969) The Williams & Wilkins Co., Baltimore.)

TABLE I   Clinical Changes in Magnesium Deficiency[a]

Change	Positive subjects/ subjects tested
Trousseau sign	5/7
Chvostek sign	2/7
Muscle fibrillation	2/7
Tremors	3/7
Spasticity, generalized	1/7
Hyporeflexia	2/7
Normoreflexia	5/7
Apathy and weakness	4/7
Anorexia, nausea, and vomiting	5/6
Electromyographic changes	5/5
Electrocardiographic changes[b]	4/7
Electroencephalographic changes	0/7

[a] Shils (1969).
[b] Nonspecific for magnesium deficiency.

of the relationships among clinical changes and magnesium and calcium levels is given in Fig. 2.

Although there are a number of interesting points demonstrated in this figure, there are five related to the subject of this paper to which attention should be directed: (1) the fall in the serum calcium that occurred as serum magnesium declined to low levels; (2) the association of the low calcium and magnesium to the onset of neurological signs; (3) administration of calcium intravenously raised the serum calcium only as long as the infusion lasted; cessation of the infusion being followed by a prompt fall in serum calcium and a prompt return of neurological signs; (4) a lag period of days before there was significant increase in the serum calcium, although serum magnesium increased rapidly with administration of magnesium; (5) most of the clinical signs cleared or improved before the calcium rose significantly.

The balance studies performed in this experiment showed clearly that the patients were absorbing calcium quite well and that they were in positive calcium balance, because the urinary calcium fell to very low levels (Fig. 3). Furthermore, the infusion of calcium intravenously did not result in a significant increase in the excretion of calcium. It was concluded that magnesium was somehow essential for the mobilization of calcium in bone, but the exact mechanism was not apparent from these studies. These experimental observations have been increasingly confirmed in patients with symptomatic magnesium deficiency of various etiologies.

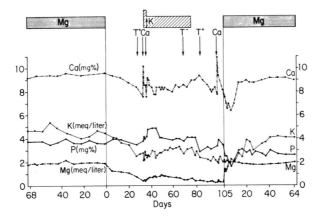

FIG. 2. The effect of magnesium depletion and repletion in man—subject C. Following onset of magnesium depletion at day 0, plasma magnesium fell progressively, and this was associated with a decline in plasma calcium. On depletion day 28, a positive Trousseau sign (T^+) appeared. Calcium gluconate (5 gm) was infused on days 33, 36, and 99 (Ca↓), with transient improvement only during the time of infusion. Increasing neurological and gastrointestinal signs developed toward the end of the depletion period, and on day 105, magnesium repletion was initiated with a rapid rise in plasma magnesium and clinical improvement. There was a striking but temporary fall in plasma Ca and P in the early repletion period followed by a return to normal, during which time remaining clinical signs and symptoms completely regressed. (From Shils, 1969.) (Permission granted by the copyright owner © (1969) The Williams & Wilkins Co., Baltimore.)

III. Observations in Other Species

Until the past few years, the rat has been the species given major attention in studies of magnesium deficiency. As increasing numbers of observations have been made with other species, it has become apparent that the rat is not a representative species with respect to serum calcium alterations. It is not even typical of other rodents in either this respect or in certain aspects of symptomatology (Alcock and Shils, 1974; Morris and O'Dell, 1969).

Table II summarizes changes noted in the level of serum calcium in experimentally induced magnesium deficiency in various species, including rodents, chick, ruminants, dog, pig, and primates, including man. I have reviewed the literature over a ten-year period and found reports from thirteen different laboratories (many having more than one published paper on the subject) reporting on serum calcium levels in the magnesium-depleted rat. Five laboratories noted either no change or variable changes as compared to control values in the deficient animals,

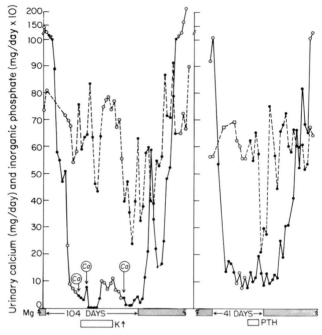

FIG. 3. Urinary calcium (solid line) and inorganic phosphate (broken line) excretion in two magnesium-depleted adult men. Note that the phosphate value is 10 times the ordinate figure. Marked hypocalciuria is consistently noted during magnesium depletion. Intravenous administration of 5 gm of calcium gluconate (Ca) did not increase calcium excretion. Urinary phosphate did not change consistently; some of the variability in the patient on the left was associated with some losses in emesis during the last week of depletion and the first few days of repletion. (From Shils, 1969.) [Permission granted by the copyright owner © (1969) The Williams & Wilkins Co., Baltimore.]

and seven observed consistent hypercalcemia; only one reported hypocalcemia. I was intrigued by this isolated report of hypocalcemia (Carillo et al., 1961) and found that the test animals were a special strain of rats raised at Cornell University in Ithaca by Maynard and Sperling. I was able to obtain some of these animals, breed them and feed them a diet that was extremely close to that used by Carillo et al. These animals did not become hypocalcemic despite the induction of severe hypomagnesemia; furthermore, the deficient animals were found to have developed renal dysfunction, as manifested by azotemia and nephrocalcinosis (M. E. Shils, unpublished data). It is possible that it was the renal failure that was responsible for the hypocalcemia reported by Carillo et al.; however, data on renal function were not reported by

TABLE II   Effect of Experimental Magnesium Depletion—Serum Calcium Levels in Various Species

Species	Effect		
	Increased Ca level	Normal Ca level[a]	Decreased Ca level[a]
Rat	+[b]	+[b]	+ (a)
Mouse		+ (b)	+ (c)
Guinea pig		+ (d)	+ (e)
Chick			+ (f,g)
Dog		+ (h–k)	+ (l–o)
Pig			+ (p)
Sheep			+ (q,r)
Cow		+ (s)	+ (t–v)
Monkey			+ (m,w)
Man		+ (x)	+ (y)

[a] *References:*   (a) Carillo et al. (1961); (b) Goldman et al. (1971); (c) Alcock and Shils (1974); (d) Morris and O'Dell (1963); (e) Morris and O'Dell (1969); (f) Breitenbach et al., (1973); (h) Hoobler et al. (1937); (i) Bunce et al. (1962b); (j) Wener et al. (1964); (k) Seta et al. (1966); (l) Bunce et al. (1962a); (m) Shils (1966; unpublished data); (n) Suh et al., (1971); (o) Levi et al. (1974); (p) Miller et al. (1965); (q) McAleese and Forbes (1959); (r) L'Estrange and Axford (1964); (s) Blaxter et al. (1960); (t) Parr (1957); (u) Smith (1958, 1961); (v) Larvor et al. (1964); (w) Dunn (1971); (x) Dunn and Walser (1966); (y) Shils (1964, 1969).
[b] Numerous references.

these investigators, so that a definitive decision cannot be made as to the etiology of the hypocalcemia. When the dietary level of calcium is severely restricted, the magnesium-deficient rat develops hypocalcemia (MacManus and Heaton, 1969; Suh et al., 1971; M. E. Shils, unpublished data).

The reports on changes in serum calcium in the deficient guinea pig and mouse are contradictory. In the report of hypocalcemia in the guinea pig, Morris and O'Dell (1969) noted a fairly marked decrease in creatinine clearance. Alcock and Shils (1974) found that deficient male Swiss mice became hypocalcemic rapidly. Goldman et al. (1971), using females of the same strain, reported normal calcium levels. In this study the dietary calcium level was high (1.2%), whereas the diet of Alcock and Shils provided 0.14%. The latter diet resulted in normocalcemia or hypercalcemia in the deficient rat, so that a true species difference unrelated to diet is apparent. The data obtained in the dog is also conflicting, but more recent studies seem to agree that hypocalcemia develops consistently, especially if the animals are not old. Experimental deficiencies in the chick, pig, sheep, calf, and monkey resulted in hypocalcemia in almost all studies.

What is the effect of raising the oral calcium intake in a hypomagnesemic, hypocalcemic animal? When hypocalcemia developed in the monkey, successive increases in dietary calcium did not prevent or overcome the hypocalcemia of magnesium-deficiency, whereas a single intramuscular injection of magnesium (17 meq) caused a marked rise in plasma calcium that persisted for a week or more (Fig. 4).

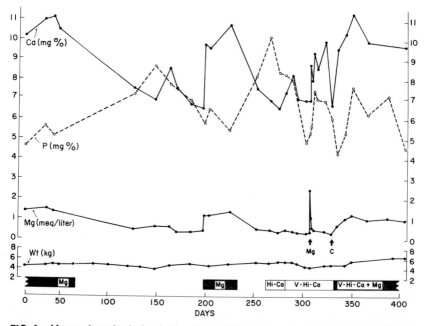

FIG. 4. Magnesium depletion in the stump-tail monkey—lack of effect of increasing calcium intake on plasma calcium. Hypomagnesemia associated with hypocalcemia and excitability occurred in each of the two indicated periods of magnesium depletion. Restoration of magnesium restored the plasma calcium to normal. During the second depletion period, the calcium content of the diet (140 mg%) was successively raised to 235 mg% (Hi-Ca) and then to 542 mg% (V-Hi-Ca). Such increases did not overcome or prevent the hypocalcemia. On day 308, while on diet V-Hi-Ca, the animal developed spasticity and tremors; 17 meq of magnesium was injected intramuscularly with a rise in plasma calcium and clinical improvement. After 1 week, plasma calcium again fell and convulsions (C) occurred on day 330. Restoration of magnesium to the diet returned the electrolytes and clinical status to normal. Serum inorganic phosphate was variable and related in part to the degree of physical activity of the animal just prior to blood sampling.

IV. INTERRELATIONSHIPS AMONG MAGNESIUM, CALCIUM, PARATHYROID HORMONE, AND BONE METABOLISM

Magnesium-deficient rats often develop hypercalcemia, hypophosphatemia, hypocalciuria, and hyperphosphaturia suggestive of a hyperparathyroid state (MacIntyre et al., 1963; Heaton, 1965; Lifshitz et al., 1967; Gitelman et al., 1968). Parathyroidectomy eliminated the relative hypercalcemia (Heaton, 1965; Gitelman et al., 1968; MacManus et al., 1971; Hahn et al., 1972) further strengthening the relationship between magnesium deficiency and increased activity of the parathyroid gland in this species. However, despite the hypercalcemia, histologic studies in intact magnesium-deficient rats have indicated that the parathyroid gland was not enlarged (Mirra et al., 1973). Furthermore, as mentioned above, restriction of dietary calcium in the magnesium-deficient rat results in hypocalcemia, revealing an important and complicated role of dietary calcium intake in the rat that does not appear to hold for other species, particularly during periods of active growth.

V. IN VITRO STUDIES RELATING MAGNESIUM TO PARATHYROID GLAND ACTIVITY

In studying the formation of parathyroid hormone in cultured explants of normal bovine parathyroid glands, Targovnik et al. (1971) found that there is a first-order relationship between hormone release from the glands and the total concentration of the divalent cations calcium and magnesium. These ions were equivalent in affecting the release of hormone; as one was decreased and the other increased so that the total divalent ion concentration was constant, parathyroid hormone secretion remained unchanged (Fig. 5). However, when magnesium concentration was very low, the hormone was diminished regardless of the total cation concentration. On the other hand, Hamilton and colleagues (1971) found a discrepancy between calcium and magnesium ions with respect to parathyroid hormone substance. They found increased incorporation of amino acids in the parathyroid hormone isolated from the tissue or from the medium when the concentration of calcium was lowered in the medium. However, changes in the magnesium concentration had no effect on the biosynthesis of parathyroid hormone. These authors suggested that calcium ions affect directly and indirectly both the synthesis and secretion of parathyroid hormone while magnesium ions affect only secretion. These apparent discrepancies remain to be resolved.

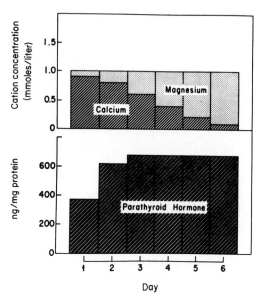

FIG. 5. Daily decreases in concentration of calcium ion and corresponding increases in magnesium ion with constancy of divalent ion concentration in incubation medium of normal bovine parathyroid glands resulted in constant release of parathyroid hormone except at the time when magnesium concentration was very low. (Targovnik *et al.,* 1971.)

Perfusion studies of goat or sheep parthyroid glands *in vivo* have suggested also that the parathyroid gland is sensitive to low magnesium concentrations with resultant increased output of the hormone. As illustrated in Fig. 6, there was a marked increase in parathyroid hormone when the perfusion fluid had a low magnesium content and the calcium level remained constant. These types of studies suggest that hypomagnesemia should result in increased hormone formation or release from the parathyroid gland. They would be consistent with the findings observed in the deficient rat, where an apparent hyperparathyroid state exists. They are not consistent with observations in the other species where hypocalcemia or an apparent hypoparathyroid state exists during magnesium depletion. However, it should be noted that the animals whose glands were perfused were not magnesium depleted and that severe depletion of magnesium in the cultured glands decreased hormone production.

Raisz and Neimann (1969) found that when parathyroid extract (PTE) was added to fetal rat bones *in vitro,* less calcium was released from the bone when the medium was low in magnesium than when

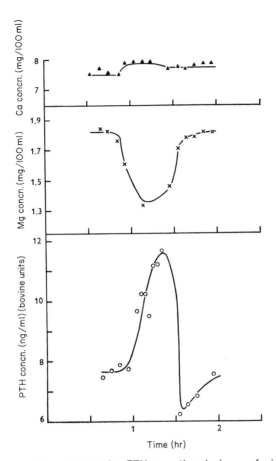

FIG. 6. Increase of immunoreactive PTH secretion during perfusion of hypomagnesemic blood into the isolated inferior parathyroid gland with thyroid lobe in an anesthetized goat. As the magnesium content of the perfusate fell, parathyroid hormone (PTH) rose. Ionized calcium increased very slightly during the procedure. (Buckle *et al.,* 1968.)

the magnesium was normal. MacManus *et al.* (1971), employing nonfetal bone derived from both magnesium-deficient and normal rats, found that when PTE was added *in vitro* it did not result in as great a release of calcium, phosphate, and hydroxyproline from bone of deficient animals as it did from that of the controls. These studies suggest that magnesium deficiency induces a degree of refractoriness of bone to the action of parathyroid hormone. If this observation holds for the intact animal, it creates an apparent contradiction, since serum calcium is higher in the deficient rat.

VI. EFFECT OF PARATHYROID EXTRACT *IN VIVO*

Because of the evidence suggesting that a hyperparathyroid state exists in the magnesium-depleted rat, various experimenters have tested the effects of PTE given to parathyroidectomized or thyroparathyroidectomized rats and other species (Table III). Heaton (1965) gave 600 units of PTE over 24 hr; when blood was sampled 6 hr later, he found large increases of serum calcium in both deficient and control animals with no significant difference. MacManus *et al.* (1971), using the thyroparathyroidectomized animals, gave only 50 units intraperitoneally, sampled blood at 2 and 6 hr, and found that the deficient animals were resistant; however, the control animals had only a relatively small rise in calcium, although this was significant. Hahn *et al.* (1972) gave 150 units per kilogram to small animals intraperitoneally with sampling 3 hr later; they found that calcium rose equally in control and deficient animals. Serum calcium rose with PTE and also with dibutyryl cyclic AMP; marked positive renal response in the deficient rats also occurred following PTE or dibutyryl cyclic AMP.

Magnesium-deficient chicks were resistant to the effects of parathyroid extract. In the study of Reddy *et al.* (1973), 50, 100, and 200 units were given subcutaneously, and calcium was determined in the blood 4 hr later. Following 3 days of magnesium repletion, the birds were

TABLE III   Effect of Parathyroid Extract Injection on Serum Calcium in Magnesium-Deficient Animals versus Controls[a]

	Surgical state[b]		
Species	Intact	PTX	T-PTX
Rat	S(a)**	S(b)	R(c)
Chick	R(d)		
	R(e)		
Dog	PR(f)		S(g)
Monkey	S(h)		

[a] *Abbreviations:* PTX = parathyroidectomized; T-PTX = thyroparathyroidectomized; S = similar response; PR = partially refractory; R = refractory.

[b] *References:* (a) Heaton (1965); (b) Hahn *et al.* (1972); (c) MacManus *et al.* (1971); (d) Breitenbach *et al.* (1973); (e) Reddy *et al.* (1973); (f) Levi *et al.* (1974); (g) Suh *et al.* (1971); (h) Dunn (1971).

again responsive to PTE. In the study of Breitenbach *et al.* (1973), 15 units of PTE were given intravenously per 100 gm body weight and calcium levels determined 15–90 min later. In the latter study, magnesium was injected into control and deficient animals sufficiently to raise the serum level to normal in 1 hr, at which time 30 units per 100 gm body weight of parathyroid extract was injected, again without response in the newly repleted animals; this study was not repeated after a longer period of repletion.

Two studies have been done on dogs. In the experiments of Suh *et al.* (1971), using dogs of various ages, no significant difference was noted in the amount of PTE required to attain normal serum calcium levels (approximately 6 meq/liter) between deficient and control animals when doses of PTE were given stepwise until the normal plasma level was reached (Suh *et al.*, 1971). Figure 7 shows that the slopes of the response curves of the two groups were identical. When 0.3 units of PTE was infused hourly beginning 6 hr after thyroparathyroidectomy and continued for 48 hr, the animals responded as well when deficient as when repleted with magnesium. Comparison of the response to PTE of magnesium-deficient thyroparathyroidectomized rats and intact deficient rats revealed no difference. This latter experiment indicates that

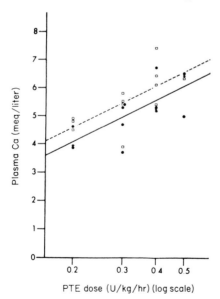

FIG. 7. Regression lines of plasma calcium concentrations and log dose of parathyroid extract (PTE) in thyroparathyroidectomized control (broken line) and magnesium depleted (solid line) groups of puppies. The dose–response relations of the two groups are similar. (Suh *et al.*, 1971.)

excess calcitonin secretion was not a factor in the hypocalcemia occurring in the deficient dogs. The authors concluded that hypocalcemia in magnesium-deficient dogs is not due to resistance of end organ (bone) to the calcium mobilizing action of PTE, but rather is a result of defective synthesis or diminished secretion of parathyroid hormone.

Levi *et al.* (1974), using adult female mongrel dogs, obtained somewhat different results. Their animals acted as their own controls in the course of control, depletion, and repletion periods. Deficiency was accelerated by the infusion of furosemide 2 or 3 days each week together with an infusion for 2 hr of a magnesium-free electrolyte solution supplying calcium, sodium, and potassium chloride and phosphate. The effect of PTE was observed by infusing two units of PTE per kilogram per hour over 8 hr with blood drawn before, during, and at the end of the infusion. Significant hypocalcemia developed with the depletion, and PTE produced an increase of serum calcium in every study in all animals. However, the magnitude of the increments in serum calcium with PTE was greater during the control and repletion period than during the depletion period. Reduced calcemic response was shown during the infusion when the serum magnesium reached 1.0 mg% or less, and there was no significant correlation between the calcemic response to PTE when serum magnesium was reduced further. As will be discussed later, immunoreactive parathyroid hormone was present in normal amounts in the two animals studied and remained stable during magnesium depletion despite the hypocalcemia. These authors concluded that there was both an impaired responsiveness to parathyroid hormone and a reduced secretion of the hormone consequent to the hypocalcemia developing during magnesium deficiency.

Dunn (1971) infused PTE into rhesus monkeys at the rate of 2 or 4 units/kg/hr for 24 hr, and serum was taken before and at 4, 7, and 24 hr after the onset of infusion; others received 15 units/kg twice daily for 2 days. The monkeys gave calcemic responses to the extract when depleted of magnesium similar to those when fed magnesium. In my own experiments using the stump-tailed monkey, I have also noted an excellent response to parathyroid hormone in hypocalcemic magnesium-deficient monkeys (M. E. Shils, unpublished data).

Thus, with the exception of the chick, the species tested—including the rat, dog, and monkey—appear to be capable of responding to PTE with respect to elevation of serum calcium levels during magnesium deficiency, although one study with dogs suggests that there may be a relative refractoriness of bone. The abnormality occurring in these magnesium-deficient mammals appears to reside primarily in the inability of the parathyroid gland to secrete an amount of hormone appropriate to the serum calcium level. However, direct evidence for this belief has been obtained only in the study of Levi *et al.* (1974), where the immunocrossreactivity between canine and bovine PTH was utilized to detect circulating PTH in canine serum.

Table IV summarizes serum calcium responses to parathyroid extract given to adult magnesium-deficient human beings. Estep *et al.* (1969) reported that magnesium-deficient individuals (primarily alcoholics who were hypocalcemic) were refractory to parathyroid extract until they had been given magnesium. Since that time, data have been published on another five patients, all of whom had malabsorption. As noted in the table, three of these appeared to respond poorly to the effects of PTE when hypomagnesemic. The patient of Connor appeared to respond more rapidly to PTE following magnesium repletion.

Note should be taken of certain methodological problems associated with most of these studies. The amount of PTE given by Muldowney *et al.* (1970) appears to have been inadequate to give positive responses in their two subjects in the repleted state; therefore, the absence of response in the depleted state has no significance and the study is invalid. Estep *et al.* (1969) and Connor *et al.* (1972) retested the effect of PTE relatively early in the repletion period, i.e., at a time where serum calcium should have been continuing to rise in response to magnesium. Hence, it is not possible to know the relative contributions of PTE and magnesium during this critical period. Chase and Slatopolsky did not retest their subjects following magnesium administration. Thus, while magnesium depletion may result in varying the degree of resistance in adults to PTE at the end organ, the data presently available do not afford a solid base for this assumption.

Data are available on the responses to PTE of five children with hypomagnesemia resulting from an isolated defect in intestinal magnesium absorption (Table V). Four of the subjects were young infants. All were treated differently and were in differing stages of deficiency, thus making comparisons hazardous. The patient of Salet *et al.* (1966) had been given magnesium therapy; this had been stopped prior to the PTE test, and serum magnesium and calcium were subnormal at that time. The patient of Paunier *et al.* (1968) was studied on two occasions when deficient; their data indicate that the serum magnesium and calcium were more depressed at the time of the first test than at the time of the second, and this may account for the differing degree of responsiveness. The patient of Strømme *et al.* (1969) had been receiving magnesium therapy until approximately 8 or 9 days prior to the PTE test; at the time of testing his serum magnesium was low, but serum calcium was at about the lower limit of normal.

TABLE IV Effect of Parathyroid Extract (PTE) Injection on Serum Calcium in Adult Man[a]

Patients[b]	Pre-Mg			Post-Mg			Reference
	PTE (units)	ΔCa[c] (mg%)	Time (hr)	PTE (units)	ΔCa[c] (mg%)	Time (hr)	
10A	200 q6h × 2d	1	48	200 q6h × 2d	3[d]	48[e]	Estep et al. (1969)
1M	200 q6h × 2d	0.3	48	200 qh6 × 2d	3.1	48[e]	Estep et al. (1969)
1M	1/kg/hr × 10 hr iv	0[d]	12 and 24	1/kg/hr × 10 hr iv	0[d]	24	Muldowney et al. (1970)
1M	1/kg/hr × 10 hr iv	<0.5[d]	12 and 24	1/kg/hr × 10 hr iv	0(?)	12	Muldowney et al. (1970)
1M	300 q6h × 3d	0.3 / 2.9	24 / 72	300 q6h × 1d	0.5 / 3.3	24 / 24[e]	Connor et al. (1972)
1M	200 q6h × 3d	2.0	72	—	—	—	Chase and Slatopolsky (1974)
1M	200 q6h × 3d	1.4	72	—	—	—	Chase and Slatopolsky (1974)

[a] Comparison of responses before and after magnesium repletion.

[b] A = alcoholic, M = malabsorber.

[c] Increase in serum calcium above baseline values at the hour indicated following initial injection of PTE.

[d] Changes estimated from graph in original publication.

[e] See text.

TABLE V   Effect of Parathyroid Extract (PTE) Injection on Serum Calcium in Children[a]

Patient age and reference	Pre-Mg			Post-Mg		
	PTE (units)	ΔCa[b] (mg%)	Time (hr)	PTE (units)	ΔCa[b] (mg%)	Time (hr)
13 weeks	400 → 100/d × 4d	3.8	24	100 → 50 d × 2d	4.2	24
(Salet et al., 1966)		3.8	72		6.3	48
12 weeks (Paunier	(a) 50 q6h × 5d	0[c]	72[d]	—	—	—
et al., 1968)		2.5[c]	120	—	—	—
	(b) 50 q6h × 2d	3.2[c]	24	—	—	—
		4.6[c]	48	—	—	—
10 weeks (Strømme	100/d × 2d	2.2[c]	24[d]	—	—	—
et al., 1969)		3.6[c]	48	—	—	—
9 weeks (Woodard	20 q6h × 2d	1.0[c]	48	20 q6h × 2d	4.7	48
et al., 1972)						
8 years (Suh et al.,	160 × 5 in 28h	5.6	28	—	—	—
1973)						

[a] Comparison of responses before and after magnesium repletion.
[b] Increase in serum calcium above baseline values at the hour indicated following initial injection of PTE.
[c] Changes estimated from graph in original publication.
[b] See text.

With the exception of the fourth patient, all responded to PTE during the deficiency period, although perhaps with a prolonged lag period in the first two patients. Only two patients were retested after magnesium repletion; both responded to PTE with more rapid rise and higher calcium levels. Unlike the adult repletion studies, these two subjects had achieved normal serum calcium levels prior to retesting.

The patients of Estep et al. (1969), Connor et al. (1972), and Muldowney et al. (1970) were refractory in their renal response to PTE. However, those of Chase and Slatopolsky (1974) had a good response as did the 8-year-old studied by Suh et al. (1973).

A resolution to the inter- and intraspecies differences and discrepancies appears to be at hand with the advent of immunoassays for parathyroid hormone (IPTH). I am aware of five studies in which circulating IPTH levels have been measured. Levi et al. (1974) compared IPTH levels in two dogs when they were normomagnesemic and normocalcemic and when they had marked hypomagnesemia and a mild hypocalcemia. The levels did not change significantly in response to the hypocalcemia. These authors conclude that there is an inappropriate response induced by magnesium depletion, with less output of parathyroid hormone than would be expected. Connor *et al.* (1972) measured IPTH in their prolonged studies on a patient with chronic magnesium depletion as the result of severe malabsorption. They concluded that, "At all times IPTH levels were found to be elevated significantly ranging from 50 to 350% above normal range for this laboratory." Anast *et al.* (1972) reported the case of a 21-year-old woman who had hypomagnesemia as the result of an isolated intestinal absorption defect (Fig. 8). IPTH was undetectable during episodes of hypomagnesemia and hypocalcemia; there was a rapid rise following injection of magnesium salts and then a decline as serum calcium rose. As hypomagnesemia recurred without therapy, hypocalcemia again developed and IPTH fell to very low levels. Essen-

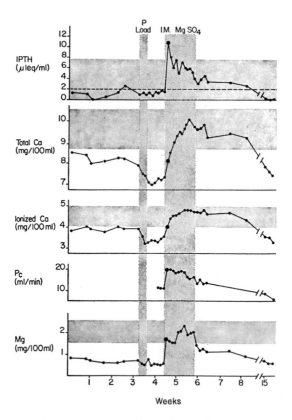

FIG. 8. The effect of magnesium deficiency and repletion on serum levels of magnesium, calcium, and immunoreactive parathyroid hormone (IPTH), and renal phosphate clearance (P_c) in a patient with isolated inability to absorb magnesium. The horizontal shaded areas indicate normal ranges. Broken line in IPTH area indicates limits of detectability of the PTH assay. A dose of 100 mg of magnesium as the sulfate was injected every 8 hr for the period indicated. (Anast *et al.*, 1972.) (Copyright 1972 by the American Association for the Advancement of Science.)

tially the same findings were found by Suh *et al.* (1973) in an 8-year-old male with the same absorptive problem.

Chase and Slatapolsky (1974) studied two adults. One had a surgically induced jejunocolic fistula for the treatment of obesity that caused marked malabsorption; the other was an alcoholic with malnutrition. Both of these patients had IPTH in the normal range during episodes of hypomagnesemia and hypocalcemia. Following administration of magnesium, the hormone levels rose to approximately twice these levels and then returned to normal as serum calcium rose to normal.

Seven of 12 hypomagnesemic-hypocalcemic patients had IPTH levels which were inappropriately low for the degree of hypocalcemia (Shils, 1975); four other had significantly elevated levels in the range 63–77 μlEq* per ml (upper normal limit 40) associated with hypocalcemia. Of the five depleted patients with levels above 40 μlEq per ml, three had a return to normal of IPTH levels while the other two continued to have elevated but lower levels when magnesium repletion occurred and serum calcium rose. The observations on one of the patients, resembling those reported by Chase and Slatapolsky (1974), are summarized in Fig. 9.

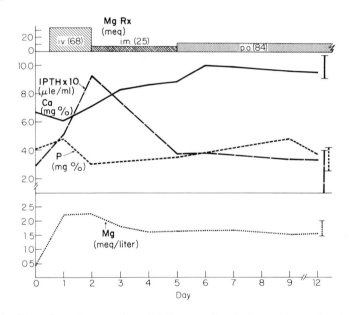

FIG. 9. The effect of magnesium deficiency and repletion on plasma levels of magnesium, calcium, phosphate, and immunoreactive parathyroid hormone (IPTH) in an adult woman with malabsorption. The normal range of each is indicated at the right, and dosage and route of administration of magnesium (as sulfate) are given at the top.

* 1 μl Eq equals 20 pg PTH.

These data indicate that magnesium depletion with its resultant hypo-calcemia can be associated with very low, normal (but inappropriately low) or elevated IPTH levels. The two patients with an isolated absorptive defect for magnesium (Anast *et al.*, 1972; Suh *et al.*, 1971, 1973) had a marked suppression of PTH production whereas the other patients who had more general malabsorption or alcoholism induced malnutrition had IPTH in the "normal" or elevated range during the deficiency period.

The explanation is not at hand for the difference in circulating IPTH levels between the two types of patients. Age is a factor to be considered, as are the differences in the nutritional effects of the underlying diseases.

The report of Connor *et al.* (1972) noted continual high circulating levels during magnesium deficiency and following repletion. These investigators were of the opinion that hypocalcemia resulted from an acquired resistance of bone to parathyroid hormone and postulated that chronic magnesium depletion and the associated intermittent hypocalcemia resulted in some degree of "autonomy" of function of the parathyroid gland with chronically elevated IPTH levels. However, the patients of Anast *et al.* (1972) and of Suh *et al.* (1971, 1973) were also chronically depleted for prolonged periods and they did not exhibit elevations in IPTH during the hypocalcemia.

VII. CONCLUSION

The following sequences of magnesium deficiency are postulated to explain most of the observations which I have mentioned.

Sequence I—The Initiation of Hypocalcemia. With an adequate intake of calcium, negative calcium balance does not occur and can be ruled out as the etiology of hypocalcemia in most species during magnesium deficiency. There must develop, as a primary factor, a failure of calcium to leave the metabolically labile bone mineral. This defect must be combined with a deposition in bone mineral or soft tissues of absorbed dietary calcium with a resultant progressive fall in serum calcium. In the rat and in older animals of certain species fed relatively large amounts of calcium, the failure to mobilize calcium from bone may be counterbalanced by increased absorption from the intestine with a resultant maintenance of serum calcium. There are at least three possible mechanisms responsible for the failure of calcium release from bone. One is a decreased heteroionic exchange of magnesium for calcium at the bone surface. Another is impairment by magnesium deficiency of the normal metabolic activity of osteocytes in maintaining mineral homeostatis by active bone resorption. This cellular change may be related, in part, to the third mechanism, the development of resistance to PTH.

Sequence II—The Perpetuation of Hypocalcemia. With the development of hypocalcemia, one would expect PTH production and secretion to increase. Data are available that indicate that at a stage of magnesium depletion some individuals do have elevated levels of the hormone. Despite this, serum calcium levels remained depressed indicating a resistance to the hormone. Other subjects had normal to low levels of hormone which were inappropriate to the circulating calcium level; this situation indicates an inadequacy of PTH production. Thus, there is a failure at two levels in the PTH mechanism designed to maintain calcium homeostasis. It is tempting to speculate that these two stages are related to the degree of deficiency with bone resistance occurring first and then being followed by a production failure as the deficiency becomes severe. Excessive calcitonin does not appear to be involved. At present there is no evidence for or against involvement of a failure of formation or function of the metabolically active form(s) of vitamin D.

Sequence III—The Regression of Hypocalcemia. Following administration of magnesium, an increase in PTH occurs after a lag period, which may extend over several days. This is consistent with the lag period in serum calcium rise following initiation of magnesium repletion. Presumably, in this interval the administered magnesium ions are entering the hydration shell of bone, permitting calcium exchange to begin; this exchange may occur early in repletion and may explain the rapid improvement that occurs in some of the neuromuscular abnormalities with little or no detectable change in circulating calcium. With the entry of magnesium into bone mineral and osteocytes, the ability to respond to PTH is regained when a degree of resistance has occurred. In this instance PTH levels may remain high or even increase until serum Ca has risen; PTH then declines. In the situation where circulating PTH has been inappropriately low, there is a rapid rise in the hormone level; bone resorption then occurs and serum calcium rises followed, in turn, by a decline in PTH.

REFERENCES

Alcock, N. W., and Shils, M. E. (1974). Comparison of magnesium deficiency in the rat and mouse. *Proc. Soc. Exp. Biol. Med.* **146**, 137–141.

Anast, C. S., Mohs, J. M., Kaplan, S. L., and Burns, T. W. (1972). Evidence for parathyroid failure in magnesium deficiency. *Science* **177**, 606–608.

Blaxter, K. L., Cowlishaw, B., and Rook, J. A. F. (1960). Potassium and hypomagnesemic tetany in calves. *Anim. Prod.* **2**, 1–15.

Breitenbach, R. P., Gonnerman, W. A., Erfling, W. L., and Anast, C. S. (1973). Dietary magnesium, calcium homeostasis, and parathyroid gland activity of chickens. *Amer. J. Physiol.* **225**, 12–17.

Buckle, R. M., Care, A. D., Cooper, C. W., and Gitelman, H. J. (1968). The influence of plasma magnesium concentration on parathyroid hormone secretion. *J. Endocrinol.* **42**, 529–534.

Bunce, G. E., Jenkins, K. J., and Phillips, P. H. (1962a). The mineral requirements of the dog. III. The magnesium requirement. *J. Nur.* **76**, 17–22.

Bunce, G. E., Chiemchaisri, Y., and Phillips, P. H. (1962b). The mineral requirement of the dog. IV. Effect of certain dietary and physiologic factors upon the magnesium deficiency syndrome. *J. Nutr.* **76**, 23–29.

Carillo, B. J., Pond, W. G., Krook, L., Lovelace, F. E., and Loosli, J. K. (1961). Response of growing rats to diets varying in magnesium, potassium, and protein content. *Proc. Soc. Exp. Biol. Med.* **107**, 793–796.

Chase, L. R., and Slatopolsky, E. (1974). Secretion and metabolic efficiency of parathyroid hormone in patients with severe hypomagnesemia. *J. Clin. Endocrinol. Metab.* **38**, 363–371.

Connor, T. B., Toskes, P., Mahaffey, J., Martin, L. G., Williams, J. B., and Walser, M. (1972). Parathyroid function during chronic magnesium deficiency. *Johns Hopkins Med. J.* **131**, 100–117.

Dunn, M. J. (1971). Magnesium depletion in the Rhesus monkey: Induction of magnesium-dependent hypocalcemia. *Clin. Sci.* **41**, 333–344.

Dunn, M. J., and Walser, M. (1966). Magnesium depletion in normal man. *Metab., Clin. Exp.* **15**, 884–895.

Estep, H., Shaw, W. A., Watlington, C., Hobe, R., Holland, W., and Tucker, S. G. (1969). Hypocalcemia due to hypomagnesemia and reversible parathyroid hormone unresponsiveness. *J. Clin. Endocrinol. Metab.* **29**, 842–848.

Flink, E. B., Stutzman, F. L., Anderson, A. R., Konig, T., and Fraser, R. (1954). Magnesium deficiency after prolonged parenteral fluid administration and after chronic alcoholism complicated by delirium tremors. *J. Lab. Clin. Med.* **43**, 169–183.

Gitelman, H. J., Kukolj, S., and Welt, L. G. (1968). The influence of parathyroid glands on the hypocalcemia of experimental magnesium depletion in the rat. *J. Clin. Invest.* **47**, 118–126.

Goldman, R. H., Kleiger, R. E., Schweizer, E., and Harrison, D. C. (1971). The effect on myocardial ^{3}H-digoxin of magnesium deficiency. *Proc. Soc. Exp. Biol. Med.* **136**, 747–749.

Hahn, T. J., Chase, L. R., and Avioli, L. V. (1972). Effect of magnesium depletion on responsiveness to parathyroid hormone in parathyroidectomized rats. *J. Clin. Invest.* **51**, 886–891.

Hamilton, J. W., Spierto, F. W., MacGregor, R. R., and Cohn, D. V. (1971). Studies on the biosynthesis *in vitro* of parathyroid hormone. II. The effect of calcium and magnesium on synthesis of parathyroid hormone isolated from bovine parathyroid tissue and incubation medium. *J. Biol. Chem.* **246**, 3224–3233.

Heaton, F. W. (1965). The parathyroid glands and magnesium metabolism in the rat. *Clin. Sci.* **28**, 543–553.

Hirschfelder, A. D. (1934). Clinical manifestations of high and low plasma magnesium. *J. Amer. Med. Ass.* **102**, 1138.

Hoobler, S. W., Kruse, H. D., and McCollum, E. V. (1937). Studies on magnesium deficiency in animals. *Amer. J. Hyg.* **25**, 86–106.

Kruse, H. D., Orent, E. R., and McCollum, E. V. (1932). Studies on magnesium deficiency in animals. I. Symptomatology resulting from magnesium deprivation. *J. Biol. Chem.* **96**, 519.

Larvor, P., Girard, A., Brochhart, M., Parodi, A., Sevestre, J., avec la collaboration technique de Chagnaud, P., Berthelol, N., and Roth, C. (1964). Etude de la carence expérimentale en magnésium chez le veau. I. observations, cliniques, biochimiques et anatomo-pathologiques. *Ann. Biol. Anim., Biochim., Biophys.* **4**, 345–369.

L'Estrange, J. L., and Axford, R. F. E. (1964). A study of magnesium and calcium metabolism in lactating ewes fed a semi-purified diet low in magnesium. *J. Agr. Sci.* **62**, 353–368.

Levi, J., Massry, S. G., Coburn, J. W., Llach, F., and Kleeman, C. R. (1974). Hypocalcemia in magnesium-depleted dogs: Evidence for reduced responsiveness to parathyroid hormone and relative failure of parathyroid gland function. *Metab., Clin. Exp.* **23**, 323–335.

Lifshitz, F., Harrison, H. C., Hull, E. C., and Harrison, H. E. (1967). Citrate metabolism and the mechanism of renal calcification induced by magnesium depletion. *Metab., Clin. Exp.* **16**, 345–357.

McAleese, D. M., and Forbes, R. M. (1959). Experimental production of magnesium deficiency on lambs on a diet containing roughage. *Nature (London)* **184**, 2025–2026.

MacIntyre, I., Boss, S., and Troughton, V. A. (1963). Parathyroid hormone and magnesium homeostasis. *Nature (London)* **198**, 1058–1060.

MacManus, J., and Heaton, F. W. (1969). The effect of magnesium deficiency on calcium homeostasis in the rat. *Clin. Sci.* **36**, 297–306.

MacManus, J., Heaton, F. W., and Lucas, P. W. (1971). A decreased response to parathyroid hormone in magnesium deficiency. *Endocrinology* **49**, 253–258.

Miller, E. R., Ullrey, D. E., Zutant, C. L., Baltzer, B. V., Schmidt, D. A., Hoefer, J. A., and Luecke, R. W. (1965). Magnesium requirement of the baby pig. *J. Nutr.* **85**, 13–20.

Mirra, J. M., Alcock, N. W., Shils, M. E., and Tennenbaum, P. J. (1973). Pathological effects of magnesium and calcium deficiencies on rat skeletal development. *Fed. Proc., Fed. Amer. Soc. Exp. Biol.* **31**, 707.

Morris, E. R., and O'Dell, B. L. (1963). Relation of excess calcium and phosphorus to magnesium requirements and toxicity in guinea pigs. *J. Nutr.* **81**, 175.

Morris, E. R., and O'Dell, B. L. (1969). Effect of magnesium deficiency in guinea pigs on kidney function and plasma ultrafiltrable ions. *Proc. Soc. Exp. Biol. Med.* **132**, 105–110.

Muldowney, F. P., McKenna, T. J., Kyle, L. H., Freaney, R., and Swan, M. (1970). Parathormone-like effects of magnesium replenishment in steatorrhea. *N. Engl. J. Med.* **28**, 61–68.

Parr, W. H. (1957). Hypomagnesaemic tetany in calves fed on milk diets. *Vet. Rec.* **69**, 71–76.

Paunier, L., Radde, I. C., Kooh, S. W., Conen, P. E., and Fraser, D. (1968). Primary hypomagnesemia in secondary hypocalcemia in an infant. *Pediatrics* **41**, 385–402.

Raisz, L. G., and Niemann, I. (1969). Effect of phosphate, calcium, and magnesium on bone resorption and hormonal responses in tissue culture. *Endocrinology* **85**, 446–452.

Reddy, C. R., Coburn, J. W., Hartenbower, D. L., Friedler, R. M., Brickman, A. S., Massry, S. G., and Jowsey, J. (1973). Studies on mechanisms of hypocalcemia of magnesium depletion. *J. Clin. Invest.* **52**, 3000–3010.

Salet, J., Polonovski, C., DeGouyon, F., Pean, G., Melekian, B., and Fournet, J. P. (1966). Tetanic hypocalcémique récidivante par hypomagnésemic congenitale: Une maladie metabolique. *Arch. Fr. Pediat.* **23**, 749–768.

Seta, K., Kleiger, R., Hellerstein, E. E., Lown, B., and Vitale, J. J. (1966). Effects of potassium and magnesium deficiency on the electrocardiogram and plasma electrolytes of purebred beagles. *Amer. J. Cardiol.* **17**, 516–519.

Shils, M. E. (1964). Experimental human magnesium depletion. *Amer. J. Clin. Nutr.* **15**, 133–143.

Shils, M. E. (1966). Species differences in electrolytes in magnesium deficiency. *Fed. Proc., Fed. Amer. Soc. Exp. Biol.* **25**, 609.

Shils, M. E. (1969). Experimental human magnesium depletion. *Medicine (Baltimore)* **48**, 61–85.

Shils, M. E. (1975). Magnesium deficiency and parathyroid hormone levels in man. *Am. J. Clin. Nutr.* **28**, 421.

Smith, R. H. (1958). Calcium and magnesium metabolism in calves. 2. Effect of dietary vitamin D and ultraviolet irradiation on milk-fed calves. *Biochem. J.* **70**, 201–205.

Smith, R. H. (1961). Importance of magnesium in the control of plasma calcium in the calf. *Nature (London)* **191**, 181–182.

Strømme, J. H., Nesbakken, R., Normann, T., Skjørten, F., Skyberg, D., and Johannessen, B. (1969). Familial hypomagnesemia. Biochemical, histological, and hereditary aspects studied in two brothers. *Acta Paediat. Scand.* **58**, 433–444.

Suh, S. M., Csima, A., and Fraser, D. (1971). Pathogenesis of hypocalcemia in magnesium depletion. Normal end-organ responsiveness to parathyroid hormone. *J. Clin. Invest.* **50**, 2668–2678.

Suh, S. M., Tashjian, A. H., Jr., Matsuo, N., Parkinson, D. K., and Fraser, D. (1973). Pathogenesis of hypocalcemia in primary hypomagnesemia: Normal end-organ responsiveness to parathyroid hormone, impaired parathyroid gland function. *J. Clin. Invest.* **52**, 153–160.

Targovnik, J. H., Rodman, J. S., and Sherwood, L. M. (1971). Regulation of parathyroid hormone secretion *in vitro:* Quantitative aspects of calcium and magnesium ion control. *Endocrinology* **898**, 1477–1482.

Wener, J., Pintar, K., Simon, M. A., Motola, R., Friedman, R., Mayman, A., and Sucher, R. (1964). Effects of prolonged hypomagnesemia on the cardiovascular system in young dogs. *Amer. Heart J.* **67**, 221–231.

Woodard, J. C., Webster, P. D., and Carr, A. A. (1972). Primary hypomagnesemia with secondary hypocalcemia, diarrhea and insensitivity to parathyroid hormone. *Amer. J. Dig. Dis.* **17**, 612–618.

28

Biochemistry and Physiology
of Magnesium

Jerry K. Aikawa

I. INTRODUCTION

Magnesium is one of the most plentiful elements on earth; in the vertebrate, it is the fourth most abundant cation. Magnesium is associated with so many different biological processes that this involvement suggests that it has some single fundametal role (Aikawa, 1971). It is the purpose of this chapter to summarize the current knowledge of the biological properties of magnesium, beginning with the genesis of life on earth and extending into molecular biology and into human physiology.

II. BIOCHEMISTRY OF MAGNESIUM

A. Role of Magnesium in Photosynthesis

1. Chloroplast

One of the greatest triumphs of early evolution was the invention of a means to harness the energy of the sun, which is transmitted as light, to drive energy-requiring synthetic processes. This process in higher plants occurs in an especially organized subcellular organelle, the chloroplast. The chloroplast is an organized set of membranes crowded with water-insoluble lipid and containing the central pigment chlorophyll. Chlorophyll is the magnesium chelate of porphyrin.

2. Chlorophyll

It is chlorophyll that produces the oxygen and the foods for all other forms of life on earth. The excess production of oxygen soon made the oxidation of organic compounds thermodynamically favorable. Under these new conditions, the desired thermodynamically uphill reactions would be the photoreduction of the oxidized organic compounds, including carbon dioxide. It is just these photoreactions that are favored by chelating a dipositive closed shell metal ion into the porphyrin ring. Mauzerall (1973) hypothesizes that the purpose of the ionically bound magnesium in the vacant hole in the porphyrin ring is to stabilize the structure so that it undergoes perfectly reversible one-electron oxidations. The redox potential of chlorophyll correlates very well with the electronegativity of the central magnesium ion. With photoactivation, the chelated magnesium makes the excited state a powerful reductant and stabilizes the resulting cation. Why magnesium rather than some other metal in the photosynthetic pigments? Fuhrhop and Mauzerall (1969) suggest that if the aim of the biological system is a minimum redox potential combined with maximum stability in a protonic solvent, then magnesium is a good minimax solution to the requirements.

3. Regulation of Photosynthesis by Magnesium

One can imagine that the chlorophyll molecule harvests light in the manner of a lightmeter. The light quantum activates the chlorophyll molecule; that is, an electron moves from the π orbitals to the exterior of an atomic shell and then is ejected, leaving behind a chlorophyll free radical. This terminates the true photochemical event, in which a light quantum is transmuted into a high-energy electron. Lin and Nobel (1971) observed an increase in the concentration of chloroplast Mg^{2+} *in vivo* caused by illuminating the plant, the first direct evidence indicating that changes in magnesium level actually occur in the plant cell. This extra magnesium in the chloroplasts enhanced the photophosphorylation rate. Thus, the increase in magnesium in chloroplasts may be a regulatory mechanism whereby light controls photosynthetic activity.

The energy of electrons is used to produce the adenosine triphosphate (ATP), which together with reduced nicotinamide adenine dinucleotide (NADH), drives the formation of carbohydrates from CO_2. Therefore, the chloroplast is a transducer that converts the electromagnetic energy from the sun into the chemical energy of ATP. This transduction does not occur in the absence of the chelated magnesium.

The chloroplast is located physically in the granum. The granum possesses a lamellar structure that is compatible with the existence of an interface between hydrophilic and hydrophobic phases, in which the chlorophyll molecule could be completely accommodated in a closely packed or monomolecular layer. From this characteristic lamellarity evolves the concept of a unit membrane held together with the assistance of magnesium. Chlorophyll functions in photosynthesis by virtue of its ability to produce and to maintain a charge separation in the highly ordered lamellar structure of the chloroplast.

4. A View of Photosynthesis

The entire photosynthetic process can be viewed as the capture of the energy of photons in the form of high-energy electrons, followed by a stepwise passage of electrons down an energy gradient in a structured membrane held together with the coordinating properties of the magnesium atom. This model is essentially the unifying concept first proposed by Szent-Györgi (1960); it is now modified to explain the role of magnesium.

The subsequent synthetic process may be summarized as follows:

$$6CO_2 + 6H_2O + 18ATP + 12NADH \rightarrow C_6H_{12}O_6 + 18ADP + 18P_i + 12NAD + 6O_2$$

ATP and chemical reducing power operate to produce carbohydrate via common intermediates, which require twelve separate enzymes. All enzyme reactions that are known to be catalyzed by ATP show an absolute requirement for magnesium.

B. Role of Magnesium in Oxidative Phosphorylation

In the absence of sunlight, plants rely on stored chemical energy to maintain life. This stored energy is released by oxidative phosphorylation, a process that occurs in the mitochondrial membrane of both plant and animal cells. The primary function of all mitochondria is to couple phosphorylation to oxidation. ATP, the main fuel of life, is produced in oxidative phosphorylation. All enzyme reactions that are known to be catalyzed by ATP show an absolute requirement for magnesium. These reactions encompass a very wide spectrum of synthetic processes.

So fundamental and widespread are the reactions involving ATP, that it must influence practically all processes of life. A host of enzymes are activated by the magnesium cation; this group includes all those utilizing ATP or catalyzing the transfer of phosphate. ATP is known to form a magnesium complex, with Mg^{2+} binding usually to the phosphate moiety. Magnesium has a single divalent state and does not form highly stable chelates with organic complexes, as do the transitional metals. It is perhaps this quality that allows it to act as a bridge in a large number of chemical reactions not requiring redox reactions but resulting in transfer of organic groups from one molecule to another. When organic phosphate takes part in a reaction, magnesium is usually its inorganic cofactor. All partners in reactions known to be dependent on ATP are capable of chelating with magnesium. The effect of magnesium chelation in such reactions is to lower the free energy of activation of the rate-determining step.

The ATP molecule is usually depicted as existing in a linear configuration, with the purine and the phosphate ends separated by the pentose. Szent-Györgi (1969) has suggested that the spacial configuration of the ATP molecule is such that it could function as a transformer as well as a storage battery. The phosphate chain can touch the purine ring; magnesium can form a very stable quadridentate chelate connecting the two ends of the ATP molecule, and energy in the form of electrons can now pass from the phosphate to the purine. The magnesium may not only actually connect the two ends of the molecule, but it may also make one single, unique electronic system of the phosphate chain and the purine with common nonlocalized electrons that could transport energy.

C. The Mitochondrion

The roles of sunlight, chlorophyll, and magnesium in the primary synthetic process on earth have already been discussed; in photosynthesis, carbon dioxide and water are synthesized into carbohydrate, and oxygen is released. In the absence of sunlight, plants rely on stored chemical energy to maintain life. This stored energy is released by oxidative phosphorylation, a process that occurs in the mitochondria of both plant and animal cells. The biosynthesis of ATP coupled to the oxidation of substrate is known as oxidative phosphorylation and takes place in the mitochondrial membrane. The primary function of all mitochondria is to couple phosphorylation to oxidation. The transduction is the conversion of chemical energy from the bond energies of certain metabolites to the bond energies of ATP. Whereas phosphorylation in the chloroplast is light-dependent, phosphorylation in the mitochondrion is dependent not on light but on oxygen. Whereas photosynthesis combines carbon dioxide and water and evolves oxygen, oxidative phosphorylation does just the reverse. It requires oxygen and evolves carbon dioxide and water, thus completing the carbon cycle on earth and returning the electrons to ground state.

ATP, the main fuel of life, is produced in both photosynthesis and oxidative phosphorylation. In both cases, ATP is produced by an electric current, that is, the energy released by "dropping" electrons.

The mitochondrion represents a general blueprint that is characteristic of all membrane systems; in fact, it is characteristic of all the energy-transforming systems of the cell (Green, 1964). The basic design of the mitochondrion is copied in all other systems in the cell that have to do with the transformation or use of energy. Under the electron microscope, the mitochondrion, just like the chloroplast, is seen to consist of a lamellar membrane. The inner membrane forms invaginations (cristae). The intermembrane and intercristal spaces are thought to be continuous and to form a central compartment. The matrix, which is surrounded by the folded inner membrane, comprises the second compartment, and the entire mitochondrion is thought to be a two-compartment system. The cristae contain a strictly regulated respiratory chain along which electrons are transferred by the difference in redox potentials. Along this respiratory chain, the oxidation–reduction energy is converted into phosphate bond energy in the form of ATP. The optimum concentration of magnesium for the process appears to be 10^{-4} to 10^{-5} M. The respiratory enzymes, cytochromes and flavoproteins, which sequentially release the energy of the electrons, may be embedded in the mitochondrial membranes that are structurally organized into respiratory units. The oxidizing enzymes in the inner mitochondrial membrane are assembled asymmetrically in a way that gives rise to a vectorial movement of protons. Racker (1974) feels that this proton current is the driving force in the production of biologically useful energy.

The traditional concept of a mitochondrion is that of small, discrete, intracellular organelle, relatively free in the cytoplasm. Recent serial section studies indicate that in the yeast (Hoffman and Avers, 1973) and in the rat liver (Brandt *et al.*, 1974) there is but one mitochondrion, consisting of a single branching tubular structure, per cell.

The mitochondrion can be made to swell and contract experimentally. Although swelling can be caused by a large variety of different chemical agents, it is significant that only ATP together with magnesium can cause contraction. ATP is always split during contraction of swollen mitochondria.

A rapid swelling of heart and liver mitochondria can be produced in rats fed a magnesium-deficient diet for 10 days, whereas no significant decrease in the magnesium content of the mitochondrion results. ATP reverses the swelling of mitochondria from heart and liver of magnesium-deficient rats.

Life could have been no more than an experiment of nature until protoorganisms developed dependable machinery to perform two basic functions: (a) generate energy in a form usable for the organisms' various requirements (ATP), and (b) reproduce themselves. It is of considerable theoretical interest that all forms of life on earth have basically the same system for these two purposes. They are summed up in the familiar initials ATP and DNA. The relationship between ATP and magnesium has already been discussed. We shall discuss next the involvement of magnesium in the biochemistry of DNA.

D. Magnesium and DNA

During the past twenty years, scientists have obtained substantial understanding of how information is stored and replicated in DNA molecules, how it is passed on to RNA molecules and finally to proteins, and how the three-dimensional structure of proteins depends upon the linear arrangement of the constituent amino acids. This information storage in molecular structure and its subsequent readout is dependent upon the presence of magnesium in optimal concentration (Krakauer, 1972). The rather complicated three-dimensional structures assumed by some polymers are a consequence of their primary sequence. The interactions of these to form even more complicated multicomponent complexes are also determined by their chemistry.

One of the most important chemical constituents of the cell is deoxyribonucleic acid (DNA); DNA is almost exclusively confined to the cell nucleus and is the carrier of genetic information.

Much of the magnesium in the cell nucleus is combined with those phosphoric groups of DNA that are not occupied by histone. The chemical factors that control the variable activity at the sites along a chromosome are largely unknown. There is a suggestion that the sites along the DNA chain at which the phosphoric acid groups are combined with histone are inactive and, conversely, that those at which they are combined with magnesium are active. The physical integrity of the DNA helix appears to be dependent upon magnesium. There is evidence to suggest that Mg^{2+} is necessary as an intermediate complexing agent during cell duplication and during the formation of ribonucleic acid (RNA) on a double-stranded DNA template.

Both magnesium and ATP are involved in the synthesis of nucleic acids. Since sections of the chromosomes in the nucleus are held together by calcium and magnesium, it seems likely that changes in the concentration of magnesium in the medium might determine the degree of chromosomal aberration. There is evidence that variations in the concentration of magnesium *in vivo* exerts control on DNA synthesis.

E. Magnesium and the Ribosome

Ribosomes are of universal occurrence in microorganisms, higher plants, and animals. The principal and probably the only function of the ribosome is the biosynthesis of protein. The rate of protein synthesis is proportionate to the number of ribosomes present. Ribosomes require magnesium ions in order to maintain their physical stability (Hughes, 1972); they dissociate into smaller particles when the magnesium concentration becomes low (Zitomer and Flaks, 1972). An optimum intracellular concentration of magnesium is required for the integrity of the macromolecules necessary for RNA synthesis (Clement et al., 1973). The physical size of the RNA aggregates is controlled by the concentration of magnesium, and polypeptide formation cannot proceed unless magnesium concentration is optimal (Willick and Kay, 1971). Magnesium ion probably acts to stabilize a favorable protein conformation (Case et al., 1973).

F. Discussion

There is very little doubt that magnesium is essential for life on earth. The exact function of magnesium in the chlorophyll molecule, as well as in maintaining the structural integrity of the granum, is conjectural; however, it seems possible that magnesium, because of its inherent atomic composition, is, in this particular situation, able to capture and transmit energy more efficiently than any other element. Moreover, the magnesium atom is able to hold reacting groups together and thus to maintain the physical configurations that are optimal either for the transfer of energy in the form of excited electrons or for the transmutation of energy into ATP. The one fundamental property of magnesium upon which all of the photosynthetic processes depends is chelation. It seems that the capture, conversion, storage, and utilization of solar energy are all dependent upon a chelating function that is unique to, and specific for, the magnesium atom.

Two of the basic functions of solar energy in living cells are genetic transcription and protein synthesis. Recent studies in molecular biology have established that interrelations exist among the three major biologic macromolecules—DNA, RNA, and proteins. Genetic information stored in DNA is transcribed into messenger RNA, which in turn translates that information into amino acid sequences in the newly synthesized protein. At literally every turn in these processes, magnesium plays a vital role. The physical integrity of the DNA helix appears to be dependent on magnesium. The physical size of the RNA aggregates is controlled by the concentration of magnesium, and polypeptide formation cannot proceed unless magnesium concentration is optimal.

Rasmussen (1974) has recently discussed the role of calcium in the "closed-loop" feedback system necessary for the mediation of hormonal action; he predicts that it is likely that Mg^{2+} will prove to be another divalent cation with a messenger function as complex as that of calcium. This messenger function of magnesium may involve chemical binding to establish physical proximity of reacting groups.

III. PHYSIOLOGY OF MAGNESIUM

A. Normal Distribution and Turnover of Magnesium in Man

1. Body Content

The limited data available from analysis of human carcasses indicate that the magnesium content of the human body ranges between 22.7 and 35.0 meq/kg wet weight of tissue (Widdowson et al., 1951). Extrapolations from tissue analyses performed on victims of accidental death indicate that the body content of magnesium for a man weighing 70 kg would be of the order of 2000 meq (24 gm) (Schroeder *et al.*, 1969).

Eighty-nine percent of all the magnesium in the body resides in bone and muscle. Bone contains about 60% of the total body content of magnesium at a concentration of about 90 meq/kg wet weight. Most of the remaining magnesium is distributed equally between muscle and nonmuscular soft tissues. Of the nonosseous tissues, liver and striated muscle contain the highest concentration, 14–16 meq/kg. Approximately 1% of the total body content of magnesium is extracellular. The levels of magnesium in serum of healthy people are remarkably constant, remaining on the average at 1.7 meq/liter and varying less than 15% from this mean value (Wacker and Parisi, 1968). The distribution of normal values for serum magnesium is identical in men and women and remains constant with advancing age (Keating *et al.*, 1969). Approximately one-third of the extracellular magnesium is bound nonspecifically to plasma proteins. The remaining 65%, which is diffusible or ionized, appears to be the biologically active component. The ratio of bound to unbound magnesium, as well as to total serum levels, is remarkably constant. The magnesium content of erythrocytes varies from 4.4 to 6.0 meq/liter (Baron and Ahmet, 1969).

2. Intake

The average American ingests daily between 20 and 40 meq of magnesium; magnesium intakes of from 0.30 to 0.35 meq/kg/day are thought to be adequate to maintain magnesium balance in normal adults (Jones *et al.*, 1967). A daily intake of 17 meq (0.25 meq/kg) may meet nutritive requirements provided that the individual remains in positive magnesium balance. Schroeder *et al.* (1969) called attention to the theoretical relationship of dietary magnesium deficiency to serious chronic diseases including atherosclerosis. The estimated daily requirement for a child is 12.5 meq (150 mg) (Coussons, 1969). The greater importance of magnesium in childhood is suggested by the relative ease with which deficiency states are produced experimentally in young animals as compared with adult animals (Coussons, 1969).

Some common foods can be ranked in order of decreasing mean concentrations of magnesium, as follows: nuts, 162 meq/kg; cereals, 66; sea foods, 29; meats, 22; legumes, 20; vegetables, 14; dairy products, 13; fruits, 6; refined sugars, 5; fats, 0.6. This order differs when the concentrations are ranked on the basis of the caloric values of the foods, as follows: vegetables, legumes, sea foods, nuts, cereals, dairy products, fruit, meat, refined sugars, and fats. Noteworthy is the very small contribution of fats and refined sugars to the total intake of magnesium. These two, the major sources of caloric energy, are virtually devoid of magnesium (Schroeder *et al.*, 1969).

3. Absorption

When a tracer dose of ^{28}Mg was administered orally to twenty-six subjects, fecal excretion within 120 hr accounted for 60–88% of the administered dose (Aikawa *et al.*, 1958). The concentration of radioactivity in the plasma was maximal at 4 hr, but the actual increase in serum magnesium concentration was negligible. When ^{28}Mg was injected intravenously into a normal human subject, only 1.8% of the radioactivity was recovered in the stool within 72 hr (Aikawa *et al.*, 1960). The fecal magnesium appears to be primarily magnesium from material that is not absorbed by the body rather than magnesium secreted by the intestine. Ingested magnesium appears to be absorbed mainly by the small intestine (Schroeder *et al.*, 1969). The factors controlling the gastrointestinal absorption of magnesium are poorly understood.

4. Secretion

There undoubtedly is considerable secretion of magnesium into the intestinal tract from bile and from pancreatic and intestinal juices. This secretion is followed by almost complete reabsorption. Parotid saliva contains about 0.3 meq/liter (Lear and Grøn, 1968) and pancreatic juice about 0.1 meq/liter of magnesium. The concentration of magnesium in other secretions varies considerably. The observation that hypomagnesemia can occur in patients suffering from large losses of intestinal fluids suggests that intestinal juices contain enough magnesium to deplete the serum when magnesium is not reabsorbed by the colon.

Studies are just beginning on the role played in the transport of divalent cations by biochemical changes in the cells of the intestinal mucosa (Szelényi, 1973). Further investigations may show that the cells of the intestinal mucosa, like those in the kidney and elsewhere in the body, may depend in part upon metabolic activity for the uptake and release of calcium and magnesium.

5. Excretion

Most of that portion of the magnesium that is absorbed into the body is excreted by the kidney; fecal magnesium represents largely the unabsorbed fraction. In subjects on a normal diet, one-third or less of the ingested magnesium (5–17 meq) is excreted by the kidney. After the intravenous injection of a tracer dose of ^{28}Mg in 12–16 meq of stable magnesium, the daily urinary excretion of magnesium in eight normal subjects ranged between 6 and 36 meq (Aikawa et al., 1960). Urinary excretion increased as the parenteral dose was increased. The maximal renal capacity for excretion is not known, but it is probably quite high, perhaps greater than 164 meq/day (Wacker and Parisi, 1968).

The diffusible magnesium in plasma is filtered by the glomeruli and is reabsorbed by the renal tubules, probably by an active process, although the control mechanisms are not known. There is some evidence that magnesium may be secreted by the renal tubule (Forster and Berglund, 1956). Both the mercurial and the thiazide diuretics increase excretion of magnesium, calcium, potassium, and sodium.

Magnesium excretion also occurs in sweat (Consolazio et al., 1963). When men are exposed to high temperature for several days, from 10 to 15% of the total output of magnesium is recovered in sweat. Acclimatization does not occur as in the case for sodium and potassium. Under extreme conditions, sweat can account for 25% of the magnesium lost daily; this factor would be important when the intake of magnesium is low.

6. Magnesium Conservation on a Low-Magnesium Diet

It is primarily the ionic fraction of the magnesium in plasma that appears in the glomerular filtrate. Any protein-bound magnesium that is filtered is probably returned to the circulation via lymph. The excretion of magnesium may be greater than normal in renal diseases associated with heavy proteinuria.

Magnesium clearance, corrected for protein binding, increases as a linear function of serum magnesium concentration and approaches the inulin clearance at high plasma levels of magnesium. There normally appears to be almost maximal tubular reabsorption of magnesium (Chesley and Tepper, 1958).

In spite of the probability of diets being low in magnesium under certain circumstances, magnesium deficiency does not occur in human beings with healthy kidneys. The explanation for this clinical observation appears to be that renal mechanisms are efficient enough to conserve all but about 1 meq of magnesium per day. Fecal losses are minimal (Barnes et al., 1958).

7. Abnormal Magnesium Levels in the Blood

Values lower than 1.1 meq/liter have been obtained in patients with congestive heart failure, cirrhosis, or renal failure after hemodialysis. All values higher than 2.0 meq/liter were found in patients with renal failure before therapy (Aikawa, 1958–1959).

B. Plasma Clearance and Tissue Uptake of Magnesium

1. Early Studies

Mendel and Benedict (1909) reviewed much of the early literature on the absorption and excretion of magnesium. These investigators showed quite clearly that rapid renal excretion of magnesium followed the subcutaneous injection of various magnesium salts, whereas intestinal excretion was minimal. However, Hirchfelder and Haury (1934) reported that in seven normal adults, 40–44% of an injected dose of magnesium appeared in the urine within 24 hr. Tibbetts and Aub (1937), by means of classic balance techniques, studied the excretion of magnesium in normal subjects; they found that individuals on an oral intake of 49–74 meq/day excreted 41–66 meq, of which slightly over one-half was in the stools. Smith et al. (1939) studied the excretion of magnesium in dogs after the intravenous administration of magnesium sulfate and concluded that the magnesium distributed itself throughout the extracellular fluid during the first 3–4 hr; during subsequent hours some of the ion appeared to be segregated from the extracellular fluid and was not excreted.

2. Tracer Studies in Human Beings

The introduction of the radioactive isotope of magnesium ^{28}Mg for clinical studies in 1957 made possible determination of the "exchangeable" pool in human subjects. When nine normal subjects were given intravenous infusions of 12–30 meq of magnesium tagged with ^{28}Mg, the material was very rapidly cleared from the extracellular fluid (Aikawa et al., 1960). The concentration of radioactivity in plasma and urine was too low to follow beyond 36 hr. Within a few hours, the volume of fluid available for the dilution of this ion, as calculated from the plasma concentration of ^{28}Mg, exceeded the volume of total body water.

The clearance curves in general showed a rapid phase during the first 4 hr, a subsequent more gradual decline up to about 14 hr, and a slow exponential slope thereafter. Biopsies of tissues contained concentrations of ^{28}Mg in liver, appendix, fat, skin, and subcutaneous connective tissue that could not be attributed solely to the extracellular components of these tissues. All of these observations suggested that ^{28}Mg rapidly entered cells of the soft tissues and that 70% or more of the infused magnesium was retained in the body for at least 24 hr.

Of interest is the observation that the 24 hr urinary excretion of stable magnesium following the infusion of ^{28}Mg approximated the amount of nonradioactive magnesium infused, whereas only 20% of the ^{28}Mg infused was recovered. Previous investigators without the benefit of the radioisotopic data have assumed that most of the infused magnesium was rapidly excreted by the kidney. The additional isotopic data indicate that the infusion of fairly large amounts of magnesium results in a compensatory renal excretion of the body store of magnesium and that the material excreted is probably not the ions that were administered.

Serial external surveys of radioactivity over the entire body revealed the maximal distribution of radioactivity at the end of infusion over the right upper quadrant of the abdomen. This finding suggests initial concentration of magnesium in the liver. At 18 hr, the specific activity in bile was equal to that of serum. This equilibration of the infused ^{28}Mg had occurred earlier in bile than in any other tissue or fluid available for study (Aikawa et al., 1960).

After about 18 hr, the specific activities in plasma and urine showed only a slight gradual increase, suggesting that the infused material had equilibrated with the stable magnesium in a rather labile pool and that further exchange was occurring very slowly in a less labile pool. The size of this labile pool in normal subjects ranged between 135 and 397 meq (2.6–5.3 meq/kg of body weight). Since the body content of magnesium is estimated to be 30 meq/kg, it appears that less than 16% of the total body content of magnesium is measured by the ^{28}Mg exchange technique.

The results of the external survey and the tissue analyses suggest that the labile pool of magnesium is contained primarily in connective tissue, skin, and the soft tissues of the abdominal cavity (such as the liver and intestine) and that the magnesium in bone, muscle, and red cells exchanges very slowly.

In another study, Silver et al. (1960) followed the turnover of magnesium for periods up to 90 hr after ^{28}Mg was injected intravenously into human subjects. Even at 90 hr, only one-third of the body's magnesium had reached equilibrium with the isotope. The results confirmed the impression that the gastrointestinal absorption of magnesium is very limited. Graphic analysis of urinary ^{28}Mg curves in terms of exponential components yielded a slow component with a half-time of 13–35 hr, which accounted for 10–15% of the injected dose, and two more rapid components with half-time of 1 and 3 hr each, which accounted for 15–25% of the injected dose. The large fraction remaining—about 25–50% of the body's total—had a turnover rate of less than 2% per day. Because approximately 25–50% of the total body content exchanges at a turnover rate of less than 2% per day, this isotopic dilution method, used so successfully with sodium and potassium, cannot be employed to quantitate the total body content of magnesium in man. In rabbits, however, the exchangeable magnesium value at 24 hr agrees well with the total carcass content of magnesium (Aikawa et al., 1959). During starvation the renal excretion of magnesium amounts to 61.7 meq/kg of weight loss (Aikawa et al., 1959).

3. Magnesium Equilibration in Bone

The reactivity of the skeleton, as measured by isotopic exchange, declines with age (Breibart et al., 1960). The exchange of ^{28}Mg, expressed as bone/serum specific activity, is much more rapid in younger animals than in older ones. ^{28}Mg accumulates in the bones of young rats about twice as fast as in the bones of adult rats (Lengemann, 1959).

The exchange of ^{28}Mg in cortical bone occurs much more rapidly in young rats than in old ones. The stable magnesium content of bone increases with age and varies inversely with the water content of bone. Magnesium-28 studies in lambs indicate that the magnesium reserve in bone is mobilized during dietary magnesium deficiency (McAleese et al., 1960).

4. Magnesium-28 Compartmental Analysis in Man

Avioli and Berman (1966) used a combination of metabolic balance and ^{28}Mg turnover techniques in order to develop a mathematical model for magnesium metabolism in man. The data thus derived were subjected to compartmental analysis using digital computer techniques.

After the intravenous administration of ^{28}Mg, the decline in the specific activity of plasma or urine can be expressed as the sum of several exponential terms by the method of graphic analysis. On the basis of such analyses, Silver et al. (1960) defined in man three exchangeable magnesium compartments with half-times of 38 hr, 3 hr, and 1 hr. MacIntyre et al. (1961) described three exchangeable magnesium compartments containing 7.3, 24.4, and 98.7 meq of magnesium. Zumoff *et al.* (1958) obtained similar data.

Multicompartmental analysis indicates that in man there are at least three exchangeable magnesium pools with varied rates of turnover (Wallach *et al.*, 1966):

Compartments 1 and 2—exemplifying pools with a relatively fast turnover, together approximating extracellular fluid in distribution.

Compartment 3—an intracellular pool containing over 80% of the exchanging magnesium with a turnover rate of one-half that of the most rapid pool.

Compartment 4—which probably accounts for most of the whole-body magnesium.

Only 15% of whole-body magnesium, averaging 3.54 meq/kg body weight, is accounted for by relatively rapid exchange processes (Avioli and Berman, 1966).

C. Gastrointestinal Absorption

1. Daily Absorption in Man

In normal individuals on regular diets, the average daily absorption of magnesium from the gastrointestinal tract is 0.14 meq/kg, an amount approximately 40% of the size of the extracellular pool. The rate of entry of magnesium into the intracellular pool would be approximately 0.0058 meq/kg/hr if one assumes that absorption occurs continuously throughout the day. This rate of entry is approximately 1% of the rate of removal of magnesium from the extracellular pool by all routes (Wallach *et al.*, 1966).

2. Factors Affecting Absorption

No single factor appears to play a dominant role in the absorption of magnesium as does vitamin D in the absorption of calcium. Several studies using ^{28}Mg suggest that the absorption of magnesium in man is influenced by the load presented to the intestinal mucosa (Aikawa, 1959; Graham *et al.*, 1960). On an ordinary diet containing 20 meq of magnesium, 44% of the ingested radioactivity was absorbed per day. On a low-magnesium diet (1.9 meq/day), 76% was absorbed. On a high-magnesium diet (47 meq/day), absorption was decreased to 24%.

Absorption begins within an hour of ingestion and continues at a steady rate for 2–8 hr; it is minimal after 12 hr. In man, absorption throughout the small intestine is fairly uniform, but little or no magnesium is absorbed from the large bowel (Graham *et al.*, 1960).

3. Site of Absorption

Evidence from a variety of animals suggests that the small intestine is the main site of magnesium absorption but that the pattern of absorption varies with the species studied (Graham *et al.*, 1960; Field, 1961). Absorption from the large intestine is negligible in the rabbit (Aikawa, 1959). In male albino rats, more than 79% of the total absorption of ^{28}Mg takes place in the colon, and excretion of endogenous magnesium occurs predominantly in the proximal gut (Chutkow, 1964). Both magnesium and calcium are bound to phosphate and to nonphosphate binding material of an unknown nature in the ileal contents of ruminating calves (Smith and McAllan, 1966) and hence are rendered nonultrafilterable.

There appears to be an interrelationship between the absorption of magnesium and calcium in the proximal part of the small intestine in the rat (Alcock and MacIntyre, 1962). The suggestion has been made that there is a common mechanism for transporting calcium and magnesium across the intestinal wall (MacIntyre, 1960; Hendrix *et al.*, 1963).

4. Role of Ionic Magnesium

At the present time, there is no unequivocal evidence that magnesium is actively transported across the gut wall (Aikawa, 1965). It seems reasonable to assume that the net amount of dietary magnesium absorbed is directly related to the intake and to the time available for absorption of the magnesium from the small intestine. Therefore, apart from a small effect from the difference in potential across the wall of the small intestine, the concentration of ionic magnesium in the digest at the absorption site must be the main factor controlling the amount absorbed in a given time (Smith and McAllan, 1966).

D. Renal Excretion

1. Control of Body Content

The kidney is the major excretory pathway for magnesium once it is absorbed into the body (Mendel and Benedict, 1909). In subjects on a normal diet, this renal excretion amounts to one-third or less of the 5–17 meq of magnesium ingested every day. The mean daily excretion of magnesium in the urine of twelve normal men on an unrestricted diet was 13.3 ± 3.5 meq (Wacker and Vallee, 1958). Following the intravenous injection of a tracer dose of ^{28}Mg in 12–16 meq of stable magnesium, the daily urinary excretion of magnesium in eight normal subjects ranged between 6 and 36 meq (Aikawa et al., 1958). Urinary excretion of magnesium increased as the parenteral dose was increased.

Metabolic balance studies in twenty-seven subjects on a self-selected diet of normal composition showed a close positive correlation between the level of dietary intake and the magnesium excretion in both the urine and the feces (Heaton, 1969). These results suggest that the absorption of magnesium from the intestinal tract is a poorly controlled process that is determined largely by the dietary intake of the element. The kidney must therefore be the organ principally responsible for regulating the total body content of magnesium. When dietary intake of magnesium is increased or decreased, urinary excretion of magnesium is increased or decreased, respectively, without any significant change in the plasma level of magnesium.

2. Effect of Dietary Restriction of Magnesium

Retention of magnesium by the kidney occurs rapidly in response to a restriction in the dietary intake (Fitzgerald and Fourman, 1956; Barnes et al., 1958). This is why it is so difficult to produce magnesium depletion in the adult without some source of abnormal loss from the body.

Diurnal variations in the urinary excretion of calcium and magnesium have been demonstrated in patients in a metabolism ward (Briscoe and Ragan, 1966). A reduction in the excretion of calcium, magnesium, sodium, and creatinine occurs at night. There are slight but constant diurnal variations in the serum concentration of calcium and magnesium, with the values being lower in the morning than in the evening. Diet and physical activity appear to play the dominant roles in this diurnal fluctuation, but there also might be an associated rhythm in the function of the parathyroid gland.

3. Mechanism of Renal Excretion

The mechanism of excretion of magnesium by the mammalian kidney is still unclear. It could involve glomerular filtration and partial reabsorption of the filtered material by the renal tubules, or the filtered material could be completely reabsorbed and the excreted magnesium appear by tubular secretion, as is believed to occur with potassium. Tubular secretion of magnesium undoubtedly occurs in the aglomerular fish

(Berglund and Forster, 1958), but stop-flow studies with radioactive magnesium in dogs have produced conflicting evidence about secretion of magnesium by the tubules (Ginn *et al.*, 1959; Murdaugh and Robinson, 1960). In the rabbit, the renal excretion of magnesium appears to be essentially glomerular; the tubular wall appears to be impermeable by magnesium throughout its length (Raynaud, 1962).

4. A Possible Renal Threshold

The amount of magnesium that is filtered at the glomerulus in an adult human is about 9.6 meq/hr, assuming a glomerular filtration rate of 130 ml/min, a total plasma magnesium concentration of 1.6 meq/liter, and an ultrafiltrable fraction comprising 75% of the total. The mean rate of magnesium excretion in the urine (about 0.33 meq/hr) therefore represents only 3.5% of the filtered load. Moreover, the whole range of excretion observed under physiological conditions in man can be explained if the tubular reabsorption of magnesium varies between 91 and 99% of the amount filtered at the glomerulus. In the rat (Averill and Heaton, 1966), sheep (Wilson, 1960), and cattle (Storry and Rook, 1962), there is evidence for the existence of a renal threshold for excretion of magnesium at a value close to the lower limit of the normal blood level. There is reduction in net tubular reabsorption of magnesium above a total serum magnesium concentration of 1.2–1.4 meq/liter; this could be due to either a decrease in the maximum capacity for tubular reabsorption or an increase in tubular secretion of magnesium.

5. Tubular Secretion

The possibility of secretion of magnesium by the renal tubules has been investigated under conditions of magnesium loading (Heaton, 1969). At serum concentrations above 6.2 meq/liter, the amount excreted exceeded twice the filtered load, thus demonstrating tubular secretion of magnesium beyond any likely experimental error. The response to the administration of 2,4-dinitrophenol suggested that magnesium is also secreted by the tubules under physiological conditions.

All the available evidence in the rat until recently has been consistent with a mechanism for magnesium excretion that involves reabsorption of the filtered material, with the excreted magnesium derived chiefly by tubular secretion. This secretion appears only to commence when the magnesium concentration in serum exceeds a critical value that is close to the lower limit of the normal range. However, studies with stop–flow techniques did not find magnesium secretion in acutely magnesium-loaded rats undergoing mannitol or sulfate diuresis (Alfredson and Walser, 1970).

In the dog (Massry et al., 1969), magnesium excretion, like sodium and calcium excretion, is determined by filtration and reabsorption alone, without evidence for tubular secretion. There is a maximal tubular reabsorptive capacity (T_m) for magnesium of approximately 11.5 μeq/min/kg body weight. The parathyroid hormone may directly enhance tubular reabsorption of magnesium.

E. Homeostasis

We do not understand yet the physiological mechanisms responsible for maintaining the plasma magnesium concentration at a constant level (MacIntyre, 1967). Both calcitonin (Littledike and Arnaud, 1971) and parathormone may be involved. Nevertheless, animals and human beings on an adequate intake of magnesium do remain in magnesium balance, and the two chief regulatory sites appear to be the gastrointestinal tract and the kidney.

1. Effects of Parathyroid Hormone

There is considerable evidence for the hypothesis that the parathyroid hormone may help to control the concentration of plasma magnesium through a negative feedback mechanism (Heaton, 1965; Gill et al., 1967; MacIntyre et al., 1963).

Magnesium deficiency in the intact rat is accompanied by hypercalcemia and hypophosphatemia, provided the parathyroid glands are intact. The concentration of ionic calcium in plasma is elevated. In the absence of the parathyroid gland, magnesium-deficient rats do not develop hypercalcemia or hypophosphatemia. Moreover, parathyroidectomized animals with magnesium deficiency develop a concentration of ionized calcium in plasma that is lower than that observed in parathyroidectomized rats on a normal diet (Gitelman et al., 1968a; Sallis and DeLuca, 1966).

These observations help to establish a relationship between an apparent increased function of the parathyroid gland and magnesium deficiency (Sallis and DeLuca, 1966). Recent studies by Anast et al. (1972) and Suh et al. (1973) suggest that magnesium depletion in man may result in impaired synthesis or release of parathyroid hormone, or both. If parathyroid regulation is influenced by the concentration of magnesium in plasma, hypermagnesemia should diminish parathyroid gland activity (Altenähr and Leonhardt, 1972).

2. Effects of Hypermagnesemia

This hypothesis was tested in intact and chronically parathyroidectomized rats that were nephrectomized to eliminate the urinary excretion of calcium as a variable in the study. Isotonic magnesium chloride was administered subcutaneously to the experimental animals, and normal saline was administered to the controls. A significant decrease in the concentration of ionic calcium was observed in the magnesium-treated animals with the intact parathyroid glands. In contrast, magnesium-treated parathyroidectomized animals failed to develop a significant change in the concentration of ionic calcium in comparison to saline-treated parathyroidectomized controls. These observations suggest that hypermagnesemia may inhibit parathyroid gland activity. The results are consistent with the hypothesis that the parathyroid regulatory mechanism, which is involved in calcium homeostatis, is modified by alterations in the concentration of plasma magnesium (Gitelman et al., 1968b).

3. Perfusion Studies

The influence of the plasma magnesium concentration on parathyroid gland function was evaluated in goats and in a sheep by perfusion of the isolated parathyroid gland with whole blood of varying magnesium concentration (Buckle et al., 1968). The concentration of parathyroid hormone in venous plasma from the gland was estimated by a specific radioimmunoassay. In each animal, the concentration of parathyroid hormone in the effluent plasma diminished when the concentration of magnesium was raised; the concentration of hormone increased when the concentration of magnesium was lowered. The response of the parathyroid hormone concentration to changes in plasma magnesium concentration occurred within minutes. Magnesium appeared to have a specific influence on the rate of release of parathyroid hormone.

4. Studies in Organ Culture

Sherwood et al. (1970) recently developed an organ culture system utilizing normal bovine parathyroid tissue. Studies with this system provide direct evidence that the release of parathyroid hormone is inversely proportional to both the calcium and the magnesium ion concentrations. These two cations are equipotent in blocking hormone release.

5. Relationship between Bone and Extracellular Magnesium

Magnesium deficiency in the rat has been shown repeatedly to cause lowering of the magnesium concentration in bone (Martindale and Heaton, 1965). The observation of a close direct relationship between the magnesium concentrations in the plasma and the femur of magnesium-deficient rats and calves supports the view that the skeleton provides the magnesium reserve in the body and suggests that there exists an equilibrium between the magnesium of the plasma and the bone. This equilibrium is apparently independent of enzymatic activity and must therefore be physicochemical in nature. The fact that the equilibrium is dependent upon the concentration of magnesium in both the medium and the bone suggests that the relationship between bone and extracellular fluid magnesium is analogous to the ionization of a poorly dissociated salt, with the magnesium in bone corresponding to the undissociated salt.

6. Effects of Parathyroid Extract *in Vitro*

Parathyroid extract increases the rate of magnesium loss from either fresh or boiled bone *in vitro* in a magnesium-low medium containing 50% bovine serum; however, the extract has no effect in a protein-free medium. These observations are consistent with the hypothesis that the physicochemical action of parathyroid preparations may involve the binding of divalent cations by a parathyroid–albumin complex (Martindale and Heaton, 1965; Gordon, 1963). This phenomenon in dead tissue, which may partially explain an important biological function, certainly is not in accord with current concepts of the mechanism of hormonal action.

F. Magnesium Deficiency in Man

1. The Clinical Syndrome

For many years there was doubt about the existence of a pure magnesium deficiency state in man. Now it is established that there is such a condition (Wacker *et al.*, 1962; Flink, 1956). It is characterized by the following features: (1) spasmophilia (Durlach *et al.*, 1967), gross muscular tremor, choreiform movements, ataxia, tetany, and, in some instances, predisposition to epileptiform convulsions (Hanna *et al.*, 1960); (2) hallucinations, agitation, confusion, tremulousness, delirium, depression, vertigo, and muscular weakness; (3) a low serum magnesium concentration associated with a normal serum calcium concentration and a normal blood pH; (4) a low-voltage T wave in the electrocardiogram (Caddell, 1967); (5) a positive Chvostek and Trousseau sign; and (6) prompt relief of the tetany when the serum magnesium concentration is restored to normal (Wacker *et al.*, 1962). Durlach recognizes the presence of other manifestations of clinical magnesium deficiency, such as phlebothrombosis, constitutional thrombasthenia and hemolytic anemia, an allergic or osseous form of the deficiency, and oxalate lithiasis (Durlach, 1967).

2. Experimental Production of a Pure Magnesium Deficiency

It is difficult to achieve a significant magnesium depletion in normal individuals by simple dietary restriction because of the exceedingly efficient renal and gastrointestinal mechanisms for conservation. The urinary magnesium in normal individuals falls to trivial amounts within 4–6 days of magnesium restriction (Fitzgerald and Fourman, 1956; Barnes *et al.*, 1960). In spite of these conservatory mechanisms, Dunn and Walser (1966) did induce in two normal subjects deficits approaching 10% of the total body content of magnesium by infusing sodium sulfate and adding calcium supplements to the magnesium-deficient diet. The concentration of magnesium in plasma and erythrocytes fell moderately. Because the muscle magnesium content remained normal, the presumption was that bone was the source of the loss. No untoward clinical effects were noted.

Randall *et al.* (1959) reported data suggesting that total body depletion of magnesium may result in psychiatric and neuromuscular symptoms. Administration of magnesium by the parenteral route or in the diet was associated with clinical improvement, which occasionally was dramatic.

The best study of magnesium deficiency in man to date is that recently reported by Shils (1964, 1969a,b). Seven subjects were placed on a magnesium-deficient diet containing 0.7 meq of magnesium per day. The concentration of magnesium in plasma declined perceptibly in all subjects within 7–10 days. Urinary and fecal magnesium decreased markedly, as did urinary calcium. At the height of the deficiency, the plasma magnesium concentration fell to a range of 10–30% of the control values, while the red cell magnesium declined more slowly and to a smaller degree. All male subjects developed hypocalcemia; the one female patient did not. Marked and persistent symptoms developed only in the presence of hypocalcemia. The serum potassium concentration decreased, and in four of the five subjects in whom the measurement was made, the ^{42}K space was decreased. The serum sodium concentration was not altered significantly. Three of the four subjects with the severest symptoms also had metabolic alkalosis.

A positive Trousseau sign, which occurred in five of the seven subjects, was the most common neurological sign observed. Electromyographic changes, which were characterized by the development of myopathic potentials, occurred in all five of the patients tested. Anorexia, nausea, and vomiting were frequently experienced. When magnesium was added to the experimental diet, all clinical and biochemical abnormalities were corrected.

3. Clinical Conditions Associated with Depletion of Magnesium

a. Fasting. Prolonged fasting is associated with a continued renal excretion of magnesium (Drenick *et al.*, 1969). After 2 months of fasting, the deficit in some subjects may amount to 20% of the total body content of magnesium. Despite evidence for depletion of magnesium in muscle, the concentration of magnesium in plasma remains unchanged. The excess acid load presented for excretion to the kidney and the absence of intake of carbohydrate might be factors contributing to the persistent loss of magnesium. The magnitude of the excretion of magnesium parallels the severity of the acidosis. The ingestion of glucose decreases the urinary loss of magnesium.

b. Excessive Loss from the Gastrointestinal Tract. Persistent vomiting or prolonged removal of intestinal secretions by mechanical suction coupled with the administration of magnesium-free intravenous infusions can induce clinical magnesium deficiency (Kellaway and Ewen, 1962; Gerst *et al.*, 1964).

c. Surgical Patients. There are postoperative changes in magnesium metabolism in patients undergoing a variety of operations involving a moderate degree of trauma (Heaton, 1964). A lowered serum magnesium concentration is observed on the day after operation in 56% of the patients, but it is usually corrected by the second or third postoperative day. Surgery is followed by a negative magnesium balance of 3 days' duration and similar changes are observed after dietary restriction in normal subjects. However, the magnitude of the magnesium loss following surgery is minimal and usually does not result in symptomatic magnesium deficiency (Macbeth and Mabbott, 1964; Monsaingeon et al., 1966; King et al., 1963).

d. *Gastrointestinal Disorders.* The intestinal tract plays a major role in magnesium homeostasis. The rate of transport of magnesium across the intestine appears to be slower than that of calcium and directly proportional to intestinal transit time (MacIntyre and Robinson, 1969). Malabsorption of magnesium therefore occurs in conditions in which intestinal transit is abnormally rapid or in which the major absorbing site, the distal small intestine, has been resected.

Hypomagnesemia is associated frequently with malabsorption due to a variety of causes. In general, there appears to be a correlation between the degree of hypomagnesemia and the severity of the underlying disease. The increased fecal loss of magnesium that has been demonstrated in this disorder may be due to steatorrhea (Gitelman and Welt, 1969).

e. *Acute Alcoholism.* The mean serum magnesium value in patients with delirium tremens in one study was 1.53 ± 0.27 meq/liter. In alcoholics without delirium tremens, it was 1.89 ± 0.22 meq/liter. In the control group of 157 nonalcoholics, the mean serum magnesium value was 1.84 ± 0.18 meq/liter. There was a tendency for the lowest serum magnesium levels to coincide with the highest values for serum glutamic oxaloacetic transaminase (Nielsen, 1963). Hypomagnesemia occurs frequently in patients with chronic alcoholism with and without delirium tremens. Patients exhibiting alcohol withdrawal signs and symptoms (Mendelson et al., 1969) have low serum and cerebrospinal fluid levels of magnesium, low exchangeable magnesium levels (Martin and Bauer, 1962; Mendelson et al., 1965), a lowered muscle content of magnesium (Jones et al., 1969), and conservation of magnesium following intravenous loading (McCollister et al., 1960). A transient decrease in serum magnesium may occur during the withdrawal state, even though prewithdrawal levels are normal. An ethanol-induced increase of magnesium in the urine occurs only when the blood alcohol level is rising. It does not persist once the subject has established high blood alcohol levels. However, in the presence of hypomagnesemia and delirium tremens, sudden death can occur as a result of cardiovascular collapse, infection, and hyperthermia (Milner and Johnson, 1965). The red cell concentration of magnesium is abnormally low in all patients with delirium tremens, whereas the plasma concentration is abnormally low in only 58% of them (Smith and Hammarsten, 1959). Intracellular fluid levels of magnesium, as reflected in the erythrocyte, correlate better with clinical symptoms and signs than do extracellular fluid levels. The predominant factor accounting for magnesium depletion in acute alcoholism is most likely an inadequate intake of magnesium, but another factor may be increased excretion of magnesium in the urine and feces (McCollister et al., 1963; Dick et al., 1969).

Independent of the phenomena described above, an abrupt and significant fall in serum magnesium levels may occur following cessation of drinking. This acute fall in serum magnesium level is associated with a transient decrease in concentration of other serum electrolytes and with respiratory alkalosis (Wolfe and Victor, 1969), and coincides with the onset of neuromuscular hyperexcitability that characterizes the withdrawal state (Mendelson et al., 1969). In most patients, there is little correlation between serum magnesium levels and such clinical findings as hallucination, tremor, and tremulous handwriting (Martin et al., 1959). A kinetic analysis of radiomagnesium turnover was performed in a group of partially repleted alcoholic subjects. Despite the continued presence of hypomagnesemia and of decreased urinary excretion of magnesium, there was little evidence of continued depletion of magnesium in the extracellular space or in the tissue pools (Wallach and Dimich, 1969).

f. Cirrhosis. The magnesium content of the liver tissue per unit weight is decreased in cirrhosis (Wilke and Spielmann, 1968). This decrease appears to be due mainly to the substitution of parenchymal tissue of high magnesium content with connective tissue of low magnesium content. There is a good relationship between histological changes (extent of fibrosis and degree of infiltration of inflammatory cells) and decrease of the magnesium concentration per number of cells. The actual changes in the concentration of magnesium in the parenchymal cells of the cirrhotic liver appear to be negligible.

IV. RESEARCH NEEDS

Almost seven decades have passed since Richard Willstatter demonstrated the central position of the magnesium atom in the chlorophyll molecule. Although much has been learned since concerning the photosynthetic process, the exact function of the magnesium atom in this process still eludes us. That magnesium is essential for photosynthesis is an established fact. There is recent evidence to suggest that magnesium may play a role in the regulation of the photosynthetic process.

Chlorophyll is a component of the chloroplast, which is located physically in the granum, which possesses a lamellar structure conducive to charge separation; the granum is the locus for photosynthesis. What is the role of magnesium at this interface of chemistry and physics to molecular biology? What about the properties of water with its low-energy bonds, as emphasized by Szent-Györgi (1971)? Can polarized water be as important as lipid in providing the living cell with its selective surface barrier (Ling, 1973)? Can all of the functions of magnesium be explained solely on the basis of the coordinating properties of the magnesium atom?

In the synthetic processes that follow the capture of solar energy, ATP plays a vital role. It is significant that all enzyme reactions known to be catalyzed by ATP have an absolute requirement for magnesium; so fundamental and widespread are the reactions involving ATP that it must influence practically all processes of life.

Is the mitochondrion a single large branching tubular structure *in vivo*, and are the small intracellular organelles the artifacts of preparation? What is the role of magnesium in this living organelle? Recent attempts to use computer graphics and computer analysis of serial section electron micrographs may supply further insight into these problems, which involve detailed studies of the tertiary structure and the spacial interrelationships of terribly complex molecules.

Energy originally derived from the sun is used by living organisms for genetic transcription and protein synthesis. It appears that magnesium plays a vital role in all of these processes—the physical integrity of the DNA helix is dependent upon magnesium; the physical size of the RNA aggregates is controlled by the concentration of magnesium; and polypeptide formation is magnesium-dependent. How can we explain this all-pervasive role of magnesium?

The first obvious fact concerning the physiology of magnesium is that most of it is located within cells. This differential concentration is of the order of 10:1 intracellular/extracellular, in the soft tissues of the body. Is metabolic energy required for the maintenance of this state, or can this be explained as due primarily to physicochemical adsorption? Can the symptoms and signs of magnesium deficiency be explained simply on the basis of the coordinating properties of the magnesium atom?

Bone contains the highest concentration of magnesium of any tissue in the body. Does this concentration require the expenditure of metabolic energy? Exactly how are the parathyroid hormone and calcitonin involved in this process?

These are all questions begging further studies.

REFERENCES

Aikawa, J. K. (1958–1959). Mg^{28} tracer studies of magnesium metabolism in animals and human beings. *Proc. U.N. Int. Conf. Peaceful Uses At. Energy, 2nd, 1958* Vol. 24, pp. 148–151.

Aikawa, J. K. (1959). Gastrointestinal absorption of Mg^{28} in rabbits. *Proc. Soc. Exp. Biol. Med.* 100, 293–295.

Aikawa, J. K. (1965). The role of magnesium in biologic processes. A review of recent developments. *In* "Electrolytes and Cardiovascular Diseases" (E. Bajusz, ed.), pp. 9–27. Karger, Basel.

Aikawa, J. K. (1971). "The Relationship of Magnesium to Disease in Domestic Animals and in Humans." Thomas, Springfield, Illinois.

Aikawa, J. K., Rhoades, E. L., and Gordon, G. S. (1958). Urinary and fecal excretion of orally administered Mg^{28}. *Proc. Soc. Exp. Biol. Med.* 98, 29–31.

Aikawa, J. K., Rhoades, E. L., Harms, D. R., and Reardon, J. Z. (1959). Magnesium metabolism in rabbits using Mg^{28} as a tracer. *Amer. J. Physiol.* 197, 99–101.

Aikawa, J. K., Gordon, G. S., and Rhoades, E. L. (1960). Magnesium metabolism in human beings: Studies with Mg^{28}. *J. Appl. Physiol.* 15, 503–507.

Alcock, N. W., and MacIntyre, I. (1962). Inter-relation of calcium and magnesium absorption. *Clin. Sci.* 22, 185–193.

Alfredson, K. S., and Walser, M. (1970). Is magnesium secreted by the rat renal tubule? *Nephron* 7, 241–247.

Altenähr, E., and Leonhardt, F. (1972). Suppression of parathyroid gland activity by magnesium. *Virchows Arch., A* 355, 297–308.

Anast, C. S., Mohs, J. M., Kaplan, S. L., and Burns, T. W. (1972). Evidence for parathyroid failure in magnesium deficiency. *Science* 177, 606–608.

Averill, C. M., and Heaton, F. W. (1966). The renal handling of magnesium. *Clin. Sci.* 31, 353–360.

Avioli, L. V., and Berman, M. (1966). Mg^{28} kinetics in man. *J. Appl. Physiol.* 21, 1688–1694.

Barnes, B. A., Cope, O., and Harrison, T. (1958). Magnesium conservation in the human being on low magnesium diet. *J. Clin. Invest.* 37, 430–440.

Barnes, B. A., Cope, O., and Gordon, E. B. (1960). Magnesium requirements and deficits. An evaluation of two surgical patients. *Ann. Surg.* 152, 518–533.

Baron, D. N., and Ahmet, S. A. (1969). Intracellular concentrations of water and of the principal electrolytes determined by analysis of isolated human leucocytes. *Clin. Sci.* 37, 205–219.

Berglund, F., and Forster, R. P. (1958). Renal tubular transport of inorganic divalent ions by the aglomerular teleost, Lophius americanus. *J. Gen. Physiol.* 41, 429–440.

Brandt, J. T., Martin, A. P., Lucas, F. V., and Vorbeck, M. L. (1974). The structure of normal rat liver mitochondria: A re-evaluation. *Fed. Proc., Fed. Amer. Soc. Exp. Biol.* 33, 603.

Breibart, S., Lee, J. S., McCoord, A., and Forbes, G. (1960). Relation of age to radiomagnesium in bone. *Proc. Soc. Exp. Biol. Med.* 105, 361–363.

Briscoe, A. M., and Ragan, C. (1966). Diurnal variations in calcium and magnesium excretion in man. *Metab., Clin. Exp.* 15, 1002–1010.

Buckle, R. M., Care, A. D., Cooper, C. W., and Gitelman, H. J. (1968). The influence of plasma magnesium concentration on parathyroid hormone secretion. *J. Endocrinol.* 42, 529–534.

Caddell, J. L. (1967). Studies in protein-calorie malnutrition. II. A double-blind clinical trial to assess magnesium therapy. *N. Engl. J. Med.* **276**, 535–540.

Case, G. S., Sinnott, M. L., and Tenu, J.-P. (1973). The role of magnesium ions in B-galactosidase-catalyzed hydrolyses. *Biochem. J.* **133**, 99–104.

Chesley, L. C., and Tepper, I. (1958). Some effects of magnesium loading upon renal excretion of magnesium and certain other electrolytes. *J. Clin. Invest.* **37**, 1362–1372.

Chutkow, J. G. (1964). Sites of magnesium absorption and excretion in the intestinal tract of the rat. *J. Lab. Clin. Med.* **63**, 71–79.

Clement, R. M., Sturm, J., and Daune, M. D. (1973). Interaction of metallic cations with DNA. VI. Specific binding of Mg^{++} and Mn^{++}. *Biopolymers* **12**, 405–421.

Consolazio, C. F., Matoush, L. O., Nelson, R. A., Harding, R. S., and Canham, J. E. (1963). Excretion of sodium, potassium, magnesium, and iron in human sweat and the relation of each to balance and requirements. *J. Nutr.* **79**, 407–415.

Coussons, H. (1969). Magnesium metabolism in infants and children. *Postgrad. Med.* **46**, 135–139.

Dick, M., Evans, R. A., and Watson, L. (1969). Effect of ethanol on magnesium excretion. *J. Clin. Pathol.* **22**, 152–153.

Drenick, E. J., Hunt, I. F., and Swendseid, M. E. (1969). Magnesium depletion during prolonged fasting of obese males. *J. Clin. Endocrinol. Metab.* **29**, 1341–1348.

Dunn, M. J., and Walser, M. (1966). Magnesium depletion in normal man. *Metab., Clin. Exp.* **15**, 884–895.

Durlach, J. (1967). Le Magnésium en pathologie humaine. Problèmes practiques et incidences diététiques. *Gaz. Med. Fr.* **74**, 3303–3320.

Durlach, J., Gremy, F., and Metral, S. (1967). La spasmophilie: Forme clinique neuro-musculaire du déficit magnésien primitif. *Rev. Neurol.* **117**, 177–189.

Field, A. C. (1961). Magnesium in ruminant nutrition. III. Distribution of Mg^{28} in the gastrointestinal tract and tissues of sheep. *Brit. J. Nutr.* **15**, 349–359.

Fitzgerald, M. G., and Fourman, P. (1956). An experimental study of magnesium deficiency in man. *Clin. Sci.* **15**, 635–647.

Flink, E. B. (1956). Magnesium deficiency syndrome in man. *J. Amer. Med. Ass.* **160**, 1406–1409.

Forster, R. P., and Berglund, F. (1956). Osmotic diuresis and its effect on total electrolyte distribution in plasma and urine of the aglomerular teleost, Lophius americanus. *J. Gen. Physiol.* **39**, 349–359.

Fuhrhop, J.-H., and Mauzerall, D. (1969). The one-electron oxidation of metalloporphyrins. *J. Amer. Chem. Soc.* **91**, 4174–4181.

Gerst, P. H., Porter, M. R., and Fishman, R. A. (1964). Symptomatic magnesium deficiency in surgical patients. *Ann. Surg.* **159**, 402–406.

Gill, J. R., Jr., Bell, N. H., and Bartter, F. C. (1967). Effect of parathyroid extract on magnesium excretion in man. *J. Appl. Physiol.* **22**, 136–138.

Ginn, H. E., Smith, W. O., Hammarsten, J. F., and Snyder, D. (1959). Renal tubular secretion of magnesium in dogs. *Proc. Soc. Exp. Biol. Med.* **101**, 691–692.

Gitelman, H. J., and Welt, L. G. (1969). Magnesium deficiency. *Annu. Rev. Med.* **20**, 233–242.

Gitelman, H. J., Kukolj, S., and Welt, L. G. (1968a). The influence of the parathyroid glands on the hypercalcemia of experimental magnesium depletion in the rat. *J. Clin. Invest.* **47**, 118–126.

Gitelman, H. J., Kukolj, S., and Welt, L. G. (1968b). Inhibition of parathyroid gland activity by hypermagnesemia. *Amer. J. Physiol.* **215**, 483–485.

Gordon, G S. (1963). A direct action of parathyroid hormone on dead bone *in vitro. Acta Endocrinol. (Copenhagen)* **44**, 481–489.

Graham, L. A., Caesar, J. J., and Burgen, A. S. V. (1960). Gastrointestinal absorption and excretion of Mg^{28} in man. *Metab., Clin. Exp.* **9**, 646–659.

Green, D. E. (1964). The mitochondrion. *Sci. Amer.* **210**, 63–74.

Hanna, S., Harrison, M., MacIntyre, I., and Fraser, R. (1960). The syndrome of magnesium deficiency in man. *Lancet* **2**, 172–176.

Heaton, F. W. (1964). Magnesium metabolism in surgical patients. *Clin. Chim. Acta* **9**, 327–333.

Heaton, F. W. (1965). The parathyroid and magnesium metabolism in the rat. *Clin. Sci.* **28**, 543–553.

Heaton, F. W. (1969). The kidney and magnesium homeostasis. *Ann. N.Y. Acad. Sci.* **162**, 775–785.

Hendrix, J. Z., Alcock, N. W., and Archibald, R. M. (1963). Competition between calcium, strontium, and magnesium for absorption in the isolated rat intestine. *Clin. Chem.* **9**, 734–744.

Hirschfelder, A. D., and Haury, V. G. (1934). Clinical manifestations of high and low plasma magnesium; dangers of epsom salt purgation in nephritis. *J. Amer. Med. Ass.* **102**, 1138–1141.

Hoffman, H.-P., and Avers, C. J. (1973). Mitochondrion of yeast: Ultrastructural evidence for one giant, branched organelle per cell. *Science* **181**, 749–751.

Hughes, M. N. (1972). "The Inorganic Chemistry of Biological Processes." Wiley, New York.

Jones, J. E., Manalo, R., and Flink, E. B. (1967). Magnesium requirements in adults. *Amer. J. Clin. Nutr.* **20**, 632–635.

Jones, J. E., Shane, S. R., Jacobs, W. H., and Flink, E. B. (1969). Magnesium balance studies in chronic alcoholism. *Ann. N.Y. Acad. Sci.* **162**, 934–946.

Keating, F. R., Jones, J. D., Elveback, L. R., and Randall, R. V. (1969). The relation of age and sex to distribution of values in healthy adults of serum calcium, inorganic phosphorus, magnesium alkaline phosphatase, total proteins, albumin, and blood urea. *J. Lab. Clin. Med.* **73**, 825–834.

Kellaway, G., and Ewen, K. (1962). Magnesium deficiency complicating prolonged gastric suction. *N. Z. Med. J.* **6**, 137–142.

King, L. R., Knowles, H. C., Jr., and McLaurin, R. I. (1963). Calcium, phosphorus, and magnesium metabolism following head injury. *Ann. Surg.* **177**, 126–131.

Krakauer, H. (1972). A calorimetric investigation of the heats of binding of Mg^{++} to Poly A, to Poly U, and to their complexes. *Biopolymers* **11**, 811–828.

Lear, R. D., and Grøn, P. (1968). Magnesium in human saliva. *Arch. Oral Biol.* **13**, 1311–1319.

Lengemann, F. W. (1959). The metabolism of magnesium and calcium by the rat. *Arch. Biochem.* **84**, 278–285.

Lin, D. C., and Nobel, P. S. (1971). Control of photosynthesis by Mg^{2+}. *Arch. Biochem. Biophys.* **145**, 622–632.

Ling, G. W. (1973). What component of the living cell is responsible for its semipermeable properties? Polarized water or lipid? *Biophys. J.* **13**, 807–816.

Littledike, E. T., and Arnaud, C. D. (1971). The influence of plasma magnesium concentrations on calcitonin secretion in the pig. *Proc. Soc. Exp. Biol. Med.* **136**, 1000–1006.

McAleese, E. M., Bell, M. C., and Forbes, R. M. (1960). Mg^{28} studies in lambs. *J. Nutr.* **74**, 505–514.

Macbeth, R. A. L., and Mabbott, J. D. (1964). Magnesium balance in the postoperative patient. *Surg., Gynecol. Obstet.* **118**, 748–760.

McCollister, R. J., Flink, E. B., and Doe, R. P. (1960). Magnesium balance studies in chronic alcoholism. *J. Lab. Clin. Med.* **55**, 98–103.

McCollister, R. J., Flink, E. B., and Lewis, M. D. (1963). Urinary excretion of magnesium in man following the ingestion of ethanol. *Amer. J. Clin. Nutr.* **12**, 415–420.

MacIntyre, I. (1960). Discussion on magnesium metabolism in man and animals. *Proc. Roy. Soc. Med.* **53**, 1037–1939.

MacIntyre, I. (1967). Magnesium metabolism. *Advan. Intern. Med.* **13**, 143–154.

MacIntyre, I., and Robinson, C. J. (1969). Magnesium in the gut: Experimental and clinical observations. *Ann. N.Y. Acad. Sci.* **162**, 865–873.

MacIntyre, I., Hanna, S., Booth, C. C., and Read, A. E. (1961). Intracellular magnesium deficiency in man. *Clin. Sci.* **20**, 297–305.

MacIntyre, I., Boss, S., and Troughton, V. A. (1963). Parathyroid hormone and magnesium homeostasis. *Nature (London)* **198**, 1058–1060.

Martin, H. E., and Bauer, F. K. (1962). Magnesium 28 studies in the cirrhotic and alcoholic. *Proc. Roy. Soc. Med.* **55**, 912–914.

Martin, H. E., McCuskey, C., Jr., and Tupikova, N. (1959). Electrolyte disturbance in acute alcoholism. With particular reference to magnesium. *Amer. J. Clin. Nutr.* **7**, 191–196.

Martindale, L., and Heaton, F. W. (1965). The relation between skeletal and extracellular fluid *in vitro. Biochem. J.* **97**, 440–443.

Massry, S. G., Coburn, J. W., and Kleeman, C. R. (1969). Renal handling of magnesium in the dog. *Amer. J. Physiol.* **216**, 1460–1467.

Mauzerall, D. (1973). Why chlorophyll? *Ann. N.Y. Acad. Sci.* **206**, 483–494.

Mendel, L. B., and Benedict, S. R. (1909). The paths of excretion of inorganic compounds. IV. The excretion of magnesium. *Amer. J. Physiol.* **25**, 1–22.

Mendelson, J. H., Barnes, B., Mayman, C., and Victor, M. (1965). The determination of exchangeable magnesium in alcoholic patients. *Metab., Clin. Exp.* **14**, 88–98.

Mendelson, J. H., Ogata, M., and Mello, N. K. (1969). Effects of alcohol ingestion and withdrawal on magnesium states of alcoholics: Clinical and experimental findings. *Ann. N.Y. Acad. Sci.* **162**, 918–933.

Milner, G., and Johnson, J. (1965). Hypomagnesaemia and delirium tremens: Report of a case with fatal outcome. *Amer. J. Psychiat.* **122**, 701–702.

Monsaingeon, A., Thomas, J., Nocquet, Y., Savel, J., and Clostre, F. (1966). Sur le role du magnesium en pathologie chirurgicale. *J. Chir. (Paris)* **91**, 437–454.

Murdaugh, H. V., and Robinson, R. R. (1960). Magnesium excretion in the dog studied by stop-flow analysis. *Amer. J. Physiol.* **198**, 571–574.

Nielsen, J. (1963). Magnesium metabolism in acute alcoholics. *Dan. Med. Bull.* **10**, 225–233.

Racker, E. (1974). Inner mitochondrial membranes: Basic and applied aspects. *Hosp. Pract.* **9**, 87–93.

Randall, R. E., Rossmeisl, E. C., and Bleifer, K. H. (1959). Magnesium depletion in man. *Ann. Intern. Med.* **50**, 257–287.

Rasmussen, H. (1974). Ions as 'second messengers.' *Hosp. Pract.* **9**, 99–107.

Raynaud, C. (1962). Renal excretion of magnesium in the rabbit. *Amer. J. Physiol.* **203**, 649–654.

Sallis, J. D., and DeLuca, H. F. (1966). Action of parathyroid hormone on mitochondria. Magnesium- and phosphate-independent respiration. *J. Biol. Chem.* **241,** 1122–1127.

Schroeder, H. A., Nason, A. P., and Tipton. I. H. (1969). Essential metals in man. Magnesium. *J. Chronic Dis.* **21,** 815–841.

Sherwood, L. M., Herrman, I., and Bassett, C. A. (1970). Parathyroid hormone secretion *in vitro:* Regulation by calcium and magnesium ions. *Nature (London)* **225,** 1056–1057.

Shils, M. E. (1964). Experimental human magnesium depletion. I. Clinical observations and blood chemistry alterations. *Amer. J. Clin. Nutr.* **15,** 133–143.

Shils, M. E. (1969a). Experimental production of magnesium deficiency in man. *Ann. N.Y. Acad. Sci.* **162,** 847–855.

Shils, M. E. (1969b). Experimental human magnesium depletion. *Medicine (Baltimore)* **48,** 61–85.

Silver, L., Robertson, J. S., and Dahl, L. K. (1960). Magnesium turnover in the human studied with Mg^{28}. *J. Clin. Invest.* **39,** 420–425.

Smith, P. K., Winkler, A. W., and Schwartz, B. M. (1939). The distribution of magnesium following the parenteral administration of magnesium sulfate. *J. Biol. Chem.* **129,** 51–56.

Smith, R. H., and McAllan, A. B. (1966). Binding of magnesium and calcium in the contents of the small intestine of the calf. *Brit. J. Nutr.* **20,** 703–718.

Smith, W. O., and Hammarsten, J. F. (1959). Intracellular magnesium in delirium tremens and uremia. *Amer. J. Med. Sci.* **237,** 413–417.

Storry, J. E., and Rook, J. A. F. (1962). The magnesium nutrition of the dairy cow in relation to the development of hypomagnesaemia in the grazing animal. *J. Sci. Food Agr.* **13,** 621–627.

Suh, S. M., Trashjian, A. H., Jr., Matsuo, N., Parkinson, D. K., and Fraser, D. (1973). Pathogenesis of hypocalcemia in primary hypomagnesemia: Normal end-organ responsiveness to parathyroid hormone, impaired parathyroid gland function. *J. Clin. Invest.* **52,** 153–160.

Szelényi, I. (1973). Magnesium and its significance in cardiovascular and gastro-intestinal disorders. *World Rev. Nutr. Diet* **17,** 189–224.

Szent-Györgi, A. (1960). "Introduction to a Submolecular Biology." Academic Press, New York.

Szent-Györgi, A. (1969). The ATP molecule. *In* "Biological Phosphorylations. Development of Concepts" (H. A. Kalckar, ed.), pp. 486–493. Prentice-Hall, Englewood Cliffs, New Jersey.

Szent-Györgi, A. (1971). Biology and pathology of water. *Perspect. Biol. Med.* **14,** 239–249.

Tibbetts, D. M., and Aub, J. C. (1937). Magnesium metabolism in health and disease. I. The magnesium and calcium excretion of normal individuals, also the effects of magnesium, chloride, and phosphate ions. *J. Clin. Invest.* **16,** 491–501.

Wacker, W. E. C., and Parisi, A. F. (1968). Magnesium metabolism. *N. Engl. J. Med.* **278,** 658–662, 712–717, and 772–776.

Wacker, W. E. C., and Vallee, B. L. (1958). Magnesium metabolism. *N. Engl. J. Med.* **259,** 431–438.

Wacker, W. E. C., Moore, F. D., Ulmer, D. D., and Vallee, B. L. (1962). Normocalcemic magnesium deficiency tetany. *J. Amer. Med. Ass.* **180,** 161–163.

Wallach, S., and Dimich, A. (1969). Radiomagnesium turnover studies in hypomagnesemic states. *Ann. N.Y. Acad. Sci.* **162,** 963–972.

Wallach, S., Rizek, J. E., Dimich, A., Prasad, N., and Siler, W. (1966). Magnesium transport in normal and uremic patients. *J. Clin. Endocrinol. Metab.* **26**, 1069–1080.

Widdowson, E. M., McCance, R. A., and Spray, C. M. (1951). The chemical composition of the human body. *Clin. Sci.* **10**, 113–125.

Wilke, H., and Spielmann, H. (1968). Untersuchungen über den Magnesiumgehalt der Leber bei der Cirrhose. *Klin. Wochenschr.* **46**, 1162–1164.

Willick, G. E., and Kay, C. M. (1971). Magnesium-induced conformational change in transfer ribonucleic acid as measured by circular dichroism. *Biochemistry* **10**, 2216–2222.

Wilson, A. A. (1960). Magnesium homeostasis and hypomagnesaemia in ruminants. *Vet. Rev.* **6**, 39–52.

Wolfe, S. M., and Victor, M. (1969). The relationship of hypomagnesemia and alkalosis to alcohol withdrawal symptoms. *Ann. N.Y. Acad. Sci.* **162**, 973–984.

Zitomer, R. S., and Flaks, J. G. (1972). Magnesium dependence and equilibrium of the *Escherichia coli* ribosomal subunit association. *J. Mol. Biol.* **71**, 263–279.

Zumoff, B., Bernstein, E. H., Imarisio, J. J., and Hellman, L. (1958). Radioactive magnesium (Mg^{28}) metabolism in man. *Clin. Res.* **6**, 260.

29

Chromium Metabolism in Man and Biochemical Effects

R. J. Doisy, D. H. P. Streeten, J. M. Freiberg, and A. J. Schneider

I. INTRODUCTION

It appears that for some trace elements, i.e., nickel, silicon, tin, and vanadium, there is little likelihood of spontaneous deficiency in man due to inadequate dietary intake. Stringent measures are required to induce deficiencies of these elements in experimental animals. On the other hand, evidence is accumulating that deficiencies of chromium and zinc do occur in some populations, presumably due to inadequate intake and/or poor availability of these two elements. Chromium nutrition in man was recently reviewed by Hambidge (1974).

Refining processes may reduce the content of chromium in some foods, e.g., sugar and flour (Czerniejewski et al., 1964; Schroeder, 1968, 1971; Schroeder et al., 1970). In sugar refining, the chromium is concentrated in the molasses fraction, and refined sugar contains less than one-tenth the concentration of chromium in molasses, i.e., refined sugar 0.08 μg/gm versus molasses 1.2 μg/gm. The geographical source of the sugar cane has a bearing on the concentration of chromium, e.g., Virgin Islands 0.07 μg/gm versus Colombia 0.35 μg/gm. In the milling of wheat, whole wheat contained 1.75 μg/gm of chromium, while white bread contained only 0.14 μg/gm. More recent analytical data (Schroeder, 1971) suggest that these levels may be too high. It should be pointed out that the determination of chromium in foodstuffs and biological samples presents formidable problems. Differences in analytical techniques, sample preparation, and possible contamination, combined with the low levels present, often lead to a divergence in reported values.

The American diet contains only small quantities of chromium—in our study, 5-115 μg per day (Levine et al., 1968), which is poorly absorbed. A high carbohydrate intake may predispose to chromium deficiency due to increased urinary excretion of chromium after carbohydrate loading (Schroeder, 1968).

II. ROLE AND STRUCTURE OF GLUCOSE TOLERANCE FACTOR (GTF)

There is no known role for chromium other than in the form of glucose tolerance factor (GTF). Various studies have shown some responses to chromium in certain enzyme systems and pathways (Mertz, 1969). Wacker and Vallee (1959) noted a high concentration of chromium in isolated nucleic acids; Mathur and Doisy (1972) noted a marked shift in the hepatic intracellular distribution of chromium in rats under conditions of increased protein synthesis. The ^{51}Cr label shifted from the nucleus to the cytoplasm in these experiments.

Schwarz and Mertz (1959) reported Cr^{3+} as an integral part of GTF. Impaired glucose tolerance in chromium-deficient animals was restored to normal by oral administration of GTF. In vitro studies suggest that GTF is required for a maximal response to insulin in insulin-sensitive tissues (Mertz, 1969). GTF was concentrated from brewers yeast, and liver and kidney were recognized as other potentially rich sources. GTF is an organic, heat-stable low molecular weight complex containing trivalent chromium.

More recently, Mertz (1974) has prepared biologically active chromium complexes that seem to be similar to but not identical with the naturally occurring GTF complex. The exact structure(s) is as yet unknown. The complex apparently contains two nicotinic acid molecules per chromium atom and may contain cysteine, glycine, and possibly glutamic acid residues. The amino acids may only be needed to convert the complex to a more water-soluble derivative, and the biological activity may be due to the chromium and nicotinic acid in a unique coordination complex.

III. EVIDENCE FOR CHROMIUM DEFICIENCY IN ANIMALS AND MAN

A. Animals

Chromium deficiency in animals has been induced both accidentally and deliberately by feeding rations low in available chromium (Mertz and Schwarz, 1959; Doisy, 1963; Schroeder, 1965; Davidson et al., 1967). The hallmark of chromium deficiency is impaired glucose tolerance. In both rats and squirrel monkeys maintained on chromium-deficient diets, restoration of a normal glucose tolerance was accomplished by oral administration of Cr^{3+} or GTF (Schwarz and Mertz, 1959; Davidson and Blackwell, 1968). In genetically diabetic mice in which hyperglycemia and hyperinsulinemia coexist, GTF administration, both acutely and chronically, reduced the elevated blood glucose levels to the normal range. In the latter experiments, inorganic Cr^{3+} was completely without effect on the elevated blood glucose levels. It was theorized that the diabetic mice were unable to convert chromium to GTF (Doisy et al., 1973).

B. Man

To date there is but indirect evidence to support the view that chromium deficiency occurs in man. There is evidence that tissue chromium levels decline with increasing age, particularly in the United States (Schroeder et al., 1962; Hambidge and Baum, 1972). Newborn and young children have higher tissue chromium levels than adults. Hepatic chromium concentration in children 0–10 years of age was 17.2 μg/gm of ash, while subjects over 30 years of age had a concentration of 1–2 μg/gm of ash. On a geographic basis, tissue chromium levels in the United States are a fraction of those reported from most, but not all, other areas studied (Schroeder et al., 1962; Schroeder, 1968). Cause and effect have not been demonstrated, but it is possible that the kind and amount of foods ingested in the United States may predispose to the observed low tissue concentrations. Decreased tissue levels of chromium are compatible with, but not proof of, deficiency.

Maturity-onset diabetics (Glinsmann and Mertz, 1966), middle-aged (Hopkins and Price, 1968), and elderly subjects (Levine et al., 1968), all in the United States, showed improvement of impaired glucose tolerance by simple addition of 150 μg of inorganic chromium (as Cr^{3+}) to their daily diets. If a suspected deficiency state exists, increasing the dietary intake of the nutrient in question should relieve the deficiency state and repair the abnormal metabolic state. Such trials have been made with subjects thought to be chromium deficient. It should be noted that the possibility exists that chromium has a pharmacological effect on carbohydrate metabolism. If this were the case, all subjects might be expected to respond in a similar fashion, if not to the same degree, when given a chromium supplement. This has not been observed to date.

Children in Jordan (Hopkins et al., 1968) suffering from kwashiorkor, and children in Turkey suffering from protein–calorie malnutrition (Gürson and Saner, 1971, 1973), received a chromium supplement (250 μg/day) to their formula. This was followed by restoration of the intravenous glucose tolerance tests to normal.

Malnourished children in Egypt (Carter et al., 1968) demonstrated no beneficial response to chromium supplementation of their diets. Chemical analysis of the diets indicated that the dietary intake of chromium was higher in Egypt than elsewhere. Analysis of Egyptian hospital diets revealed a mean daily intake of chromium of 129 μg/day, with a range of 76–1057 μg/day (Maxia et al., 1972), which contrasts with the estimated United States intake of 52 μg/day (Levine et al., 1968). It should be noted that there are obviously many causes for impaired glucose tolerance including intercurrent infection, emotional stress, antecedent diet, etc., but only in chromium-deficient subjects would one expect to see a beneficial response with chromium supplementation (unless the response is a pharmacological one).

A growing body of evidence based primarily on improved glucose tolerance tests after chromium supplementation suggests that chromium deficiency does occur in man, most probably due to inadequate intake.

TABLE I   Effect of Chromium on Mean Glucose Tolerance Tests[a]

Subject	Age	Cr[b]	Plasma glucose concentration (mg/dl)					No. of tests
			0 min	30 min	60 min	90 min	120 min	
Elderly								
GF		−	84	143	149	163	170	2
	79	+	82	138	129	125	106	2
HH		−	67	122	186	197	167	2
	78	+	83	132	139	126	123	2
Ech		−	82	153	180	165	153	2
	88	+	81	136	157	140	131	3
FW		−	98	148	181	152	135	2
	96	+	101	142	152	111	100	3
Young								
AG		−	90	161	192	151	115	2
	22	+	91	161	126	82	104	3
LS		−	81	146	194	127	120	2
	24	+	81	160	147	132	118	3
With hemochromatosis		−	111	209	225	166	125	2
	49	+	97	155	170	150	139	2

[a] Reprinted by permission of publisher. Doisy et al., Effects and metabolism of chromium in normals, elderly subjects, and diabetics. In "Trace Substances in Environmental Health" (D. D.Hemphill, ed.) Vol. II, pp. 75–82. University of Missouri, Columbia, 1968.

[b] Supplement: 50 μg of Cr three times daily ($CrCl_3 \cdot 6H_2O$).

Table I shows glucose tolerance tests in subjects with impaired glucose tolerance before and after inorganic chromium supplementation of their diets. The subjects include four institutionalized elderly subjects, two young volunteers originally considered to be normal, and one subject with hemochromatosis. Plasma glucose levels while on the chromium supplement, particularly at 60, 90, and 120 min, are considerably reduced compared to the baseline control tests in all subjects. Thus, inorganic chromium was effective in restoring the impaired glucose tolerance tests (GTTs) to normal in these seven subjects. It should be noted that of ten elderly subjects who received chromium supplement, only four displayed an improved glucose tolerance (Levine et al., 1968).

More recently, we have studied other elderly subjects living in the City of Syracuse Public Housing units. They were active, in good health, and prepared their own meals with complete freedom of choice (as

TABLE II   Effect of GTF Supplementation on Glucose Tolerance Tests in Elderly Subjects with Impaired Tolerance[a]

	Mean plasma glucose levels (mg/dl)			Cholesterol (mg/dl)[b]	Triglyceride (mg/dl)
	0 hr	1 hr	2 hr		
Before GTF (11)*	106 ± 4	201 ± 7	178 ± 8	245 ± 9	121 ± 8
After GTF (9)	99 ± 4	162 ± 11	132 ± 5	205 ± 10	112 ± 12
Significance	NS	<0.01	<0.001	<0.01	NS

	Mean serum insulin levels (microunits/ml)		
	0 hr	1 hr	2 hr
Before GTF	24 ± 6	78 ± 17	118 ± 17
After GTF	26 ± 12	70 ± 8	83 ± 8

[a] Mean ± SE; number of tests in parentheses. *Supplement:* 4 gm Yeastamin/day. *GTT:* 100 gm oral load.
[b] Using paired t test, difference is significant.

contrasted with the institutionalized subjects). Food costs did not appear to be restrictive at the time of his study (i.e., 1971-1972).

Thirty-one persons over the age of 65 were screened, and fourteen (45%) had impaired GTTs. Of the fourteen, twelve volunteered to go on a commercial brewer's yeast extract containing GTF (4 gm of extract per day).* The extract, Yeastamin, was shown by Mertz and Schwarz (1959) to contain potent GTF activity. After 1 and/or 2 months on the oral supplement, six of the twelve subjects showed glucose tolerance improved to values within the normal limits. (Note that our criteria for abnormality are a peak plasma glucose value above 185 mg/dl and a 2 hour value above 140 mg/dl.) The results on the six subjects who responded are shown in Table II.

Again, only 50% of the subjects tested responded to the GTF supplement, but this is not surprising. It is in agreement with the earlier studies with trivalent chromium, where 40% of the subjects tested responded with improved GTTs. The cholesterol, triglyceride, and insulin levels will be discussed in Section VI.

* Yeastamin Powder 95, Vico Asmus Division of A. E. Staley Co., Chicago, Illinois.

IV. CHROMIUM CONTENT OF THE DIET

A. Foodstuffs

Analyses of various foodstuffs have been made by a number of researchers (Schroeder *et al.*, 1962; Gormican 1970; Maxia *et al.*, 1972; Toepfer *et al.*, 1973). There are few foodstuffs with appreciable amounts of chromium. Spices in general have the highest concentrations with lesser amounts in meats, vegetables, and fruits (exceptions are liver and kidney). The use of spices is usually based primarily on personal preference and nationality. Determination of the chromium content of foodstuffs gives but limited information bearing on dietary adequacy. Availability of the chromium for absorption, and how much is in the form of GTF are important considerations.

Toepfer *et al.* (1973) attempted in an exhaustive study to correlate chromium content and GTF activity of various foodstuffs. In terms of relative biological values for GTF activity, the following data were obtained: brewers yeast 44.88, black pepper 10.21, calf's liver 4.52, chicken leg muscle 1.89, haddock 1.86, patent flour 1.86, and skim milk 1.59. It is obvious that a marked variability in the biologically active chromium occurs in natural foodstuffs. Much additional work in this area is needed before one can recommend a diet that would supply adequate chromium or GTF. Mertz (1971) has tentatively suggested a daily intake of 10–30 μg of GTF–chromium per day as enough to meet man's daily requirement.

It should be noted that stainless steel cooking ware might contribute chromium to the diet if acidic foodstuffs are prepared. Stainless steel is high in chromium content, and chromium has been found to leach out during the cooking process (Schroeder *et al.*, 1962).

In our study (Levine *et al.*, 1968), the daily intake of chromium ranged from a low of 5 μg/day to a high of 115 μg/day, with an average intake of 52 μg/day. Diets on three representative days are shown in Table III. Though the diets appear to be usual ones, the low content of chromium in seafoods results in the very low daily intake observed on day 3. It is apparent that a diet low in chromium could inadvertently be selected.

B. Drinking Water

Analyses by Durfor and Becker (1962) of drinking water in the United States reveals that the water supplies provide only small amounts of chromium. The mean chromium content of 100 selected cities was 0.43 ng/ml, with the range from nondetectable to 35 ng/ml. The city of

TABLE III   Composition of Elderly Subjects' Diet[a]

Day 1—115 µg Cr/day

    Breakfast: Orange juice, farina, toast, milk, coffee
    Lunch: Cream of tomato soup, egg souffle, tossed salad, applesauce, tea
    Dinner: Meat loaf with gravy, mashed potato, beets, cottage cheese, cookies, milk, tea

Day 2—47 µg Cr/day

    Breakfast: Prune juice, oatmeal, 1 egg, 2 slices toast, 1 cup milk, coffee
    Lunch: Chicken noodle soup, roast beef hash, crushed pineapple, 1 cup tea
    Dinner: Baked chicken, dressing, gravy, mashed potato, 1 slice bread, peas, fruit gelatin, milk, tea

Day 3—5 µg Cr/day

    Breakfast: Prune juice, farina, egg, toast, milk, coffee
    Lunch: Clam chowder, tuna fish sandwich, white cake, tea
    Dinner: Creamed cod fish, mashed potato, peas, apricots, 1 slice bread, milk

[a] Levine et al. (1968), reprinted by permission of publisher.

Milwaukee, Wisconsin had water with the highest observed chromium level, but has been retested and the chromium content is no longer high. The water treatment and purification methods may add or remove chromium depending on the nature of the purification processes.

V. ABSORPTION, TRANSPORT, AND EXCRETION OF CHROMIUM

Little work has been done on the intestinal absorption of chromium in man. Animal studies suggest that chromium is absorbed in the upper small intestines (Donaldson and Barreras, 1966).

A. Absorption of Chromium

Inorganic trivalent chromium salts are poorly absorbed by man and animals. Chromates are better absorbed, but the preferred valence state for chromium is 3+, and it is likely that any chromates present in the diet are reduced in the gastrointestinal tract from 6+ to 3+ valence.

Using ^{51}Cr-labeled chromic chloride, we observed that only 0.69% of an orally administered dose was absorbed by human subjects (Doisy et al., 1968). This agrees well with the value of 0.5% reported by Donaldson and Barreras (1966). Absorption in the elderly subjects was not significantly different from young normal adults (Doisy *et al.,* 1971). Thus, decreased ability to absorb chromium with age does not appear to account for the decreased tissue chromium concentrations with age.

The only group of persons studied to date that display an abnormal rate of chromium absorption are insulin-requiring diabetics (see Fig. 1). During the first 24 hours after a single oral dose of chromium, they (in contrast to maturity-onset diabetics) absorb two to four times more chromium than do normal subjects. Parallel with the increased rate of absorption, there is an increased urinary excretion of chromium (see Fig. 2). A tentative thesis is that insulin-requiring diabetics are chromium deficient and develop an adaptive increase in absorption to help offset the deficiency. In addition, if insulin-requiring diabetics are given ^{51}Cr-labeled chromic chloride intravenously, there is an increased urinary

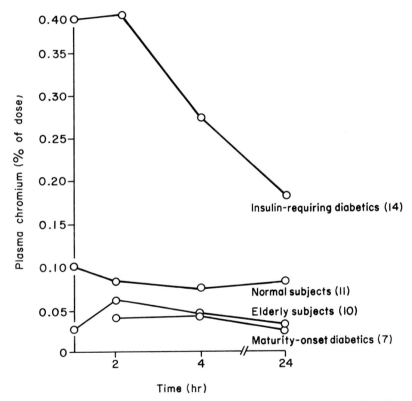

FIG. 1. Plasma chromium concentrations in normal, elderly, and diabetic sujbects after oral administration of ^{51}Cr. Dosage: 100 μCi (about 10 μg) ^{51}Cr administered orally with breakfast. Sterile sodium chromate was reduced with excess ascorbic acid immediately prior to administration. Number of subjects is given in parentheses. Reprinted from Doisy *et al.* (1971, p. 158), by courtesy of Marcel Dekker, Inc.

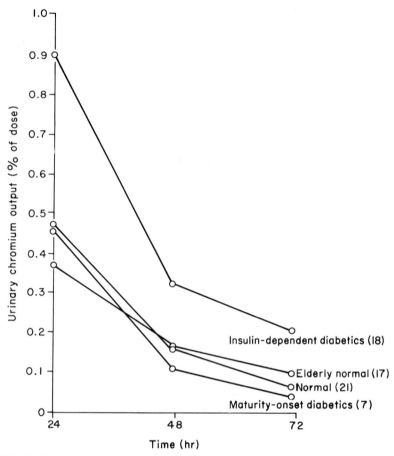

FIG. 2. Urinary chromium output in normal, elderly, and diabetic subjects after oral administration of ^{51}Cr. Number of subjects is given in parentheses. Reprinted from Doisy *et al.* (1971, p. 159), by courtesy of Marcel Dekker, Inc.

excretion as compared to normal subjects (Doisy *et al.*, 1971). Thus, diabetics may be unable to utilize chromium in a normal manner. Morgan (1972) demonstrated that the hepatic chromium content in diabetic autopsy material was 8 μg/gm of ash as compared to 12 μg/gm for control subjects. These values are higher than those reported by Schroeder *et al.* (1962), but Morgan states that background corrections were not made. Hambidge *et al.* (1968) found that insulin-requiring diabetic children have lower hair chromium levels than do normal children. Average values for the former and latter, respectively, were 0.56 and 0.85 μg/gm. It is of interest that both diabetic liver and hair concentrations of chromium are proportionately decreased, i.e., by 33%.

B. Transport of Chromium

It seems clear that at least two forms of chromium circulate in the plasma compartment. Some chromium is bound to transferrin (sidero-philin) in the β-globulin fraction and is thought to be trivalent chromium, based on studies by Hopkins and Schwarz (1964). The other form is presumably GTF-bound chromium, but definite studies on this point have yet to be done.

Earlier reports by Glinsmann et al. (1966) and Levine et al. (1968) suggested a rise in serum chromium levels after glucose or insulin administration. With recent advances in atomic absorption techniques, it now appears that the serum chromium values reported in those earlier papers were too high by a factor of 20–40-fold.

Present analytical techniques employed by a number of investigators suggest that serum or plasma chromium levels in normal subjects in the United States are in the range of 1–5 ng/ml. Various investigators, their techniques, and results are shown in Table IV. As of this writing, there is no consensus of opinion, but it appears that a rise in serum chromium levels after oral glucose loading is not a prerequisite to normal glucose tolerance. Recent values reported by Behne and Diel (1972) from Germany suggest an increase during glucose loading. It is of interest that fasting serum chromium levels were of the order of 10 ng/ml. It is possible that geographical differences will be documented in the fu-

TABLE IV Reported Average Plasma/Serum Chromium Levels[a]

Investigator	Analytical technique[b]	Chromium concentration (ng/ml)
Davidson	Atomic absorption	4.7
Doisy	Atomic absorption	1.3
Hambidge	Emission arc	1–3
Pekarek	Atomic absorption	1.5
Pierce	Neutron activation	1.4

[a] Some values are unpublished results presented at a chromium workshop held at University of Missouri, Columbia, Missouri, April 1974, sponsored by USDA, W. Mertz, Chairman.

[b] The values with atomic absorption by all three investigators were obtained using a heated graphite atomizer that increases detection limits over the conventional flame techniques.

ture. This further points up the need for standardization of our present analytical techniques.

Pekarek *et al.* (1973a,b) have demonstrated that during an induced infectious disease, serum chromium levels fell and glucose tolerance became impaired. We have observed that a young insulin-requiring diabetic while under good control has a fasting serum chromium level of 0.6 ng/ml. During an infectious attack, while spilling 4+ sugar in the urine, his serum chromium concentration fell to nondetectable levels. On the other hand, intravenous administration of glucose or insulin appears to cause a rapid decline in serum chromium concentration in normal subjects (Davidson and Burt, 1973; Burt and Davidson, 1973).

C. Placental Transport

Studies by Mertz and Roginski (1971) suggest that inorganic chromium does not cross the placenta to any significant extent, while chromium in the form of GTF is readily transported. The ^{51}Cr-labeled GTF appears to be concentrated mainly in the fetal liver. Schroeder *et al.* (1962) demonstrated that postpartum female rats may have nondetectable tissue chromium levels.

Impaired glucose tolerance in pregnancy is a common finding, but whether this is due to GTF deficiency or not is unknown. Davidson and Burt (1973) have shown that pregnant women have a lower circulating plasma chromium level than nonpregnant subjects of the same age (2.9 versus 4.7 ng/ml, respectively). Hambidge (1971) demonstrated that hair chromium concentrations of the newborn exceeded corresponding maternal hair levels (average values 974 versus 382 ng/gm), suggesting that the fetus extracts chromium from the maternal stores.

D. Urinary Excretion of Chromium

Orally absorbed chromium appears to be excreted mainly by the kidneys. The daily urinary excretion of chromium runs from 3 to 50 μg/24 hr (Hambidge, 1971; Davidson and Secrest, 1972; Wolf *et al.*, 1974). Of this quantity, it is not known how much is inorganic chromium and/or GTF chromium. Schroeder (1968) demonstrated that glucose loading caused an increased chromium excretion in the urine during the first 2 hr after loading. Recent evidence by Wolf *et al.* (1974) suggests that there is a volatile form of chromium in urine that may be lost, depending on the method of sample preparation. We have recently reported that insulin-requiring diabetics display a markedly reduced incidence of volatile chromium in the urine as compared to normal subjects

(Canfield and Doisy, 1975). This observation is compatible with the suggestion that diabetics may have an impaired ability to convert chromium to GTF.

VI. BIOLOGICAL EFFECTS OF GTF SUPPLEMENTATION OF THE DIET

A. Normal and Elderly Subjects

1. Serum Insulin Response

The function of GTF in mammalian systems is slowly beginning to unfold. As documented earlier, chromium, in the form of GTF, appears to act in concert with insulin and thus helps dispose of ingested carbohydrate. GTF appears to be active only in the presence of insulin. Subjects with impaired GTTs due to inadequate GTF or chromium respond to supplementation of the diet with a return to normal tolerance and a reduction in the amount of endogenous insulin released (see Table II).

As shown in Fig. 3, young subjects (20–25 years of age) who have GTTs within normal limits also show a reduction in endogenous insulin output during the GTTs. Plasma glucose levels during the tests are unchanged, but while on the GTF-containing supplement, decreased insulin levels are required to maintain normal glucose tolerance. This could be interpreted to mean that even in "normal" subjects the dietary intake of chromium (or GTF) is marginal. Reduction in the work load of the β cells of the pancreas seems likely to be beneficial. It further raises the question of what is a normal insulin response during GTTs. If insulin determinations from different laboratories can be compared directly, then the following conclusions may be reached. After oral glucose loading, the peak insulin response is lowest and appears most rapidly (30 min) in childhood. Young adults have intermediate responses, while middle aged and elderly subjects have higher and most delayed peaks (see Table V). The magnitude of the insulin response appears to be inversely correlated with tissue chromium levels. The older the subjects tested, the lower the chromium content of their tissues and the greater is their insulin response to a glucose load. Perhaps the body stores of chromium influence the magnitude of the insulin response during GTTs.

2. Serum Lipid Levels

In addition to the reduction in insulin levels, some subjects with impaired GTTs also show a reduction in the fasting serum cholesterol

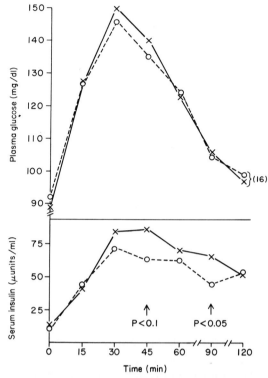

FIG. 3. Effect of a daily brewer's yeast supplement on plasma glucose and serum insulin levels in young normal subjects during GTTs. *Supplement:* 10 gm of brewer's yeast daily for 1 month. *GTTs:* 100 gm oral load. *Subjects:* Sixteen male subjects 20–25 years of age. *Key:* X = before supplement; O = after supplement.

TABLE V   Time and Magnitude of Peak Insulin Response with Age

Subject	Age (years)	Time of peak after loading (min)	Average peak insulin level (μunits/ml)	References
Children	5–15	30	59	Jackson *et al.* (1973)
Young adults (see Fig. 3), this chapter	20–25	45	86	Doisy *et al.* and Section VA, this chapter
Adults	Not stated	45–60	143	Yalow and Berson (1960)
Elderly	>65	60–120	118	Doisy *et al.* and Section IIB, this chapter

Impaired GTTs—See Table II, this chapter

and triglyceride levels while on the GTF supplement (see Table II). Fasting serum cholesterol levels in the young normal subjects show a mean decrease of 36 mg/dl after 1 month of supplementation of the diet with brewer's yeast. One subject showed an increase of 5 mg/dl, while the other fifteen showed decreases ranging from 3 to 107 mg/dl. It is apparent that if the fasting serum cholesterol level is above 240 mg/dl, the decrement is likely to be greater than if the fasting level is 240 mg/dl or below (54 versus 17 mg/dl) (see Table VI). These results are in agreement with Schroeder (1968), who demonstrated that trivalent chromium administration in humans caused a mean reduction of 14% in the serum cholesterol levels.

TABLE VI Serum Cholesterol Levels in Young Normal Subjects Receiving a Daily Dietary Supplement[a] of Brewer's Yeast

Subject	Serum cholesterol level (mg/dl) Pre-GTF	Post-GTF	Change in level (mg/dl)	Decrease
				(Mean value, Subjects 1-8)
1	350	306	−44	
2	286	243	−43	
3	282	175	−107	
4	253	211	−42	
5	250	230	−20	−54 mg/dl
6	250	206	−44	
7	243	201	−42	
8	243	151	−92	
				(Mean value, Subjects 9-16)
9	235	206	−29	
10	233	201	−32	
11	227	203	−24	
12	203	179	−24	
13	199	204	+5	−17 mg/dl
14	191	169	−22	
15	190	178	−12	
16	141	138	−3	
Mean ± SE	236.0 ± 11.9[b]	200.0 ± 9.9	−36	

[a] Supplement: 10 gm of brewer's yeast once daily for 1 month.
[b] Using paired t test, difference is significant $p < 0.001$.

Triglyceride levels were normal and unchanged while on the supplement. Some subjects with elevated triglycerides do show a reduction in triglyceride levels while on the supplement (Table VII).

It is possible that the observed fall in serum cholesterol is due to the nicotinic acid content of brewer's yeast, but it seems more likely that it is due to the chromium content of the yeast. The usual dosage of nicotinic acid for reduction of elevated cholesterol levels is 1–2 gm three times daily. Nicotinic acid may be effective by conversion to GTF if adequate tissue stores of chromium are available. This lot (#052273H, Philadephia Dry Yeast Co., Philadelphia, Pennsylvania) of brewer's yeast has not been assayed for nicotinic acid, but brewers yeast usually contains approximately 1.0 mg/gm, which would thus provide a daily intake of 10 mg in these studies. Of course, it is possible that the cholesterol-lowering effect resulting from brewers yeast supplementation is unrelated to the chromium content of the yeast.

Curran (1954) implicated chromium in fatty acid and cholesterol synthesis, while Schroeder and Balassa (1965) and Staub et al. (1969) found in rats that chromium supplementation of certain diets resulted in a reduction in serum cholesterol levels. In addition, Schroeder et al. (1965a) observed a decreased incidence of aortic plaques in animals on a chromium supplement.

B. Insulin-Requiring Diabetics

Evidence presented earlier indicated that insulin-requiring diabetics have an abnormal pattern in their absorption and excretion of chromium. To date, we have studied only a few insulin-requiring diabetics in terms of their response to brewer's yeast (GTF) supplementation of the diet. A reduction in the daily insulin requirement has been observed. Preliminary results in five diabetics whose daily insulin requirement ranged from 60 to 130 units/day showed reductions of 20–45 units in their daily requirements over a 1–2 month period. This observation confirms a report by McCay (1952), who recommended a daily brewer's yeast supplement for elderly people. McCay also suggested that supplementation might lessen the insulin requirement in elderly diabetics. Elimination of the daily insulin requirement has not been achieved, and would not be expected in these subjects, since in all likelihood they have little endogenous insulin production based on the magnitude of their daily insulin requirement. It has been estimated by Yalow and Berson (1960) that a normal adult makes approximately 40 units of insulin per day. It is possible that elimination of the exogenous insulin requirement may occur in subjects who are still capable of making insulin and require

TABLE VII Effect of GTF Supplement on Glucose Tolerance[a]

Date	Time (min)	Glucose (mg/dl)	Insulin (μunits/ml)	Cholesterol (mg/dl)	Triglycerides (mg/dl)
8/10/73	0	117	35	194	265
	30	251	>200		
	60	267	>200		
	120	150	95		
	180	96	27		
8/23/73	0	108	38	198	256
	15	176	200		
	30	220	>200		
	45	206	183		
	60	167	163		
	90	158	138		
GTF 8/24/73	120	97	39		
9/27/73	0	110	14	—	167
	15	198	90		
	30	250	155		
	45	268	150		
	60	270	>200		
	90	225	143		
	120	188	80		
	150	118	31		
	180	85	15		
11/3/73	0	113	63	198	96
	15	135	158		
	30	260	>200		
	45	253	>200		
	60	245	>200		
	90	160	150		
	120	93	28		
	150	65	0		
	180	78	23		
1/4/74	0	112	5	150	68
	15	162	52		
	30	212	110		
	45	204	125		
	60	185	166		
	90	156	130		
	120	85	25		
	150	73	12		
	180	76	12		
4/19/74	0	92	10	206	134
	30	154	57		
	60	131	52		
	90	126	44		
	120	117	35		
	150	75	22		
	180	63	10		

[a] *Subject:* Sibling of diabetic, male, age 30. Subject gained 8 pounds between 1/4/74 and 4/19/74. *Supplement:* 4 gm of Yeastamin per day 8/24/73–11/9/73; 8 gm of Yeastamin per day 11/10/73–4/19/74.

only modest amounts, i.e., 5–20 units/day. An attendant risk of hypo-glycemia when initiating the supplement should be emphasized. The insulin requirement is usually decreased within 24 hr and progressively declines 1–2 units every 48–72 hr.

C. Siblings and/or Offspring of Known Diabetics

The incidence of impaired glucose tolerance in the siblings of diabetics is higher than in the general population. This suggested a large body of clinical material that could be brought under fruitful study. Our studies in genetically diabetic mice showed that inorganic chromium was without effect on the elevated blood glucose levels that accompany the genetic diabetic state. GTF preparations caused a reduction in glucose levels to within normal limits in these mice, in which an inability to convert chromium to GTF was postulated (Doisy *et al.*, 1973).

Starting in 1969, the opportunity for studying the four offspring of an insulin-requiring diabetic was available. The son had mild chemical diabetes as judged from his elevated glucose and insulin levels during GTTs. Glucose tolerance became progressively more impaired from 11/3/1969 to 8/3/1971, by which time daily insulin injections were required. This progression took place in spite of the daily administration of tolbutamide and a daily dietary supplement of 150 µg of inorganic chromium per day. Thus, inorganic chromium was ineffective in this subject as in the diabetic mice. The other three sisters all had some impairment in glucose tolerance, as judged by both glucose and insulin levels, and two of the girls were started on a daily supplement of GTF in the form of brewer's yeast (10 gm/day). The third sister served as a control for 6 months and then received the supplement. After 15 months, all three subjects displayed normal glucose tolerances. Initially, the two sisters on the supplement had fasting serum chromium levels of 2.5 and 2.8 ng/ml, respectively, while the control sister had a value of 1.5 ng/ml. Thus, the supplement caused a sizable percentage increase in circulating chromium levels.

Figures 4 and 5 depict average glucose and insulin levels before and after supplementation of the diet with brewer's yeast for the indicated number of tests. Biphasic responses for insulin were observed with a delayed elevation in insulin output in both subjects. Peak insulin and glucose levels as shown demonstrate a reduction in both parameters while on the supplement. The third sister (not shown) displayed a similar response. Biphasic responses appear to be relatively common in the offspring of diabetics and perhaps may be indicative of problems

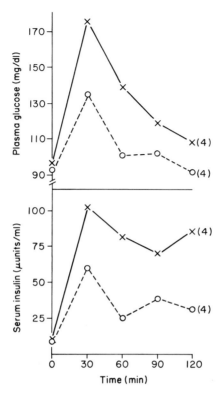

FIG. 4. Effect of a daily oral brewer's yeast supplement on plasma glucose and serum insulin levels during GTTs. *Subject:* sibling of a diabetic, female, age 20. *Supplement:* 10 gm brewer's yeast daily over 8-month period. *GTTs:* 100 gm oral load; tests repeated at approximately 2-month intervals. *Key:* X = before supplement; O = after supplement; number of tests is given in parentheses.

to arise later in life. The improvement of glucose tolerance in these subjects was not associated with weight loss.

The glucose tolerance and lipid levels of an additional subject are shown in Table VII. The subject appears to have a familial hyperlipoproteinemia (carbohydrate-induced). After approximately 8 months of supplementation of the diet with 4–8 gm of Yeastamin daily, glucose tolerance has returned to normal; more importantly, fasting triglyceride levels have fallen to within normal limits. A marked reduction in glucose-induced increments in serum insulin concentrations was observed on the last test (4/19/1974) with normalization of plasma levels in spite of an 8 pound weight gain.

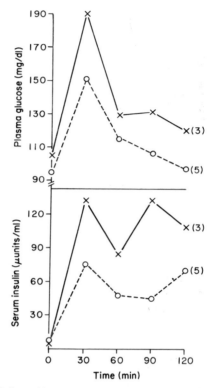

FIG. 5. Effect of a daily oral brewer's yeast supplement on plasma glucose and serum insulin levels during GTTs. *Subject:* sibling of a diabetic, female, age 22. *Supplement:* 10 gm brewer's yeast daily over 15-month period. *GTTs:* 100 gm oral load; tests repeated at approximately 2–3 month intervals. *Key:* ✕ = before supplement; ○ = after supplement; number of tests is given in parentheses.

At present, approximately eighty subjects have received a dietary supplement containing GTF. The majority show improvement in glucose tolerance, but not all respond in this manner. The length of time after which improvement has been seen varies with the individual subject. The elderly subjects who responded (Table II), and who were presumably only chromium-deficient, did so in 1–2 months time. In some siblings of diabetics, 6–8 months had elapsed before normalization of both glucose and insulin levels occurred.

Brewer's yeast contains many substances but is the richest known source of GTF. Until synthetic GTF or a brewer's yeast preparation free of GTF activity becomes available for testing, the assertion that improvement in carbohydrate and lipid metabolism was due to GTF remains uncertain.

VII. UNSOLVED PROBLEMS AND RESEARCH NEEDS

A. Structure and Function of GTF

The structure of GTF may be known soon. Until then, elucidation of the function of GTF must wait. It has been shown that GTF and insulin interact and form a complex, and Mertz (1967) has postulated that GTF was required to bind insulin to the cell surface through exposed sulfhydryl groups. GTF may be considered a hypoglycemic agent effective in lowering plasma glucose levels, particularly if glucose is elevated above the normal fasting range.

Using GTF concentrates (kindly supplied by Dr. Mertz), both normal and diabetic fed mice displayed a decrease in plasma glucose levels after a single intraperitoneal injection of GTF. However, fasted normal mice showed no such response. Fasting presumably would shut off endogenous insulin production, and perhaps for this reason GTF was ineffective in the fasting state. That is to say, if glucose levels were elevated along with circulating insulin, GTF administration would lower the plasma glucose concentration. The maximal response to GTF occurred 4–8 hr after injection. If the function of GTF is related to insulin binding, an immediate response might be expected. The delayed response actually observed seems inconsistent with a binding mechanism. The possibility exists that insulin is the vehicle that permits GTF to penetrate the cell and produce the physiological effects that have been observed. When adequate supplies of ^{51}Cr-labeled GTF become available, definite studies can be carried out on the mechanism and site of action of GTF.

B. Physiological Mechanisms for Conversion of Chromium to Glucose Tolerance Factor

Currently, one can but speculate about the importance of GTF and chromium relationship in man. It is of interest to speculate, however, in order to indicate potential directions for fruitful investigations. Chromium in the form of GTF appears to be essential for normal carbohydrate metabolism in man. Toepfer et al. (1973) suggested that varying amounts of GTF occur in natural foodstuffs. Some foods contain chromium but little or no biological (GTF) activity.

Can chromium be converted to GTF in man? The fact that children respond with improved GTT to inorganic chromium supplementation of the diet within 24 hr (Hopkins et al., 1968; Gürson and Saner, 1971, 1973) suggests that they (children) can convert chromium to GTF.

Elderly subjects required 1–3 months to respond to inorganic chromium. This suggests a possibility that with advancing age the ability to convert chromium to GTF may diminish.

Is it possible that some individuals (i.e., insulin-requiring diabetics) completely lose the ability to convert chromium to GTF? The daily dietary intake of chromium and GTF is quite variable depending on the nature of the diet selected. If it is true, as suggested, that the insulin-requiring diabetic is unable to convert chromium to GTF, then the insulin-requiring diabetic would be dependent solely on the exogenous GTF in the diet. This could explain the so called "brittle diabetics." If GTF intake is high one day, the insulin requirement is reduced. Conversely, if GTF intake is low, then the insulin requirement is increased. By feeding brewer's yeast daily, the daily GTF intake is more constant and thus insulin dosage may remain more constant. It may be worthy of mention that a few of the insulin-requiring diabetics have reported a greater stability of blood sugar, with less tendency to spill sugar in the urine and a reduced incidence of hypoglycemic reactions while on the brewers yeast supplement.

If chromium must be converted to GTF, where does synthesis take place—in the liver, pancreas, gut, or elsewhere? Is there a pool of GTF in the body, or is GTF utilized like other B vitamins? Can a recommended dietary allowance (RDA) be established? How can chromium deficiency be overcome? These are some of the unanswered questions that face workers in this field.

C. Pregnancy and Plasma Chromium Levels

As indicated, pregnancy appears to lower maternal body stores of chromium as judged by plasma and hair chromium levels. It would be interesting to learn whether supplementation of the diet during pregnancy would maintain normal plasma chromium levels and reduce the incidence of impaired glucose tolerance during pregnancy.

D. Quantitative Aspects of GTF Determination

If GTF supplements are beneficial for asymptomatic subjects with abnormal GTTs, then identification of these people at the earliest possible age is necessary. Plasma or serum chromium levels may not be useful in determining one's status with respect to GTF stores in the body. Urinary chromium (or GTF) will probably reflect and be complicated by the amount in the diet and the nature of the diet consumed in the previous 24 hr (i.e., high carbohydrate diets leading to increased chromium excretion). Would standard glucose tolerance tests with a 12 or 24 hr urine collection for GTF assay be a useful diagnostic tool? If after a glucose load, the urinary GTF excretion were below a certain limit, the subject might be considered GTF and/or chromium deficient, and supplementation of the diet could be instituted. A specific assay for urinary GTF is needed, and such work is underway in this laboratory.

Only long-term studies will determine if GTF supplementation of the diet can prevent potential diabetics from progressing to overt diabetics. Likewise, it appears that subjects with elevated cholesterol and triglyceride levels might benefit from brewer's yeast or GTF supplementation of the diet. In view of our present state of knowledge, reduction of elevated serum cholesterol and triglyceride levels seems desirable.

VIII. SUMMARY

Evidence is accumulating that chromium deficiency does occur in man. It is suggested that a deficiency in the United States may occur due to inadequate intake because of losses of chromium in processing of foodstuffs, e.g., flour and sugar.

At some point, it may be that public health measures to insure adequate chromium intake will be desirable, but implementation of any such measure will demand careful thought as to the safety of the procedure, the toxicity of excessive levels, and appropriate safeguards against undesirable excesses.

ACKNOWLEDGMENT

This investigation was supported by USPHS Grants AM 15,100 and RR 229. The technical assistance of Anne B. Holden, Mary Kearney, and the nursing staff of the Clinical Research Center is gratefully acknowledged. The elderly subjects were arranged for through the help of Dr. William A. Harris, Onondaga County Health Commissioner, and Miss Audrey Byrnes, Supervisor of Nurses. The siblings of diabetics were provided to us by Dr. Arthur H. Dube.

REFERENCES

Behne, D., and Diel, F. (1972). Relations between carbohydrate and trace-element metabolisms investigated by neutron activation analysis. In "Nuclear Activation Techniques in the Life Sciences," IAEA-SM-157/11, pp. 407–413. IAEA, Vienna.
Burt, R. L., and Davidson, I. W. F. (1973). Carbohydrate metabolism in pregnancy: A possible role of chromium. Acta Diabetol. Lat. 10, 770–778.
Canfield, W. K., and Doisy, R. J. (1975). Evidence for an unrecognized metabolic defect in diabetic subjects. Diabetes 24(2), 406 (Abstract).

Carter, J. P. Kattob, A., Abd-El-Hodi, Davis, J. T., EL Cholmy, A., and Patwardhan, V. N. (1968). Chromium III in hypoglycemia and in impaired glucose utilization in Kwashiorkor. *Amer. J. Clin. Nutr.* 21, 195–202.

Curran, G. L. (1954). Effect of certain transition group elements on hepatic synthesis of cholesterol in the rat. *J. Biol. Chem.* 210, 765–770.

Czerniejewski, C. P., Shank, C. W., Bechtel, W. G., and Bradley, W. B. (1964). The minerals of wheat, flour, and bread. *Cereal Chem.* 41, 65–72.

Davidson, I. W. F., and Blackwell, W. L. (1968). Changes in carbohydrate metabolism of squirrel monkeys with chromium dietary supplementation. *Proc. Soc. Exp. Biol. Med.* 127, 66–72.

Davidson, I. W. F., and Burt, R. L. (1973). Physiological changes in plasma chromium of normal and pregnant women: Effect of glucose load. *Amer. J. Obstet. Gynecol.* 116, 601–608.

Davidson, I. W. F., and Secrest, W. L. (1972). Determination of Chromium in biological materials by atomic absorption spectrometry using a graphite furnace atomizer. *Anal. Chem.* 44, 1808–1813.

Davidson, I. W. F., Lang, C. M., and Blackwell, W. L. (1967). Impairment of carbohydrate metabolism of the squirrel monkey. *Diabetes* 16, 395–401.

Doisy, R. J. (1963). Plasma insulin assay and adipose tissue metabolism. *Endocrinology* 72, 273–278.

Doisy, R. J., Streeten, D. H. P., Levine, R. A., and Chodos, R. B. (1968). Effects and metabolism of chromium in normals, elderly subjects, and diabetics. *In* "Trace Substances in Environmental Health" (D. D. Hemphill, ed.), Vol. II, p. 75. University of Missouri, Columbia.

Doisy, R. J., Streeten, D. H. P., Souma, M. L., Kalafer, M. E., Rekant, S. L., and Dalakos, T. G. (1971). Metabolism of ^{51}chromium in human subjects. *In* "Newer Trace Elements in Nutrition" (W. Mertz and W. E. Cornatzer, eds.), Chapter 8. Dekker, New York.

Doisy, R. J., Jastremski, M. S., and Greenstein, F. L. (1973). Metabolic effects of glucose tolerance factor and trivalent chromium in normal and genetically diabetic mice. *Excerpta Med. Found. Int. Congr. Ser.* 280, 155 (abstr.).

Donaldson, R. M., and Barreras, R. F. (1966). Intestinal absorption of trace quantities of chromium. *J. Lab. Clin. Med.* 68, 484–493.

Durfor, C. N., and Becker, E. (1962). Public water supplies of the 100 largest cities in the United States. U.S. Government Printing Office, Washington, D.C. Geological Survey Water Supply Paper 1812.

Glinsmann, W. H., and Mertz, W. (1966). Effect of trivalent chromium on glucose tolerance. *Metab., Clin. Exp.* 15, 510–520.

Glinsmann, W. H., Feldman, F. J., and Mertz, W. (1966). Plasma chromium after glucose administration. *Science* 152, 1243–1245.

Gormican, A. (1970). Inorganic elements in foods used in hospital menus. *J. Amer. Diet. Ass.* 56, 397–403.

Gürson, C. T., and Saner, G. (1971). Effect of chromium on glucose utilization in marasmic protein-calorie malnutrition. *Amer. J. Clin. Nutr.* 24, 1313–1319.

Gürson, C. T., and Saner, G. (1973). Effect of chronium supplementation on growth in marasmic protein-calorie malnutrition. *Amer. J. Clin. Nutr.* 26, 988–991.

Hambidge, K. M. (1971). Chromium nutrition in the mother and the growing child. *In* "Newer Trace Elements in Nutrition" (W. Mertz and W. E. Cornatzer, eds.), Chapter 9. Dekker, New York.

Hambidge, K. M. (1974). Chromium nutrition in man. *Amer. J. Clin. Nutr.* **27,** 505–514.

Hambidge, K. M., and Baum, J. D. (1972). Hair chromium concentrations of human newborn and changes during infancy. *Amer. J. Clin. Nutr.* **25,** 376–379.

Hambidge, K. M., Rodgerson, D. O., and O'Brien, D. (1968). The concentration of chromium in the hair of normal and children with juvenile diabetes mellitus. *Diabetes* **17,** 517–519.

Hopkins, L. L., Jr., and Price, M. G. (1968). Effectiveness of Chromium III in improving the impaired glucose tolerance of middle-aged Americans. *Proc. West. Hemisphere Nutr. Congr., 2nd, 1968* Abstract, Vol. 2, pp. 40–41.

Hopkins, L. L., Jr., and Schwarz, K. (1964). Chromium binding to serum proteins, specifically siderophilin. *Biochim. Biophys. Acta* **90,** 484–491.

Hopkins, L. L., Jr., Ransome-Kuti, O., and Majaj, A. S. (1968). Improvement of impaired carbohydrate metabolism by Chromium III in malnourished infants. *Amer. J. Clin. Nutr.* **21,** 203–211.

Jackson, R. L., Guthrie, R. A., and Murthy, D. Y. N. (1973). Oral glucose tolerance tests and their reliability. *Metab., Clin. Exp.* **22,** 237–245.

Levine, R. A., Streeten, D. H. P., and Doisy, R. J. (1968). Effects of oral chromium supplementation on the glucose tolerance of elderly human subjects. *Metab., Clin. Exp.* **17,** 114–125.

McCay, C. M. (1952). Chemical aspects of aging and the effect of diet upon aging. *In* "Cowdry's Problems of Aging" (A. J. Lansing, ed.), 3rd ed., Chapter 6. Williams & Wilkins, Baltimore, Maryland.

Mathur, R. K., and Doisy, R. J. (1972). Effect of diabetes and diet on the distribution of tracer doses of chromium in rats. *Proc. Soc. Exp. Biol. Med.* **139,** 836–38.

Maxia, V., Meloni, S., Rollier, M. A., Brandone, A., Patwardhan, V. N., Waslien, C. I., and Said-El-Shami. (1972). Selenium and chromium assay in Egyptian foods and blood of Egyptian children by activation analysis. *In* "Nuclear Activation Techniques in the Life Sciences," IAEA-SM 157/67, pp. 527–550. IAEA, Vienna.

Mertz, W. (1967). Biological role of chromium. *Fed. Proc., Fed. Amer. Soc. Exp. Biol.* **26,** 186–193.

Mertz, W. (1969). Chromium occurrence and function in biological systems. *Physiol. Rev.* **49,** 169–239.

Mertz, W. (1971). Human requirements: Basic and optimal. *Ann. N.Y. Acad. Sci.* **199,** 191–199.

Mertz, W. (1974). Biological function of chromium nicotinic acid-complexes. *Fed. Proc., Fed. Amer. Soc. Exp. Biol.* **33,** 659 (abstr.).

Mertz, W., and Roginski, E. E. (1971). Chromium metabolism: The glucose tolerance factor. *In* "Newer Trace Elements in Nutrition" (W. Mertz and W. E. Cornatzer, eds.), Chapter 7. Dekker, New York.

Mertz, W., and Schwarz, K. (1959). Relation of glucose tolerance factor to impaired glucose tolerance in rats on stock diets. *Amer. J. Physiol.* **196,** 614–618.

Morgan, J. M. (1972). Hepatic chromium content in diabetic subjects. *Metab., Clin. Exp.* **21,** 313–316.

Pekarek, R. S., Hauer, E. C., Wannemacher, R. W., Jr., and Beisel, W. R. (1973a). Serum chromium concentrations and glucose utilization in healthy and infected subjects. *Fed. Proc., Fed. Amer. Soc. Exp. Biol.* **32,** 930 (abstr.).

Pekarek, R. S., Hauer, E. C., Wannemacher, R. W., Jr., and Beisel, W. R. (1973b).

The direct determination of serum chromium by an atomic absorption spectrophotometer with a heated graphite atomizer. *Anal. Biochem.* **59**, 283–292.

Schroeder, H. A. (1965). Diabetic-like serum glucose levels in chromium-deficient rats. *Life Sci.* **4**, 2057–2062.

Schroeder, H. A. (1968). The role of chromium in mammalian nutrition. *Amer. J. Clin. Nutr.* **21**, 230–244.

Schroeder, H. A. (1971). Losses of vitamin and trace minerals resulting from processing and preservation of foods. *Amer. J. Clin. Nutr.* **24**, 562–573.

Schroeder, H. A., and Balassa, J. J. (1965). Influence of chromium, cadmium, and lead on rat aortic lipids and circulating cholesterol. *Amer. J. Physiol.* **209**, 433–437.

Schroeder, H. A., Balassa, J. J., and Tipton, I. H. (1962). Abnormal trace metal in man: Chromium. *J. Chronic Dis.* **15**, 941–964.

Schroeder, H. A., Balassa, J. J., and Vinton, W. H., Jr. (1965a). Chromium, cadmium and lead in rats: Effects on life span, tumors, and tissue levels. *J. Nutr.* **86**, 51–66.

Schroeder, H. A., Nason, A. P., and Tipton, I. H. (1970). Chromium deficiency as a factor in atherosclerosis. *J. Chronic Dis.* **23**, 123–142.

Schwarz, K., and Mertz, W. (1959). Chromium III and the glucose tolerance factor. *Arch. Biochem. Biophys.* **85**, 292–295.

Staub, H. W., Reussner, G., and Thiessen, R. T., Jr. (1969). Serum cholesterol reduction by chromium in hypercholesterolemic rats. *Science* **166**, 746–747.

Toepfer, E. W., Mertz, W., Roginski, E. E., and Polansky, M. M. (1973). Chromium in foods in relation to biological activity. *J. Agr. Food Chem.* **21**, 69–73.

Wacker, W. E. C., and Vallee, B. L.(1959). Nucleic acids and metals. I. Chromium, manganese, nickel, iron, and other metals in ribonucleic acid from diverse biological sources. *J. Biol. Chem.* **234**, 3257–3262.

Wolf, W., Greene, F. E., and Mitman, F. W. (1974). Determination of urinary chromium by low temperature ashing-flameless atomic absorption. *Fed. Proc., Fed. Amer. Soc. Exp. Biol.* **33**, 659 (abstr.).

Yalow, R. S., and Berson, S. A. (1960). Immunoassay of endogenous plasma insulin in man. *J. Clin. Invest.* **39**, 1157–1175.

30
Selenium in Man

Raymond F. Burk

I. INTRODUCTION

Selenium occupies an awkward place in a monograph on human aspects of trace elements, because while its importance in animals is undisputed and its biochemical aspects are exciting, no human disease conditions have been rigorously proven to be causally related to it. It has been shown to be essential for several animal species (McCoy and Weswig, 1969; Thompson and Scott, 1970), and although essentiality has not been proven for man, several lines of reasoning from existent data suggest it: (1) selenium has been shown to be an essential constituent of erythrocyte glutathione peroxidase in several species (Rotruck et al., 1973), and such an enzyme is known to be present in human red cells (Steinberg and Necheles, 1971); (2) some of the same urinary metabolites of selenium seem to be produced by man (see below) and

105

by the rat, a species in which selenium is known to be essential; (3) accumulated evidence suggests that there is homeostatic regulation of blood selenium level (see below); (4) finally, there is evidence that selenium binds specifically to certain human plasma proteins (Burk, 1974).

There have been major recent advances in our basic knowledge of selenium in addition to its discovery as part of glutathione peroxidase. The protective effect against mercury toxicity in animals (Ganther *et al.*, 1972) could be extremely important if found to be operative in man. Two bacterial enzyme systems (Turner and Stadtman, 1973; Andreesen and Ljungdahl, 1973) and a sheep muscle cytochrome (Whanger *et al.*, 1973) have been shown to contain selenium. These important discoveries permit the prediction that selenium will be found to be part of several more enzyme systems including some in human beings. Furthermore, these rapid strides in basic research should stimulate studies at a clinical level.

Applied research on widespread selenium deficiency in farm animals has culminated in the approval of selenium as a feed additive in this country. This has implications for human medicine. Since it affects animals, does selenium deficiency occur in human beings? What will be the impact on human selenium status of adding selenium to animal feeds?

Answers to these and other pertinent questions will depend upon more complete knowledge of selenium metabolism in man. It will be apparent from this review and other similar ones (Hopkins and Majaj, 1967; Cooper, 1967; Shapiro, 1973) that the information on selenium in man has been accumulated haphazardly with important areas left unstudied. The tremendous advances in the knowledge of the basic functions of selenium and in applied animal science must be matched now by systematic studies of selenium in man. Information gained from those studies will provide the basis for a rational approach to the use of selenium in human medicine.

II. DIETARY INTAKE

A. Chemical Form and Availability

Selenium occurs in a number of forms in food. Only limited information about these forms and their biological availability has been published. The forms present in wheat have recently been investigated (Olson *et al.*, 1970). Ion-exchange chromatography of pronase hydrolyzates of gluten and seeds from wheat grown in soil containing

[75Se]selenate indicated that over 40% of the 75Se was present as protein-bound selenomethionine. No other major 75Se-containing peak was identified. Thus, if wheat can be regarded as representative of plants eaten by human beings, about half of the element in plant food sources is present as selenomethionine. The nature of the other half is unknown. Certain selenium-indicator plants accumulate high levels of selenium in nonprotein amino acids (Shrift, 1969). These plants are not used as food but are important causes of selenium toxicity in animals (see below).

Very little is known about the form of selenium in animal tissues. The original recognition of the nutritional significance of selenium was its identification as the essential component of factor 3 against dietary liver necrosis (Schwarz and Foltz, 1957). This factor can be extracted from animal tissues and is a biologically highly active form of selenium, but its chemical structure has never been elucidated. Recent work with the selenoenzyme glutathione peroxidase demonstrates that selenium is present in it in a low molecular weight organic prosthetic group (Oh et al., 1974). This group could be related to factor 3.

Selenoamino acids can be incorporated into animal protein (Ochoa-Solano and Gitler, 1968), but their origin is probably in plants, since presently available evidence suggests that mammals and birds are unable to make them (Cummins and Martin, 1967; Jenkins, 1968). Another form of selenium, the selenotrisulfide, has been found in animal tissues (Jenkins, 1968), but more recent work suggests that this form may be present only in situations of selenium excess (Burk, 1973a); it may not be found in significant amounts in food. An association of selenium with mercury in certain fish and marine mammals has been noted (Ganther et al., 1972; Koeman et al., 1973), and evidence that a chemical bond exists between selenium and mercury in animal tissues has been presented (Burk et al., 1974). Thus, many foods containing mercury will also contain appreciable quantities of selenium.

From the above considerations, it can be postulated that in the presence of adequate selenium a relatively fixed amount of the element in animals will be present in selenoenzymes. The amount present as selenoamino acids will depend on the ingestion of this form, and selenotrisulfide formation will result from intake of excess amounts of selenium. The presence of selenium in association with mercury will depend on mercury intake. Thus a number of factors can influence the form of selenium found in animal tissues used for food by human beings.

Several factors modify the biological availability of dietary selenium. Extensive studies have been reported by Schwarz and co-workers (Schwarz and Foltz, 1958; Schwarz et al., 1972) on the biological effectiveness of dozens of selenium compounds in the prevention of dietary liver necrosis. From these studies it is clear that some forms of selenium are more available than others. To mention the most important ones, selenium as selenite, DL-selenomethionine, and DL-selenocystine were all found about equally effective in preventing liver necrosis, but factor 3 selenium was three times more effective than these (Schwarz and Foltz, 1958).

It is likely that selenium associated with mercury is a relatively un-available form. This is based on the report of low availability of selenium in fish meal (Miller *et al.*, 1972) and the knowledge that selenium is sometimes associated with mercury in fish (Ganther *et al.*, 1972). There is some evidence that high dietary sulfate levels decrease selenium avail-ability, at least in selenium toxicity (Halverson and Monty, 1960). Tri-*o*-cresyl phosphate (Shull and Cheeke, 1973) and silver (Swanson *et al.*, 1974) in the diet are known antagonists of selenium.

B. Quantity in Foods

Food selenium content is related to protein content and geographical origin. In most biological material, selenium is found largely in the protein fraction (Olson *et al.*, 1970; Burk, 1973a); indeed, foods low in protein, such as fruits, have been shown to contain very little of the element (Morris and Levander, 1970). Geographic areas have been delineated where the soil content of selenium is high, intermediate, or low; selenium content of plant and animal products from those areas generally corresponds to the soil selenium levels (Allaway, 1973; Millar *et al.*, 1973b). Cooking has been shown not to cause major losses of selenium from most foods (Higgs *et al.*, 1972). However, up to 23% loss was noted when cereals were dry heated, and a few vegetables lost even more selenium than this.

No attempt is made in this review to list all the known food selenium contents, since such a list has been published recently (Scott, 1973). In that compilation, various fish and fish products contained by far the greatest quantity of selenium—generally greater than 1 μg/gm. Grains from seleniferous areas contained around 1 μg selenium per gram, but the same products from low-selenium areas were selenium poor. Animal meats contained about 0.2 μg/gm.

Selenium content of tap water must be low in most areas, since the author has had no trouble producing selenium deficiency in rats given tap water in three different regions of the United States. Also, Jaffé *et al.* (1972) found that selenium in municipal water supplies was very low and almost the same in seleniferous and nonseleniferous areas of

Venezuela. Thus, it appears that food is the only significant source of selenium for man.

Several authors have provided values for daily selenium intake. No selenium could be detected in five total diet samples collected in Baltimore in 1963 and 1964 (Hopkins, and Majaj, 1967). Analysis of a hospital diet in Vermont indicated a daily selenium intake of 31 μg (Schroeder et al., 1970). Measurement of dietary selenium intake of thirteen New Zealand women revealed a range of 6–70 μg/day (Griffiths, 1973). All of these measurements were made in low-selenium areas. It is likely, then, that significantly higher selenium intakes could be recorded elsewhere. Significantly lower selenium intakes could also be expected in people eating little meat and obtaining their food supply from low-selenium areas. Consideration of the factors known to affect selenium availability should also be part of an assessment of selenium intake.

III. METABOLISM

A. Effect of Chemical Form

Knowledge of the effect of the chemical form of selenium on its metabolism is important with respect both to the bioavailability of the element (see above) and to the interpretation and comparison of experimental data. It has been documented that ^{75}Se from selenite and selenomethionine can share a common fate in producing urinary trimethylselenonium ion (Palmer et al., 1970). Also, binding of ^{75}Se to rat plasma and tissue proteins as determined by gel filtration and electrophoresis 24 hr or more after administration of either form was similar (Millar et al., 1973a), and after the first week, ^{75}Se whole-body retention decreased at a similar rate in rats given ^{75}Se either as selenite or as selenomethionine (Thomson and Stewart, 1973). These recent studies are supported by previous work showing that the elimination of ^{75}Se originally administered to rats as selenomethionine could not be hastened by raising dietary methionine but could be by increasing selenium intake (Said and Hegsted, 1970).

All those studies emphasize the similarities between selenium supplied as selenite and as selenomethionine, but differences can also be shown. The incorporation of selenomethionine into ovalbumin has been shown by amino acid analysis (Ochoa-Solano and Gitler, 1968). Selenomethionine has been shown to cause higher rat muscle selenium levels than selenite when they are supplied at levels above the minimal selenium requirement (Cary et al., 1973). The presumptive mechanism would be direct incorporation of the amino acid into muscle protein.

Based on these data, it seems logical to conclude that selenium supplied as selenomethionine can have two major fates, that of methionine and, when the selenomethionine is catabolized, that of selenium. Thus, experiments utilizing this form of selenium can be extremely difficult to interpret. In general, the methionine effect will predominate shortly after administration. As selenomethionine is catabolized, the released selenium will be reutilized via the regular selenium metabolic pathways so that predominantly selenium metabolism will be observed at later times.

B. Homeostasis

1. Whole-Body Retention

Animal experiments have demonstrated that retention of a dose of ^{75}Se is inversely related to the dietary selenium level (Ewan *et al.*, 1967; Burk *et al.*, 1972). Although this variable has not yet been studied in human beings, some whole-body retention data are available. A study of three cancer patients using [^{75}Se]selenite gave a biological half-life of 65 days (Cavalieri *et al.*, 1966). The corresponding figure for [^{75}Se]selenomethionine was 70 days as calculated from data collected from twenty-four subjects (Lathrop *et al.*, 1972).

2. Absorption

Comparatively little attention has been paid to the intestinal absorption of selenium. There is evidence that selenomethionine is absorbed via the methionine carrier (McConnell and Cho, 1967). Selenite is better absorbed in monogastric animals than in ruminants (Wright and Bell, 1966), but in rats, at least, the selenium status of the animal seems to have no influence on absorption (Brown *et al.*, 1972). Human absorption of [^{75}Se]selenite has been reported to be 70%, 64%, and 44% in three healthy subjects, which compares with over 90% absorption by rats (Thomson and Stewart, 1972). On the basis of the limited data available, it appears likely that selenium absorption is less efficient in man than in the rat.

3. Excretion

Experiments with rats have established that under physiological conditions selenium homeostasis is achieved by the regulation of urinary selenium excretion (Burk *et al.*, 1972). When large quantities of selenium are ingested, some of the element is lost in the breath as dimethyl selenide, but in other circumstances this route of excretion is negligible. Fecal losses are not governed by selenium intake in the same way as is urinary selenium.

Available human data show that 11.2% of the ^{75}Se in an intravenous dose of [^{75}Se]L-selenomethionine appeared in the urine in the 120 hr after administration, while 2.5% appeared in the feces (Lathrop *et al.*, 1972); when [^{75}Se]selenite was given intravenously, urinary excretion was 11% in 24 hr and 16.5% in 72 hr in one study (Cavalieri *et al.*, 1966) and 5.5–9.4% in 24 hr in another (Burk, 1974).

Measurement of urinary selenium content has long been used in screening studies, especially for identifying groups at risk of selenium toxicity (Smith and Westfall, 1937; Mondragón and Jaffé, 1971). Urinary selenium has been estimated to account for about half the dietary intake (Thomson, 1972), but this is based on data obtained from only four subjects consuming from 7.8 to 15.7 μg of selenium per day and thus may not be valid for higher intakes. The determination of selenium in urine is more difficult than in blood, because some of the urinary selenium resists digestion.

Urinary selenium in the rat consists largely of trimethylselenonium ion and an unidentified substance called U-2 (Palmer *et al.*, 1969). These substances can be separated by two-dimensional paper chromatography and quantitated (Kiker and Burk, 1974). Such a chromatogram of urine from a young man with a testicular tumor who had been given [^{75}Se]selenite is shown in Fig. 1.* The R_f values of authentic trimethylselenonium ion† were found to be 0.90:0.40 (phenol front:butanol front) in this system, and this closely matches a major ^{75}Se spot in the human urine (Fig. 1). U-2, with R_f values of 0.88:0.61 in rat urine (Kiker and Burk, 1974), is likely to be the other major spot in Fig. 1. Urine samples collected from this patient during three periods were chromatographed in this manner, and the results in Table I indicate that the percentage of urinary ^{75}Se appearing in the trimethylselenonium ion and U-2 areas increased with time. These data are not conclusive proof of trimethylselenonium ion production by man but do strongly suggest it.

4. Summary

Rat studies indicate that selenium absorption and fecal excretion are not regulated by the selenium status of the animal. Homeostasis is main-

* This work was carried out while the author was a member of the Bioenergetics Division, U.S. Army Medical Research and Nutrition Laboratory, Denver, Colorado.
† This was kindly supplied by Dr. I. S. Palmer, South Dakota State University, Brookings, South Dakota.

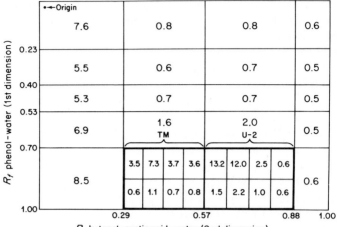

FIG. 1. Two-dimensional paper chromatogram of urine collected between 5 and 10.5 hr after intravenous injection of 200 μCi of [75Se]selenite (1 μg selenium) in a 19-year-old man with a testicular tumor. Details of the method are published elsewhere (Kiker and Burk, 1974). Numbers inside the boxes indicate the percentage of the recovered 75Se found in that area. Trimethylselenonium ion and U-2 areas are shown as heavy boxes.

tained by urinary excretion of selenium metabolites, including trimethyl-selenonium ion and U-2. The excretion of these two metabolites is directly proportional to dietary selenium level. When large quantities of selenium are supplied, dimethyl selenide is excreted in expired air.

Data available from human studies suggest that urinary selenium is controlled by dietary selenium as in the rat, and new data presented here suggest that the same major urinary selenium metabolites are found in man and the rat. Thus, although knowledge of human selenium homeostasis is incomplete, what is known indicates similarity to the rat.

TABLE I   **Percentage of Urinary Selenium-75 Appearing as Trimethylselenonium Ion and U-2 in Human Urine as a Function of Time**

Hours postinjection urine collected	Trimethyl-selenonium ion (%)	U-2 (%)
0–3	14.0	19.4
3–5	16.2	33.2
5–10½	21.3	33.6

C. Distribution of [75]Se

The distribution of ^{75}Se from a single dose has been studied in rats and was found to be highly dependent on dietary selenium intake, amount of selenium injected with the ^{75}Se, and time between ^{75}Se administration and study (Hopkins *et al.*, 1966; Atkins *et al.*, 1971; Burk *et al.*, 1972; Brown and Burk, 1973). No ^{75}Se distribution studies in human beings have adequately controlled or characterized the selenium intake, and their results should be interpreted with care.

Human tissue distribution of ^{75}Se after [^{75}Se]L-selenomethionine administration has been reviewed by Lathrop *et al.* (1972). Early concentration of the ^{75}Se by the liver and pancreas was found. Pancreas ^{75}Se decreased to blood level by 2 days, but liver ^{75}Se concentration remained about twice the blood level at 100 days. Skin and muscle never had a ^{75}Se concentration as high as blood.

Penner (1966) demonstrated incorporation of ^{75}Se into hemoglobin following [^{75}Se]selenomethionine administration. He was able to study red cell turnover by measuring ^{75}Se content of red cells and also demonstrated significant reutilization of the label, which could have been incorporation of ^{75}Se into glutathione peroxidase.

Fewer data are available on the distribution of ^{75}Se after its administration as inorganic selenium, and all of these are in cancer patients. After [^{75}Se]selenite injection, liver [75]Se (monitored externally) rose for 2 hr and then fell gradually, while muscle ^{75}Se fell throughout observation in three patients (Cavalieri *et al.*, 1966). In a similar study of six patients, biological half-times of 100 days for muscle, 70 days for tumor, 50 days for liver, 32 days for kidney, and 28 days for serum were obtained (Wenzel *et al.*, 1971). Eight days after [^{75}Se]selenate injection in a patient with a hepatoma, the greatest ^{75}Se concentrations of the ten tissues studied were found in the kidney and liver (Hirooka and Galambos, 1966b).

D. Protein Binding

The usual state of selenium in animal tissues is protein bound. The voluminous and extremely important literature on protein-bound forms of selenium in animals is expanding rapidly. Although a discussion of this general topic is beyond the range of this review, some available data on selenium binding to human plasma proteins will be considered.

Binding of ^{75}Se to human plasma proteins after incubation of [^{75}Se]selenite with plasma is very small; however, if the incubation is done using whole blood, a substantial amount of the ^{75}Se will bind to the plasma proteins after having entered the red cells and been extruded from them (Lee *et al.*, 1969). Dialysis of these proteins against a bath containing cysteine caused release of the ^{75}Se. This suggests that the ^{75}Se was associated with protein sulfhydryl groups.

Selenium-75 incorporation into plasma proteins has been shown following [^{75}Se]selenomethionine injection (Awwad *et al.*, 1966). Virtually all the plasma ^{75}Se was trichloroacetic acid-precipitable 10 hr after injection. The decline in plasma protein specific activity was shown to follow a multiexponential pattern during the 25 days of observation.

Paper electrophoresis of serum from patients with liver disease who had received [^{75}Se]selenate showed that the α_2- and β-globulins had the greatest affinity for ^{75}Se (Hirooka and Galambos, 1966b). The plasma lipoproteins of these patients were separated in one fraction and those from patients with alcoholic liver disease were found to contain more ^{75}Se than those from normal subjects and one patient with postnecrotic cirrhosis. These results may indicate a derangement of selenium metabolism in patients with alcoholic liver disease.

After intravenous injection of [^{75}Se]selenite into patients with various forms of cancer, plasma ^{75}Se decreased rapidly during the first hour and then rose slightly between 1 and 6 hr due to a marked increase in protein-bound ^{75}Se (Cavalieri *et al.*, 1966; Burk, 1974). Gel filtration of the human plasma (Fig. 2) showed that large amounts of the ^{75}Se was unbound in the early samples, but by 6 hr, about 85% was protein-

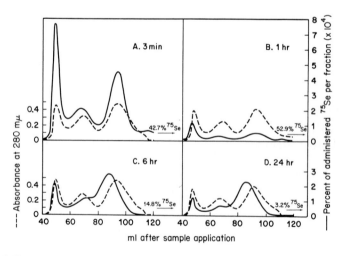

FIG. 2.   Gel filtration chromatograms of plasma from the patient whose urine chromatogram is shown in Fig. 1. Sephadex G-200 was used, and column conditions were the same for all experiments. The figure is taken from Burk (1974).

bound. A ^{75}Se peak seen at 48 ml in Fig. 2C was due mostly to lipopro-
tein-bound ^{75}Se, but the peak at 86 ml was similar in position to a
peak previously reported to occur in rat plasma (Millar, 1972; Burk,
1973b). These studies suggest that selenium is bound to specific human
plasma proteins.

Significant amounts of the ^{75}Se were associated with very low-density
and low-density lipoproteins, especially shortly after injection, but very
little was found in the high-density lipoproteins (Burk, 1974). The very
low-density lipoprotein ^{75}Se activity declined more rapidly than low-density lipoprotein ^{75}Se activity. These findings are intriguing, since it is
known that very low-density lipoproteins are catabolized to low-density
lipoproteins (Bilheimer et al., 1972). Selenium has not been found in
rat lipoproteins under similar conditions (Burk, 1973a). It will remain
for further studies to establish whether selenium is a natural constituent
of human very low-density and low-density lipoproteins.

IV. TISSUE LEVELS

A. Blood Levels

The human tissue in which selenium has been most frequently measured is blood. A full understanding of selenium blood levels is not
presently possible, however, due to lack of knowledge of the nature
of selenium in human blood. Some information is available about the
element in animal blood, and it may be pertinent in man. Recent work
has shown that over 75% of ovine red cell selenium is in the enzyme
glutathione peroxidase (Oh et al., 1974). Since the red cells present
at any one time were produced up to 120 days previously, red cell
selenium content might be expected to drop more slowly than that in
plasma and tissues such as liver under conditions of acute selenium
deprivation. Plasma selenium has not been qualitatively well characterized, but some glutathione peroxidase is present in plasma in animals
(Noguchi et al., 1973).

A study of Cohn fractions of human plasma showed that most selenium
was in the α- and β-globulins (Dickson and Tomlinson, 1967). Recent
studies have shown an association of selenium with human plasma lipoproteins (see above) and at least one other unidentified human plasma
protein fraction (Fig. 2).

Three large series of blood selenium contents in normal individuals
are available. Dickson and Tomlinson (1967), using a neutron activation

method, found 18.2 μg selenium per 100 ml of blood, 23.6 μg per 100 ml of cells, and 14.4 μg per 100 ml of plasma in 253 subjects in Canada. They noted a gradual decline in both plasma and cell selenium with age. Allaway *et al.* (1968) studied the selenium content of blood from blood banks across the United States using a fluorimetric method. They found slightly higher values in blood from seleniferous areas, but the range of their 210 samples was only 10–34 μg per 100 ml blood, with a mean of 20.6. Kasperek *et al.* (1972) studied serum selenium levels in 184 normal persons using neutron activation analysis and found a mean value of 9.8 μg/100 ml. They noted a gradual rise of serum selenium to age 35 and then a gradual decline in older individuals.

Blood selenium levels in a few pathological conditions have been measured. Plasma but not cell selenium was markedly depressed in three patients with extensive burns (Dickson and Tomlinson, 1967). Guatemalan children with kwashiorkor had a mean blood selenium content of 11 μg/100 ml compared to 23 μg/100 ml in controls (Burk *et al.*, 1967). Plasma but not red cell selenium was also significantly depressed. Thai infants with kwashiorkor and marasmus were also found to have lower blood selenium contents than controls due to lower plasma selenium levels (Levine and Olson, 1970). Jaffé *et al.* (1972) reported 81.3 μg selenium per 100 ml blood in Venezuelan children living in a seleniferous zone and 35.5 μg per 100 ml blood in a control group in Caracas.

In a study of the association of blood selenium content and cancer, Shamberger *et al.* (1973) found 22.9 μg selenium per 100 ml blood in forty-eight normal subjects. Patients with colonic (15.8 μg selenium per 100 ml), gastric (15.3 μg/100 ml), and pancreatic (13.2 μg/100 ml) cancer all had significantly lower levels than controls as did patients with cirrhosis (13.6 μg/100 ml) and hepatitis (14.5 μg/100 ml). Blood selenium levels were normal in patients with a number of disorders, including rectal cancer and diabetes.

The human blood selenium level seems to be regulated in the vicinity of 20 μg/100 ml. Low blood selenium levels seem to be associated with low plasma levels and no fall in cell selenium content. Therefore, measurement of plasma or serum selenium level may be a more sensitive indicator of selenium status than whole blood measurement.

B. Organ Levels

Reports of organ selenium content have been mostly anecdotal and values have varied widely. Kidney and liver generally have had the highest concentrations of selenium (Dickson and Tomlinson, 1967; Schroeder *et al.*, 1970). Dickson and Tomlinson (1967) measured liver,

TABLE II   Selenium Content of Three Tissues from Ten Individuals[a]

Subject	selenium content in μg/g whole tissue		
	Liver	Skin	Muscle
1	0.44	0.30	0.32
2	0.42	0.30	0.25
3	0.18	0.19	0.26
4	0.66	0.12	0.40
5	0.53	0.62	0.32
6	0.48	0.17	0.44
7	0.44	0.37	0.48
8	0.43	0.29	0.59
9	0.30	0.22	0.28
10	0.45	0.12	0.35

[a] From Dickson and Tomlinson (1967).

skin, and muscle selenium in tissues from ten autopsies, and the values are shown in Table II to illustrate the variation found in this kind of data. No consistent relationships among different tissues from an individual are noted in this undefined autopsy series. Animal studies have yielded more consistent values for tissue selenium, and this emphasizes the need to define more carefully the human population whose tissue levels are being measured. Such studies could be helpful in determining relationships of tissue selenium levels in health and disease.

V. DEFICIENCY

Experimental selenium deficiency has been produced in several animal species by prolonged feeding of rations low in selenium. Selenium-deficient rats grow slowly, develop cataracts, lose their hair, and have aspermatogenesis (Sprinker *et al.*, 1971). Pancreatic degeneration is the dominant selenium-deficiency lesion in the chick (Gries and Scott, 1972).

A report of possible selenium deficiency in a primate, the squirrel monkey, is of great interest, even though it is of a preliminary nature (Muth *et al.*, 1971) and confirmation has not appeared. Seven adult monkeys were fed a selenium-deficient diet for 9 months until one animal died. Hair on the others had become sparse and they were losing weight and becoming listless. Survivors were paired by weight and one animal of each pair received selenium by injection. Animals receiving selenium responded with weight gain, hair growth, and return to normal physical activity. The other three monkeys died and were found to have "hepatic necrosis, cardiac and skeletal muscle degeneration and nephrosis." Without supporting data or corroboration, this study cannot be accepted uncritically as a report of pure selenium deficiency in the monkey for several reasons, including: (1) in no other instance has selenium deficiency been produced in an adult animal that matured eating a selenium-adequate diet; (2) some of the pathology produced is more typical of combined vitamin E–selenium deficiency; furthermore, although adequate vitamin E was added to the diet, no plasma vitamin E levels were reported to show that the monkeys were not also vitamin E-deficient.

Conditions under which human dietary selenium deficiency is likely to occur can be inferred from what is known about selenium in food (see above) and animal studies. Since selenium is associated with protein in food, a low-protein diet is probably also low in selenium. Crops produced in areas with low soil selenium are low in selenium, so people in such an area subsisting on locally grown foods are likely to have a low selenium intake. Finally, growing animals have been shown to be more susceptible to development of selenium deficiency than mature ones, so children might be more prone to develop it than adults. It is also possible that human selenium deficiency might occur as a consequence of an acquired or inherited metabolic defect analogous to copper deficiency in the kinky hair syndrome (Danks et al., 1972).

Based on these considerations, a logical group to study for the occurrence of selenium deficiency would be children with protein–calorie malnutrition. Schwarz (1961) reported a weight gain in response to feeding selenium to such children. Two children with protein–calorie malnutrition who were not gaining weight in response to apparently adequate treatment were given 25 μg of selenium daily as γ,γ'-diselenodivaleric acid. They then gained 450 and 660 gm over 10 and 14 days of treatment.

Hopkins and Majaj (1967) reported similar results in three infants given 25 μg of selenium as sodium selenite daily, and demonstrated a reticulocyte response following the institution of selenium treatment in three of five anemic infants. Unfortunately, neither of these studies included nontreated control patients, so no firm conclusions about selenium therapy in protein–calorie malnutrition can be drawn.

Decreased plasma and whole blood selenium contents have been reported in protein–calorie malnutrition (Burk et al., 1967; Levine and Olson, 1970). Figure 3 shows blood selenium values from five children

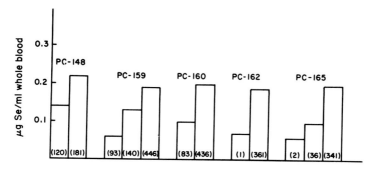

FIG. 3. Blood selenium levels of five Guatemalan children hospitalized with kwashiorkor. The numbers in parentheses indicate the day of hospitalization on which the blood sample was obtained. The figure is from Burk *et al.* (1967).

followed for up to a year after hospital admission. They received no supplemental selenium. Blood selenium levels rose slowly to reach the normal range only after many months. In contrast, plasma proteins rapidly returned to normal after the institution of an adequate diet. These findings imply that selenium stores were severely depleted in these children.

Protein–calorie malnutrition is a condition that by its nature should predispose to selenium deficiency; indeed, there is good indication that in this condition selenium stores may be reduced. Furthermore, some evidence suggests that some children with the condition benefit from selenium administration. More studies of selenium's role in this condition are needed.

The role of selenium in causation and prevention of cancer has been widely debated, and a recent review is available (Shapiro, 1972). There has been an attempt to link cancer incidence with low crop selenium content from specific areas in the United States (Shamberger and Willis, 1971). This type of study suffers from failure to evaluate all area differences such as rainfall, pollution, and population type, and therefore cannot be regarded as conclusive. However, another report has demonstrated lower blood selenium levels in people with certain types of cancer than in healthy individuals (see above). It is not known, however, whether the low selenium levels existed before the cancer developed or were a consequence of it.

Selenium–vitamin E deficiency has been proposed as a cause of crib death (Money, 1971). Another report has shown low vitamin E levels but normal selenium levels in blood from infants dying of that cause (Rhead *et al.*, 1972), suggesting that selenium does not play a role in it.

VI. TOXICITY

The toxic effects of selenium have been recognized much longer than the nutritional ones. The discovery in the 1930s that certain geographical areas are seleniferous and produce plants with high selenium content explained observations dating back centuries that food grown in these areas caused sickness in man and beast consuming it. In addition to the generalized increase of selenium in vegetation from such areas, a few species of plants were identified that thrived there and were called selenium indicator plants (Rosenfeld and Beath, 1964). These plants characteristically accumulate selenium to extremely high levels in the form of nonprotein selenoamino acids such as Se-methylselenocysteine (Nigam and McConnell, 1969) and produce acute toxicity in animals consuming them.

A number of syndromes of selenium toxicity in animals have been described (Rosenfeld and Beath, 1964). The pathology in acute toxicity is widespread necrosis and hemorrhage, and death is probably due to hypoxia secondary to these lesions in the lungs. Manifestations of chronic toxicity are often species-dependent and related to the form and amount of selenium ingested. In almost all species the liver is affected and cirrhosis develops. Frequently a cardiomyopathy is found. Loss of hair and sloughing of hoofs occurs.

The biochemical mechanism of selenium toxicity has not been established. Recent *in vitro* studies have demonstrated glutathione-dependent inhibition of amino acid incorporation into polyribosomes by nanomole quantities of selenite (Vernie *et al.*, 1974). The implication is that the mixed selenotrisulfide of a critical enzyme sulfhydryl group and glutathione formed, rendering the enzyme inactive. Further studies of this mechanism are merited.

Several moderating influences on selenium toxicity are known. Increasing dietary protein generally decreases toxicity (Lewis *et al.*, 1940). The combination of methionine and vitamin E apparently facilitates excretion of the element (Levander and Morris, 1970), while a nonprotein factor in linseed oil meal increases tissue levels of selenium but decreases toxicity (Levander *et al.*, 1970). Arsenic protects by increasing biliary excretion of selenium (Levander and Baumann, 1966).

Although selenium toxicity has had a tremendous impact on animals in seleniferous areas, very little effect on human populations has been demonstrated. Smith and his colleagues (1936; Smith and Westfall, 1937) surveyed rural populations of seleniferous areas in South Dakota and Nebraska. They found high concentrations of selenium in urine from many subjects but were unable to demonstrate signs or symptoms that could be confidently attributed to selenium toxicity because their study lacked a control population.

Jaffé et al. (1972) reported a clinical and biochemical study of Venezuelan children, comparing a group living in a seleniferous area with a control group. Some of the results are seen in Table III. Blood and urinary selenium were much higher in the seleniferous area. The liver function tests, serum glutamic oxaloacetic transaminase (SGOT) and alkaline phosphatase, were normal in both groups. Pathological symptoms, such as history of nausea and vomiting, skin depigmentation, and hair loss, were more frequent and hemoglobin values were lower in the group exposed to selenium, but the authors felt that this was due to population differences as evidenced in the different incidence of intestinal parasites. They concluded that this level of selenium intake was not likely to pose severe health hazards in children.

An isolated instance of selenium poisoning by well water containing 9 ppm selenium has been reported (Rosenfeld and Beath, 1964). The Indian family affected had alopecia, abnormal nails, and lassitude, and recovered when use of the contaminated water was stopped.

Selenium is widely used in the electronics, glass, and paint industries, and safeguards against worker exposure must be employed. Glover (1970) had the opportunity to observe for 15 years men exposed to selenium in their work and concluded on the basis of a statistical study that selenium exposure did not alter the death rate or affect the cause of death. He pointed out that an early sign of excessive selenium exposure is garlicky breath due to dimethyl selenide excretion.

Dental caries has been attributed to high selenium intake, and several epidemiological studies have indicated a slightly higher overall caries

TABLE III   Study of Children Living in a Seleniferous Area of Venezuela and a Control Group[a]

Parameter	Control group	Seleniferous group
Number	50	111
Hemoglobin (gm)	14.8	12.8
μg selenium/100 ml blood	35.5	81.3
μg selenium/mg creatinine in urine	0.224	0.636
SGOT (U/ml)	17	14
Alkaline phosphatase (sigma U/ml)	4	4
Pathological symptoms (%)	14	40
Intestinal parasites found (%)	15	79

[a] Adapted from Jaffé et al. (1972).

incidence in seleniferous areas than in control areas (Hadjimarkos, 1965; Ludwig and Bibby, 1969). Animal studies have not yielded consistent production of caries except when selenium was administered during tooth development (Bowen, 1972). The conclusion that selenium is cariogenic for human beings cannot yet be made.

Selenium has known teratogenic effects in chickens (Moxon and Rhian, 1943), and recently it was reported that a higher number of abortions than expected were noted in a group of laboratory technicians handling selenite (Robertson, 1970). No differences in urinary selenium levels between the technicians and nonexposed individuals was found. This report indicates a need for a controlled study of women of childbearing age exposed to selenium.

Recently, the Food and Drug Administration approved the use of selenite as an animal feed additive in an amount of up to 0.2 ppm selenium. This was done to combat widespread selenium deficiency in farm animals. Although this level of selenium in organic forms has been shown to cause accumulation of more selenium in muscle tissue with each increment of dietary selenium, such does not occur with selenite (Cary et al., 1973), so meat from these animals is unlikely to cause selenium toxicity in humans consuming them.

No specific treatment for selenium toxicity exists except the removal from selenium exposure. BAL (British anti-Lewisite), penicillamine, and bromobenzene have all been evaluated for use in selenium toxicity but found ineffective or impractical for one reason or another (Rosenfeld and Beath, 1964; Levander, 1972).

Selenium toxicity in animals has been a major problem in the past, and a few cases of selenium toxicity in human beings have been reported. But although large land areas contain excessive quantities of the element and selenium is extensively used in industry, there is no firm evidence of a significant selenium toxicity problem in human beings.

VII. MEDICAL APPLICATIONS

A. Therapeutic Uses

Because of selenium's widely recognized toxicity and imputed carcinogenicity, therapeutic agents containing the element have found little use in medicine. Many selenium-containing compounds and selenium analogs of sulfur-containing drugs and biological compounds have been synthesized and tested, and a recent review is available on this subject

(Klayman, 1973). No really promising drugs have emerged from these studies.

Selenium sulfide is incorporated into shampoos and ointments and sold for the treatment of seborrheic dermatitis. It and zinc pyrithione shampoos were found to be equally effective and better than an unmedicated shampoo in the treatment of dandruff (Orentreich et al., 1969). Selenium sulfide is water-insoluble and possesses a very low toxicity when compared with selenite (Cummins and Kimura, 1971). However, toxicity due to prolonged use of the agent on open skin lesions has been reported, and elevated urinary selenium levels were documented (Ransone et al., 1961). Symptoms included a tremor and loss of appetite. It seems reasonable to avoid the use of this compound when the integument is not intact.

Since selenium is very likely an essential element for man, deficiency may occur either due to lack of biologically available selenium in the diet or secondary to another disease state (see above). Should such a deficiency be discovered, it will be necessary to administer microgram quantities of a biologically active form such as selenite.

B. Diagnostic Uses

Selenium in the form [^{75}Se]selenomethionine is used to scan the pancreas and the parathyroid glands. A recent critical review of pancreatic scanning techniques concluded that the concept is basically sound but that in practice many pancreatic lesions are not detected and many normal pancreases give abnormal scans (Bachrach et al., 1972). It was recommended that the use of these scans be restricted to major research centers for further evaluation and improvement. Parathyroid scans with [^{75}Se]selenomethionine are infrequently used because of the difficulty in obtaining an adequate image and lack of accuracy (Giulio and Morales, 1969).

Several reports of the use of [^{75}Se]selenomethionine in the diagnosis and staging of lymphoma have appeared (Herrera et al., 1965; Ferrucci et al., 1970). The latter report concluded that a negative study was not a reliable indicator of the absence of disease, but that an abnormal study indicated a 70–80% probability that disease was present. These authors felt that [^{75}Se]selenomethionine scans might be useful in patients who could not undergo lymphangiography and in detection of reactivation of disease.

Reduced brain uptake of [^{75}Se]selenomethionine has been reported in phenylketonuria (Oldendorf et al., 1971). This was felt to be due to saturation of the blood–brain barrier carrier system for selenomethionine by the elevated blood phenylalanine. Even though differences between patients and normal subjects were highly significant, more specific tests are available for the diagnosis of phenylketonuria.

The use of [^{75}Se]selenite as a scanning agent for a variety of tumors has been recommended. Cavalieri and Steinberg (1971) advocate using it in conjunction with another isotope to take advantage of selenium's greater uptake in rapidly metabolizing cells. Thus, it can be used with strontium in bone. They feel that a positive strontium scan with a negative [^{75}Se]selenite scan would suggest a noncancerous lesion while ^{75}Se uptake in the area would suggest cancer. These authors apply similar arguments to the use of [^{75}Se]selenite with another isotope in brain scanning and scanning the chest. Detection of lung cancer (Jereb et al., 1972) and many other tumors (Thiemann et al., 1971) has been accomplished with [^{75}Se]selenite, but not enough control data are available to make recommendations on these uses.

[^{75}Se]Selenomethionine has been used to measure erythrocyte life-span (Penner, 1966), but this use of the compound has not been widespread due to the greater radiation exposure than with ^{51}Cr. Attempts have been made to use it to study protein turnover in human beings (Waterlow et al., 1969), but these have failed, probably because of the reutilization of the ^{75}Se after catabolism of the amino acid (see above).

Measurement of extracellular fluid volume with [^{75}Se]selenate has been tried (Nelp and Blumberg, 1965) but was unsuccessful due to tissue uptake and metabolism of the ^{75}Se.

When excess selenium as selenite or selenate is injected, a certain percentage of it is exhaled as dimethyl selenide. Most of the methylation presumably takes place in the liver. Hirooka and Galambos (1966a) studied the effect of experimental liver injury in rats on ^{75}Se exhaled after injection of [^{75}Se]selenate with the aim of developing a liver function test. They found no impairment of ^{75}Se excretion in choline deficiency-induced fatty liver. Even if they had been able to show depressed ^{75}Se exhalation in liver damage, such a test would not be applicable to man because large doses of selenium must be given that might prove toxic.

VIII. ASSESSMENT OF SELENIUM STATUS

Adequate means of assessing selenium status of individuals are needed for population surveys and to diagnose selenium deficiency and toxicity in individual patients. A number of methods have been used in animal and human studies.

Blood levels of selenium have been widely used as an index of selenium status since the development of sensitive fluorimetric assays. Many studies have demonstrated that blood selenium levels were lower in animals fed a selenium-deficient diet than in controls. It has been shown that when rats are fed a selenium-deficient diet, blood selenium concentration falls in the same way liver selenium does, although not quite as precipitously (Burk et al., 1968). This suggests that blood selenium level may mirror tissue stores when they are subnormal. However, studies suggest that once adequate selenium intake is achieved, the blood level does not continue to rise with further increases in dietary selenium until toxic selenium intake occurs unless organic forms of selenium such as selenomethionine are ingested (Burk et al., 1968; Scott and Thompson, 1971).

Studies in human beings suggest that blood selenium is under homeostatic control and that plasma or serum levels may be a more sensitive indicator of selenium status than whole blood levels (see above). No studies have been reported in which human beings were fed selenium-deficient diets to study changes in selenium levels.

The in vitro uptake of [^{75}Se]selenite by ovine red cells has been shown to increase with the length of time the animals were fed a selenium-deficient diet (Wright and Bell, 1963). This technique has been used in a study of children with protein–calorie malnutrition and the results correlated inversely with the blood selenium concentration as shown by Fig. 4 (Burk et al., 1967). This is a simple procedure but needs further evaluation before it can be accepted as being useful in assessing selenium status.

Urinary selenium excretion in rats seems to reflect dietary intake of the element until pulmonary excretion begins at high selenium intakes (see above). Attempts to correlate urinary excretion of the element with dietary intake in man is warranted. Twenty-four hour urine collections, not spot checks of urine, should be used, as they are not subject to error from meal and dilution effects.

Erythrocyte glutathione peroxidase activity in rats has been shown to fall in response to a selenium-deficient diet and rise in response to a diet containing mildly toxic amounts of the element (Hafeman et al., 1974). If this can be shown to happen in man also, it could eventually prove to be the most sensitive and useful indicator of human selenium status.

Measurement of selenium in hair and nails has been seldom reported (Hadjimarkos and Shearer, 1973), but should be evaluated in view of its usefulness in assessing status with respect to other trace elements.

Animal studies have shown that the percentage of an injected dose

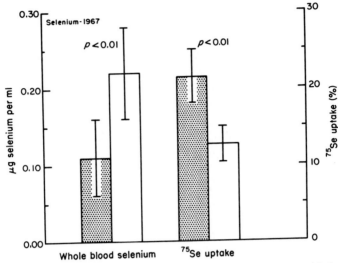

FIG. 4. Blood selenium levels and *in vitro* red blood cell uptake of [^{75}Se]selenite of Guatemalan children with kwashiorkor (shaded) and controls (unshaded). Data are from Burk *et al.* (1967).

of [^{75}Se]selenite appearing in the urine is a sensitive indicator of the concentration of selenium in the diet (Burk *et al.*, 1972). Human application of this method is precluded, however, by the necessity of administering ^{75}Se.

Presently, blood or plasma selenium levels would seem to be the best method for diagnosing human selenium deficiency and toxicity. Urinary selenium excretion should, in most cases, be the best measure of dietary intake of the element. Even though the author feels these methods to be the best available at the present time, they need more evaluation to assure their specificity and reliability.

IX. RESEARCH NEEDS

Research efforts should be directed to learning whether selenium plays a role in human health and disease and, if so, what that role is. As a basis for further clinical studies, evaluation of the methods available for assessment of selenium status needs to be performed. This will involve monitoring many of the measurements discussed in Section VIII in subjects fed specially prepared diets of known selenium content. This should at least allow identification of those tests that are sensitive to changes in dietary selenium intake. Since human selenium deficiency is not likely to be produced in this manner, continued reliance on results of animal studies for guidance in interpreting data from human studies will be necessary.

Homeostatic mechanisms for selenium are important to guard against accumulation of toxic levels of the element and to insure retention of enough to meet the body's needs. These mechanisms need careful study, since they involve the liver and kidneys in the rat. Both these organs are frequently the site of pathology in human disease, and in many cases, organ failure develops. It is entirely possible that selenium could play a role in hepatic or renal insufficiency.

Beyond these specific areas of need, it can be recommended that other studies of selenium metabolism in man, such as its presence in erythrocyte glutathione peroxidase and its binding to plasma proteins, discussed in Section III, be pursued. It is from such studies that clues to involvement of selenium in specific disease processes may come, as well as better ways of assessing selenium status. Once adequate means of selenium status assessment are available, wideranging studies of selenium status in human disease states should be carried out.

ADDENDUM

Since the submission of this manuscript several publications of importance have appeared. Selenium has been proved an essential nutrient for man by Awasthi *et al.* (1975). They purified human erythrocyte glutathione peroxidase and found that 3.5 gram-atoms of selenium were present per mole of protein. Thompson *et al.* (1975) have provided data on selenium intake by Canadians. Their data indicate an average daily intake of 197 μg with a range of 113 to 220 μg.

Human blood selenium levels in New Zealand have been reported (Watkinson, 1974). They were 0.069 μg/ml or about one-third those in North America. This was explained by the low selenium content of food in New Zealand. Future studies such as this can yield more information if glutathione peroxidase is measured.

Absorption of 1 mg doses of selenium as selenite by human beings was studied by Thomson (1974). She found 90–95% absorption of the dose when the selenite was dissolved in water, but only 20–40% absorption of solid sodium selenite. The virtually complete absorption of this large dose of selenium strongly suggests that selenium absorption is not controlled in human beings.

ACKNOWLEDGMENTS

The author acknowledges the technical assistance of Mr. Kenneth W. Kiker in the study of human urinary selenium metabolites and thanks Mrs. Dorothy Bass for help in the preparation and typing of the manuscript.

REFERENCES

Allaway, W. H. (1973). Selenium in the food chain. *Cornell Vet.* **63**, 151–170.

Allaway, W. H., Kubota, J., Losee, F., and Roth, M. (1968). Selenium, molybdenum, and vanadium in human blood. *Arch. Environ. Health* **16**, 342–348.

Andreesen, J. R., and Ljungdahl, L. G. (1973). Formate dehydrogenase of *Clostridium thermoaceticum:* Incorporation of selenium-75, and the effects of selenite, molybdate, and tungstate on the enzyme. *J. Bacteriol.* **116**, 867–873.

Atkins, H. L., Hauser, W., and Klopper, J. F. (1971). Effect of carrier on organ distribution of ^{75}Se-selenomethionine. *Metab., Clin. Exp.* **20**, 1052–1056.

Awasthi, Y. C., Beutler, E., and Srivastava, S. K. (1975). Purification and properties of human erythrocyte glutathione peroxidase. *J. Biol. Chem.* **250**, 5144–5149.

Awwad, H. K., Potchen, E. J., Adelstein, S. J., and Dealy, J. B. (1966). Se^{75}-selenomethionine incorporation into human plasma proteins and erythrocytes. *Metab., Clin. Exp.* **15**, 626–640.

Bachrach, W. H., Birsner, J. W., Izenstark, J. L., and Smith, V. L. (1972). Pancreatic scanning: A review. *Gastroenterology* **63**, 890–910.

Bilheimer, D. W., Eisenberg, S., and Levy, R. I. (1972). The metabolism of very low density lipoprotein proteins. I. preliminary *in vitro* and *in vivo* observations. *Biochim. Biophys. Acta* **260**, 212–221.

Bowen, W. H. (1972). The effect of selenium and vanadium on caries activity in monkeys (*M. Irus*). *J. Ir. Dent. Ass.* **18**, 83.

Brown, D. G., and Burk, R. F. (1973). Selenium retention in tissues and sperm of rats fed a torula yeast diet. *J. Nutr.* **103**, 102–108.

Brown, D. G., Burk, R. F., Seely, R. J., and Kiker, K. W. (1972). Effect of dietary selenium on the gastrointestinal absorption of ^{75}SeO$_3^{2-}$ in the rat. *Int. J. Vitam. Nutr. Res.* **42**, 588–591.

Burk, R. F. (1973a). ^{75}Se-binding by rat plasma proteins after injection of ^{75}SeO$_3^{2-}$. *U.S. Army Med. Res. Nutr. Lab., Rep. 334.*

Burk, R. F. (1973b). Effect of dietary selenium level on ^{75}Se binding to rat plasma proteins. *Proc. Soc. Exp. Biol. Med.* **143**, 719–722.

Burk, R. F. (1974). *In vivo* ^{75}Se binding to human plasma proteins after administration of ^{75}SeO$_3^{2-}$. *Biochim. Biophys. Acta* **372**, 255–265.

Burk, R. F., Pearson, W. N., Wood, R. P., and Viteri, F. (1967). Blood-selenium levels and *in vitro* red blood cell uptake of ^{75}Se in kwashiorkor. *Amer. J. Clin. Nutr.* **20**, 723–733.

Burk, R. F., Whitney, R., Frank, H., and Pearson, W. N. (1968). Tissue selenium levels during the development of dietary liver necrosis in rats fed torula yeast diets. *J. Nutr.* **95**, 420–428.

Burk, R. F., Brown, D. G., Seely, R. J., and Scaief, C. C. (1972). Influence of dietary and injected selenium on whole-body retention, route of excretion, and tissue retention of ^{75}SeO$_3^{2-}$ in the rat. *J. Nutr.* **102**, 1049–1056.

Burk, R. F., Foster, K. A., Greenfield, P. M., and Kiker, K. W. (1974). Binding of simultaneously administered inorganic selenium and mercury to a rat plasma protein. *Proc. Soc. Exp. Biol. Med.* **145**, 782–785.

Cary, E. E., Allaway, W. H., and Miller, M. (1973). Utilization of different forms of dietary selenium. *J. Anim. Sci.* **36**, 285–292.

Cavalieri, R. R., and Steinberg, M. (1971). Selenite (Se^{75}) as a tumor-scanning agent. *J. Surg. Oncol.* **3**, 617–624.

Cavalieri, R. R., Scott, K. G., and Sairenji, E. (1966). Selenite (^{75}Se) as a tumor-localizing agent in man. *J. Nucl. Med.* **7**, 197–208.

Cooper, W. C. (1967). Selenium toxicity in man. *In* "Selenium in Biomedicine" (O. H. Muth, ed.), pp. 185–199. Avi Publ., Westport, Connecticut.

Cummins, L. M., and Kimura, E. T. (1971). Safety evaluation of selenium sulfide antidandruff shampoo. *Toxicol. Appl. Pharmacol.* **20**, 89–96.

Cummins, L. M., and Martin, J. L. (1967). Are selenocystine and selenomethionine synthesized *in vivo* from sodium selenite in mammals? *Biochemistry* **6**, 3162–3168.

Danks, D. M., Campbell, P. E., Walker-Smith, J., Stevens, B. J., Gillespie, J. M., Blomfield, J., and Turner, B. (1972). Menkes' kinky hair syndrome. *Lancet* **1**, 1100–1104.

Dickson, R. C., and Tomlinson, R. H. (1967). Selenium in blood and human tissues. *Clin. Chim. Acta* **16**, 311–321.

Ewan, R. C., Pope, A. L., and Baumann, C. A. (1967). Elimination of fixed selenium by the rat. *J. Nutr.* **91**, 547–554.

Ferrucci, J. T., Berke, R. A., and Potsaid, M. S. (1970). Se^{75}-selenomethionine isotope lymphography in lymphoma: Correlation with lymphangiography. *Amer. J. Roentgenol.* **109**, 793–802.

Ganther, H. E., Goudie, C., Sunde, M. L., Kopecky, M. J., Wagner, P., Oh, S. H., and Hoekstra, W. G. (1972). Selenium: Relation to decreased toxicity of methylmercury added to diets containing tuna. *Science* **175**, 1122–1124.

Giulio, W. D., and Morales, J. O. (1969). The value of the selenomethionine Se 75 scan in preoperative localization of parathyroid adenomas. *J. Amer. Med. Ass.* **209**, 1873–1880.

Glover, J. R. (1970). Selenium and its industrial toxicology. *Ind. Med. Surg.* **39**, 50–54.

Gries, C. L., and Scott, M. L. (1972). Pathology of selenium deficiency in the chick. *J. Nutr.* **102**, 1287–1296.

Griffiths, N. M. (1973). Dietary intake and urinary excretion of selenium in some New Zealand women. *Proc. Univ. Otago Med. Sch.* **51**, 8–9.

Hadjimarkos, D. M. (1965). Effect of selenium on dental caries. *Arch. Environ. Health* **10**, 893–899.

Hadjimarkos, D. M., and Shearer, T. R. (1973). Selenium content of human nails: A new index for epidemiologic studies of dental caries. *J. Dent. Res.* **52**, 389.

Hafeman, D. G., Sunde, R. A., and Hoekstra, W. G. (1974). Effect of dietary selenium on erythrocyte and liver glutathione peroxidase in the rat. *J. Nutr.* **104**, 580–587.

Halverson, A. W., and Monty, K. J. (1960). An effect of dietary sulfate on selenium poisoning in the rat. *J. Nutr.* **70**, 100–102.

Herrera, N. E., Gonzalez, R., Schwartz, R. D., Diggs, A. M., and Belsky, J. (1965). ^{75}Se methionine as a diagnostic agent in malignant lymphoma. *J. Nucl. Med.* **6**, 792–804.

Higgs, D. J., Morris, V. C., and Levander, O. A. (1972). Effect of cooking on selenium content of foods. *J. Agr. Food Chem.* **20**, 678–680.

Hirooka, T., and Galambos, J. T. (1966a). Selenium metabolism. I. Respiratory excretion. *Biochim. Biophys. Acta* **130**, 313–320.

Hirooka, T., and Galambos, J. T. (1966b). Selenium metabolism. III. Serum proteins, lipoproteins, and liver injury. *Biochim. Biophys. Acta* **130**, 321–328.

Hopkins, L. L., and Majaj, A. S. (1967). Selenium in human nutrition. *In* "Selenium in Biomedicine" (O. H. Muth, ed.), pp. 203–211. Avi Publ., Westport, Connecticut.

Hopkins, L. L., Pope, A. L., and Baumann, C. A. (1966). Distribution of microgram quantities of selenium in the tissues of the rat, and effects of previous selenium intake. *J. Nutr.* **88**, 61–65.

Jaffé, W. G., Ruphael-D., M., Mondragon, M. C., and Cuevas, M. A. (1972). Estudio clínico y bioquímico en niños escolares de una zona selenífera. *Arch. Latinoamer. Nutr.* **22**, 595-611.

Jenkins, K. J. (1968). Evidence for the absence of selenocystine and selenomethionine in the serum proteins of chicks administered selenite. *Can. J. Biochem.* **46**, 1417–1425.

Jereb, M., Jereb, B., and Unge, G. (1972). Radionuclear selenite (⁷⁵Se) for scintigraphic demonstration of lung cancer and metastases in the mediastinum. *Scand. J. Resp. Dis.* **53**, 331–337.

Kasperek, K., Shicha, H., Siller, V., and Feinendegen, L. E. (1972). Normalwerte von Spurenelementen im menschlichen Serum und Korrelation zum Lebensalter und zur Serum-Eiweiss-Konzentration. *Strahlentherapie* **143**, 468–472.

Kiker, K. W., and Burk, R. F. (1974). Production of urinary selenium metabolites in the rat following ⁷⁵SeO₃²⁻ administration. *Amer. J. Physiol.* **227**, 643–646.

Klayman, D. L. (1973). Selenium compounds as potential chemotherapeutic agents. *In* "Organic Selenium Compounds: Their Chemistry and Biology" (D. L. Klayman and W. H. H. Günther, eds.), pp. 727–761. Wiley (Interscience), New York.

Koeman, J. H., Peeters, W. H. M., Koudstaal-Hol, C. H. M., Tjioe, P. S., and deGoeij, J. J. M. (1973). Mercury-selenium correlations in marine mammals. *Nature* (*London*) **245**, 385–386.

Lathrop, K. A., Johnston, R. E., Blau, M., and Rothschild, E. O. (1972). Radiation dose to humans from ⁷⁵Se-L-selenomethionine. *J. Nucl. Med.* **13**, Suppl. 6, 7–30.

Lee, M., Dong, A., and Yano, J. (1969). Metabolism of ⁷⁵Se-selenite by human whole blood *in vitro*. *Can. J. Biochem.* **47**, 791–797.

Levander, O. A. (1972). Metabolic interrelationships and adaptations in selenium toxicity. *Ann. N.Y. Acad. Sci.* **192**, 181–192.

Levander, O. A., and Baumann, C. A. (1966). Selenium metabolism. VI. Effect of arsenic on the excretion of selenium in the bile. *Toxicol. Appl. Pharmacol.* **9**, 106–115.

Levander, O. A., and Morris, V. C. (1970). Interactions of methionine, vitamin E, and antioxidants in selenium toxicity in the rat. *J. Nutr.* **100**, 1111–1117.

Levander, O. A., Young, M. L., and Meeks, S. A. (1970). Studies on the binding of selenium by liver homogenates from rats fed diets containing either casein or casein plus linseed oil meal. *Toxicol. Appl. Pharmacol.* **16**, 79–87.

Levine, R. J., and Olson, R. E. (1970). Blood selenium in Thai children with protein-calorie malnutrition. *Proc. Soc. Exp. Biol. Med.* **134**, 1030–1034.

Lewis, H. B., Schultz, J., and Gortner, R. A. (1940). Dietary protein and the toxicity of sodium selenite in the white rat. *J. Pharmacol. Exp. Ther.* **68**, 292–299.

Ludwig, T. G., and Bibby, B. G. (1969). Geographic variations in the prevalence of dental caries in the United States of America. *Caries Res.* **3**, 32–43.

McConnell, K. P., and Cho, G. J. (1967). Active transport of selenium in the everted intestine of the hamster. *In* "Selenium in Biomedicine" (O. H. Muth, ed.), pp. 329–343. Avi Publ., Westport, Connecticut.

McCoy, K. E. M., and Weswig, P. H. (1969). Some selenium responses in the rat not related to vitamin E. *J. Nutr.* **98**, 383–389.

Millar, K. R. (1972). Distribution of ^{75}Se in liver, kidney, and blood proteins of rats after intravenous injection of sodium selenite. N.Z. J. Agr. Res. 15, 547–564.

Millar, K. R., Gardiner, M. A., and Sheppard, A. D. (1973a). A comparison of the metabolism of intravenously injected sodium selenite, sodium selenate, and selenomethionine in rats. N.Z. J. Agr. Res. 16, 115–127.

Millar, K. R., Craig, J., and Dawe, L. (1973b). α-tocopherol and selenium levels in pasteurized cows' milk from different areas of New Zealand. N.Z. J. Agr. Res. 16, 301–303.

Miller, D., Soares, J. H., Bauersfeld, P., and Cuppett, S. L. (1972). Comparative selenium retention by chicks fed sodium selenite, selenomethionine, fish meal, and fish solubles. Poultry Sci. 51, 1669–1673.

Mondragón, M. C., and Jaffé, W. G. (1971). Selenio en alimentos y en orina de escolares de diferentes zonas de Venezuela. Arch. Latinoamer. Nutr. 21, 185–195.

Money, D. F. L. (1971). Cot deaths and deficiency of vitamin E and selenium. Brit. Med. J. 4, 559.

Morris, V. C., and Levander, O. A. (1970). Selenium content of foods. J. Nutr. 100, 1383–1388.

Moxon, A. L., and Rhian, M. (1943). Selenium poisoning. Physiol. Rev. 23, 305–337.

Muth, O. H., Weswig, P. H., Whanger, P. D., and Oldfield, J. E. (1971). Effect of feeding selenium-deficient ration to the subhuman primate (Saimiri sciureus). Amer. J. Vet. Res. 32, 1603–1605.

Nelp, W. B., and Blumberg, F. (1965). A comparison of the selenate and sulfate ions in man and dog. J. Nucl. Med. 6, 822–830.

Nigam, S. N., and McConnell, W. B. (1969). Seleno amino compounds from Astragalus bisulcatus. Isolation and identification of γ-L-glutamyl-Se-methyl-seleno-L-cysteine and Se-methylseleno-L-cysteine. Biochim. Biophys. Acta 192, 185–190.

Noguchi, T., Cantor, A. H., and Scott, M. L. (1973). Mode of action of selenium and vitamin E in prevention of exudative diathesis in chicks. J. Nutr. 103, 1502–1511.

Ochoa-Solano, A., and Gitler, C. (1968). Incorporation of ^{75}Se-seleno-methionine and ^{35}S-methionine into chicken egg white proteins. J. Nutr. 94, 243–248.

Oh, S. H., Ganther, H. E., and Hoekstra, W. G. (1974). Selenium as a component of glutathione peroxidase isolated from ovine erythrocytes. Biochemistry 13, 1825–1829.

Oldendorf, W. H., Sisson, W. B., and Silverstein, A. (1971). Brain uptake of seleno-methionine Se 75. II. Reduced brain uptake in phenylketonuria. Arch. Neurol. (Chicago) 24, 524–528.

Olson, O. E., Novacek, E. J., Whitehead, E. I., and Palmer, I. S. (1970). Investigations on selenium in wheat. Phytochemistry 9, 1181–1188.

Orentreich, N., Taylor, E. H., Berger, R. A., and Auerbach, R. (1969). Comparative study of two antidandruff preparations. J. Pharm. Sci. 58, 1279–1280.

Palmer, I. S., Fischer, D. D., Halverson, A. W., and Olson, O. E. (1969). Identification of a major selenium excretory product in rat urine. Biochim. Biophys. Acta 177, 336–342.

Palmer, I. S., Gunsalus, R. P., Halverson, A. W., and Olson, O. E. (1970). Trimethylselenonium ion as a general excretory product from selenium metabolism in the rat. Biochim. Biophys. Acta 208, 260–266.

Penner, J. A. (1966). Investigation of erythrocyte turnover with selenium-75-labeled methionine. J. Lab. Clin. Med. 67, 427–438.

Ransone, J. W., Scott, N. M., and Knoblock, E. C. (1961). Selenium sulfide intoxication. N. Engl. J. Med. 264, 384–385.

Rhead, W. J., Schrauzer, G. N., Saltzstein, S. L., Cary, E. E., and Allaway, W. H. (1972). Vitamin E, selenium, and the sudden infant death syndrome. *J. Pediat.* 81, 415–416.

Robertson, D. S. F. (1970). Selenium—a possible teratogen? *Lancet* 1, 518–519.

Rosenfeld, I., and Beath, O. A. (1964). "Selenium: Geobotany, Biochemistry, Toxicity and Nutrition." Academic Press, New York.

Rotruck, J. T., Pope, A. L., Ganther, H. E., Swanson, A. B., Hafeman, D. G., and Hoekstra, W. G. (1973). Selenium: Biochemical role as a component of glutathione peroxidase. *Science* 179, 588–590.

Said, A. K., and Hegsted, D. M. (1970). ^{75}Se-selenomethionine in the study of protein and amino acid metabolism of adult rats. *Proc. Soc. Exp. Biol. Med.* 133, 1388–1391.

Schroeder, H. A., Frost, D. V., and Balassa, J. J. (1970). Essential trace metals in man: Selenium. *J. Chronic Dis.* 23, 227–243.

Schwarz, K. (1961). Development and status of experimental work on Factor 3-selenium. *Fed. Proc., Fed. Amer. Soc. Exp. Biol.* 20, 666–673.

Schwarz, K., and Foltz, C. M. (1957). Selenium as an integral part of factor 3 against dietary necrotic liver degeneration. *J. Amer. Chem. Soc.* 79, 3292–3293.

Schwarz, K., and Foltz, C. M. (1958). Factor 3 activity of selenium compounds. *J. Biol. Chem.* 233, 245–251.

Schwarz, K., Porter, L. A., and Fredga, A. (1972). Some regularities in the structure-function relationship of organoselenium compounds effective against dietary liver necrosis. *Ann. N.Y. Acad. Sci.* 192, 200–214.

Scott, M. L. (1973). Nutritional importance of selenium. In "Organic Selenium Compounds: Their Chemistry and Biology" (D. L. Klayman and W. H. H. Günther, eds.), pp. 629–661. Wiley (Interscience), New York.

Scott, M. L., and Thompson, J. N. (1971). Selenium content of feedstuffs and effects of dietary selenium levels upon tissue selenium in chicks and poults. *Poultry Sci.* 50, 1742–1748.

Shamberger, R. J., and Willis, C. E. (1971). Selenium distribution and human cancer mortality. *CRC Crit. Rev. Clin. Lab. Sci.* 2, 211–221.

Shamberger, R. J., Rukovena, E., Longfield, A. K., Tytko, S. A., Deodhar, S., and Willis, C. E. (1973). Antioxidants and cancer. I. selenium in the blood of normals and cancer patients. *J. Nat. Cancer Inst.* 50, 863–870.

Shapiro, J. R. (1972). Selenium and carcinogenesis: A review. *Ann. N.Y. Acad. Sci.* 192, 215–219.

Shapiro, J. R. (1973). Selenium and human biology. In "Organic Selenium Compounds: Their Chemistry and Biology" (D. L. Klayman and W. H. H. Günther, eds.), pp. 693–726. Wiley (Interscience), New York.

Shrift, A. (1969). Aspects of selenium metabolism in higher plants. *Annu. Rev. Plant Phys.* 20, 475–494.

Shull, L. R., and Cheeke, P. R. (1973). Antiselenium activity of tri-o-cresyl phosphate in rats and Japanese quail. *J. Nutr.* 103, 560–568.

Smith, M. I., and Westfall, B. B. (1937). Further field studies on the selenium problem in relation to public health. *Pub. Health Rep.* 52, 1375–1384.

Smith, M. I., Franke, K. W., and Westfall, B. B. (1936). The selenium problem in relation to public health. A preliminary survey to determine the possibility of selenium intoxication in the rural population living on seleniferous soil. *Pub. Health Rep.* 51, 1496–1505.

Sprinker, L. H., Harr, J. R., Newberne, P. M., Whanger, P. D., and Weswig,

P. H. (1971). Selenium deficiency lesions in rats fed vitamin E supplemented rations. *Nutr. Rep. Int.* 4, 335–340.

Steinberg, M. H., and Necheles, T. F. (1971). Erythrocyte glutathione peroxidase deficiency. *Amer. J. Med.* 50, 542–546.

Swanson, A. B., Wagner, P. A., Ganther, H. E., and Hoekstra, W. G. (1974). Antagonistic effects of silver and tri-o-cresyl phosphate on selenium and glutathione peroxidase in rat liver and erythrocytes. *Fed. Proc., Fed. Amer. Soc. Exp. Biol.* 33, 693 (abstr.).

Thiemann, G., Holldorf, M., and Schwartz, K. D. (1971). Ergebnisse der Se^{75}-selenit-tumorszintigraphie. *Radiobiol. Radiother.* 12, 109–116.

Thompson, J. N., and Scott, M. L. (1970). Impaired lipid and vitamin E absorption related to atrophy of the pancreas in selenium-deficient chicks. *J. Nutr.* 100, 797–809.

Thompson, J. N., Erbody, P., and Smith, D. C. (1975). Selenium content of food consumed by Canadians. *J. Nutr.* 105, 274–277.

Thomson, C. D. (1972). Urinary excretion of selenium in some New Zealand women. *Proc. Univ. Otago Med. Sch.* 50, 31–33.

Thomson, C. D. (1974). Recovery of large doses of selenium given as sodium selenite with or without vitamin E. *N.Z. Med. J.* 80, 163–168.

Thomson, C. D., and Stewart, R. D. H. (1972). Measurement of intestinal absorption of selenium. *Proc. Univ. Otago Med. Sch.* 50, 63–64.

Thomson, C. D., and Stewart, R. D. H. (1973). Metabolic studies of [^{75}Se] selenomethionine and [^{75}Se] selenite in the rat. *Brit. J. Nutr.* 30, 139–147.

Turner, D. C., and Stadtman, T. C. (1973). Purification of protein components of the clostridial glycine reductase system and characterization of protein A as a selenoprotein. *Arch. Biochem. Biophys.* 154, 366–381.

Vernie, L. N., Bont, W. S., and Emmelot, P. (1974). Inhibition of *in vitro* amino acid incorporation by sodium selenite. *Biochemistry* 13, 337–341.

Waterlow, J. C., Garrow, J. S., and Millward, D. J. (1969). The turnover of [^{75}Se] selenomethionine in infants and rats measured in a whole body counter. *Clin. Sci.* 36, 489–504.

Watkinson, J. H. (1974). The selenium status of New Zealanders. *N.Z. Med. J.* 80, 202–205.

Wenzel, M., Otto, R., and Riehle, I. (1971). Der Einbau von ^{75}Se nach Applikation von radioaktivem Natriumselenit in Normalgewebe und in Tumoren *in vitro* und *in vivo*. *Int. J. Appl. Radiat. Isotop.* 22, 361–369.

Whanger, P. D., Pedersen, N. D., and Weswig, P. H. (1973). Selenium proteins in ovine tissue. II. spectral properties of a 10,000 molecular weight selenium protein. *Biochem. Biophys. Res. Commun.* 53, 1031–1035.

Wright, P. L., and Bell, M. C. (1963). Selenium and vitamin E influence upon the *in vitro* uptake of Se^{75} by ovine blood cells. *Proc. Soc. Exp. Biol. Med.* 114, 379–382.

Wright, P. L., and Bell, M. C. (1966). Comparative metabolism of selenium and tellurium in sheep and swine. *Amer. J. Physiol.* 211, 6–10.

31

Selected Aspects of the Comparative Metabolism and Biochemistry of Selenium and Sulfur

Orville A. Levander

I. INTRODUCTION

When one considers the chemical and physical characteristics of selenium and sulfur, the similarities in the properties of these two elements are readily observed (Table I). For example, selenium and sulfur have similar electronic configurations in their outermost valence shells, although the completely filled $3d$ shell of the former should not be ignored. Also, the sizes of the atoms of these two elements are very much the same, no matter whether they are in the covalent or the ionic state. The bond energies, ionization potentials, and electron affinities of selenium and sulfur are quite similar, and the electronegativities and polarizabilities are essentially identical.

But our experience with living systems tells us that these two elements, which appear to have so much in common chemically and physically, can not substitute for one another *in vivo*. Then what chemical or physical difference accounts for this lack of biologic interchangeability? One

TABLE I   Selected Chemical and Physical Properties of the Group VIA Elements

Property	O	S	Se	Te
Electron configuration	$2s^2 2p^4$	$3s^2 3p^4$	$4s^2 3d^{10} 4p^4$	$5s^2 4d^{10} 5p^4$
Covalent radius (Å)	0.66	1.04	1.17	1.37
Ionic radius (M^{2-}) (Å)	1.45	1.90	2.02	2.22
Ionic radius (M^{6+} in $MO_4{}^{2-}$) (Å)	—	0.34	0.40	—
Bond energy (M-M) (kcal/mole)	33	63	44	33
Bond energy (M-H) (kcal/mole)	111	88	67	57
Ionization potential (eV)	13.61	10.36	9.75	9.01
Electron affinity (eV)	−7.28	−3.44	−4.21	—
Electronegativity (Pauling)	3.5	2.5	2.4	2.1
Polarizability (M^{-2})(cm^3 × 10^{-25})	39	102	105	140
pK_a				
MO(OH)$_2$, aqueous	—	1.9	2.6	2.7
MO$_2$(OH)$_2$, aqueous	—	−3	−3	—
(H$_2$M), aqueous	16	7.0	3.8	2.6
(HM$^-$), aqueous	—	12.9	11.0	11.0

clue can perhaps be obtained from the following equation:

$$H_2SeO_3 + 2H_2SO_3 \rightarrow Se + 2H_2SO_4 + H_2O \qquad (1)$$

which states that the quadrivalent selenium in selenite tends to undergo reduction, whereas the quadrivalent sulfur in sulfite tends to undergo oxidation (Rosenfeld and Beath, 1964). This chemical difference in the ease of reduction of selenite versus the ease of oxidation of sulfite is reflected in the metabolic fate of these two oxyanions as well, since in mammals selenium compounds generally tend to be reduced while sulfur compounds generally tend to be oxidized. The implications of this metabolic divergence will be discussed in Section II.

Another chemical distinction between selenium and sulfur can be seen in the relative strengths of the acids H$_2$Se and H$_2$S. Although the analogous oxyacids of selenium and sulfur are of similar strength (Table I), H$_2$Se is a much stronger acid than H$_2$S. This difference in the acidic strengths of the hydrides of selenium and sulfur is also seen in the difference in the dissociation behavior of the selenohydryl group of selenocysteine compared to that of the sulfhydryl group of cysteine. The pK of the former is 5.24, whereas the pK of the latter is 8.25 (Huber and Criddle, 1967a). The biological significance of this is the fact that at physiological pH, the sulfhydryl group in cysteine (or other thiols) exists mainly in the protonated form, while the selenohydryl group in selenocysteine (or other selenols) exists largely in the dissociated form. The implications of this chemical difference will be discussed in Section III.

Although there are several superficial similarities in the metabolism of selenium and sulfur, it is the opinion of this reviewer that the physiological role of selenium will be fully understood only when the chemical differences between these two elements are taken into account. Therefore, the purpose of this review will be to focus on some metabolic and chemical peculiarities of selenium that promise to increase our knowledge about the biological importance of this element. No special attempt will be made to discuss selenium in relation to man, the interactions of selenium with other trace elements, or the role of selenium in glutathione peroxidase, since these aspects are thoroughly covered elsewhere in this volume.

II. COMPARATIVE METABOLISM OF SELENIUM AND SULFUR

A. Microorganisms

Microbial systems offer several opportunities to study the comparative metabolism of selenium and sulfur under a wide variety of conditions. Although there are certain similarities in the metabolism of selenium and sulfur by microorganisms, the research discussed below calls attention to the metabolic individuality of these two elements.

1. Competitive Transport Phenomena

The competitive transport phenomena seen with certain selenium and sulfur analogs in microorganisms provide some of the best examples of the apparent inability of biological systems to differentiate between similar compounds of these two elements. The uptake of sulfate by *Penicillium chrysogenum* was blocked by selenate, and this inhibition was felt to be mediated through the sulfate permease (Yamamoto and Segal, 1966). Such competition for transport is not limited to inorganic compounds of selenium and sulfur. Shrift (1954a,b) showed that not only did sulfate interfere with selenate uptake by *Chlorella vulgaris*, but that methionine also inhibited the uptake of selenomethionine. Metabolic antagonisms of this kind are relatively easy to comprehend because of the strong chemical similarities of the two interacting species.

In some situations, however, the basis for the antagonism between sulfur and selenium is not quite so obvious. For example, selenate toxicity in yeast could be decreased by methionine as well as by sulfate (Fels and Cheldelin, 1949b, 1950). This relief of selenate toxicity by methionine is understandable when one realizes that the toxicity was due to a competitive inhibition between sulfate and selenate, which resulted in a blockade of methionine biosynthesis. On the other hand, selenate toxicity in *Escherichia coli* was not affected by methionine, although cysteine and glutathione were able to reverse such toxicity (Fels and Cheldelin, 1949a). In this case, the sulfhydryl compounds may have aided in the formation of nontoxic elemental selenium. Finally, Bonhorst (1955) has found that the inhibition of yeast respiration by selenite can be diminished by several nonsulfur anions such as phosphate, arsenate, or arsenite, which seem to have little chemical resemblance to selenite. The biochemical basis for these antagonisms is very poorly understood.

2. Reductive *versus* Oxidative Pathways

The reductive and oxidative pathways of selenium metabolism seen in microorganisms illustrate very well the principle that selenium tends to be reduced rather than oxidized in living systems. There are several examples of selenium reduction in the literature but few, if any, well-documented cases of selenium oxidation. Woolfolk and Whiteley (1962) showed that *Micrococcus lactilyticus* could use molecular hydrogen to reduce selenite, but not selenate, to selenide. *Salmonella heidelberg* reduces selenite to the insoluble elemental selenium, and this may be the basis for the tolerance of *Salmonella* spp. to selenite (McCready *et al.*, 1966). Cell-free preparations of yeast also are able to reduce selenite to elemental selenium, but this process appears to require a flavin moiety for adequate electron flow (Nickerson and Falcone, 1963). A similar flavin requirement for optimal reduction of selenite to elemental selenium was reported for cell-free extracts of *Streptococcus faecalis* or *S. faccium* (Tilton *et al.*, 1967). In some instances, adaptation of microorganisms to selenium toxicity may be due to an increased level of "selenoreductase" in the selenium-tolerant strains (Letunova, 1970).

Although, as shown above, there are numerous situations in which microbial systems can readily bring about the reduction of selenium compounds, such is not the case for the oxidation of selenium (see, e.g., the comments of Shrift, 1973).

3. Amino Acid Metabolism

a. Biosynthesis of Selenomethionine and Selenocystine. Several workers have shown that microorganisms can biosynthesize selenomethionine from inorganic selenium salts, and this point appears to be well established (Tuve and Williams, 1961; Huber *et al.*, 1967; Blau, 1961). However, Paulson *et al.* (1968) investigated the incorporation of inorganic selenium into the protein of mixed rumen bacteria cultures and found that dialysis of the trichloroacetic acid-insoluble fraction of rumen fluid against glutathione removed most of the selenium. Since the selenium in this fraction was released by thiols, it was concluded that very little or none of the selenium was present as selenomethionine. These results suggest that non-amino acid forms of selenium may exist in proteins (see Section II,C,3c).

Although some workers have claimed to have found selenocystine in microbial proteins (see, for example, Weiss *et al.*, 1965), reports such as these have to be regarded with caution because of the extreme chemical instability of this selenoamino acid (see Section II,C,3c).

b. Substitution of Methionine by Selenomethionine. There seems to be little question but that selenomethionine can effectively replace methionine in a number of biochemical processes. For example, a yeast methionine-activating enzyme could convert selenomethionine to Se-adenosylselenomethionine, which then was a functional methyl donor for the enzymatic formation of creatine from guanidoacetic acid (Mudd and Cantoni, 1957). Wu and Wachsman (1971) found that selenomethionine was as efficient a methyl donor as methionine for nucleic acid methylation in both *Bacillus megaterium* and *E. coli*.

In addition to substituting for methionine in transmethylation reactions, selenomethionine also can substitute for methionine in all of the known reactions of methionine during polypeptide chain initiation and synthesis in *E. coli* (McConnell and Hoffman, 1972a; Hoffman *et al.*, 1970). But there appears to be significant disagreement concerning the ultimate metabolic consequences of selenomethionine substituting for methionine in microbial protein. Selenomethionine could completely replace methionine for the normal exponential growth of a methionine-requiring mutant of *E. coli* (Cowie and Cohen, 1957), whereas selenomethionine only partially satisfied the methionine requirement of methionineless strains of *E. coli* WWU or *B. megaterium* KM (Wu and Wachsman, 1970). β-Galactosidase isolated from strains of *E. coli* that were relatively resistant to selenium toxicity had up to 75% of its methionine residues replaced by selenomethionine with little or no effect on the catalytic activity of the enzyme, although increased instability of the enzyme to heat and urea was noted (Coch and Greene, 1971; Huber and Criddle, 1967b).

4. Dimethyl Selenide

The formation of the volatile dimethyl selenide by certain molds from inorganic selenium salts (see Challenger, 1955, for a general review) provides an important example of the metabolic nonequivalence of selenium and sulfur. Challenger and North (1934) showed that *Scopulariopsis brevicaulis* could convert selenite or selenate to dimethyl selenide, but attempts to produce dimethyl sulfide from sulfite, thiosulfate, thiourea, elemental sulfur, or thiodiglycolic acid were all negative. However, dimethyl sulfide could be produced when dimethyl sulfoxide, but not the sulfone, was added to cultures of the mold. A species difference was noted, since *Schizophyllum commune* was able to convert inorganic sulfate to a variety of volatile sulfur compounds, including hydrogen sulfide, methyl mercaptan, dimethyl sulfide, and dimethyl disulfide (Challenger and Charlton, 1947). In addition to synthesizing dimethyl selenide from inorganic selenium salts, *S. brevicaulis* could produce trimethylarsine and dimethyl telluride from inorganic arsenic and tellurium salts, respectively. Challenger postulated a mechanism which consisted of alternate methylation and reduction steps to account for the biosynthesis of dimethyl selenide from selenite:

$$H_2SeO_3 \rightarrow HSeO_3^- \xrightarrow{CH_3^+} CH_3SeO_3H \xrightarrow{reduction}$$
$$CH_3SeO_2^- \xrightarrow{CH_3^+} (CH_3)_2SeO_2 \xrightarrow{reduction} (CH_3)_2Se \quad (2)$$

The plausibility of this mechanism is discussed in Section II,C,4.

5. Specific Roles in Enzymes

The existence of specific roles for selenium in certain microbial enzyme systems represents one of the most compelling arguments against the metabolic equivalence of selenium and sulfur.

a. Formate Dehydrogenase. Perhaps the first report of a "nutritional" effect of selenium was the demonstration by Pinsent (1954) that, in a purified culture medium, traces of selenite were needed for the production of formate dehydrogenase in *E. coli*. The presence of iron and molybdate was also shown to be required for the activity of this enzyme. Pinsent's results were confirmed many years later by Fukuyama and Ordal (1965), and more recently, Lester and DeMoss (1971) showed that protein biosynthesis apparently is essential to demonstrate the response to selenium. Selenite and selenocystine were about equal in stimulating the synthesis of formate dehydrogenase, but selenomethionine was much less active (Enoch and Lester, 1972). These workers suggested that the selenium might be present in the enzyme as nonheme iron selenide (see Section III,A). The relative differences in the potencies of different forms of selenium in inducing formate dehydrogenase have been substantiated by Shum and Murphy (1972), who also found a coincidence of ^{75}Se incorporation and formate dehydrogenase activity after sucrose gradient centrifugation of a partially purified enzyme preparation. Although all of the studies discussed above were carried out with *E. coli*, Andressen and Ljungdahl (1973) noted similar effects of selenite and molybdate on the activity of the formate dehydrogenase of *Clostridium thermoaceticum*.

b. *Glycine Reductase.* One of the most fascinating unexpected twists in the field of selenium research was the recent finding by Turner and Stadtman (1973) that their "protein A" of the clostridial glycine reductase system is a selenoprotein. These workers noted that the yield of protein A was strongly influenced by the age of the cells at the time of harvest. Cells harvested from relatively young cultures were good sources of protein A, whereas cells from old cultures were poor sources of this protein. Others had shown that only very young cultures of *Clostridium thermoaceticum* contain detectable levels of formate dehydrogenase under the usual growth conditions, but that the microbe continues to synthesize this enzyme throughout the entire log phase of growth when selenite and molybdate are added to the culture medium. This observation suggested that inorganic micronutrients might be important in glycine reductase, and when selenite was added to the medium used for culture of *C. sticklandii*, there was a marked stimulatory effect on the activity of the enzyme. Little or no effect of the addition of molybdate was observed, which suggested either that there was already an ample supply of this nutrient in the growth medium or that molybdate was not required for the synthesis of this enzyme. A direct quotation of a paragraph from this paper could be instructive:

> It, perhaps, is of some general interest that in the 1950's, when the water supply in the Bethesda area was of quality that permitted the use of tap water for the large-scale culture of anaerobic bacteria, the glycine reductase activity of *C. sticklandii* was generally higher. In retrospect, this was probably related to the fact that selenium was supplied in the tap water. In the 1960's when fastidious organisms such as *Methanococcus vannielii* could no longer be cultured in the Bethesda tap water (or even in deionized Bethesda tap water), we began to use distilled water for media for other anaerobic bacteria as well. Although even the more complex media were frequently supplemented with iron, cobalt, magnesium, and manganese, *it was not suspected that rich tryptone-yeast extract media such as those used for C. sticklandii would be deficient in nutrients required only in trace amounts* [italics added for emphasis].

Nutritionists perhaps do not have to address themselves to the commentary regarding the quality of our domestic water supply, but the implications for nutrition of the italicized lines of the above should be clear.

As with formate dehydrogenase, the precise chemical nature of the selenium at the active site of protein A is not known, but the selenium-containing moiety may be an aromatic substance or heterocyclic compound that yields a selenol group after borohydride reduction (Stadtman, 1974a,b). The specific nature of the incorporation of selenium into protein A was emphasized by Stadtman when she pointed out that ferredoxin, a protein that contains substantial amounts of sulfur, contained only slight amounts of selenium.

B. Plants

The comparative metabolism of selenium and sulfur in plants has recently been extensively discussed by Shrift (1973), and since many of the comments that could be made are analogous to those already brought out in the previous section on microorganisms, no detailed discussion about plant metabolism will be offered here. It should be pointed out, however, that one of the most important findings that helps to establish the metabolic nonequivalence of selenium and sulfur in microorganisms and animals—a specific role for selenium in an enzyme system—has yet to be discovered in plants.

C. Animals

1. Competitive Transport Phenomena

Few studies have been carried out on the transport of selenium compounds in mammalian systems. McConnell and Cho (1965) showed that selenomethionine was actively transported by everted hamster intestinal sacs, but selenite and selenocystine were not. This transport of selenomethionine was blocked by methionine, although sulfite and cystine did not inhibit the transport of selenite or selenocystine, respectively. Perhaps the ability of high protein diets to decrease selenium toxicity might be related to such a methionine/selenomethionine transport antagonism at the intestinal level (McConnell and Cho, 1967). But a similar mechanism apparently does not operate in the protection of sulfate against selenate toxicity, since sulfate causes an increased urinary excretion rather than a decreased intestinal absorbtion of selenium (Ganther and Baumann, 1962b). The work of McConnell and associates, however, does show that selenium analogs of sulfur compounds can compete effectively for sulfur transport mechanisms in animal as well as in microbial and plant systems.

2. Reductive *versus* Oxidative Pathways

Diplock and associates have contributed an important series of papers that bear directly on the problem of reductive versus oxidative pathways of selenium metabolism (Diplock *et al.*, 1971, 1973; Caygill *et al.*, 1971). In these studies, radioselenite was administered, usually orally, to rats under different nutritional conditions. Liver subcellular organelle fractions were prepared, and the oxidation state of the radioselenium present was characterized by the following criteria: acid-volatile selenium, assumed to be selenide; $Zn + HCl$-reducible selenium, assumed to be selenite; and residual nonvolatile selenium, called selenate for convenience. (This latter choice of nomenclature was somewhat unfortunate, since it could leave the reader with the impression that selenate had indeed been formed *in vivo* from selenite. Since this process is highly unlikely thermodynamically, the nonvolatile fraction of selenium more likely represents organic selenium derivatives that were not readily cleaved by the $Zn + HCl$ treatment. Rhead *et al.* (1974) have recently reported that selenate, as well as selenite, is reduced to H_2Se by treatment with zinc and HCl). Diplock and co-workers found that 36 and 43% of the radioselenium present in the liver mitochondria and microsomes, respectively, was in the form of selenide. The proportion of selenide present was dependent upon the vitamin E status of the animals, since mitochondria and microsomes isolated from vitamin E-deficient rats contained only 26 and 30% of the selenium, respectively, as selenide. Omission of antioxidants from the homogenization medium (mercaptoethanol and α-tocopherol) led to a further decrease in the percentage of selenide present, since under these conditions mitochondria and microsomes from vitamin E-deficient rats contained only 11 and 17% selenide, respectively. These results were interpreted by the authors to be consistent with their hypothesis that the biologically active form of selenium may be selenide in a nonheme iron protein (see Section III,A for additional discussion of this hypothesis). However, these workers were fully cognizant of the fact that "investigations on sulphur metabolism, which may be similar to the metabolism of selenium, indicate that the reduction of sulphite to sulphide does not occur in animal tissues, and indeed reduced sulphur is generally acquired in the form of the thiol groups of amino acids, and their subsequent metabolic fate is oxidative." Diplock felt that it was ". . . necessary to suppose, therefore, that a specific, unique mechanism exists in animal tissues for the reduction of selenite, administered orally, to the selenide that we have detected in liver subcellular fractions." Thus, we have here again a distinct difference in the manner by which selenium and sulfur are metabolized.

Diplock and his group then went on to carry out experiments that essentially ruled out the possibility that the intestinal microorganisms were responsible for the reduction of selenite to selenide. Additional work with different trapping agents for the volatile selenium liberated from tissues by acid treatment established that this material was not dimethyl selenide and most probably was hydrogen selenide. The possibility that the selenide found in rat liver subcellular organelles might be an artifact formed *in vitro* as a decomposition product of selenotrisulfide generated by reaction between selenite and the mercaptoethanol added to the homogenization medium seemed to be eliminated by studies that showed that a similar proportion of the selenium was found to be present in the selenide form regardless of whether or not the thiol was added to the solution used for homogenization (Diplock *et al.*, 1973). It appears, however, that the rat livers were first chilled in a medium that contained mercaptoethanol even if subsequent homogenization was carried out in a medium devoid of the thiol. The possibility, therefore, still exists that some thiol diffused into the liver during the cooling process, which means that artifactual production of selenide cannot be completely discounted.

3. Amino Acid Metabolism

a. Biosynthesis. Although early investigations concerned with the nature of selenium in the tissues of animals poisoned with the element established that most of the selenium was associated with protein, the precise form of selenium in proteins was not determined by these experiments (Smith *et al.*, 1938). Later, McConnell and co-workers used a combination of radioactive tracer and chromatographic techniques in an attempt to characterize the selenium present in tissue proteins (McConnell and Wabnitz, 1957). These workers found radioactive selenium spots on paper chromatograms in those areas that would correspond to cystine or selenocystine and methionine or selenomethionine. The method employed by McConnell to prepare tissue protein hydrolyzates, however, is now known to destroy both selenocystine (Huber and Criddle, 1967a) and selenomethionine (Shepherd and Huber, 1969). More recently, a possible explanation of the results of McConnell has been provided by Schwarz and Sweeney (1964), who found that selenite could bind to a variety of sulfur compounds *in vitro* to give adducts with chromatographic properties similar to the parent sulfur compound. Thus, the use of chromatographic criteria as the sole means of characterizing selenium compounds was challenged. Cummins and Martin (1967) designed a study specifically to answer the question "Are selenocystine and selenomethionine synthesized *in vivo* from sodium selenite in mammals?" These workers fed quite high levels of selenium as radioselenite to a rabbit for a period of 35 days. One day before sacrifice, the animal in addition received orally and by injection rather large doses of radioactivity as selenite. A postnuclear supernate was prepared from the liver and dialyzed at pH 11 for a period of 2 weeks. The hepatic protein purified in this relatively harsh manner was then subjected to a mild enzymatic hydrolysis. Ion exchange chromatography of the hydrolyzate revealed that there was no radioactivity in those fractions that would correspond to the elution volumes of the selenium amino acids. Ion exchange chromatography also was used to characterize the urinary selenium metabolites of a rabbit that had been injected 24 hr previously with radioselenite. Although the presence of selenocystine and selenomethionine could have been inferred by the appearance of two radioselenium peaks that eluted at the appropriate volumes, similar radioactive peaks could be obtained merely by adding radioselenite either to a normal urine sample *in vitro* or to a chemically defined mixture of sulfur compounds. The results of this study once again underscored the danger in relying exclusively on chromatographic criteria for the identification of selenium compounds. The final conclusion from this work was that at least in the rabbit there was no biosynthetic pathway by which selenium as selenite could replace sulfur in cystine or methionine.

In a related study, Godwin and Fuss (1972) claimed to have found that a very small proportion (0.5%) of a dose of radioselenite given orally to rabbits was apparently converted to selenocystine. These authors commented on the fact that it was not possible to say whether this conversion was of physiological significance. Also, the rather large dose of selenium used in this study (0.5 mg) plus the rather short time period of the experiment (2 days) raises serious questions regarding the relevance of the results to the metabolism of physiological levels of selenium. One might reasonably expect to find various selenide derivatives in the tissues of animals shortly after they had been given relatively large doses of selenite just as a result of the nonspecific reaction of selenite with sulfhydryl groups (see Section II,C,3c). Millar (1972) found that there was a transient appearance of radioselenium in several liver proteins of rats that had been dosed with even submicrogram quantities of the element, but that after 2 weeks the radioactivity was limited to only one or two different proteins.

b. Substitution. A close relationship between the metabolism of selenomethionine and methionine has been shown in a variety of mammalian systems. For example, selenomethionine could inhibit the transport of methionine by hamster intestine and vice versa (already discussed in Section II,C,1). Also, selenomethionine is incorporated into polypeptides via the methionine pathway in an *in vitro* rat liver protein-synthesizing system (McConnell and Hoffman, 1972b). Moreover, McConnell *et al.* (1974) have found that there are certain parallels in the metabolism of selenium and sulfur amino acids in the skin of zinc-deficient rats.

Because of this apparent metabolic similarity between selenomethionine and methionine, Yousef and Johnson (1970) felt that the total body turnover rate of radioselenomethionine might be a convenient index for protein metabolism during growth and aging in rats. Said and Hegsted (1970), however, found that this technique was of no value in assessing overall changes in protein metabolism in animals fed different amounts of protein or methionine, since changes in body radioactivity were not affected by changes in these dietary variables but rather were greatly affected by the selenium content of the diet. Additional evidence for the metabolic nonequivalence of selenomethionine and methionine derives from the work of Millar and Sheppard (1973), who injected rats with a mixture of [^{75}Se]selenomethionine and [^{35}S]methionine and found that the distribution of ^{75}Se and ^{35}S in the proteins of liver and kidney supernatant fractions after gel filtration was quite different, particularly in proteins of intermediate molecular weight. Moreover, a comparison of the metabolism of intravenously injected sodium selenite, sodium selenate, and selenomethionine in rats revealed such a similarity in the ^{75}Se distribution patterns, that Millar *et al.* (1973) concluded that "some breakdown of the selenomethionine occurs and that selenium is released in a form which is metabolized in a manner indistinguishable from that of selenite or selenate."

Thus, the hypothesis that selenomethionine necessarily follows the same course as methionine in protein metabolism appears to be false, and the old caveat of Schwarz (1961a) still holds: "While it is likely that selenium when given in large amounts may travel with sulfur in its metabolic channels, available evidence suggests that it follows pathways of its own when supplied at small physiological levels." The comments regarding the metabolic differences between methionine and selenomethionine also apply for cystine versus selenocystine, only more so, since, as pointed out by Huber and Criddle (1967a), the chemical differences between the latter two amino acids are so great that substitution of one by the other would cause vast alterations in the properties of any proteins containing them.

   c. Form of Selenium in Tissue Proteins. If one then makes the assumptions that (a) the endogenous biosynthesis of selenomethionine or selenocystine from selenite or other inorganic forms of selenium by monogastric mammalians is only a minor or nonexistent pathway of selenium metabolism and (b) the metabolism of exogenously supplied selenomethionine obtained in the diet as from wheat (Olson *et al.*, 1970) consists largely of catabolism to the selenite, what possibilities exist for the form of selenium in tissue proteins? One possibility arises from the reaction first postulated by Painter (1941):

$$4RSH + H_2SeO_3 \rightarrow RSSeSR + RSSR + 3H_2O \qquad (3)$$

Several compounds of the RSSeSR family (selenotrisulfides) have been characterized by Ganther (1968) after reacting selenious acid nonenzymatically with cysteine, 2-mercaptoethanol, or coenzyme A. Under physiological conditions of pH and reactant concentrations, the selenotrisulfide derivative of glutathione (GSSeSG) reacted further to form the glutathione selenopersulfide (Ganther, 1971):

$$GSSeSG + GSH \rightarrow GSSeH + GSSG \qquad (4)$$

Such selenopersulfides may play a role in the biological function of selenium (see Section III,B). Selenotrisulfide derivatives of sulfhydryl proteins can also be prepared, since reduced pancreatic ribonuclease can be cross-linked with selenite *in vitro* to form an intramolecular R—S—Se—S—R linkage in place of a disulfide bridge (Ganther and Corcoran, 1969). Circumstantial evidence for the *in vivo* incorporation of selenium into proteins by selenotrisulfide formation was furnished by Jenkins and Hidiroglou (1971), who found a good correlation between the cysteine content of several proteins and their ability to take up selenium.

Although selenotrisulfide formation provides a reasonable rationale for the initial binding of selenite by tissue proteins, the nature of the binding changes with time in a way that is not understood (Jenkins, 1968; Millar, 1972). Thus, over 70% of the radioactivity from serum proteins taken from chicks 4 hr after dosing with radioselenite could be released by reduction with thiols, sulfitolysis, or treatment with alkali. Much less ^{75}Se was removed, however, by reduction or sulfitolysis 4 days after radioselenite administration, whereas the alkali treatment remained equally effective. Since the average half-life of chick serum proteins is too long to allow for this relatively rapid change in the susceptibility of protein-bound selenium to release, the formation of seleno amino acids was not considered a plausible explanation for this phenomenon. Rather, an influence of the amino acid residues adjacent to the selenium binding site on the strength of binding of the selenium was thought to be a more likely reason. Thus, the selenium in the more labile binding sites would be lost quickly at first, and then a greater proportion of the more resistant complexes would remain.

Another possibility concerning the nature of selenium in tissue proteins is that the selenium may exist in a unique and hitherto unsuspected form. Recent work with glutathione peroxidase, for example, has suggested that the selenium at the active site may be present as a seleninic or selenenic acid derivative (Ganther et al., 1974). Such a concept, of course, is in agreement with the leitmotiv of this review, namely that the metabolism of physiologically relevant amounts of selenium is unrelated to the metabolism of sulfur.

4. Methylated Metabolites

a. Volatile Compounds. Hofmeister (1894) first suggested that animals given inorganic selenium salts can produce volatile methylated selenium compounds that are eliminated via the lungs. Generally, the formation of such volatile metabolites assumes importance only when the animals are challenged with subacute doses of the element (Olson et al., 1963). McConnell and Portman (1952a) characterized the volatile selenium as dimethyl selenide, but more recent work using gas chromatographic techniques suggests that some dimethyl diselenide may also be formed (Vlasáková et al., 1972). This methylation of selenium is usually regarded as a highly effective mechanism for detoxifying the element, since dimethyl selenide is about five hundred times less toxic than selenite (McConnell and Portman, 1952b). However, the generally presumed innocuousness of dimethyl selenide may have to be reconsidered because of its pronounced synergistic toxicity with mercury (Pařízek et al., 1971) and arsenic (Obermeyer et al., 1971). The amount of volatile selenium produced depends upon the form of selenium given (McConnell and Roth, 1966) and can be increased by certain dietary variables, such as supplemental methionine, high protein level, previous exposure to selenium, and unknown "volatilization factors" present in some crude diets (Ganther et al., 1966). Formation of volatile selenium can be blocked by arsenic, mercury, cadmium, and thallium, but lead had no such inhibitory effect (Levander and Argrett, 1969; Ganther and Baumann, 1962a).

That the biosynthesis of volatile selenium might be an enzymatic process was first suggested by the work of Rosenfeld and Beath (1948), who showed that although fresh bovine liver minces could convert selenite into volatile selenium, liver minces that had been autoclaved could not. The enzymatic synthesis of volatile selenium from sodium selenite in mouse liver extracts was studied in detail by Ganther (1966). He found that the 9000 g liver fraction was more active than either the 165,000 g supernatant fraction or the washed microsomes alone. S-Adenosyl-L-methionine was thought to be the probable methyl donor, and other factors needed for optimal activity included reduced nicotinamide adenine dinucleotide phosphate (NADPH), coenzyme A, adenosine 5'-triphosphate, and magnesium. Dithiol blockers such as arsenite and cadmium were effective inhibitors of volatile selenium formation, whereas monothiol reagents such as N-ethylmaleimide and p-mercuribenzoate were much less effective. The biosynthesis of volatile selenium had a specific requirement for glutathione that could not be satisfied by other thiols or by dithiothreitol. On the basis of these results and the fact that glutathione can react with selenious acid to form the selenotrisulfide derivative of glutathione (Ganther, 1968):

$$4GSH + H_2SeO_3 \rightarrow GSSeSG + GSSG + 3H_2O \tag{5}$$

a reaction pathway was postulated (Ganther, 1971) whereby the selenotrisulfide would be reduced further either by NADPH via glutathione reductase or by an excess of glutathione to yield glutathione selenopersulfide:

$$\text{GSSeSG} \xrightarrow[\substack{\text{NADPH} \quad \text{NADP}^+ \\ \text{glutathione} \\ \text{reductase}}]{\substack{\text{GSH} \quad \text{GSSG}}} \text{GSSeH} \tag{6}$$

The selenopersulfide would give rise to hydrogen selenide, which would then be methylated by S-adenosylmethionine to dimethyl selenide. This mechanism for the biosynthesis of dimethyl selenide is quite different from that proposed by Challenger (discussed in Section II,A,4), since in the former no methylation occurs until the selenium is first reduced to the 2− oxidation state, whereas in the latter the pathway consists of alternate methylation and reduction steps. The Ganther hypothesis seems reasonable, since certain compounds that contain selenium in the 2− valence state are readily methylated by microsomal systems from rat liver (Bremer and Natori, 1960). Moreover, the first step of the Challenger scheme of dimethyl selenide formation (methylation of the biselenite anion to yield methaneselenonic acid) seems to require an oxidation of selenium from a 4+ to a 6+ state, which appears to be a highly unlikely process. Although one cannot deny the possibility that the selenopersulfide may act as the methyl acceptor in Ganther's scheme rather than the highly toxic hydrogen selenide (Diplock et al., 1973), the overall idea of reduction of selenium to the selenide level followed by methylation seems to be the most plausible mechanism available to explain dimethyl selenide production, at least in mammalian systems.

b. Urinary Compounds. Identification of trimethylselenonium ion, $(CH_3)_3Se^+$, a major urinary metabolite of selenite, was reported independently by two different research groups in 1969 (Byard, 1969; Palmer et al., 1969). These results represented the first chemical characterization of any urinary organoselenium compound. Trimethylselenonium ion was also found to be a general excretory product of selenium metabolism in the rat, since this compound was a major urinary metabolite when a variety of sources of selenium was tested (Palmer et al., 1970). As in the case of dimethyl selenide, trimethylselenonium ion may be a detoxification product of selenium, since it is less than one-tenth as toxic as selenite (Obermeyer et al., 1971). Trimethylselenonium ion is also rather inactive biologically in a nutritional sense, since the compound has little or no ability to prevent the liver necrosis due to selenium deficiency (Tsay et al., 1970). However, both dimethyl selenide and trimethylselenonium ion exhibit a synergistic toxicity with arsenic (Obermeyer et al., 1971). Although an appreciable amount of radioactivity was found in the urine of rats given small doses of dimethyl [^{75}Se]selenide (Pařízek et al., 1971), only very small amounts of radioselenium were excreted in the urine of rats given large doses of this compound (Obermeyer et al., 1971). Therefore, a product–precursor relationship between dimethyl selenide and trimethylselenonium ion cannot be stated with certainty at this time.

The excretion of [^{75}Se]trimethylselenonium ion in the urine of rats injected with radioselenomethionine appears to be another example of the lack of parallelism in the metabolism of selenium and sulfur, since no trimethylsulfonium ion was found in the urine of rats injected with methionine (Palmer, 1973).

5. Specific Roles in Enzymes

Although specific roles for selenium have been proposed in cytochromes (Whanger et al., 1973) and nonheme iron proteins (see Section III,A), the only fully documented role for selenium in a protein with enzymatic activity in mammalians as of June 1974 was in glutathione peroxidase, which is discussed elsewhere in this volume.

III. COMPARATIVE BIOCHEMISTRY OF SELENIUM AND SULFUR

A. Iron–Sulfur Proteins

Several research groups have now shown that selenium can be chemically substituted for the labile sulfur of certain nonheme iron proteins, such as putidaredoxin (Tsibris *et al.*, 1968), adrenodoxin (Orme-Johnson *et al.*, 1968), and ferredoxin (Fee and Palmer, 1971). The selenium homologs have physical properties that are similar to those of the native proteins, and in many instances, the selenoproteins have been shown to possess biological activity. In the case of parsley ferredoxin, for example, the selenium derivative was prepared by reconstituting the apoprotein in the presence of selenious acid and excess dithiothreitol under anaerobic conditions (Fee and Palmer, 1971). Apparently, the selenious acid first reacted with dithiol to yield a compound of the RS—Se—SR type. The excess dithiol then presumably reduced the selenotrisulfide to RS^- and Se^{2-}, and the latter was incorporated into the protein. The selenium-substituted parsley ferredoxin had spectroscopic properties very similar to those of the native protein, and the selenium-containing protein was about 80% as active as the native material in the ferredoxin-mediated reduction of cytochrome c by NADPH in the presence of ferredoxin–NADP reductase. The selenium homolog, however, was not very stable and spontaneously decomposed in the presence of oxygen (Fee *et al.*, 1971). The selenium derivative of adrenal iron–sulfur protein also was shown to possess biological activity, since the selenoprotein had 75% of the NADPH–cytochrome c reductase activity and 60% of the steroid-11β-hydroxylase activity of the native protein (Mukai *et al.*, 1974).

The fact that biologically active selenium derivatives of some iron–sulfur proteins can be prepared chemically lends support to the recent hypothesis of Diplock and Lucy (1973) that a biochemically active form of selenium may be as selenide in the active site of certain as yet uncharacterized nonheme iron proteins. These workers first showed that a portion of the selenium in the liver organelles of rats given small doses of the element behaved as acid-labile protein-bound selenide (discussed in Section II,C,2). The proportion of selenium present as selenide was greater when vitamin E was included in the diet than when the vitamin was absent.

Experiments with the zonal centrifugation technique indicated that the acid-labile selenide was particularly associated with the mitochondria and the smooth endoplasmic reticulum (Caygill *et al.*, 1971). This association was absent in vitamin E-deficient rats but could be restored by refeeding the vitamin to deficient rats for 5 days. Further work from this group showed that the large increase in selenide noted in the smooth reticulum of rats treated with phenobarbital was not seen in animals deficient in vitamin E (Caygill *et al.*, 1973). Moreover, the initial rate and extent of microsomal aminopyrine demethylation was very depressed in rats deficient in vitamin E and selenium, and full restoration of activity occurred only when both nutrients were available together (Giasuddin *et al.*, 1975). The conclusion from these studies was that there may be a specific vitamin E-dependent role for selenium as selenide in the smooth endoplasmic reticulum whereby the selenide forms a part of the active site of a nonheme iron-containing protein "X" that functions between the flavoprotein and cytochrome P450 in the NADPH-dependent electron-transfer chain of rat liver microsomal fractions. Recent work, which demonstrated that selenium was an effective catalyst for the reduction of cytochrome *c* by thiols (Levander *et al.*, 1973b, and see Section III,B), lends credence to this concept.

An important feature of the Diplock–Lucy hypothesis is that any *in vivo* antioxidant effects of vitamin E would be largely directed toward oxygen-labile selenide-containing proteins rather than toward polyunsaturated lipids. The extreme sensitivity of selenium-substituted parsley ferredoxin to oxygen was already pointed out above, and experiments by Caygill and Diplock (1973) suggest the existence of oxidant-labile nonheme iron in rat liver microsomes that is dependent on the presence of dietary vitamin E and selenium. On the other hand, the well-known nutritional relationship between vitamin E and polyunsaturated lipids would be explained by the formation of specific tocopherol–phospholipid complexes that would be necessary for normal membrane permeability and stability. The Diplock–Lucy conceptualization of vitamin E and selenium function has several pleasing aspects, but ultimate proof of this idea must await isolation and characterization of a selenononheme iron protein.

B. Selenopersulfide as an Electron Transfer Catalyst

Early in 1971, a series of experiments was initiated in our laboratory in an attempt to clarify on a biochemical level the well-established nutritional interrelationship between vitamin E and selenium. Schwarz (1961b) had previously shown that weanling male rats fed diets lacking both vitamin E and selenium developed a massive acute hepatic necrosis in 3–4 weeks. When we began our studies, the only known prenecrotic metabolic lesion in the livers of rats fed such doubly deficient diets was the so-called respiratory decline of rat liver slices (Chernick *et al.*, 1955). At that time, the prevailing, albeit controversial, hypothesis of the mode of action of vitamin E was that tocopherol acted as a fat-soluble antioxidant (Tappel, 1972; Green, 1972) and that selenium also exerted its biological effect somehow through its antioxidant properties (Tappel and Caldwell, 1967).

As an experimental model, we chose to study the *in vitro* swelling of rat liver mitochondria for 2 reasons:

1. Any breakdown in respiration as seen in the liver slices prepared from rats fed diets devoid of vitamin E and selenium obviously involved the mitochondrion.

2. Since other workers had shown that vitamin E could protect against the mitochondrial swelling induced by various chemical agents that initiated lipoperoxidation (Hunter *et al.*, 1963, 1964a,b), selenium might be expected to do the same if it acted as an antioxidant *in vivo*.

We found that dietary vitamin E did indeed protect against the swelling of rat liver mitochondria caused by ferrous ion, ascorbate, and thiols, but dietary selenium had no such protective effect (Levander *et al.*, 1973a, 1974a). In fact, dietary selenium seemed to have a pronounced accelerating effect on the mitochondrial swelling caused by sulfide or by certain thiols, such as cysteine. When liver mitochondria were prepared from rats deficient in selenium (selenium-deficient mitochondria), selenite added *in vitro* also was found to enhance cysteine-induced swelling. Various selenium compounds had similar relative abilities to accelerate the swelling of selenium-deficient mitochondria caused by either cysteine or glutathione (GSH). Selenite was the most active form of selenium in this regard, followed by selenocystine and then selenate or selenomethionine. The specificity of selenium compounds was illustrated by the inability of a wide variety of other oxyanions or cations to promote GSH-induced *in vitro* mitochondrial swelling.

The swelling of selenium-deficient mitochondria caused by the addition of 10^{-2} M GSH plus 10^{-5} M selenite to the incubation medium was strongly inhibited by dithiol reagents such as Hg^{2+}, Cd^{2+}, or arsenite at 10^{-5} M, but was inhibited by thiol reagents such as iodoacetate or N-ethylmaleimide only at concentrations of 10^{-2}–10^{-3} M. Uncoupling agents such as dinitrophenol or dicoumarol had little or no effect on swelling induced by GSH plus selenite. The respiratory inhibitors antimycin A and amytal only partially blocked the swelling caused by GSH plus selenite, whereas cyanide completely blocked such swelling. This latter observation suggested that the swelling might be at least partially mediated at the cytochrome c level, and selenite was shown to be an effective catalyst for the reduction of cytochrome c by thiols in model chemical systems (Levander *et al.*, 1973b). Other forms of selenium that were catalytically active in this system included selenocystine and to a lesser extent selenate, but selenomethionine was essentially inactive. The selenite-catalyzed reduction of cytochrome c by GSH required levels of 10^{-3} M Cd^{2+} or Hg^{2+} for full inhibition, and arsenite had little inhibitory effect even at 10^{-2} M. On the other hand, cyanide at $5 \times 10^{-5}M$ caused a 50% inhibition of the selenite-catalyzed reduction of cytochrome c by GSH. Selenocyanate was found to be a relatively poor catalyst for reduction of the cytochrome. These results were interpreted by a series of reactions in which the selenite in the presence of excess GSH formed the selenopersulfide derivative of glutathione (Ganther, 1971) [see also Eqs. (5) and (6) above]. The glutathione selenopersulfide was considered to be the active species in bringing about reduction of the cytochrome:

$$GSSeSG + GS^- \rightleftharpoons GSSe^- + GSSG \tag{7}$$
$$2GSSe^- + 2cyt\ c^{3+} \rightarrow 2GSSe\cdot + 2cyt\ c^{2+} \tag{8}$$
$$2GSSe\cdot \rightleftharpoons GSSeSeSG \tag{9}$$
$$GSSeSeSG + GS^- \rightleftharpoons GSSeSG + GSSe^- \tag{10}$$

$$Net:\quad 2GS^- + 2cyt\ c^{3+} \rightarrow GSSG + 2cyt\ c^{2+} \tag{11}$$

The inhibitory effect of cyanide was thought to be due to the destruction of the catalytically active glutathione selenotrisulfide and formation of the relatively inactive selenocyanate:

$$GSSeSG + CN^- \rightarrow GSSG + SeCN^- \tag{12}$$

Rhead and Schrauzer (1974) have recently completed a kinetic analysis of the selenium-catalyzed reduction of methylene blue by a variety of thiols. These workers concluded that under conditions whereby [RS-] $\gg$ [Se], the selenopersulfide may undergo further reactions with RS- to form a diselenide species:

$$RSSe^- + RS^- \rightleftharpoons Se^{2-} + RSSR \tag{13}$$

The Se^{2-} anion was then considered to reduce the methylene blue by way of a one- or two-electron transfer process. In agreement with the results of Levander and associates, Rhead and Schrauzer found that the selenium-catalyzed reduction of methylene blue could be inhibited by cyanide, Hg^{2+}, or Cd^{2+}, but that arsenite was without noticeable effect. This lack of effect of arsenite in blocking the selenium-catalyzed reduction of either cytochrome c or methylene blue by thiols is in sharp contrast to the pronounced inhibitory effect of arsenite against the mitochondrial swelling caused by GSH plus selenite. This discrepancy suggests that the swelling phenomenon induced by GSH plus selenite is not due merely to a direct reduction of the cytochrome. Rather, a dithiol group may serve as an intermediate electron carrier in this process. Rhead and Schrauzer also showed that selenium could catalyze the reduction of a variety of dyes other than methylene blue by thiols. Moreover, the rate of reduction correlated well with the reduction potentials of the dyes. The observation that selenium can act as a catalyst for the transfer of electrons from thiols to a number of acceptors, plus the fact that selenium is an effective catalyst for the reduction of central metal ions in cytochromes by thiols, suggests that a selenopersulfide may function *in vivo* as an electron transfer catalyst.

More recent work carried out by Levander and co-workers (1974b) has been an attempt to characterize chemically the form of selenium in rat liver mitochondria. The approach taken in these studies was to give young rats a vitamin E-supplemented but selenium-deficient diet and physiologically relevant levels of radioselenium (0.1 ppm) in the drinking water for a period of several weeks. After that time, liver mitochondria were prepared by standard techniques and then subjected to various extraction procedures. The fractionation techniques used initially were those that had been applied successfully by others for the isolation of cytochrome c from mitochondria, since we had shown that selenium was a good catalyst for cytochrome c reduction and since Whanger *et al.* (1973) had claimed the existence of a selenium-containing cytochrome. But no appreciable quantities of radioselenium were found to be associated with the cytochrome c that was isolated from rat liver mitochondria. Rather, the 60% of the mitochondrial radioselenium that was solubilized by the extraction procedure used was shown by chromatographic methods to be largely associated with glutathione peroxidase (this selenoenzyme is discussed in detail elsewhere in this volume). If the selenium associated with the enzyme glutathione peroxidase is the form of selenium in mitochondria directly responsible for the enhanced thiol-induced swelling, these studies may tell us two things about the enzyme:

1. The selenium in the active site of glutathione peroxidase is in a chemical form that can react with thiols; i.e., the selenium in the enzyme is not, for example, in the selenide valence state singly bonded to two different carbon atoms as in selenomethionine, since this form of selenium was shown to be inactive in promoting the reduction of cytochrome c by GSH.

2. Although glutathione peroxidase is thought to be located in the mitochondrial matrix, the enzyme apparently is accessible to the thiols that promote mitochondrial swelling.

Another example of a possible role for selenium in mitochondrial metabolism via glutathione peroxidase is as a component of "contraction factor," a substance required in reversal of GSH-induced swelling by adenosine triphosphate (Neubert *et al.*, 1962). Of course, there is a reasonable possibility that the form of selenium that is actually the most important as far as thiol-induced mitochondrial swelling is concerned exists in that fraction of mitochondrial selenium that has yet to be characterized. A likely form for this selenium might be as selenide in a nonheme iron protein as discussed in Section III,A. Additional work on characterizing the forms of selenium in mitochondria and various other subcellular organelles needs to be carried out in order to determine whether or not glutathione peroxidase can account for all of the protein-bound selenium under normal circumstances.

IV. RESEARCH NEEDS

In spite of much time and effort spent on the problem, the form(s) of selenium in animal proteins still cannot be described with precision. Although certain similarities between the metabolism and biochemistry of selenium and sulfur might lead to the conclusion that selenium merely replaces sulfur in some crucial metabolite, evidence is now accumulating that suggests that the selenium associated with, for example, glutathione peroxidase, exists in a form that could not have been anticipated on the basis of known sulfur biochemistry. Clearly, more research is needed to establish with certainty the chemical form(s) that selenium can assume in tissues.

Although much of the mystery surrounding the selenium problem appears to have been swept aside with the discovery of the role of selenium in glutathione peroxidase, there remains a reasonable likelihood that selenium may play a role in other enzymes as well. Surely the precedent found in microbial enzymology is encouraging in this respect, since selenium has been shown to be involved in at least two enzymes in microorganisms other than glutathione peroxidase. The existence of still other selenoproteins in both the plant and animal kingdoms would not be surprising, and additional work to characterize these proteins should be encouraged.

The possibility that selenium compounds of low molecular weight may be important in intermediary metabolism should not be overlooked. The physiological role of glutathione remains rather vague, and the relative ease with which selenium can either catalyze the oxidation of glutathione or form selenopersulfide derivatives with glutathione tempts one to speculate about the significance of such reactions in cellular biochemistry. For example, Kosower et al. (1972) have shown that oxidized glutathione can block protein biosynthesis and have suggested that a rise in the level of oxidized glutathione may be responsible for the diminution of initiation of protein synthesis during mitosis. Also, Vernie *et al.* (1974) found that selenite was a potent inhibitor of polyribosomal amino acid incorporation and that the maximal inhibitory effect required glutathione. Moreover, a reaction product between glutathione and selenite was likewise inhibitory and this product was thought to be glutathione selenotrisulfide. Research to determine whether or not selenium modulates the intracellular SH/SS ratio, which apparently is involved in the regulation of cell division, is admittedly somewhat adventurous, but the payoff may warrant the gamble.

Researchers should keep an open mind concerning possible roles for selenium in biomolecules other than proteins, peptides, or amino acids. There is some recent evidence (Saelinger *et al.*, 1972; Hoffman *et al.*, 1974) to suggest that selenium may be incorporated into the transfer RNA of microorganisms, although the physiological importance of such minor "selenobases" is not clear at present. Pioneering efforts such as these may uncover hitherto unsuspected implications for selenium in living systems.

REFERENCES

Andressen, J. R., and Ljungdahl, L. G. (1973). Formate dehydrogenase of *Clostridium thermoaceticum:* Incorporation of selenium-75, and the effects of selenite, molybdate, and tungstate on the enzyme. *J. Bacteriol.* 116, 867–873.

Blau, M. (1961). Biosynthesis of [^{75}Se] selenomethionine and [^{75}Se]selenocystine. *Biochim. Biophys. Acta* 49, 389–390.

Bonhorst, C. W. (1955). Anion antagonisms in yeast as indicators of the mechanism of selenium toxicity. *J. Agr. Food Chem.* 3, 700–703.

Bremer, J., and Natori, Y. (1960). Behavior of some selenium compounds in transmethylation. *Biochim. Biophys. Acta* 44, 367–370.

Byard, J. L. (1969). Trimethyl selenide. A urinary metabolite of selenite. *Arch. Biochem. Biophys.* 130, 556–560.

Caygill, C. P. J., and Diplock, A. T. (1973). The dependence on dietary selenium and vitamin E of oxidant-labile liver microsomal non-haem iron. *FEBS (Fed. Eur. Biochem. Soc.) Lett.* 33, 172–176.

Caygill, C. P. J., Lucy, J. A., and Diplock, A. T. (1971). The effect of vitamin E on the intracellular distribution of the different oxidation states of selenium in rat liver. *Biochem. J.* 125, 407–416.

Caygill, C. P. J., Diplock, A. T., and Jeffery, E. H. (1973). Studies on selenium incorporation into, and electron-transfer function of, liver microsomal fractions from normal and vitamin E-deficient rats given phenobarbitone. *Biochem. J.* 136, 851–858.

Challenger, F. (1955). Biological methylation. *Quart. Rev., Chem. Soc.* 9, 255–286.

Challenger, F., and Charlton, P. T. (1947). Studies of biological methylation. Part X. The fission of the mono- and disulfide links by molds. *J. Chem. Soc., London* pp. 424–429.

Challenger, F., and North, H. E. (1934). The production of organometalloidal com-

158 ORVILLE A. LEVANDER

pounds by microorganisms. II. Dimethylselenide. *J. Chem. Soc., London* pp. 68–71.

Chernick, S. S., Moe, J. G., Rodnan, G. P., and Schwarz, K. (1955). A metabolic lesion in dietary necrotic liver degeneration. *J. Biol. Chem.* **217,** 829–843.

Coch, E. H., and Greene, R. C. (1971). The utilization of selenomethionine by *Escherichia coli. Biochim. Biophys. Acta* **230,** 223–236.

Cowie, D. B., and Cohen, G. N. (1957). Biosynthesis by *Escherichia coli* of active altered proteins containing selenium instead of sulfur. *Biochim. Biophys. Acta* **26,** 252–261.

Cummins, L. M., and Martin, J. L. (1967). Are selenocystine and selenomethionine synthesized *in vivo* from sodium selenite in mammals? *Biochemistry* **6,** 3162–3168.

Diplock, A. T., and Lucy, J. A. (1973). The biochemical modes of action of vitamin E and selenium: A hypothesis. *FEBS (Fed. Eur. Biochem. Soc.) Lett.* **29,** 205–210.

Diplock, A. T., Baum, H., and Lucy, J. A. (1971). The effect of vitamin E on the oxidation state of selenium in rat liver. *Biochem. J.* **123,** 721–729.

Diplock, A. T., Caygill, C. P. J., Jeffrey, E. H., and Thomas, C. (1973). The nature of the acid-volatile selenium in the liver of the male rat. *Biochem. J.* **134,** 283–293.

Enoch, H. G., and Lester, R. L. (1972). Effects of molybdate, tungstate, and selenium compounds on formate dehydrogenase and other enzyme systems in *Escherichia coli. J. Bacteriol.* **110,** 1032–1039.

Fee, J. A., and Palmer, G. (1971). The properties of parsley ferredoxin and its selenium-containing homolog. *Biochim. Biophys. Acta* **245,** 175–195.

Fee, J. A., Mayhew, S. G., and Palmer, G. (1971). The oxidation-reduction potentials of parsley ferredoxin and its selenium-containing homolog. *Biochim. Biophys. Acta* **245,** 196–200.

Fels, I. G., and Cheldelin, V. H. (1949a). Selenate inhibition studies. II. The reversal of selenate inhibition in *Escherichia coli. Arch. Biochem. Biophys.* **22,** 323–324.

Fels, I. G, and Cheldelin, V. H. (1949b). Selenate inhibition studies. III. The role of sulfate in selenate toxicity in yeast. *Arch. Biochem. Biophys.* **22,** 402–405.

Fels, I. G., and Cheldelin, V. H. (1950). Selenate inhibition studies. IV. Biochemical basis of selenate toxicity in yeast. *J. Biol. Chem.* **185,** 803–811.

Fukuyama, A. T., and Ordal, E. J. (1965). Induced biosynthesis of formic hydrogenlyase in iron-deficient cells of *Escherichia coli. J. Bacteriol.* **90,** 673–680.

Ganther, H. E. (1966). Enzymic synthesis of dimethyl selenide from sodium selenite in mouse liver extracts. *Biochemistry* **5,** 1089–1098.

Ganther, H. E. (1968). Selenotrisulfides. Formation by the reaction of thiols with selenious acid. *Biochemistry* **7,** 2898–2905.

Ganther, H. E. (1971). Reduction of the selenotrisulfide derivative of glutathione to a persulfide analog by glutathione reductase. *Biochemistry* **10,** 4089–4098.

Ganther, H. E., and Baumann, C. A. (1962a). Selenium metabolism. I. Effects of diet, arsenic, and cadmium. *J. Nutr.* **77,** 210–216.

Ganther, H. E., and Baumann, C. A. (1962b). Selenium metabolism. II. Modifying effects of sulfate. *J. Nutr.* **77,** 408–414.

Ganther, H. E., and Corcoran, C. (1969). Selenotrisulfides. II. Cross-linking of reduced pancreatic ribonuclease with selenium. *Biochemistry* **8,** 2557–2563.

Ganther, H. E., Levander, O. A., and Baumann, C. A. (1966). Dietary control of selenium volatilization in the rat. *J. Nutr.* **88,** 55–60.

Ganther, H. E., Oh, S. H., Chitharanjan, D., and Hoekstra, W. G. (1974). Studies on selenium in glutathione peroxidase. *Fed. Proc., Fed. Amer. Soc. Exp. Biol.* 33, 694 (abstr.).

Giasuddin, A. S. M., Caygill, C. P. J., Diplock, A. T., and Jeffrey, E. H. (1975). The dependence on vitamin E and selenium of drug demethylation in rat liver microsomal fractions. *Biochem. J.* 146, 339–350.

Godwin, K. O., and Fuss, C. N. (1972). The entry of selenium into rabbit protein following the administration of Na₂⁷⁵SeO₃. *Aust. J. Biol. Sci.* 25, 865–871.

Green, J. (1972). Vitamin E and the biological antioxidant theory. *Ann. N.Y. Acad. Sci.* 203, 29–44.

Hoffman, J. L., McConnell, K. P., and Carpenter, D. R. (1970). Aminoacylation of *Escherichia coli* methionine tRNA by selenomethionine. *Biochim. Biophys. Acta* 199, 531–534.

Hoffman, J. L., McConnell, K. P., and Warick, R. (1974). Identification of 4-seleno-uridine in ⁷⁵Se-labelled tRNA from *E. coli. Fed. Proc., Fed. Amer. Soc. Exp. Biol.* 33, 1364 (abstr.).

Hofmeister, F. (1894). Ueber Methylirung im Thierkoerper. *Arch. Exp. Pathol. Pharmakol.* 33, 198–215.

Huber, R. E., and Criddle, R. S. (1967a). Comparison of the chemical properties of selenocysteine and selenocystine with their sulfur analogs. *Arch. Biochem. Biophys.* 122, 164–173.

Huber, R. E., and Criddle, R. S. (1967b). The isolation and properties of β-galactosidase from *Escherichia coli* grown on sodium selenate. *Biochim. Biophys. Acta* 141, 573–586.

Huber, R. E., Segal, I. H., and Criddle, R. S. (1967). Growth of *Escherichia coli* on selenate. *Biochim. Biophys. Acta* 141, 573–586.

Hunter, F. E., Jr., Gebicki, J. M., Hoffsten, P. E., Weinstein, J., and Scott, A. (1963). Swelling and lysis of rat liver mitochondria induced by ferrous ions. *J. Biol. Chem.* 238, 828–835.

Hunter, F. E., Jr., Scott, A., Hoffsten, P. E., Guerra, F., Weinstein, J., Schneider, A., Schutz, B., Fink, J., Ford, L., and Smith, E. (1964a). Studies on the mechanism of ascorbate-induced swelling and lysis of isolated liver mitochondria. *J. Biol. Chem.* 239, 604–613.

Hunter, F. E., Jr., Scott, A., Hoffsten, P. E., Gebicki, J. M., Weinstein, J., and Schneider, A. (1964b). Studies on the mechanism of swelling, lysis, and disintegration of isolated liver mitochondria exposed to mixtures of oxidized and reduced glutathione. *J. Biol. Chem.* 239, 614–621.

Jenkins, K. J. (1968). Evidence for the absence of selenocystine and selenomethionine in the serum proteins of chicks administered selenite. *Can. J. Biochem.* 46, 1417–1425.

Jenkins, K. J., and Hidiroglou, M. (1971). Comparative uptake of selenium by low cystine and high cystine proteins. *Can J. Biochem.* 49, 468–472.

Kosower, N. S., Vanderhoff, G. A., and Kosower, E. M. (1972). Glutathione. VIII. The effects of glutathione disulfide on initiation of protein synthesis. *Biochim. Biophys. Acta* 272, 623–637.

Lester, R. L., and DeMoss, J. A. (1971). Effect of molybdate and selenite on formate and nitrate metabolism in *Escherichia coli. J. Bacteriol.* 105, 1006–1014.

Letunova, S. V. (1970). Geochemical ecology of soil microorganisms. *In* "Trace Element Metabolism in Animals" (C. F. Mills, ed.), pp. 432–437. Livingstone, Edinburgh.

Levander, O. A., and Argrett, L. C. (1969). Effects of arsenic, mercury, thallium, and lead on selenium metabolism in rats. *Toxicol. Appl. Pharmacol.* **14**, 308–314.

Levander, O. A., Morris, V. C., and Higgs, D. J. (1973a). Acceleration of thiol-induced swelling of rat liver mitochondria by selenium. *Biochemistry* **12**, 4586–4590.

Levander, O. A., Morris, V. C., and Higgs, D. J. (1973b). Selenium as a catalyst for the reduction of cytochrome *c* by glutathione. *Biochemistry* **12**, 4591–4595.

Levander, O. A., Morris, V. C., and Higgs. D. J. (1974b). Characterization of the selenium in rat liver mitochondria as glutathione peroxidase. *Biochem. Biophys. Res. Commun.* **58**, 1047–1052.

Levander, O. A., Morris, V. C., and Higgs, D. J. (1974a). Selenium catalysis of swelling of rat liver mitochondria and reduction of cytochrome *c* by sulfur compounds. *In* "Protein-Metal Interactions" (M. Friedman, ed.). Plenum, New York 405–423.

McConnell, K. P., and Cho, G. J. (1965). Transmucosal movement of selenium. *Amer. J. Physiol.* **208**, 1191–1195.

McConnell, K. P., and Cho, G. J. (1967). Active transport of L-seleno-methionine in the intestine. *Amer. J. Physiol.* **213**, 150–156.

McConnell, K. P., and Hoffman, J. L. (1972a). Methionine-selenomethionine parallels in *Escherichia coli* polypeptide chain initiation and synthesis. *Proc. Soc. Exp. Biol. Med.* **140**, 638–641.

McConnell, K. P., and Hoffman, J. L. (1972b). Methionine-selenomethionine parallels in rat liver polypeptide chain synthesis. *FEBS (Fed. Eur. Biochem. Soc.) Lett.* **24**, 60–62.

McConnell, K. P., and Portman, O. W. (1952a). Excretion of dimethyl selenide by the rat. *J. Biol. Chem.* **195**, 277–282.

McConnell, K. P., and Portman, O. W. (1952b). Toxicity of dimethyl selenide in the rat and mouse. *Proc. Soc. Exp. Biol. Med.* **79**, 230–231.

McConnell, K. P., and Roth, D. M. (1966). Respiratory excretion of selenium. *Proc. Soc. Exp. Biol. Med.* **123**, 919–921.

McConnell, K. P., and Wabnitz, C. H. (1957). Studies on the fixation of radioselenium in proteins. *J. Biol. Chem.* **226**, 765–776.

McConnell, K. P., Hsu, J. M., Herrman, J. L., and Anthony, W. L. (1974). Parallelism between sulfur and selenium amino acids in protein synthesis in the skin of zinc deficient rats. *Proc. Soc. Exp. Biol. Med.* **145**, 970–974.

McCready, R. G. L., Campbell, J. N., and Payne, J. I. (1966). Selenite reduction by *Salmonella heidelberg. Can. J. Microbiol.* **1**, 703–714.

Millar, K. R. (1972). Distribution of Se[75] in liver, kidney, and blood proteins of rats after intravenous injection of sodium selenite. *N.Z.J. Agr. Res.* **15**, 547–564.

Millar, K. R., and Sheppard, A. D. (1973). A comparison of the metabolism of methionine and selenomethionine in rats. *N.Z.J. Agr. Res.* **16**, 293–300.

Millar, K. R., Gardiner, M. A., and Sheppard, A. D. (1973). A comparison of the metabolism of intravenously injected sodium selenite, sodium selenate, and selenomethionine in rats. *N.Z.J. Agr. Res.* **16**, 115–127.

Mudd, S. H., and Cantoni, G. L. (1957). Selenomethionine in enzymatic transmethylations. *Nature (London)* **180**, 1052.

Mukai, K., Huang, J. J., and Kimura, T. (1974). Studies on adrenal steroid hydroxylases. Chemical and enzymatic properties of selenium derivatives of adrenal iron-sulfur protein. *Biochim. Biophys. Acta* **336**, 427–436.

Neubert, D., Wojtczak, A. B., and Lehninger, A. L. (1962). Purification and enzymatic identity of mitochondrial contraction factors I and II. *Proc. Nat. Acad. Sci. U.S.* **48**, 1651–1658.

Nickerson, W. J., and Falcone, G. (1963). Enzymatic reduction of selenite. *J. Bacteriol.* **85**, 763–771.

Obermeyer, B. D., Palmer, I. S., Olson, O. E., and Halverson, A. W. (1971). Toxicity of trimethylselenonium chloride in the rat with and without arsenite. *Toxicol. Appl. Pharmacol.* **20**, 135–145.

Olson, O. E., Schulte, B. M., Whitehead, E. I., and Halverson, A. W. (1963). Effect of arsenic on selenium metabolism in rats. *J. Agr. Food Chem.* **11**, 531–534.

Olson, O. E., Novacek, E. J., Whitehead, E. I., and Palmer, I. S. (1970). Investigations on selenium in wheat. *Phytochemistry* **9**, 1181–1188.

Orme-Johnson, W. H., Hansen, R. E., Beinert, H., Tsibris, J. C. M., Bartholomaus, R. C., and Gunsalus, I. C. (1968). On the sulfur components of iron-sulfur proteins. I. The number of acid-labile sulfur groups sharing an unpaired electron with iron. *Proc. Nat. Acad. Sci. U.S.* **60**, 368–372.

Painter, E. P. (1941). The chemistry and toxicity of selenium compounds with special reference to the selenium problem. *Chem. Rev.* **28**, 179–213.

Palmer, I. S. (1973). An example of the lack of parallelism in the metabolism of sulfur and selenium. *Proc. S. Dak. Acad. Sci.* **52**, 108–111.

Palmer, I. S., Fischer, D. D., Halverson, A. W., and Olson, O. E. (1969). Identification of a major selenium excretory product in rat urine. *Biochem. Biophys. Acta* **177**, 336–342.

Palmer, I. S., Gunsalus, R. P., Halverson, A. W., and Olson, O. E. (1970). Trimethylselenonium ion as a general excretory product from selenium metabolism in the rat. *Biochim. Biophys. Acta* **208**, 260–266.

Pařízek, J., Oštádalová, I., Kalousková, J., Babický, A., and Beneš, J. (1971). The detoxifying effects of selenium: interrelations between compounds of selenium and certain metals. *In* "Newer Trace Elements in Nutrition" (W. Mertz and W. E. Cornatzer, eds.), pp. 85–122. Dekker, New York.

Paulson, G. D., Baumann, C. A., and Pope, A. L. (1968). Metabolism of ^{75}Se-selenite, ^{75}Se-selenate, ^{75}Se-selenomethionine, and ^{35}S-sulfate by rumen microorganisms *in vitro. J. An. Sci.* **27**, 497–503.

Pinsent, J. (1954). The need for selenite and molybdate in the formation of formic dehydrogenase by members of the coli-aerogenes group of bacteria. *Biochem. J.* **57**, 10–16.

Rhead, W. J., and Schrauzer, G. N. (1974). The selenium catalyzed reduction of Methylene Blue by thiols. *Bioinorg. Chem.* **3**, 225–242.

Rhead, W. J., Evans, G. A., and Schrauzer, G. N. (1974). Selenium in human plasma: Levels in blood proteins and behavior upon dialysis, acidification, and reduction. *Bioinorg. Chem.* **3**, 217–223.

Rosenfeld, I., and Beath, O. A. (1948). Metabolism of sodium selenite by the tissues. *J. Biol. Chem.* **172**, 333–341.

Rosenfeld, I., and Beath, O. A. (1964). "Selenium: Geobotany, Biochemistry, Toxicity and Nutrition." Academic Press, New York.

Saelinger, D. A., Hoffman, J. L., and McConnell, K. P. (1972). Biosynthesis of selenobases in transfer RNA by *Escherichia coli. J. Mol. Biol.* **69**, 9–17.

Said, A. K., and Hegsted, D. M. (1970). ^{75}Se-selenomethionine in the study of protein and amino acid metabolism of adult rats. *Proc. Soc. Exp. Biol. Med.* **133**, 1388–1391.

Schwarz, K. (1961a). Nutritional significance of selenium (Factor 3): Introduction. *Fed. Proc., Fed. Amer. Soc. Exp. Biol.* 20, 665.

Schwarz, K. (1961b). Development and status of experimental work on Factor 3—selenium. *Fed. Proc., Fed. Amer. Soc. Exp. Biol.* 20, 666–673.

Schwarz, K., and Sweeney, E. (1964). Selenite binding to sulfur amino acids. *Fed. Proc., Fed. Amer. Soc. Exp. Biol.* 23, 421 (abstr.).

Shepherd, L., and Huber, R. E. (1969). Some chemical and biochemical properties of selenomethionine. *Can J. Biochem.* 47, 877–881.

Shrift, A. (1954a). Sulfur-selenium antagonism. I. Antimetabolite action of selenate on the growth of *Chlorella vulgaris. Amer. J. Bot.* 41, 223–230.

Shrift, A. (1954b). Sulfur-selenium antagonism. II. Antimetabolite action of selenomethionine on the growth of *Chlorella vulgaris. Amer. J. Bot.* 41, 345–352.

Shrift, A. (1973). Metabolism of selenium by plants and microorganisms. In "Organic Selenium Compounds: Their Chemistry and Biology" (D. L. Klayman and W. H. H. Gunther, eds.), pp. 763–814. Wiley-Interscience, New York.

Shum, A. C., and Murphy, J. C. (1972). Effects of selenium compounds on formate metabolism and coincidence of selenium-75 incorporation and formic dehydrogenase activity in cell-free preparations of *Escherichia coli. J. Bacteriol.* 110, 447–449.

Smith, M. I., Westfall, B. B., and Stohlman, E. F. (1938). Studies on the fate of selenium in the organism. *Pub. Health Rep.* 53, 1199–1216.

Stadtman, T. C. (1974a). Selenium biochemistry. *Science* 183, 915–922.

Stadtman, T. C. (1974b). Composition and some properties of the selenoprotein of glycine reductase. *Fed. Proc., Fed. Amer. Soc. Exp. Biol.* 33, 1291 (abstr.).

Tappel, A. L. (1972). Vitamin E and free radical peroxidation of lipids. *Ann. N.Y. Acad. Sci.* 203, 12–28.

Tappel, A. L., and Caldwell, K. A. (1967). Redox properties of selenium compounds related to biochemical function. In "Selenium in Biomedicine" (O. H. Muth, J. E. Oldfield, and P. H. Weswig, eds.), pp. 345–361. Avi Publ., Westport, Connecticut.

Tilton, R. C., Gunner, H. B., and Litsky, W. (1967). Physiology of selenite reduction by enterococci. I. Influence of environmental variables. *Can. J. Microbiol.* 13, 1175–1185.

Tsay, D. T., Halverson, A. W., and Palmer, I. S. (1970). Inactivity of dietary trimethylselenonium chloride against the necrogenic syndrome of the rat. *Nutr. Rep. Int.* 2, 203–207.

Tsibris, J. C. M., Namtvedt, M. J., and Gunsalus, I. C. (1968). Selenium as an acid labile sulfur replacement in putidaredoxin. *Biochem. Biophys. Res. Commun.* 30, 323–327.

Turner, D. C., and Stadtman, T. C. (1973). Purification of protein components of the clostridial glycine reductase system and characterization of protein A as a selenoprotein. *Arch. Biochem. Biophys.* 154, 366–381.

Tuve, T., and Williams, H. H. (1961). Metabolism of selenium by *Escherichia coli:* Biosynthesis of selenomethionine. *J. Biol. Chem.* 236, 597–601.

Vernie, L. N., Bont, W. S., and Emmelot, P. (1974). Inhibition of *in vitro* amino acid incorporation by sodium selenite. *Biochemistry* 13, 337–341.

Vlasáková, V., Beneš, J., and Pařízek, J. (1972). Application of gas chromatography for the analysis of trace amounts of volatile ^{75}Se metabolites in expired air. *Radiochem. Radioanal. Lett.* 10, 251–258.

Weiss, K. F., Ayres, J. C., and Kraft, A. A. (1965). Inhibitory action of selenite on *Escherichia coli, Proteus vulgaris,* and *Salmonella thompson. J. Bacteriol.* **90,** 857–862.

Whanger, P. D., Pedersen, N. D., and Weswig, P. H. (1973). Selenium proteins in ovine tissues. II. Spectral properties of a 10,000 molecular weight selenium protein. *Biochem. Biophys. Res. Commun.* **53,** 1031–1036.

Woolfolk, C. A., and Whiteley, H. R. (1962). Reduction of inorganic compounds with molecular hydrogen by *Micrococcus lactilyticus. J. Bacteriol.* **84,** 647–658.

Wu, M., and Wachsman, J. T. (1970). Effect of selenomethionine on growth of *Escherichia coli* and *Bacillus megaterium. J. Bacteriol.* **104,** 1393–1396.

Wu, M., and Wachsman, J. T. (1971). Selenomethionine, a methyl donor for bacterial nucleic acids. *J. Bacteriol.* **105,** 1222–1223.

Yamamoto, L. A., and Segal, I. H. (1966). The inorganic sulfate transport system of *Penicillium chrysogenum. Arch. Biochem. Biophys.* **114,** 523–538.

Yousef, M. K., and Johnson, H. D. (1970). ^{75}Se-selenomethionine turnover rate during growth and aging in rats. *Proc. Soc. Exp. Biol. Med.* **133,** 1351–1353.

32
Selenium and Glutathione Peroxidase in Health and Disease—A Review

H. E. Ganther, D. G. Hafeman, R. A. Lawrence,
R. E. Serfass, and W. G. Hoekstra

I. INTRODUCTION

Glutathione peroxidase (GSH-Px) was discovered by Mills (1957), who demonstrated the presence of a peroxidase in bovine erythrocytes that catalyzed the breakdown of hydrogen peroxide, with glutathione serving as the hydrogen donor. Mills (1959) later purified the enzyme and confirmed that the peroxidase and catalase activities of the red cell could be attributed to two different enzymes. Cohen and Hochstein (1963) compared the role of erythrocyte GSH-Px and catalase in hydrogen peroxide destruction and concluded that under physiological conditions, the major pathway of hydrogen peroxide destruction involved GSH-Px. Through the investigations of Little and O'Brien (1968; O'Brien and Little, 1969) and Christophersen (1968, 1969), the important discovery was made that GSH-Px also catalyzed the reduction of hydroperoxides formed from fatty acids or from other substances, as well as hydrogen peroxide, so that the general reaction catalyzed by the enzyme could be described by

$$ROOH + 2GSH \rightarrow R\text{---}OH + HOH + GSSG \tag{1}$$

Thus, a broad role for GSH-Px in protecting tissues from oxidative damage was apparent.

Major contributions to the knowledge about the chemistry and biological function of GSH-Px have come from the work of Flohe and his co-workers in Germany. By the early 1970s this group had succeeded for the first time in isolating weighable quantities of the pure enzyme (Flohe et al., 1971a). Flohe (1971) thoroughly reviewed the knowledge of GSH-Px from 1957 to the early 1970s.

In the early 1970s, Rotruck, Hoekstra, and co-workers at the University of Wisconsin began an investigation of GSH-Px in relation to the overlapping nutritional roles of selenium, vitamin E, and sulfur amino acids (Hoekstra, 1974). By an interesting coincidence, in the same year that GSH-Px was discovered, selenium was found to be a beneficial trace element for animals (Schwarz and Foltz, 1957; Patterson et al., 1957). The work of Schwarz demonstrated that selenium, as the active component of factor 3, could prevent liver necrosis in rats, a nutritional disorder also prevented by vitamin E and delayed by the sulfur-containing amino acids (reviewed by Schwarz, 1961, 1965). By the late 1960s, the essentiality of selenium, even in the presence of vitamin E in the diet, had been firmly established (Thompson and Scott, 1969), but no specific biochemical role had been discovered. The trail that led to the discovery of a role for selenium in erythrocyte GSH-Px, culminating in its identification in 1973 as a selenoprotein, has been published and was reviewed by Hoekstra (1974). Thus, after a period of a decade and a half, when selenium and GSH-Px were being intensively but independently investigated, these trails of research converged, opening up numerous and significant opportunities for research in both the basic and clinical areas.

The purpose of this chapter is to discuss the biochemistry of selenium and GSH-Px, bring together the present knowledge of this topic with regard to man, and point out some areas needing further study. No attempt has been made to cite every paper concerning GSH-Px, but a reasonably thorough review of its properties and functions has been attempted because the only previous review (Flohe, 1971) is in German. A search of the more recent literature through mid-1974 has been made using the MEDLINE service. The interesting function of GSH-Px as related to mitochondrial swelling is not discussed, since the subject has been reviewed in depth by Flohe (1971) and elsewhere in Chapter 21 by Levander. The information about selenium in man is well covered elsewhere in this volume by Burk. For those readers who desire a further knowledge of selenium, the subject of its nutritional essentiality has recently been reviewed by Scott (1973) and the biochemistry of selenium is covered by Stadtman (1974) and Ganther (1974).

II. PROPERTIES OF GLUTATHIONE PEROXIDASE

A. Physical and Chemical Properties

Estimates of the molecular weight of GSH-Px, using gel filtration, sedimentation equilibrium, or gel electrophoresis techniques are summarized in Table I. The purified erythrocyte enzyme has a molecular

TABLE I Molecular Weight of Glutathione Peroxidase and Its Subunits

Enzyme source	Method	Molecular weight Native enzyme	Subunits	Reference
Bovine erythrocytes	Gel filtration	85,000	—	Schneider and Flohe (1967)
Human erythrocytes	Gel filtration	100,000	—	Paglia and Valentine (1967)
Bovine lens	Gel filtration	96,600	—	Holmberg (1968)
Bovine erythrocytes	Sedimentation equilibrium	83,800	—	Flohe et al. (1971a)
Bovine erythrocytes	Electrophoresis in SDS[a]	—	21,000	Flohe et al. (1971a)
Pig aorta	Gel filtration	about 84,000	—	Smith et al. (1973)
Ovine erythrocytes	Gel filtration	88,000	—	Oh et al., (1974a)
Ovine erythrocytes	Electrophoresis in SDS[a]	—	22,000	Oh et al. (1974a)

[a] Sodium dodecyl sulfate (plus dithiothreitol).

weight of 84,000 (cattle) or 88,000 (sheep), while a somewhat greater value was estimated for the partially purified enzyme from bovine lens. Upon acrylamide gel electrophoresis after treatment with sodium dodecyl sulfate (SDS) and dithiothreitol at elevated temperatures, a single band of protein having a molecular weight of 21,000 (Flohe et al., 1971a) or 22,000 (Oh et al., 1974a) was obtained. Flohe et al. (1971a) found that dissociation was not complete at 37°C. Even in the absence of reducing substances, the enzyme at least partially dissociates into subunits in the presence of guanidine (unpublished results of L. Flohe and B. Eisele, 1970, cited by Flohe et al., 1971c). Flohe et al. (1971a) also observed subunits upon electrophoresis in 8 M urea, apparently in the absence of reducing agents. These results indicate that disulfide bridges or other covalent bonds are not responsible for holding the subunits together.

There is no evidence for heterogeneity of the subunits in the erythrocyte enzyme. Gel electrophoresis in SDS (where the mobility is determined primarily by the size of the polypeptide chain and not by intrinsic charge) shows that the subunits have an identical size. Although this finding does not rule out the possibility of the subunits differing in their intrinsic charge by virtue of variations in amino acid composition, this possibility is not supported by additional studies of Flohe et al. (1971a), where only one major band was found upon electrophoresis of GSH-Px in 8 M urea. Thus, in the absence of evidence to the contrary, it appears that native GSH-Px consists of four identical subunits joined by noncovalent bonds.

The isoelectric point of bovine erythrocyte GSH-Px determined by zone electrophoresis ranged from 5.6 to 6.0, depending on ionic strength of the buffer (Flohe, 1969), while a value of 6–6.5 was obtained by isoelectric focusing of the enzyme from ovine erythrocytes (Oh et al., 1974a).

Spectral studies of the purified enzyme (Flohe et al., 1971c) show no absorption bands in the visible region, ruling out the presence of heme, flavins, and other colored substances. The ultraviolet spectrum of the enzyme from bovine erythrocytes shows a maximum at 281 nm (Flohe et al., 1971c). An extinction coefficient ($E_{1\%}^{280}$) of 7.41 was obtained (Flohe et al., 1971a). From this value, a molar extinction coefficient of 6.21×10^4 can be calculated for the bovine erythrocyte enzyme, assuming that the reported absorbance was obtained for the usual path length of 1 cm. A value of 7.06×10^4 has been obtained for the erythrocyte enzyme from sheep based on a microbiuret analysis for protein (S. H. Oh, unpublished data, 1973).

Circular dichroism studies have been carried out on the bovine erythrocyte enzyme (Flohe et al., 1971c). An α-helix content of approximately 25% was estimated. Marked shifts in both the circular dichroism and ultraviolet spectra are observed upon reduction of the enzyme with glutathione; these changes are attributed to an altered tertiary structure (Flohe et al., 1971c).

GSH-Px from bovine blood has recently been crystalized from 1.2 M potassium phosphate buffer (Flohe et al., 1973).

The amino acid composition of the erythrocyte enzyme has never been published.* From its isoelectric point of approximately 6, as well as its behavior on ion exchange columns, there is nothing unusual in regard to its content of acidic or basic amino acids. Its spectrum provided no evidence for the presence of other than the usual amino acids, but this does not rule out the possible presence of modified amino acid residues containing essential selenium. Titration of the native enzyme with [^{203}Hg]p-mercuribenzoate (Flohe et al., 1971c) followed by gel filtration indicated the presence of three mercury-binding groups per mole (84,000 gm), while an additional three to four mercury-binding sites were detected following reduction of the enzyme with substrate levels of glutathione. These results were interpreted in terms of mercury binding to sulfhydryl groups formed by reduction of disulfide bonds, but now must be reconsidered in regard to the possible binding of mercury to selenium in the enzyme.

Following the discovery that the formation of GSH-Px activity in animals was dependent on selenium (Rotruck et al., 1971, 1972) and that radioactive selenium was extensively incorporated into the rat erythrocyte enzyme (Rotruck et al., 1973), fluorometric analysis of the 4000-fold purified enzyme showed a selenium content of 0.34%, equivalent to approximately 4 gm atoms of selenium per mole of ovine erythrocyte GSH-Px (Hoekstra et al., 1973; Oh et al., 1974a). This stoichiometry was independently confirmed by Flohe et al. (1973) following activation analysis of the crystalline GSH-Px from bovine erythrocytes. Since the enzyme is composed of four subunits and the subunits are alike, the presence of one selenium in each subunit is assumed, although this has not yet been established. The γ-spectrum of the irradiated enzyme sample revealed that no other metal detectable by neutron activation was present in the enzyme (Flohe et al., 1973).

The form of selenium in GSH-Px has not been established. It remains tightly bound to the enzyme during isolation, but preliminary studies (Ganther et al., 1974) indicate that much of the selenium is released

---

* The amino acid composition and other physicochemical data for rat liver GSH-Px have recently been published by Nakamura et al. (1974).

from the enzyme in a low molecular weight form after long storage. The released selenium had anionic properties but did not appear to be selenite. Whether this form of selenium represents a degradation product of the selenium in GSH-Px or a dissociable cofactor released during denaturation is not known.

B. Substrate Specificity

GSH-Px is highly specific for the donor substrate glutathione. For the erythrocyte enzyme, Mills (1959) found little activity with other tissue thiols such as cysteine, cysteinylglycine, and ergothioneine. GSH-Px did not catalyze the breakdown of hydrogen peroxide in the presence of o-tolidine, guaiacol, or pyrogallol, even though these compounds are widely used as hydrogen donors for other peroxidases. Flohe et al. (1971b), in a systematic study of the purified erythrocyte enzyme with twenty-nine thiols, also concluded that glutathione is the only substrate having physiological significance for this enzyme. Only γ-L-glutamyl-L-cysteine methyl ester and mercaptoacetic acid methyl ester gave more than 10% of the activity obtained with glutathione under the conditions employed. The possible importance of the α-carboxyl of the γ-glutamyl moiety of glutathione in substrate orientation was indicated by greatly decreased rates for derivatives having the carboxyl group esterified or having the γ-glutamyl substituted by β-aspartyl or acetyl radicals. For the enzyme obtained from rat liver supernatant fractions, Flohe et al. (1970) observed relative activities similar to that for the erythrocyte enzyme, using hydrogen peroxide as the other substrate; in contrast, Little and O'Brien (1968), who used linoleic acid hydroperoxide as the substrate for the liver enzyme, observed substantial activity for cysteine and cysteamine relative to glutathione. The specificity for the enzyme from liver mitochondria or tissues other than erythrocytes and liver does not appear to have been investigated. It should also be mentioned that many sulfhydryl compounds inhibit GSH-Px (Flohe et al., 1971b). Coenzyme A is a poor substrate and an especially potent inhibitor (Little et al., 1970b), as discussed in a subsequent section.

GSH-Px shows a rather low specificity for the peroxide substrate. For ten years following the discovery of the enzyme, it appears that hydrogen peroxide was exclusively employed, but since that time a wide variety of hydroperoxides was found to be decomposed by the enzyme at rates comparable to that of hydrogen peroxide. Little and O'Brien (1968), following their initial studies with linoleic acid hydroperoxide, demonstrated in addition the suitability of cumene hydroperoxide, t-butylhydroperoxide, and ethyl linolenate hydroperoxide as substrates for rat liver GSH-Px. Similar results were obtained by Holmberg (1968) for the enzyme from bovine lens. Gunzler et al. (1972) have described the kinetic behavior of the bovine erythrocyte enzyme with various hydroperoxides. Christophersen (1969) reported the reduction of thymine hydroperoxide and peroxidized DNA by rat liver GSH-Px.

The list of hydroperoxides that serve as substrates has been extended to steroids by the work of Little (1972). Steroid hydroperoxides may be formed as intermediates in steroid hydroxylations, and thus might be regarded as "normal" or "physiological" compounds, suggesting effects for GSH-Px beyond the protection of cell membranes from oxidative damage. Little (1972) tested six steroid hydroperoxides and found the rate of glutathione oxidation with progesterone-17α-hydroperoxide to be nearly as fast as with hydrogen peroxide. Three other steroid hydroperoxides showed definite activity as substrates, while cholesterol-25-hydroperoxide was inactive, the first hydroperoxide reported that could not be metabolized by GSH-Px. Rapid denaturation and precipitation of the enzyme occurred with 6-ketocholestanol-5α-hydroperoxide.

The relative activity of partially purified GSH-Px from pig aorta with various lipid hydroperoxides was found to vary widely, possibly influenced by solubility effects (Smith et al., 1973). The cholesteryl hydroperoxyoctadecadienoates present in atheromatous tissue were reduced to the hydroxy esters, but relatively slowly.

Recent studies of prostaglandin metabolism raise interesting questions in regard to the substrate specificity of GSH-Px. Hamberg et al. (1974) have demonstrated the formation of two intermediates in the biosynthesis of prostaglandin PGE_2 and $PGF_{2\alpha}$ from arachidonic acid. Both compounds have a peroxide bridge between ring carbons 9 and 11, and thus are called endoperoxides. One of these, named PGG_2, also has a hydroperoxy group at carbon 15 and appears to be the first stable compound formed from arachidonate. The other compound (PGH_2) has a hydroxy group at carbon 15. Whether GSH-Px might catalyze reduction of the hydroperoxy group at carbon fifteen of PGG_2 to the hydroxyl group, forming PGH_2, is not known. It also is not known whether or not the endoperoxide class of compounds can serve as substrates for the enzyme. In view of the high biological potency of these prostaglandin peroxides in stimulating platelet aggregation or aorta contraction (Hamberg et al., 1974; J. B. Smith et al., 1974), studies of their suitability as substrates for GSH-Px might have significance beyond the field of enzyme chemistry.

C. Inhibitors

Unlike heme proteins, neither the erythrocyte GSH-Px nor the liver enzyme (Little and O'Brien, 1968) is inhibited by cyanide or azide

(Mills, 1957; Mills and Randall, 1958). These substances are frequently added to suppress catalase in the assay for GSH-Px in crude systems.

A variety of classic thiol or dithiol reagents was tested as inhibitors of liver GSH-Px (Little and O'Brien, 1968). It was found that 3 mM p-mercuribenzoate or N-ethylmaleimide caused 60–70% inhibition but that the same concentration of iodoacetate, iodoacetamide, cadmium chloride, or sodium arsenite gave no inhibition. These results apparently were obtained on the native (probably oxidized) form of the enzyme without prior reduction with glutathione. Khandwala and Gee (1973) have reported that GSH-Px from alveolar macrophages is inhibited 50% by 5×10^{-5} M N-ethylmaleimide.

Schneider and Flohe (1967) found a weak, readily reversible inhibition of the erythrocyte enzyme with 2×10^{-4} M mercuric chloride following preincubation with 10^{-4} M glutathione, but in the presence of ethylene-diaminetetraacetic acid (EDTA), the same concentration of mercuric chloride caused more than 90% inhibition. It was postulated that EDTA formed a complex with mercuric chloride that was inhibitory to the enzyme, perhaps as a result of EDTA serving as a carrier to transport mercury to the active site. Examples of such a phenomenon with other enzymes are known (Wu, 1965). The enzyme was slightly and reversibly inhibited by sodium sulfite. Further studies with classic sulfhydryl inhibitors following reduction of the enzyme might be beneficial in regard to the possibility of an active-site selenol (E-SeH) being involved in catalysis.

A number of substances related to the glutathione substrate have been tested as inhibitors. Ophthalmic acid, a close relative of glutathione having a methyl group in place of the sulfhydryl group, does not inhibit the enzyme from lens (Holmberg, 1968) or erythrocytes (Flohe et al., 1971b) even at a severalfold molar ratio to glutathione. Cysteine had no effect on the enzyme from lens (Holmberg, 1968), but cysteine and several other thiols and disulfides were found to be inhibitory to erythrocyte GSH-Px (Flohe et al., 1971b), possibly as a result of mixed disulfide formation involving an enzyme sulfhydryl group, as suggested by Flohe et al. (1971b), or perhaps involving an enzyme–SeH group.

A number of substances unrelated to glutathione, except for their anionic character, are known to inhibit GSH-Px. High concentrations of multivalent anions, including phosphate, sulfate, and maleate, caused reversible inhibition of GSH-Px (Flohe and Brand, 1970). Holmberg (1968) reported that GSH-Px had a lower specific activity when assayed in phosphate than in tris buffer, but did not specify what anion was used with the tris. Flohe and Brand (1970) found no significant difference in activity with various cations (Na^+, K^+, $tris^+$). Beyond these rather nonspecific effects of anions, interesting effects of certain nucleo-tides on GSH-Px activity have been described. Little *et al.* (1970a) found a wide range of nucleotides such as reduced nicotinamide adenine dinucleotide phosphate (NADPH) to be more inhibitory than phosphate. The inhibitory effect increased with the number of phosphate groups in the nucleotide. The possibility of an allosteric type of inhibition of GSH-Px was supported by evidence for differential loss of catalytic activ-ity and nucleotide sensitivity after various physical or chemical treat-ments. Further study (Little *et al.*, 1970b) showed that coenzyme A was a much more potent inhibitor than other nucleotides, causing 50% inhibition at 6×10^{-5} M. Although blocking the sulfhydryl group of coenzyme A considerably decreased the inhibitory effect, the major effect was apparently related to the nucleotide moiety. The low levels of coen-zyme A in the erythrocyte preclude a physiologically significant type of inhibition there, but levels in liver are sufficiently high for the inhibi-tion to have possible physiological relevance.

D. Kinetics

The kinetic properties of GSH-Px are rather complicated, and no at-tempt at a detailed treatment of the subject will be undertaken here. The earlier literature was reviewed by Flohe (1971), and an extensive reinvestigation of the subject was subsequently published by Flohe *et al.* (1972), who used rapid reaction stopped-flow techniques to obviate technical problems.

Although three molecules of substrates are involved in the GSH-Px reaction, the general rate equation for the reaction reduces to a fairly simple expression, because many terms equal or approach zero (Flohe *et al.*, 1972). This mechanism, using the nomenclature of Cleland, is a ter uni ping pong mechanism; ternary complexes are not formed. The maximum velocity and limiting Michaelis constants are indeterminate; the apparent K_m for hydrogen peroxide increases with increasing glutathi-one but is only 8.8 μM at 2 mM glutathione (Flohe *et al.*, 1972). In practice, one does not see a dependency of the reaction rate on peroxide concentration under commonly used assay conditions (see Sec-tion III). The apparent K_m for glutathione is calculated to vary between 10^{-7} and 10^{-4} M when the concentration of hydrogen peroxide is in the nanomolar to micromolar range. Under physiological conditions, the enzyme should be present largely in the reduced state. The rate constant for the reaction of the reduced enzyme with hydrogen peroxide at physio-logical concentrations of substrates is estimated by Flohe *et al.* (1972) to be comparable to that observed with catalase.

Although the activity of GSH-Px is usually assayed near neutrality, its activity increases with increasing pH (Mills, 1959; Holmberg, 1968) and shows a distinct optimum at pH 8.8 (Flohe et al., 1972). According to the latter authors, denaturation of the enzyme does not seem to be a significant factor in the decline of activity below pH 10. The pH dependency of the enzyme is apparently not related to charge effects in the binding of the glutathione substrate, since mercaptoethanol methyl ester gave similar results. Although the nonenzymatic reaction rate is dependent on the acidity of the sulfhydryl group in various thiols, suggesting the importance of the RS⁻ concentration, this effect is not seen for the enzymatic reaction (Flohe et al., 1972), contrary to an earlier suggestion (Flohe, 1971). Unlike many other peroxidases of plant or animal origin, GSH-Px has no activity below pH 6 (Mills, 1959).

E. Possible Mechanisms

Based on their kinetic study, Flohe et al. (1972) concluded that the most probable general reaction mechanism involved an initial oxidation of the reduced enzyme by peroxide and a subsequent two-step reduction of the oxidized enzyme by glutathione. Such a sequence of three bimolecular oxidation–reduction steps involving oxidized and reduced forms of the enzyme seems to be more consistent with the kinetic data than the mechanism proposed by Little et al. (1970a) involving ternary complexes of enzyme, peroxide, and glutathione.

The explicit chemical reactions occurring at the active site of GSH-Px are not known. Prior to the discovery of selenium in GSH-Px, Flohe (1971) developed a detailed model and compared it to the tentative mechanism offered by Little et al. (1970a). Both of these mechanisms were based on the presence of a sulfhydryl group at the active site that formed a mixed disulfide intermediate with glutathione during the reaction. Flohe rejected the mechanism of Little et al., primarily on kinetic grounds, and proposed that the enzyme cycled between a dithiol form and a disulfide form (Scheme 1A). Participation of an active site disulfide could explain the finding that treatment with sulfite caused reversible inhibition of the enzyme (Flohe et al., 1971c). The fact that three to four additional moles of p-mercuribenzoate became bound per mole (84,000 gm) of GSH-Px following reduction of the enzyme with glutathione was attributed to reduction of the disulfide to a pair of sulfhydryls. However, such a mechanism requires that eight sulfhydryl groups be liberated from four active-site disulfides if the enzyme contains one active site per subunit, but only four at most were titrated. The discrepancy was attributed to the additional sulfhydryls being in an unaccessible form (despite the use of 5 M guanidine in some cases).

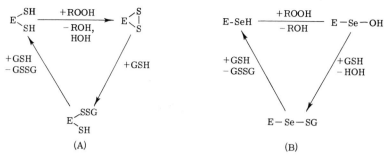

Scheme 1. Proposed mechanisms for glutathione peroxidase. (A) Flohe (1971); (B) Ganther et al. (1974).

The possibility of two active sites formed by linking two subunits together through disulfide bonds was not a plausible alternative, since there do not appear to be covalent bonds holding the subunits together. Also, there was no evidence for heterogeneous subunits, making it unlikely that only two subunits would have active sites.

The failure of arsenite and cadmium to inhibit GSH-Px (Little and O'Brien, 1968) further weakened the case for a vicinal dithiol moiety. Flohe et al. (1971c) felt that the sulfhydryl groups might be too far apart as a result of marked conformational change upon reduction of the enzyme, but the sulfhydryl groups would have to be brought close together at some stage of catalysis to form the disulfide, even if they were far apart at other times, so this is probably not a satisfactory explanation.

With the discovery that GSH-Px contains 4 gm atoms of selenium per mole, it is appropriate to reconsider the reaction mechanism. Although the selenium atoms have not yet been shown to function in catalysis, the unique chemical properties of selenium and its presence in stoichiometric amounts with the number of subunits make it attractive to propose a mechanism based on selenium functioning at the active site (Ganther et al., 1974). The first step in the proposed mechanism (Scheme 1B) begins with an active site selenol (E—SeH) undergoing oxidation with peroxide to a selenenic acid. The observed uptake of four additional moles of p-mercuribenzoate upon reduction of the enzyme (Flohe et al., 1971c) can be attributed to the complexing of four selenol groups, one per subunit. Unlike sulfenic acids, some selenenic acids are fairly stable, especially the aromatic types (Klayman, 1973). Since a single atom of selenium can undergo a two-election oxidation to a stable form, it is unnecessary to postulate an additional electron acceptor atom as is the case with sulfur in the dithiol–disulfide mechanism. In the second step of the mechanism, the oxidized form of the enzyme reacts with the first glutathione, forming the mixed selenosulfide

(E—Se—SG) and a molecule of water. In the third step, the selenosulfide linkage is cleaved by a second molecule of glutathione, similar to a sulfhydryl–disulfide interchange reaction, producing oxidized glutathione and restoring the enzyme to the selenol form. It is known that selenenic acids are reduced by thiols to selenols (Klayman, 1973). It is also known that the S—Se type of linkage is cleaved by thiols even more readily than the disulfide linkage (Walter et al., 1969; Ganther and Corcoran, 1969). This series of reactions is in accord with the series of three bimolecular reactions postulated by Flohe et al. (1972) on kinetic grounds. An analogous set of reactions can also be written in which the selenium cycles between selenenic (E—Se—OH) and seleninic (E—SeO₂H) forms (Ganther et al., 1974), but the sensitivity of the enzyme to N-ethylmaleimide and p-mercuribenzoate is more readily accounted for by a mechanism based on a selenol.

F. Variant Forms

Beutler and West (1974) subjected freshly prepared lysates of blood from 351 individuals to starch gel electrophoresis and detected a fast moving variant of GSH-Px in five cases. The variant was present in 4 out of 91 Negro subjects and 1 out of 255 Caucasians. The GSH-Px activities of lysates containing the fast moving form were normal. Although genetic studies suggested that the affected individuals were heterozygotes, only a single band could be distinguished on electrophoresis, and this overlapped only slightly with the normal band. A fast moving band of enzyme activity, as well as an additional slow band, developed in blood samples aged for several days. The fast band disappeared from aged samples after the addition of 1 mM glutathione or 2-mercaptoethanol, suggesting that it resulted from the formation of a mixed disulfide between glutathione and the protein, but the slow band persisted. The variant band observed in freshly drawn blood samples was unaffected by thiols, however.

Although Little et al. (1970a) raised the possibility of separate catalytic and regulatory sites in the enzyme in relation to allosteric regulation, the subunits of GSH-Px purified from erythrocytes appear to be homogeneous upon electrophoresis, and so the existence of catalytic subunits and regulatory subunits appears unlikely (Flohe et al., 1971c; Oh et al., 1974a). GSH-Px from sources other than erythrocytes has not been examined for possible isoenzyme forms, so the isolation and study of the enzyme from different tissues, or a comparison of cytosol and mitochondrial forms in tissues such as liver, would be desirable in this regard, as well as studies of the enzyme in various individuals.

III. ASSAY OF GLUTATHIONE PEROXIDASE

In his review of GSH-Px, Flohe (1971) listed four difficulties encountered in assaying the enzyme: (1) nonenzymatic reaction of the substrates, (2) reaction of substrates with other substances in biological materials, (3) inhibition of the enzyme by certain anions, and (4) lack of a definite pH optimum. In a subsequent paper, Flohe et al. (1972) were able to find a pH optimum for the enzyme at pH 8.8 using organic buffers and rapid reaction techniques. The nonenzymatic reaction, however, increases with pH and is quite substantial at this pH. In addition, these investigators found that the reaction mechanism is such that the limiting Michaelis constants and maximum velocities for both substrates are indeterminate. The apparent K_m for each substrate is proportional to the concentration of the other, so that both cannot be made saturating at the same time.* This means that when the enzyme is assayed by direct measurement of product formed or reactant remaining, the reaction is first order with respect to one of the substrates. This type of assay has most often been done by running the reaction at first order with respect to glutathione, stopping the reaction at intervals, and measuring the glutathione remaining by different methods (Flohe, 1971; Hafeman et al., 1974).

When the enzyme activity is assayed in this direct manner, the units of activity are expressed by different investigators as various multiples of K, the first-order reaction rate constant. Since this constant is independent of the initial concentrations of the substrates, these units can be compared directly when the multiplying factors are taken into account, provided that the buffer type and concentration, the pH, and the temperature of the reaction mixtures are the same.

It is possible to make the GSH-Px reaction pseudo zero order with respect to glutathione at saturating* concentrations of peroxide by continuously regenerating glutathione by means of the glutathione reductase-catalyzed reaction with NADPH. This method was first developed by

---

* In the coupled assay, the reaction shows apparent zero-order kinetics. In this case, the glutathione is continuously regenerated, so its concentration does not decline during the reaction. Peroxide concentration does decline, but with the relatively low level of glutathione and relatively high level of peroxide substrates employed (typically 1 mM glutathione and 0.1 mM peroxide), the K_m for peroxide (Flohe et al., 1972) is well below the peroxide concentration at all times, thus the enzyme is "saturated." At any rate, the continuously recorded decline in A_{340} shows no tendency for a slowing of the reaction until the NADPH (needed for glutathione reductase) is nearly exhausted.

Paglia and Valentine (1967) for assay of enzyme activity in red blood cells and has been variously adapted by different investigators for use in many different tissues. It is considerably more sensitive than the direct method (Emerson et al., 1972). The linearity of the curve obtained when absorbance is plotted against time during the initial phase of the coupled assay, in contrast to the nonlinearity for the same type of plot for the direct method, can be seen in the paper by Emerson et al. (1972) comparing the two methods. These authors unfortunately did not appreciate the necessity to plot the log of the absorbance change against time to obtain a linear curve in the direct procedure. Flohe and Brand (1969) have criticized the coupled method on the basis of lack of specificity of the reaction and inhibition of glutathione reductase by high concentrations of glutathione. They claim that glutathione reacts with many other substances in biological materials, including hemoglobin, and they present data showing catalysis of the reaction between hydrogen peroxide and glutathione by various hemoglobin derivatives. We have found, however, that there is no appreciable decrease in NADPH concentration when NADPH is incubated in the presence of various tissue homogenates, glutathione, and glutathione reductase without hydrogen peroxide, nor when the complete reaction mixture is incubated without GSH (A. A. Swanson, R. A. Lawrence, and W. G. Hoekstra, unpublished data). Furthermore, Flohe and Brand (1970) concede that conversion of hemoglobin to cyanmethemoglobin as described by Paglia and Valentine (1967) lowers the rate of the reaction catalyzed by hemoglobin considerably, and examination of their data shows that at the hemolyzate concentrations used routinely in the authors' laboratory to get easily measurable reaction rates for GSH-Px, the rate of the reaction catalyzed by cyanmethemoglobin is negligible. High concentrations of glutathione do cause product inhibition of glutathione reductase, and this fact makes the reaction unsuitable for kinetic studies in this range; reports of limiting K_m values for glutathione (Paglia and Valentine, 1967; Hochstein and Utley, 1968; Demus-Oole et al., 1969) using the coupled assay cannot be relied upon. This is not a problem for routine assays, provided that enough glutathione reductase is used so that it is not rate-limiting.

Centrifugation of samples to remove particulate matter before using the coupled assay method may lead to errors in some tissues, since appreciable amounts of enzyme activity may be associated with the particulate fraction, especially the mitochondria, if the usual mild homogenizing procedures are used (see Section IV,A). Furthermore, in samples where peroxidation of the mitochondria membrane has occurred, there is the possibility that more GSH-Px activity will appear in the cytosol, giving an apparent "adaptive" increase in GSH-Px. These potential errors should be evaluated for each tissue before using the coupled assay on that tissue.

With the coupled assay method, units of activity may be expressed as change in $A_{340 \text{ nm}}$ per minute, amount of NADPH oxidized per minute, amount of glutathione oxidized per minute, or, according to Flohe and Brand (1970), can be expressed in units equivalent to the K units of the direct assay as 0.5 [NADPH]/min [GSH]$_0$, where [GSH]$_0$ is the initial glutathione concentration. It must be emphasized that units of activity measured with different assays cannot be directly compared unless they are expressed in equivalent units and the reactions are run under the same conditions of pH, temperature, and buffer concentrations.

The activity of purified GSH-Px is strongly enhanced by preincubation with glutathione (Little et al., 1970a). We have found that this activation is readily observed during the first few minutes when the activity of GSH-Px is continuously recorded using the coupled assay, and is not seen when the enzyme is preincubated with glutathione for 5 min before peroxide addition. Flohe et al. (1972) also have noted this effect and find that the range of activation varies between 0 and 300% depending on purity of the enzyme and storage conditions. Highly purified samples show the greatest effect, typically a two- to threefold activation. Flohe et al. (1972) state that other thiols can substitute for glutathione but that their efficiency seems to be related to their suitability as substrates, mercaptoacetic acid ethyl ester being good and 2-mercaptoethanol poor.

It is to be noted that in assay procedures based on glutathione disappearance, the first portion for glutathione determination is usually taken 1 min after starting the reaction. This delay was not customary in the coupled assay of Paglia and Valentine (1967), which was developed for assaying GSH-Px in relatively crude hemolyzate preparations. Flohe and Brand (1970) failed to obtain a constant rate of reaction during the first minute of the reaction when using the method of Paglia and Valentine with purified enzyme. In retrospect, this result may have been caused by a failure to take into account the necessity for reactivating the purified enzyme.

For clinical screening purposes, where time, technical skills, or equipment are not available to conduct one of the previously mentioned assays, the spot test developed by Boguslawska-Jaworska and Kaplan (1969) or a similar test seems to be adequate. A method for the detection of GSH-Px activity on starch gels after electrophoresis of red cell lysates, based on the decrease in fluorescence of NADPH in a coupled procedure using glutathione reductase, has been developed by Beutler and West (1974).

IV. DISTRIBUTION OF GLUTATHIONE PEROXIDASE

A. General Distribution and Dependence on Dietary Selenium

Although originally discovered in erythrocytes, GSH-Px has since been shown to occur in many body organs, tissues, cells, subcellular components, and fluids. It has not been successfully demonstrated in plant tissues (Flohe, 1971), and apparently no attempt has been made to study extensively its occurrence in microorganisms. However, its presence in *Candida lipolytica* has been reported (Grosch *et al.*, 1972), and preliminary unpublished work (R. Sunde and W. G. Hoekstra, 1974) has suggested a low level of such catalytic activity in extracts of *Neurospora crassa*. However, it has not been demonstrated that such catalysis in *Neurospora* results from a specific isolatable GSH-Px.

Mills (1960) first compared the GSH-Px activity of various organs or tissues of the rat and found liver to be highest with moderately high activity in erythrocytes, heart, lung and kidneys and only slight, possibly insignificant, activity in intestinal tract and skeletal muscle. The most extensive recent surveys of GSH-Px activity in various tissues have been those conducted in relation to the effects of selenium deficiency on GSH-Px. Because of the different experimental conditions, methods of assay, definitions of enzyme units and bases for expressing the data, values reported in different studies for a tissue can not often be compared directly. However, the relative GSH-Px activities of various tissues determined in a single study should give a reasonable comparison for the different body components.

Table II presents examples of some of the more recent comparisons of GSH-Px activities of various tissues of animals that have received presumably adequate quantities of selenium (at least 0.1 ppm selenium) with those for animals fed selenium-deficient diets (usually 0.02 ppm selenium or less). The reader is cautioned to compare directly only values within a given study and to refer to the conditions and method of expressing the results that are briefly outlined in the table. The two basically different methods of assay that have been used, i.e., the direct determination of glutathione disappearance and the enzymatically coupled method (see Section III), may not give an identical pattern of GSH-Px distribution; however, the ranking of tissues in decreasing order should be similar.

A number of general conclusions can be drawn from the data presented in Table II. For selenium-adequate rats, the body components can be arbitrarily separated into three general categories with respect to GSH-Px

TABLE II Recent Data on the Glutathione Peroxidase Activities of Various Body Components and Their Response to Dietary Selenium Intake

Species, conditions, and reference	Body component	Glutathione peroxidase activity		
		+Se	−Se	−Se/+Se × 100
Rat—0.5 ppm selenium supplied as sodium selenite versus basal selenium-deficient diet. Males only. Assays made when weanling rats had been fed respective diets for 13–28 weeks. Tissue homogenates assayed by direct determination of GSH disappearance. Values are enzyme units (a decrease in log[GSH] of 0.001 per min is 1 EU) per mg protein. Hoekstra (1974)	Liver	49	3.0	7
	Kidney	48	11	22
	Heart	24	1.0	4
	Adrenal gland	14	4.0	36
	Lung	9.0	0.9	10
	Brain	2.3	1.5	65
	Testis	1.9	0.8	42
Rat—0.1 ppm selenium supplied as sodium selenite versus basal selenium-deficient diet. Males only. Assays made when weanling rats had been fed the respective diets for the time indicated in next column. Samples assayed by direct determination of GSH disappearance. Values are enzyme units (see first listing) per gm fresh tissue for liver and enzyme units per mg hemoglobin for erythrocytes. Hafeman et al. (1974).	Liver			
	10 days	6,310	1490	24
	134 days	8,260	0	0
	Erythrocytes			
	17 days	34	20	59
	66 days	34	9	24
Rat—0.1 ppm selenium supplied as sodium selenite versus basal selenium-deficient diet. Females only, except testis. Assays made on rats fed the diets to 6–9 months of age born from dams that had been fed the respective diets from weaning. Samples assayed by direct determination of GSH disappearance. Values are enzyme units (see first listing) per gm fresh tissue. Lawrence et al. (1974).	Liver	16,000	0	0
	Erythrocytes	9,600	2630	27
	Kidney	5,050	1760	35
	Adrenal gland	4,220	2250	53
	Heart	2,180	51	2
	Lung	1,620	132	8
	Testis	183	98	54
	Brain	132	82	62
	Lens	84	12	14
Rat—0.2 ppm selenium supplied as selenomethionine versus basal selenium-deficient diet. Males only. Assays made when weanling rats had been fed	Plasma	700	50	14
	Liver	210	70	33
	Heart	100	10	10
	Erythrocytes	90	40	44
	Kidney	90	20	25

TABLE II   (Continued)

Species, conditions, and reference	Body component	Glutathione peroxidase activity		
		+Se	−Se	−Se/+Se × 100
respective diets for 5 weeks. Soluble, or cytosolic, fraction assayed by the coupled method and values expressed as nmoles NADPH oxidized per min per mg protein (or per ml for plasma). Values estimated from published graphs. P. J. Smith et al. (1974).	Lung	60	15	22
	Skeletal muscle	<10	?	?
Rat—1-month-old normal male rats (designated as +Se) versus the same rats following 28 days depletion on a −Se diet. Plasma, lysed erythrocytes, and soluble or cytosolic fraction of tissues assayed by the coupled method and values expressed as nmoles NADPH oxidized per min per mg protein. Values estimated from published graphs and percentage figures in text. The values for plasma have been divided by 35 to correct an error in the original publication where plasma values were mistakenly reported as units/mg protein. (Chow and Tappel estimate rat plasma contained 35 mg protein/ml) Chow and Tappel (1974).	Plasma	31	2	6
	Liver	310	165	53
	Erythrocytes	170	170	100
	Heart	125	60	47
	Kidney	110	50	45
	Lung	57	35	61
	Testis	45	90	200
Rat—2.0 ppm selenium supplied as selenomethionine versus basal selenium-deficient diet. Males only. All rats at 1-month of age were depleted for 2 weeks on the −Se diet and then fed for 4 weeks the respective −Se or +Se diet. Plasma, lysed erythrocytes and soluble, or cytosolic, fraction of tissues assayed by the coupled method and values expressed as nmoles NADPH oxidized per min per mg protein. Values for rats fed peroxidized corn oil are not included. Reddy and Tappel (1974).	Liver	540	75	14
	Erythrocytes	333	74	22
	Stomach mucosa	91	8	9
	Paraepididymal adipose tissue	83	15	18
	Plasma	35	3	9
	Small intestine mucosa			
	Upper thrid	18	9	50
	Middle third	15	8	53
	Lower third	19	5	26
	Cecum mucosa	18	6	33

TABLE II (Continued)

Species, conditions, and reference	Body component	Glutathione peroxidase activity		
		+Se	−Se	−Se/+Se × 100
Chick—0.1 ppm selenium supplied as sodium selenite versus basal selenium-deficient diet. Females only. Assays were made when newly hatched chicks had been fed the respective diets for the time indicated in next column. Samples assayed by direct determination of GSH disappearance. Values are enzyme units (1% of GSH disappearance per min is 1 EU) per mg N. Values estimated from published graphs. Noguchi et al. (1973).	Plasma 6 days 11 days Liver 6 days 11 days Erythrocytes 6 days 11 days	12 14 10 9 14 13	2 <1 5 3 13 10	17 <7 50 33 93 77
Chick—0.1 ppm selenium (+Se) supplied as selenomethionine (values for 0.1 ppm selenium as sodium selenite in parenthesis). Males only. Assays were made when newly hatched chicks had been fed the diets for 20–24 days. Plasma, lysed erythrocytes and soluble, or cytosolic, fraction of tissues assayed by the coupled method and values expressed as nmoles NADPH oxidized per min per mg protein. Omaye and Tappel (1974a).	Liver Heart Erythrocytes Plasma Pancreas Lung Skeletal muscle	51(64) 14(24) 12(16) 12(10) 10(11) 9(10) 5(3)	—[a] —[a] —[a] 1.2 — — —	—[a] —[a] —[a] 10 — — —
Lamb—0.1 ppm selenium supplied as sodium selenite versus basal selenium-deficient diet. Data includes that for males and females (except testis). Assays made when newborn lambs had been fed the respective diets for 8 weeks. Samples assayed by direct determination of GSH disappearance. Values are enzyme units (a decrease in log[GSH] of 0.001 is 1 EU) per gm fresh tissue. S. H. Oh, A. L. Pope, and W. G. Hoekstra (Oh, 1975).	Erythrocytes Kidney Lung Heart Adrenal gland Testis Pancreas Liver Plasma Skeletal muscle	21,700 2,710 1,720 1,470 1,430 575 (2 lambs) 438 348 261 140	7810 298 289 130 391 658 (1 lamb) 37 4 3 13	36 11 17 9 27 114? 8 1 1 9

[a] All body components studied had GSH-Px activity in proportion to the log of the selenium intake (from 0.013 to 14.0 ppm. selenium). The magnitude of this relationship (slope) was in the order plasma > liver > heart > lung > pancreas > skeletal muscle.

activity. Those components that are usually highest in GSH-Px activity in the rat include liver and erythrocytes; those usually moderate or intermediate in activity include heart, kidney, lung, adrenal glands, stomach mucosa, pancreas, and adipose tissue. Those of low GSH-Px activity include brain, testis, eye lens, and skeletal muscle. For the chick, a generally similar pattern appears to exist; however, all values appear to be lower than for the rat—e.g., compare Omaye and Tappel (1974a) with Chow and Tappel (1974). For the lamb, some marked differences from the rat exist; in particular, lamb erythrocytes are very high in GSH-Px, while liver is among the organs lowest in GSH-Px. It is abundantly clear that one cannot extrapolate from one species to another with respect to GSH-Px activities of specific body components or the relative distribution of GSH-Px within the body. Studies to determine the biological causes and physiological significances of such species differences and their relation to (a) selenium- and vitamin E-responsive diseases, (b) sites and amounts of peroxide production or other oxidant stressors, and (c) other mechanisms of protection against oxidant damage (e.g., catalase and superoxide dismutase) should be interesting and worthwhile.

In addition to the body components listed in Table II, GSH-Px activity has been found in apparently large amounts in phagocytic cells such as leukocytes and macrophages (see Section V,A,2) and blood platelets (see Section V,A,3) and in small but detectable amounts in aorta (Smith et al., 1973), in parts of the eye in addition to lens (Reim et al., 1974), and in uterus (Little, 1972). In the case of human subjects, studies on GSH-Px have so far been almost entirely confined to blood components (see Section V,A). From the studies to date, it can be stated that GSH-Px is present in a large variety of body components of animals (perhaps all tissues), but in grossly different amounts in different tissues and with substantial differences between animal species.

Data on blood plasma GSH-Px are confusing. GSH-Px activity has been found in plasma, but various studies indicate amounts from high to low, compared to other tissues (see Table II). The nature of plasma GSH-Px is a needed area of study. How much of the activity has arisen from blood platelets or possibly leakage from other cellular components of blood? To what extent does GSH-Px activity in plasma represent leakage from other tissues, and what are the primary tissues of origin? Does free enzyme exist in blood plasma in vivo, and does it carry out a physiological function as proposed by Noguchi et al. (1973)? Plasma GSH-Px is further discussed in Section V,A,4.

Another major conclusion that can be drawn from Table II is that selenium intake dramatically affects the GSH-Px activity of body components and the relative body distribution of the enzyme. In studies of long-term selenium deficiency, some decrease in GSH-Px activity is observed in all body components studied, but the magnitude of decrease varies greatly for different tissues. Short-term studies show rapid depletion of GSH-Px in some components such as plasma and liver, but little or no depletion in tissues such as testis and lens. For a given species, the relative GSH-Px activities of tissues of selenium-supplemented versus selenium-deficient animals undoubtedly depends on the extent and duration of selenium deficiency, on the actual levels of selenium intake compared, and perhaps on other dietary or environmental conditions. Thus, some variation between studies in the extent of GSH-Px depletion induced by selenium deficiency is apparent. However, the body components in which GSH-Px activity has been most extensively depleted due to dietary selenium deficiency include plasma, liver, heart, lungs, stomach mucosa, skeletal muscle, and lens. Components showing at least moderate decreases in GSH-Px include kidney, adrenal glands, and erythrocytes, and those that appear least subject to GSH-Px depletion are testis and brain. The smaller response of GSH-Px to dietary selenium intake in organs such as testis and brain may in part be a reflection of slow turnover; however, there appears to be in addition an adaptive mechanism for allowing a limited selenium intake to be preferentially utilized by certain tissues. In the case of testis, it is interesting that this organ has the ability to retain a surprisingly large part of an administered tracer dose of ^{75}Se when the rat is deficient in selenium (Brown and Burk, 1973), but whether GSH-Px accounts for a substantial part of the testicular selenium and is of special significance to testicular tissue or spermatozoa is presently unknown.

According to the results of Tappel and co-workers with the rat (P. J. Smith et al., 1974) and the chick (Omaye and Tappel, 1974a), the activity of GSH-Px is considered to increase in proportion to the logarithm of the dietary selenium concentration, even to chronically toxic levels of selenium. A similar response has been observed for rat erythrocytes by Hafeman et al. (1974), but liver did not respond in a like manner. Liver showed a plateau of GSH-Px activity in the range of the selenium requirement, and GSH-Px actually decreased per unit of liver weight (or liver protein), with a chronically toxic dose of 5 ppm selenium provided as selenite, which apparently was the result of liver damage. Studies with lambs (Oh et al., 1974b; Hoekstra, 1974, and unpublished data), which employed various levels of dietary selenium (up to 0.5 ppm) supplied as selenite, showed a continuous increase in GSH-Px up to the highest level of selenium for erythrocytes and pancreas, but eight other tissues assayed showed a plateau of GSH-Px activity at about 0.1 ppm selenium, which is considered to be in the range of the selenium requirement. One might reason that an enzyme level should plateau when the requirement for its trace element constituent is met; however, this does not hold for some components, such as erythrocytes, and perhaps all body tissues if a sufficiently wide range of selenium intakes is studied. Hafeman *et al.* (1974) suggested that the continued increase of erythrocyte GSH-Px with increasing dietary selenite may reflect an adaptive change to the "oxidant stressor" effect of an excess of selenite, which may also occur in other tissues if the selenium intake exceeds a certain point. Stated another way, the homeostatic regulation of selenium may be limited to a rather narrow range above the selenium requirement, and in this range, plateauing of GSH-Px in relation to selenium intake may be observed in some organs, but when effective homeostatic regulation is exceeded, adaptive increases in GSH-Px may occur. Further studies are needed to clarify the relation of selenium intake, particularly excessive levels, to GSH-Px activity.

Information on the subcellular localization of GSH-Px is available for liver. Green and O'Brien (1970) found that of the nuclei-free homogenate of rat liver, 60% of the total GSH-Px was recovered in the soluble or cystosolic fraction and 28% in the mitochondrial fraction. The soluble fraction had a specific activity for GSH-Px of 31 units/mg protein, while the mitochondrial fraction had 17 units/mg protein, and the microsomal and lysosomal fractions had much lower amounts, which could be accounted for by contamination. No values were given for the nuclear fraction. From studies of the release of mitochondrial GSH-Px in response to various agents, the conclusion was drawn that within the mitochondria GSH-Px was located within the mitochondrial matrix and may be responsible for protecting the inner membrane, while cytosolic GSH-Px may protect the outer membrane. Flohe and Schlegel (1971) has also concluded that the noncytosolic, particulate portion of liver GSH-Px must be attributed almost quantitatively to the miotochondria. Recent studies of Levander *et al.* (1974) have shown that GSH-Px accounts for a large fraction (at least 60%) of the total mitochondrial selenium of rats fed 0.1 ppm dietary selenium. Reports in which rather large amounts of GSH-Px activity are associated with other particulate fractions, such as the nuclear fraction (Demus-Oole and Swierczewski, 1969a; Noguchi *et al.*, 1973), must be viewed with caution until more highly purified and carefully characterized preparations are studied. In the case of erythrocytes, some GSH-Px activity is found in the isolated membrane (or ghost) fraction, but it appears to be loosely bound, as is the case for hemoglobin (Duchon and Collier, 1971).

B. Factors Other Than Selenium That Affect Glutathione Peroxidase Activities in Tissues

The association between selenium intake and tissue GSH-Px activity documented in the previous section is easily explainable by the presence of selenium in the active enzyme. However, selenium intake is not the only factor influencing tissue GSH-Px activity. A number of other dietary, physiological, pathological, and environmental factors have been shown to either increase or decrease GSH-Px activity. Usually, it is not known how these factors alter tissue GSH-Px; some may act through alterations of selenium metabolism or by altering the "oxidant stress" to the cell. The interaction between selenium intake and the response of GSH-Px to most of these factors has not yet been assessed, but such studies are obviously of interest. Some of these factors will be briefly reviewed.

1. Age and Sex

Studies on the effects of age and sex on GSH-Px have focused on liver and erythrocytes. Age and sex effects on rat liver GSH-Px were demonstrated by Pinto and Bartley (1969a). GSH-Px activity of fetal male rat liver was about 35% of the adult male value, and there was a steady and rather rapid increase in liver GSH-Px from birth to 55 days of age, at which time the young adult value was essentially reached. However, aged male rats (18 months of age) had a liver GSH-Px that was 40% above the young adult values. Female rats were similar at birth, but by 45 days of age, their liver GSH-Px had begun to rise above the male value, and by 4 months of age was 80% above male values. These changes in GSH-Px were unrelated to the dietary change that took place at weaning. Still greater but qualitatively similar age and sex effects on rat liver GSH-Px were found by Demus-Oole and Swierczewski (1969b) for liver soluble fraction; however, they showed that the increase in activity did not begin until more than 8 days of age, with a rapid increase between 8 days and 1 month of age. The sex difference was shown by Pinto and Bartley (1969b) to be the result of increased liver GSH-Px caused by the female hormones estrogens and progesterone, and to reflect a greater susceptibility of female liver to peroxidation *in vitro*, which was due in part to greater unsaturation of liver lipids. Such sex effects have been repeatedly confirmed, but the difference observed in liver apparently does not hold for other tissues, such as kidney and adrenal glands (Little, 1972).

Studies on the effects of age on erythrocyte GSH-Px in humans have usually, but not invariably, shown a lower level of GSH-Px in erythro-cytes of the newborn compared to the adult. This is discussed in Section VI,A. Such differences between studies may relate to differences in sele-nium status, but this has not yet been studied.

2. Oxidant Stressors

Recent evidence has suggested that GSH-Px may be an "adaptive enzyme," often increasing in response to oxidant stressors. Chow and Tappel (1972, 1973) have shown that in rats exposed to ozone there is an increase in lung cytosolic GSH-Px. Similarly, Reddy and Tappel (1974) have demonstrated an increased GSH-Px activity in several tis-sues of rats fed peroxidized corn oil; such an increase was observed when selenium in the diet was limiting (basal, low-selenium diet), but not when selenium was present at a more than adequate level (2 ppm). Presumably there was an "excess" of the enzyme in the latter situation and "induction" was not observed. Vitamin E deficiency also tends to increase tissue GSH-Px (Chow et al., 1973), apparently because of the greater susceptibility of the tissues to peroxidation. Ethanol has been shown to increase liver GSH-Px activity, which may relate to lipid peroxi-dation induced by ethanol (MacDonald, 1973). It is of interest that animals with genetically-induced muscular dystrophy have increased GSH-Px activity in muscle tissue, suggesting an increased susceptibility to peroxidation (Omaye and Tappel, 1974b) or possibly an increased production of oxidant stressors in the tissue.

3. Other Toxicants

A number of additional toxicants that cannot be considered as obvious oxidant stressors or antioxidants have been shown to alter tissue GSH-Px activity. Some of these appear to exert their effect through an influence on selenium metabolism, particularly on its utilization for synthesis of GSH-Px. Silver and tri-o-cresyl phosphate are in this category. Silver has been shown to precipitate in rats and chicks the defects characteristic of selenium–vitamin E deficiency (Bunyan et al., 1968). We have recently demonstrated that inclusion of 750 ppm silver supplied as silver acetate in the water supply of rats fed a liberal amount of selenium (0.5 ppm) supplied as selenite produces a profound depression of liver GSH-Px and smaller but major decreases in GSH-Px activity in other tissues, such as erythrocytes and kidney (Wagner et al., 1975; Wagner, 1975; Swanson et al., 1974; Hoekstra, 1975). The pattern of decrease in GSH-Px suggests that silver induced a conditioned selenium deficiency by causing an almost complete block in the utilization of selenite for the ultimate synthesis of GSH-Px. The exact mechanism of reaction between silver and selenite or its metabolites is not known, but it does not appear to be through inhibited absorption. Rat tissues can reduce selenite to hydrogen selenide (Ganther and Hsieh, 1974), which might form insoluble silver selenide. Feeding additional selenite to counteract the effects of silver causes an increase in silver concentration in the liver, suggesting that slowly metabolizable "complexes" of silver and selenium may be formed that may explain the interaction between the two elements. Mercury, as methylmercury, did not depress liver GSH-Px as did silver; in fact, an increase in liver GSH-Px from methylmercury has been consistently observed (P. Wagner, H. E. Ganther, and W. G. Hoekstra, unpublished data). However, methylmercury did cause decreases in GSH-Px of some other body organs (P. Wagner, H. E. Ganther, and W. G. Hoekstra, unpublished data), and mercury has been shown to precipitate signs of selenium deficiency in pigs (Froseth et al., 1974). The ability of selenite to decrease methylmercury toxicity (Ganther et al., 1972) is well established.

Tri-o-cresyl phosphate (TOCP) also produces toxicity effects that are alleviated, at least in part, by vitamin E and selenium, with selenium reported to be the more effective of the two nutrients (Shull and Cheeke, 1973). Recent work in our laboratory (Swanson et al., 1974, and Swanson, 1975) has shown a dramatic decrease in liver GSH-Px and a smaller decrease in liver selenium as a result of feeding 0.2% tri-o-cresyl phosphate in the diet of rats. Effects on GSH-Px and selenium in other organs were less dramatic. Metabolism of ^{75}Se supplied as selenite is grossly altered by tri-o-cresyl phosphate, as evidenced by greater urinary and fecal excretion of ^{75}Se and a dramatically altered body distribution of ^{75}Se. The mechanism whereby tri-o-cresyl phosphate or its metabolites interfere with selenium metabolism, and particularly with its incorporation into GSH-Px, remains to be discovered. This may become clearer as a better understanding of the steps involved in selenium incorporation into the enzyme evolves. Diethylnitrosamine, a potent carcinogen, has also been shown to depress liver GSH-Px activity in rat liver while increasing liver glutathione reductase (Pinto and Bartley, 1973). Such effects of drugs and other dietary factors on liver GSH-Px are not explained by decreased food intake, since work in our laboratory (R. A. Lawrence, 1975) has shown no decrease in liver GSH-Px with greatly restricted feed intakes (paired-feeding technique). However, Pinto and Bartley (1973) have shown that complete starvation of duration greater than 4 days does cause an ultimate decrease in liver GSH-Px activity.

4. Iron-Deficiency Anemia and Other Anemias

Recent reports show that iron-deficiency anemia is accompanied by decreased erythrocyte GSH-Px activity, and supplementation with iron causes a rapid increase in GSH-Px (MacDougall, 1972; Hopkins and Tudhope, 1973; Rodvien et al., 1974). While the studies in humans suggest that the decrease in GSH-Px parallels the decrease in hemoglobin (MacDougall, 1972; Hopkins and Tudhope, 1973), a study with rabbits demonstrated that the decrease in GSH-Px was manifest even when expressed per unit of hemoglobin (Rodvien et al., 1974). This depressed erythrocyte GSH-Px was suggested as the possible cause of the shortened life-span of erythrocytes in iron deficiency. The effect of iron deficiency on GSH-Px was not caused by anemia per se, since anemia induced by bleeding or phenylhydrazine did not cause a decreased GSH-Px (Rodvien et al., 1974), and pernicious anemia in man (a conditioned vitamin B_{12} deficiency) was accompanied not by a decreased, but an increased level of erythrocyte GSH-Px (Hopkins and Tudhope, 1973). The relation of iron to GSH-Px remains to be clarified. Iron is apparently not a component of GSH-Px, so that its effect must be by some other mechanism. Studies on the effect of iron deficiency on GSH-Px in tissues other than erythrocytes are lacking. Iron-containing enzymes may be involved in selenium metabolism (i.e., in GSH-Px synthesis), or perhaps some feedback effect from lack of hemoglobin depresses the amount of GSH-Px synthesized by the developing erythrocyte.

V. CELLULAR FUNCTIONS OF GLUTATHIONE PEROXIDASE

A. Blood

1. Erythrocytes

The role of GSH-Px in the erythrocyte is discussed in Flohe's review (1971) of the enzymology and biological aspects of the enzyme and is also a part of several reviews on the more general topic of drug-induced hemolytic anemias associated with enzyme deficiencies and their detection and treatment (Beutler, 1972a,b; Fairbanks and Fernandez, 1969; Jaffe, 1970; Keitt, 1971; Neely and Kraus, 1972; Kaplan, 1971; Swanson, 1973; Valentine, 1972). In this paper we will attempt only to correlate the more recent observations on the topic and suggest directions for further research.

The glutathione-dependent pathway concerned with the protection of the red blood cell from oxidative damage due to hydrogen peroxide

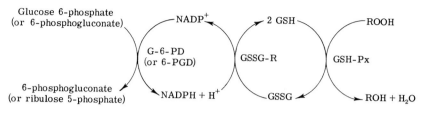

Scheme 2. Glutathione peroxidase-dependent peroxide decomposition in relation to hexose monophosphate shunt. G-6-PD = glucose-6-phosphate dehydrogenase; 6-PGD = 6-phosphogluconate dehydrogenase; GSSG-R = glutathione reductase; GSH-Px = glutathione peroxidase.

and other peroxides is shown schematically in Scheme 2. The preferential oxidation of glutathione by peroxides is catalyzed by GSH-Px. The oxidized glutathione is then reduced by NADPH in a reaction catalyzed by glutathione reductase. The only known mechanism for the reduction of NADP in the mature erythrocyte is by oxidation of glucose via the hexose monophosphate shunt pathway. Decreased activity of any of the four enzymes in the pathway or the enzymes of glutathione synthesis due to genetic deficiency, the presence of inhibitors, deficiency of dietary factors necessary for their synthesis or activity (certain amino acids, riboflavin, selenium), or deficiency of any of the building blocks of the substrates involved (niacin, sulfur amino acids) might be expected to result in impaired functioning of this protective pathway, leading to oxidative damage to hemoglobin, precipitation of Heinz bodies, and hemolytic anemia subsequent to oxidative challenge.

Genetic deficiencies of each of the enzymes in the pathway as well as the enzymes of glutathione synthesis have been implicated as causes for increased sensitivity to oxidant drugs. Glucose-6-phosphate dehydrogenase (G-6-PD) deficiency is by far the most common of these (Beutler, 1965, 1969a; Carson and Frischer, 1966) and results in lack of sufficient NADPH to reduce the oxidized glutathione produced in oxidative stress. Reports of oxidant sensitivity with 6-phosphogluconate dehydrogenase deficiency have also appeared (Brewer, 1969; Scialom et al., 1966; Lausecker et al., 1965). Deficiency of this activity would not only block another NADP-reducing step but also could cause accumulation of 6-phosphogluconate, leading to product inhibition of G-6-PD. Glutathione reductase deficiency was originally thought to be a genetic disorder (Carson et al., 1961; Waller, 1968), but subsequent reports (Glatzle et al., 1968; Beutler, 1969a,b) have indicated that in a majority of cases glutathione reductase deficiency is due to mild riboflavin deficiency and that animals and human subjects made deficient in glutathione reductase by a partial riboflavin deficiency do not show increased sensitivity to oxidant drugs (Beutler and Srivastava, 1970; Jaffe et al., 1968; Paniker *et al.,* 1970). Likewise, GSH-Px deficiency, although previously attributed to genetic causes, could be due in part to selenium deficiency. Several clinical cases of GSH-Px deficiency associated with hemolysis have been described (Gharib *et al.,* 1969; Necheles *et al.,* 1967, 1969, 1970; Boivin *et al.,* 1969; Steinberg *et al.,* 1970; Steinberg and Necheles, 1971; Nishimura *et al.,* 1972), and when the deficiency is sufficiently severe, extensive hemolysis has resulted even in the absence of external oxidative challenge (see Section VI,A). A lack of reduced glutathione caused by deficiency of glutathione synthesis has also been reported to result in severe drug-induced anemia (Waller and Gerok, 1964) or congenital hemolytic anemia (Prins *et al.,* 1966; Boivin *et al.,* 1966).

The presence of relatively large amounts of catalase in the red blood cell raises some question about the essentiality of the glutathione-dependent pathway for the removal of hydrogen peroxide. Nicholls, in his earlier publication on the subject (1965) discounted the role of GSH-Px in protecting hemoglobin from peroxidation but later modified his position (Nicholls, 1972) and now maintains that both are important. Paniker and Iyer (1965, 1969, 1972), Aebi *et al.* (1964a,b), Aebi and Suter (1966), and Jacob *et al.* (1965) all favor nearly equal roles for the two, with GSH-Px being more important at low concentrations and catalase at high concentrations of hydrogen peroxide, but with either being capable of protecting adequately in the absence of the other. Cohen and Hochstein (1963) and Tudhope and Leece (1971), on the other hand, maintain that GSH-Px is the primary agent for eliminating hydrogen peroxide at the low concentrations found *in vivo.* In support of the latter view, erythrocytes having normal levels of catalase but deficient in G-6-PD are more susceptible to oxidant drugs than are normal erythrocytes. Many of these drugs, however, have been shown to inhibit catalase to varying degrees (Tudhope and Leece, 1971), and glutathione may function in other ways to enhance the stability of the erythrocyte and its hemoglobin. GSH-Px activity of erythrocytes has been shown to vary with species (see Section IV,A), and the relative amounts of GSH-Px and catalase and hence their relative importance in removing hydrogen peroxide may vary widely in different species.

In addition to catalyzing the destruction of hydrogen peroxide, GSH-Px catalyzes the reduction of a wide variety of hydroperoxides other than hydrogen peroxide (see Section II,B) against which catalase is inactive. The role of these other hydroperoxides in promoting the destruction of red cells and hemoglobin is unclear. In a recent re-evaluation of the kinetics of GSH-Px, Flohe *et al.* (1972) have concluded that catalase and GSH-Px are equally effective in competing for hydrogen peroxide and that the increased sensitivity of GSH-Px-deficient erythrocytes to oxidation in the presence of catalase and the essential role of the glutathione-dependent pathway in the red blood cell are due to the ability of GSH-Px to reduce hydroperoxides of nearly any structure, such as might be produced by free radical reactions (Pryor, 1973) involving the oxidant drugs known to produce hemoylsis.

Very little has appeared on possible physiologically important inhibitors of GSH-Px or the other enzymes in the glutathione pathway with regard to promoting erythrocyte hemolysis (Little et al., 1970a; Vetrella and Barthelmai, 1972). More work needs to be done to determine if enzyme inhibition by some drugs either of the natural form of the enzyme or a more susceptible genetic variant can account for their effects in increasing hemolysis.

2. Phagocytic Cells

Because GSH-Px functions to protect cells from hydrogen peroxide and lipid hydroperoxides through its catalysis of the glutathione-dependent reduction of these compounds, the enzyme is of particular interest in regard to phagocytic cells, which greatly increase their peroxide production and lipid turnover during particle ingestion (phagocytosis). These cells include granulocytes (neutrophils, basophils, eosinophils) and monocytes in the blood, as well as specialized tissue macrophages such as alveolar and peritoneal macrophages. Following the ingestion of foreign objects, oxygen consumption increases markedly (respiratory burst), hydrogen peroxide is formed, and hexose monophosphate shunt activity increases (Klebanoff, 1971). Highly reactive forms of oxygen such as singlet oxygen and the superoxide radical also appear to be generated and may be directly or indirectly involved in the killing process (Allen et al., 1972; Babior et al., 1973; Curnutte and Babior, 1974). Although the ingested object is completely enclosed in a membranous structure (the phagolysosome), peroxides and other substances may diffuse from the phagolysosomes into the surrounding cytoplasm. Thus, the phagocytic cell may bring about its own destruction in the process of attacking the foreign particle. It is possible, as Fridovich (1974) has suggested, that phagocytic cells are expendable. On the other hand, they might also have developed defensive mechanisms to prolong their lifetime. Catalase (Baehner, 1972) and superoxide dismutase (Fridovich, 1974) are present in phagocytic cells and also are present in many bacteria. GSH-Px, however, has been demonstrated with certainty only in animal cells (Flohe, 1971) and has not been reported to occur in bacteria. Conceivably, the presence of GSH-Px in phagocytic cells of the host organism but not in bacteria could be an advantage for the host.

In discussing the occurrence and cellular function of GSH-Px in phago-cytic cells, we will review its well-established role in linking increased peroxide production to increased glucose oxidation by the hexose mono-phosphate shunt, as well as more limited information bearing on its possible importance to the survival of phagocytic cells.

There is a comparatively high activity of GSH-Px in most phagocytic cells. It is difficult to compare the results of different investigators who have employed different preparative methods, assays, and expression of results. Rat peritoneal polymorphonuclear leukocytes (PMNs) (Reed, 1969; Noseworthy and Karnovsky, 1972), rabbit alveolar macrophages (Vogt *et al.*, 1971), and rat alveolar and peritoneal macrophages (Serfass *et al.*, 1974) show high cytosolic GSH-Px activities. Human peripheral polymorphonuclear leukocytes have moderately high cytosolic activity (Holmes *et al.*, 1970; Bracci *et al.*, 1970a; Nishimura *et al.*, 1972; Nose-worthy and Karnovsky, 1972). Guinea pig peritoneal PMNs are reported to contain GSH-Px (Strauss *et al.*, 1969), but the cytosolic activity is very low (Noseworthy and Karnovsky, 1972). Particle-associated GSH-Px activity is reported to be less than one-fourth of the cytosolic activity in rat peritoneal PMNs (Reed, 1969). Where studies permit a reasonably direct comparison of erythrocyte and phagocyte activities, human leukocytes possess the higher specific activity (units per milligram of protein) by a factor of about 2 (Holmes *et al.*, 1970), and rat macro-phages twofold the specific activity of erythrocytes (Serfass *et al.*, 1974).

Because of its requirement for reducing equivalents in the form of glutathione, GSH-Px is coupled to the hexose monophosphate shunt via glutathione reductase (Scheme 1), which oxidizes NADPH to $NADP^+$. The rate of glucose oxidation by the hexose monophosphate shunt is controlled by the amount of $NADP^+$ present (Beck, 1958). Thus, the oxidation of glutathione by GSH-Px will cause a certain amount of NADPH to be oxidized to $NADP^+$, and glucose oxidation will take place in order to restore the $NADPH/NADP^+$ ratio to its initial level. The results of several investigations (Reed, 1969; Strauss *et al.*, 1969; Baehner *et al.*, 1970; Mandell, 1972) confirm the importance of the GSH-Px-dependent coupled system for hexose monophosphate shunt stimulation in normal PMNs from various species. Also, in several cases of hereditary GSH-Px deficiency in human leukocytes, hexose monophosphate shunt stimulation was greatly diminished during phagocytosis (Holmes *et al.*, 1970; Nishimura *et al.*, 1972).

Some *in vitro* hexose monophosphate shunt enzyme inhibition studies suggest that stimulation of the shunt enzymes above resting levels is not required for the actual killing process (DeChatelet *et al.*, 1971; Strauss *et al.*, 1968). Although resting levels of NADPH and hexose monophosphate shunt activity may suffice for the initial phase of killing, additional shunt activity may be needed to maintain an adequate level of glutathione for the destruction of lipoperoxides and hydrogen peroxide produced as a consequence of the killing process. Thus, in order for the cell to kill maximal numbers of bacteria before its own demise, hexose monophosphate shunt stimulation may be vital to maintain glutathione levels so that GSH-Px can provide sustained protection of the cell. Support for this view comes from studies of PMNs incubated with N-ethylmaleimide. Mandell (1972) showed that incubation with 10^{-4} M N-ethylmaleimide decreased glutathione levels by a factor of 15 and decreased protein sulfhydryl levels. The treated PMNs were able to ingest small numbers of bacteria (bacteria/PMN = 5) normally, but N-ethylmaleimide interfered with phagocytosis at higher bacteria:PMN ratios (100:1). The hexose monophosphate shunt stimulation was impaired, even though high levels of peroxide were generated. The killing of bacteria was also impaired in the N-ethylmaleimide-treated cells. A study by Khandwala and Gee (1973) showed that 5×10^{-5} M linoleic acid hydroperoxide caused a 60% decrease in bacteria uptake by alveolar macrophages and a corresponding decrease in the hexose monophosphate shunt stimulation. GSH-Px in the supernate from the sonicated alveolar macrophages was inhibited 50% with 5×10^{-5} M N-ethylmaleimide. An impairment in the killing of yeast cells ingested by GSH-Px deficient leukocytes from rats depleted of selenium was observed (Serfass and Ganther, 1975); ingestion of the cells was not affected.

GSH-Px thus appears to be important for the hexose monophosphate shunt stimulation initiated by phagocytosis and may be essential for optimal microbicidal capacity under some circumstances. Whether or not phagocytic GSH-Px deficiency necessarily leads to increased susceptibility of the host to infection is a more complicated subject because of the variety of host defense mechanisms. Inconsistent effects of selenium deficiency on the survival of rats or mice injected intravenously with *Salmonella enteriditis*, var. *typhimurium* were observed (Serfass *et al.*, 1974; Serfass, 1975). The limited data on apparent genetic deficiency of GSH-Px in humans are discussed in Section VI,C.

3. Platelets

A single study describing relatively high levels of glutathione and GSH-Px in platelets has been published (Karpatkin and Weiss, 1972). These authors noted that a deficiency of platelet GSH-Px was associated with a defect in platelet function in three patients having Glanzmann's thrombasthenia, a bleeding disorder (see Section VI,B,1). To the authors' knowledge there have been no previous studies carried out on platelet function in experimental animals made deficient in GSH-Px by selenium depletion. Bleeding disorders have not been generally associated with nutritional deficiencies of selenium and vitamin E, but the little-noticed report of DeWitt (1957) concerning dietary effects on parasite infections does describe some studies of blood coagulation in mice fed a *Torula* yeast diet deficient in selenium, vitamin E, and cystine. Compared to a "control" group fed a semipurified casein diet, the deficient mice had increased blood clotting time, increased prothrombin time, and decreased fibrinogen levels, along with a decrease in total plasma protein. The author states in a summary that supplementation of the *Torula* yeast diet with either a concentrate of factor 3 (an unidentified organic form of selenium) or a combination of vitamin E and cystine gave results comparable to those obtained with mice fed an adequate diet, but he does not specifically indicate whether these treatments were effective with regard to the abnormalities in blood coagulation.

In the absence of direct experimental studies, one cannot evaluate the possible importance of platelet GSH-Px in a glutathione-dependent system protecting platelets from oxidative damage analogous to the case of erythrocytes. Platelets have neither the presence of hemoglobin nor the copious production of peroxides to contend with, in contrast to erythrocytes and phagocytic cells. Nevertheless, as Beutler (1972c) has commented, the observations of Karpatkin and Weiss (1972) have focused attention on platelet glutathione and GSH-Px, an aspect of platelet metabolism that has not been explored in depth. Beutler suggests that if glutathione levels do affect platelet function, riboflavin deprivation should cause abnormalities if platelet glutathione reductase is dependent on riboflavin intake as in the case of erythrocyte glutathione reductase. Certainly, an even more direct approach for experimentally investigating the cellular role of the glutathione GSH-Px system in platelets would be to deplete platelet GSH-Px levels by feeding animals a selenium deficient diet. Besides GSH-Px, hereditary defects affecting the formation of other components linking glucose metabolism to glutathione-dependent peroxide destruction might conceivably lead to altered platelet function, in analogy to erythrocytes and phagocytic cells. In males with complete erythrocyte glucose-6-phosphate dehydrogenase deficiency, platelets had about 25% of the normal level of this enzyme; glutathione levels were not determined. No bleeding disorders were observed in such persons, but several platelet function tests were abnormal (Schwartz *et al.*, 1974). Platelet aggregation with adenosine diphosphate, collagen, and adrenalin was normal, unlike the case in persons with platelet

GSH-Px deficiency (see Section VI,B,1). The platelet function abnormalities in partial glucose-6-phosphate dehydrogenase deficiency may result from a lack of sufficient NADPH for synthesis of phospholipids involved in platelet function, as suggested by Schwartz et al. (1974), rather than a failure to maintain adequate glutathione levels for the prevention of oxidative damage, as in the classic case of erythrocyte hemolysis in hereditary glucose-6-phosphate dehydrogenase deficiency. Perhaps a more severe deficiency of the enzymes like glucose-6-phosphate dehydrogenase, which are indirectly involved in glutathione-dependent functions, may be required in order to affect the glutathione-linked processes in platelets, in contrast to GSH-Px, which is more directly involved.

In view of the importance of the membrane of platelets in relation to the critical platelet aggregation functions, it is reasonable to suggest that lipid peroxidation of the platelet membrane may lead to altered platelet function. This and other types of oxidative damage were suggested as the cause of Glanzmann's thrombasthenia in persons deficient in GSH-Px (Karpatkin and Weiss, 1972). In a system as complex as platelet aggregation, however, alternative explanations might be developed. Recent studies of platelet aggregation in relation to prostaglandin biosynthesis need to be discussed in relation to the possible connection between GSH-Px deficiency and platelet function. Hamberg et al. (1974) have described the isolation and structure of two prostaglandin endoperoxides that cause platelet aggregation. These compounds have a peroxide bridge between carbons 9 and 11 and either a hydroxy or hydroperoxy group at carbon 15 (PGH_2 and PGG_2, respectively). It was shown that PGG_2 and/or PGH_2 are formed during thrombin-induced aggregation and that they are powerful aggregating agents, the relative potency of PGG_2 and PGH_2 being about 3:1. The effect of these compounds is in contrast to the inhibitory effect of PGE_1 on the initial phase of platelet aggregation (Marquis et al., 1969).

J. B. Smith et al. (1974) have similarly found that a labile intermediate in prostaglandin synthesis is associated with platelet aggregation. Earlier it was shown (Vargaftig and Zirinis, 1973) that the precursor of PGE_2 and PGF_2, arachidonic acid, induces platelet aggregation; indeed, arachidonate injection causes sudden death in rabbits through the formation of platelet thrombi in the lungs (Silver et al., 1974). Aspirin, which inhibits prostaglandin synthesis in platelets, blocked these effects of arachidonate. J. B. Smith et al. (1974) present evidence that the link between prostaglandin formation and aggregation of platelets is the release of adenosine diphosphate triggered by the endoperoxide intermediates.

In view of the nonspecificity of GSH-Px for the peroxide substrate, one might expect that some of the intermediates in prostaglandin synthesis would be metabolized by platelet GSH-Px. It follows that more of the prostaglandin peroxide intermediates would accumulate in GSH-Px-deficient platelets, leading to increased platelet aggregation. However, this is opposite to the effect observed in GSH-Px-deficient platelets, so some other mechanism must be sought involving prostaglandins. Reduction of the hydroperoxide (PGG_2) to the hydroxy derivative (PGH_2) might be catalyzed by GSH-Px, but the hydroperoxide has three times the platelet aggregating activity of the hydroxy product, so a block in this step would not explain the observation of decreased platelet aggregation with platelet GSH-Px deficiency. A qualitatively satisfactory explanation might be developed on the basis that the higher level of glutathione in GSH-Px-deficient platelets (Karpatkin and Weiss, 1972) alters prostaglandin metabolism. For example, glutathione increases PGE formation at the expense of PGF, and PGE_1 inhibits aggregation of platelets by stimulating adenylcyclase activity (see review by Hinman, 1972).

An important factor limiting the biosynthesis of prostaglandins is the concentration of free essential fatty acid precursors (Hinman, 1972). Thus, increased peroxidation of unsaturated fatty acids such as arachidonate caused by GSH-Px deficiency might limit the production of prostaglandins required for stimulating platelet aggregation. A lack of arachidonate might also affect the synthesis of phospholipids involved in platelet function (Marcus, 1969). Finally, peroxidation of the platelet membrane might alter its properties enough to prevent the formation and release of prostaglandins thought to occur in response to a variety of stimuli that disturb cell membranes (Piper and Vane, 1971).

4. Plasma

The first reported study of plasma GSH-Px appears to be that of Noguchi *et al.* (1973), who were investigating the possible role of GSH-Px in the development of exudative diathesis in chicks. This condition, which is prevented by selenium (or vitamin E under some conditions), is a severe edema characterized by accumulation of a viscous subcutaneous fluid and was shown long ago to be associated with an increase in capillary permeability (Dam and Glavind, 1940).

In day-old chicks fed a diet containing 0.1 ppm selenium as sodium selenite for 6–12 days, the specific activity (units per milligram of nitrogen) of plasma GSH-Px was as high as erythrocytes and liver (Noguchi *et al.* 1973). In chicks fed the same diet lacking selenium, plasma GSH-Px had decreased to nearly zero after only 5 days of depletion, while GSH-Px in liver had decreased about 50% in this period and erythrocytes showed little change. Plasma GSH-Px levels were roughly proportional to dietary selenium levels between 0 and 0.06 ppm.

Tappel and collaborators have measured erythrocyte and plasma GSH-Px both in chicks and in rats, as well as cytosolic activities of GSH-Px in various tissues (see Section IV,A). The specific activity of GSH-Px in plasma was approximately 60–100% that of erythrocytes. In chicks, the specific activity of plasma glutathione reductase ranged from 27 to 47% of that for erythrocytes. Omaye and Tappel (1974a) also observed that plasma GSH-Px (but not glutathione reductase) was strongly influenced by the dietary selenite level and was fivefold higher when 14 ppm selenium was fed compared to the activity obtained with a level of selenium (0.1 ppm) comparable to the nutritional requirement. In rats fed 0 or 2 ppm selenium as selenomethionine, Chow and Tappel (1974) found that plasma showed the greatest variation in GSH-Px specific activity compared to other tissues. Although plasma in selenium-supplemented rats was reported in the paper by Chow and Tappel (1974) to have a considerably higher specific activity than other tissues, this proved not to be the case upon checking these results with the authors. The values for plasma in their paper were mistakenly reported to be units per milligram of protein, but actually were units per milliliter of plasma.

A primary role of plasma GSH-Px in preventing peroxidation of the plasma membrane of capillary endothelial cells was proposed by Noguchi et al. (1973), who observed that a drop in plasma GSH-Px to almost zero levels, occurred just before the onset of exudative diathesis in chicks. They developed a hypothesis involving the action of GSH-Px in plasma together with vitamin E in the plasma membrane and GSH-Px in the cytosol of capillary endothelial cells to explain the mechanism of selenium and vitamin E in preventing exudative diathesis.

The presence of GSH-Px in plasma and the suggestion that it has a primary protective function raise interesting questions. From the historical standpoint, interest was always focused on the erythrocyte fraction of blood. The apparent absence of data on plasma GSH-Px prior to 1973 is surprising in itself. In this laboratory, a limited study of sheep blood samples has generally shown a preponderance of activity in erythrocytes, and it may be that GSH-Px is elevated in plasma only under certain circumstances. The fact that total selenium level sets an upper limit on the amount of GSH-Px in a given tissue allows some information to be inferred from plasma selenium levels. Dickson and Tomlinson (1967) found 14 μg of selenium per 100 ml of plasma, 24 μg per 100 ml of cells, and 19 μg per 100 ml of blood in 253 Canadian subjects. Schrauzer *et al.* (1973) found a similar selenium level in plasma of normal subjects. Plasma selenium levels change in various diseases (Burk, Chapter 30). A large part of the selenium in ovine red cells is accounted for as GSH-Px (Oh *et al.*, 1974a).

It would be highly desirable to establish whether or not the apparent plasma GSH-Px activity is truly GSH-Px, preferably by isolation of the enzyme from plasma. Indeed, isolation from plasma would be easier than isolation from hemolyzates, where removal of hemoglobin is a major step. It has not been shown that the plasma activity is associated with the protein fraction, although Chow and Tappel (1974) did state that dialysis of "tissue samples" did not remove the activity. Many low molecular weight selenium compounds such as selenite or derivatives of glutathione (Ganther, 1971) catalyze thiol oxidation. The feeding of high levels of selenite might elevate plasma selenite levels enough to catalyze glutathione oxidation. This factor would be less important in cases (Chow and Tappel, 1974) where selenomethionine was fed. Erythrocytes actively transport to the plasma a form of selenium that may be selenodiglutathione (GSSeSG) following the incubation of erythrocytes with selenite (Lee *et al.*, 1969; Jenkins and Hidiroglou, 1972).

If the plasma activity is associated with a protein, it is possible that various other plasma proteins that bind selenium might catalyze glutathione oxidation nonspecifically, and for this reason, a characterization of the protein(s) responsible should be undertaken.

If the plasma activity is indeed GSH-Px, then the question arises concerning the availability of glutathione as a substrate in the plasma. Although numerous studies indicating a substantial erythrocyte glutathione level can be cited, data on plasma glutathione levels could not be located in standard reference works. The fact that glutathione in erythrocytes turns over rapidly and is actively transported to plasma in the form of oxidized glutathione (Srivastava and Beutler, 1969) and that plasma contains glutathione reductase in significant amounts (Chow and Tappel, 1974) suggests that glutathione could be formed if NADPH were present in plasma. The concentration that glutathione would have to attain in plasma to be physiologically significant is not known, but GSH-Px is catalytically active even with low levels of glutathione and peroxide substrates; thus, low substrate levels would not necessarily rule out an important function, particularly if potent agents such as prostaglandin derivatives were the substrates involved. Perhaps it would be interesting to investigate prostaglandin-mediated enhancement of capillary permeability in relation to plasma, GSH-Px, and exudative diathesis.

B. Liver

1. Catabolism of Hydrogen Peroxide

GSH-Px is present in the liver of some species in rather large amounts (Mills, 1960) (Table II). Since liver is also a rich source of catalase, controversy arose as to whether GSH-Px played a role in destroying intracellularly generated hydrogen peroxide. Hochstein and Utley (1968) demonstrated that GSH-Px and catalase competed equally for the hydrogen peroxide produced at a low steady state level by glucose oxidase and glucose. However, when hydrogen peroxide was present in high concentration, catalase was mainly responsible for its decomposition. Sies *et al.* (1972) showed that perfusion of hydrogen peroxide into intact liver resulted in metabolic changes associated with glutathione oxidation. Oxidized glutathione appeared in the perfusate, and utilization of NADPH for the maintainance of reduced glutathione was indicated by decreased pyridine nucleotide-specific surface fluorescence. These changes were not attributed to membrane damage caused by hydrogen peroxide, since they could be reversed by discontinuing hydrogen peroxide infusion. The authors pointed out that since hepatic catalase is predominantly localized in peroxisomes (deDuve and Baudhuin, 1966), GSH-Px is likely to have an appreciable role in utilizing extraperoxisomally generated hydrogen peroxide.

2. Lipid Peroxides

The major role of GSH-Px may not be its role in hydrogen peroxide metabolism, but rather its ability to catalyze the decomposition of lipid hydroperoxides. Catalase has no activity toward these substrates, although it can act on low molecular weight organic peroxides such as methyl and ethyl hydroperoxides (O'Brien, 1969; Nicholls and Schonbaum, 1963). GSH-Px in comparison reacts with many organic peroxides with very little specificity (see Section II,B). Reaction of lipid hydroperoxides with glutathione either enzymatically or nonenzymatically converts them to their corresponding hydroxyl compounds. The latter no longer sustain autocatalytic lipid peroxidation, since they cannot participate in free radical attack on other lipid double bonds. Lipid peroxides are generated as a product of microsomal enzyme activity, as first shown by Hochstein and Ernster (1963). This activity, although present in tissues such as muscle, brain, and kidney, is exceptionally high in liver (McCay *et al.*, 1971). The system requires peroxide and NADPH plus Fe^{2+} or Fe^{3+} complexed with adenosine di- or triphosphate or pyrophosphate (Hochstein et al., 1964; Poyer and McCay, 1971). NADPH and oxygen are consumed, while lipid peroxidation can be monitored by the release of malondialdehyde. Polyunsaturated fatty acids situated in β-acyl position of phosphatidylcholine and phosphatidylethanolamine are oxidized and disappear from the microsomal membrane (May and McCay, 1968). Early during the course of peroxidation there is a rapid decrease in microsomal turbidity (Tam and McCay, 1970).

The final result of this process is membrane fragmentation and dissociation of protein from the endoplasmic reticulum (Ernster and Nordenbrand, 1967; Arstila et al., 1972; Hogberg et al., 1973). These physical disturbances are accompanied by alteration of membrane-bound enzyme activity. Some enzymes, such as glucose-6-phosphate dehydrogenase, decrease in activity, while others such as nucleotide diphosphatase and adenosine triphosphatase undergo activation. In general, changes parallel those observed after treatment of microsomes with detergents, e.g., deoxycholate, suggesting that disruption of membrane integrity is responsible for altered enzyme properties (Ernster and Nordenbrand, 1967; Wills, 1971).

α-Tocopherol, chelating agents, and antioxidants such as diphenyl-p-phenylenediamine (DPPD) and ethoxyquin effectively prevent microsomal lipid peroxidation (Gram and Fouts, 1966; Ernster and Nordenbrand, 1967; May and McCay, 1968). Liver supernatant fraction also gives protection. Glutathione is one protective component found in the liver soluble fraction, but in the absence of the complete supernate, it provides only partial protection (Gram and Fouts, 1966). GSH-Px although present in mitochondrial preparations, is predominantly a soluble enzyme (see Section IV,A). Very little activity is found in microsomes (Demus-Oole and Swierczeski, 1969a; Green and O'Brien, 1970). GSH-Px, along with glutathione and the enzymes necessary for its maintenance in the reduced state, may represent the major protective factors present in liver supernate. This hypothesis can be tested, since GSH-Px declines to very low levels or disappears from liver tissue in selenium-deficient rats (see Section IV,A). If this hypothesis is correct, selenium deficiency would greatly diminish protection by liver supernatant fraction, and addition of purified GSH-Px should restore protection.

3. Liver GSH-Px and Pathological Changes in Selenium Deficiency

The nutritional benefit of selenium was first realized because of its ability to prevent liver necrosis in rats fed a diet suboptimal in the sulfur-containing amino acids and deficient in vitamin E (Schwarz and

Foltz, 1957). The disease becomes fatal after feeding the diet for 3–4 weeks to weanling rats. It is characterized by massive hepatic necrosis; degeneration of the endoplasmic reticulum and mitochondrial swelling can be observed by electron microscopy (Piccardo and Schwarz, 1958). Liver tissue from rats deficient in vitamin E and selenium fails to maintain normal respiration *in vitro*, a phenomenon called respiratory decline (Chernick *et al.*, 1955; Schwarz, 1965). Lack of liver GSH-Px when vitamin E is also absent may be responsible for this liver disease. Work in our laboratory showed that rat liver GSH-Px declined to 20% of that found in selenium-supplemented controls after feeding the deficient diet for only 10 days to weanling rats. The enzyme was undetectable (<1% of the control level) by the twenty-fourth day of the deficiency (Hafeman *et al.*, 1974). Others have reported less severe, although still highly significant, declines in rat liver GSH-Px caused by selenium-deficiency (J. B. Smith *et al.*, 1974; Chow and Tappel, 1974; Reddy and Tappel, 1974). A possible explanation for the different liver GSH-Px levels reported in selenium deficiency could be variable selenium levels in the deficient diets used by individual investigators. Another explanation could be contamination of the liver enzyme with GSH-Px of erythrocyte origin. Erythrocytes become depleted only very slowly. In the latter studies, where selenium deficiency caused less severe declines in GSH-Px, blood cells were not flushed from the livers prior to homogenization and enzyme determination.

Either dietary selenium or vitamin E prevents liver necrosis as well as respiratory decline in liver slices *in vitro*. In homogenates of the same tissue, only vitamin E affords protection against respiratory failure (Schwarz, 1962). It is possible that the lack of protection by selenium in homogenates results from dilution of cytosolic GSH-Px and glutathione in the homogenate medium. Glutathione, when present in adequate concentration, can protect in the absence of vitamin E or dietary selenium (Schwarz, 1962). The effect of glutathione may be attributed to non-enzymatic reduction of hydrogen peroxide by glutathione. This reaction is appreciable at neutral or elevated pH and is also promoted by high levels of glutathione (Flohe, 1971).

4. Liver GSH-Px and Carbon Tetrachloride Toxicity

Certain environmental factors apparently can increase the need for cellular agents preventing peroxidation. Carbon tetrachloride is an example of one such factor. Ethanol is another compound that has been postulated to induce peroxidation (DiLuzio, 1968).

The mechanism of carbon tetrachloride toxicity has received considerable study. It causes fatty liver due to inhibition of triglyceride transport out of this organ (Recknagel, 1967). Centrolobular necrosis is also observed, and if the dosage is sufficiently high, death is the final result. One of the earliest changes seen in carbon tetrachloride toxicity is an increase in diene conjugation of microsomal lipids (Recknagel and Ghoshal, 1966). Diene conjugation of polyunsaturated fatty acids results from rearrangement of the double bonds during peroxidation. The metabolism of carbon tetrachloride appears to be a necessary prerequisite for its toxicity and for lipid peroxidation. Free radicals generated during carbon tetrachloride oxidation to carbon dioxide and inorganic chloride are believed to initiate lipid peroxidation, ultimately leading to disruption of cellular membranes and inhibited protein synthesis (Recknagel, 1967; Slater, 1972; Ugazio et al., 1973).

Vitamin E, synthetic antioxidants. selenium, and the sulfur-containing amino acids all give some degree of protection against carbon tetrachloride poison (Hove, 1948; Muth, 1960; Gallager, 1962; Fodor and Kemeny, 1965; Seward et al., 1966). Vitamin E reduces the amount of lipid diene conjugation in liver microsomes and also decreases carbon tetrachloride-induced steatosis (Comporti and Benedetti, 1972). Whether selenium and the sulfur-containing amino acids protect by reducing lipid peroxidation has not yet been proven. It is plausible that GSH-Px mediates selenium's protective effect by inhibiting the lipid peroxidation reaction. The sulfur-containing amino acids may similarly protect by increasing the level of liver glutathione (Linden and Work, 1953) to serve as substrate for the reduction of lipid peroxides.

C. Lens

The effects that peroxides and free radicals may have on lens tissue have not been thoroughly investigated. It seems likely, however, that they could cause oxidation of protein components and peroxidation of membrane lipids with disruption of membrane function, both of which have been postulated as possible mechanisms of cataract formation (Barber, 1973). Hydrogen peroxide is produced in the aqueous humor of the eye by a photocatalyzed oxidation of ascorbate involving riboflavin (Pirie, 1965a,b), in aqueous humor and corneal epithelium extracts by autoxidation of ascorbate (Pirie, 1965b; Anderson and Spector, 1971), and in various parts of the eye by 1,2-dihydroxynaphthalene (Rees and Pirie, 1967; van Heyningen and Pirie, 1967), a metabolite of naphthalene that is a known cataractogenic agent. Pirie (1965b) has also demonstrated that hydrogen peroxide can diffuse into the lens in vitro.

The lens fibers are similar to red blood cells in many respects (Kinoshita, 1964; Jacob, 1971), including the lack of mitochondria and therefore the citrate cycle enzymes. The same glutathione-dependent pathway for destruction of peroxides that is operative in erythrocytes (Section V,A,1) is also responsible for their removal in the lens (Kinoshita, 1955, 1964; van Heyningen and Pirie, 1953; Pirie, 1965b). The same conditions that result in precipitation of the hemoglobin into Heinz bodies and hemolysis of red cells might therefore be expected to result in cataract formation. The existence of this pathway in lens may explain the importance of the extremely high glutathione content of lens tissue.

In support of this hypothesis, cataracts have been observed in patients with severe glucose-6-phosphate dehydrogenase deficiency (Westring and Pisciotta, 1966; Harley et al., 1966; Helge and Barness, 1966). Glutathione peroxidase activity has been demonstrated in the lenses of various animal species (Pirie, 1965b; Holmberg, 1968; Lawrence et al., 1974) and has been partially purified from cattle lens (Holmberg, 1968). This activity decreases to very low levels with selenium deficiency (Lawrence et al., 1974), and cataracts have been observed in the second- and third-litter offspring of selenium-deficient female rats (Sprinker et al., 1971; R. A. Lawrence, 1975). In addition, Swanson and Truesdale (1971) present data showing that selenium concentration increased about fourfold in normal human lenses between birth and age eighty-five, while in cataractous lenses the selenium concentration was less than one-sixth that of normal lenses from the same age groups.

Catalase activity in whole lenses is very low (Zeller, 1953), but recent reports have indicated high activity in the capsule-epithelium portion of the lens (Bhuyan and Bhuyan, 1970). Bhuyan et al. (1973) have also reported that catalase activity is inhibited during amizol-induced cataract formation, while GSH-Px activity remains unchanged, and they postulate that catalase has a significant role in lens metabolism. It would seem that this catalase activity in the epithelium may be important in impeding diffusion of hydrogen peroxide from the aqueous humor into the lens interior, but it could not protect the lens from hydrogen peroxide diffusion via the vitreous humor or that produced inside the lens, nor could it protect against other peroxides.

Cataractogenic drugs and chemicals may exert their effects by producing peroxides in amounts too great to be handled by the GSH-Px protective mechanism, or by impairing the ability of this mechanism to protect against endogenously produced peroxides, or both. Naphthalene (Pirie, 1965b) and many of the antimalarials (Bernstein, 1967; Cohen and Hochstein, 1964) have been shown to produce peroxides in the course of their metabolism in the body. A rather large group of cataractogenic chemicals is known as radiomimetics (Paterson, 1971; van Heyningen,

1969; Kuck, 1970); these chemicals, like ionizing radiation, probably produce free radicals or are themselves metabolized to free radicals (e.g., see Pirie et al., 1970). Free radicals can cause peroxidation of unsaturated lipids, nucleic acids, and other cell components (Pryor, 1973; Meyers, 1973), and these may be produced in amounts sufficient to overwhelm the protective mechanisms, especially if these mechanisms are in some way defective.

Certain N-substituted phenothiazines and other drugs belong to a class of cataractogenic agents known as photosensitizers. They cause cataracts in lenses exposed to ultraviolet radiation and may produce hydrogen peroxide in a manner analogous to the light-catalyzed reaction of ascorbate and riboflavin mentioned previously (Pirie, 1965b). Light in the range of 494–551 nm has also been reported to cause free radical peroxidation of the lipids in the rod outer segments of frog retina in the presence of rhodopsin as sensitizer (Kagan et al., 1973), and the action of the N-substituted phenothiazines has been postulated to be mediated by their free radicals (Karremann et al., 1959; Gooley et al., 1969).

In addition to their role as photosensitizers the N-substituted phenothiazines may act as riboflavin antagonists in inhibiting glutathione reductase activity. It has been reported that riboflavin protects against the hemolytic action of chlorpromazine (Popov et al., 1970). Methionine sulfoximine produces cataracts, presumably by blocking glutathione synthesis (Bagchi, 1959); sulfhydryl reagents such as iodoacetate (Cibis et al., 1957; Tieri and Vecchione, 1963) also produce cataracts, presumably by blocking the sulfhydryl groups of glutathione or of sulfhydryl-containing enzyme. No evidence is available that the many other cataractogenic drugs produce peroxides or interfere with the glutathione-dependent pathway for their removal, but some of them may be found to act in this manner.

In addition to selenium deficiency, deficiencies of several other essential nutrients have been implicated in cataract formation. Riboflavin deficiency cataracts were reported by Day et al. (1931), but later work showed that if the diet was adequate to support normal growth, no cataracts were formed despite riboflavin deficiency (Day and Darby, 1936). It has also been shown that riboflavin deficiency combined with other adverse factors can produce cataracts where neither alone will suffice (Bourne and Pyke, 1935; Srivastava and Beutler, 1970, 1972). The role of riboflavin as a precursor of the cofactor in glutathione reductase has already been mentioned (see Section V,A,1).

Deficiency of vitamin E has been shown to cause cataracts in turkey embryos (Ferguson et al., 1954, 1956), and it has been reported that congenital cataracts seen in the progeny of rats fed a specific cataracto-genic diet could be prevented by feeding either vitamin E or a combina-tion of tryptophan, methionine, and niacin (Bunce et al., 1972). The interrelationship between vitamin E and selenium in preventing oxidative damage is well known (Sondegaard, 1967).

Some degree of lens damage has been attributed to a deficiency of each of the essential amino acids in the rat except arginine (Hall et al., 1948). Of these, cataracts due to tryptophan deficiency are by far the best documented (Albanese and Buschke, 1942; Curtis et al., 1932; Pike, 1951; Schaeffer and Murray, 1950; Totter and Day, 1942; Cart-wright et al., 1945; von Sallman et al., 1959). The special case of methio-nine as a precursor of glutathione and its antagonism by methionine sulfoximine have already been mentioned. In addition, deficiency of any of the essential amino acids could result in a deficiency of any of the enzymes of the glutathione-dependent pathway for removal of peroxides and make the lens vulnerable to peroxidative damage.

Although high galactose 1-phosphate concentrations have been re-ported to inhibit glucose-6-phosphate dehydrogenase activity (Lerman, 1959, 1965), there is little evidence that galactose cataracts or any of the other types of cataracts not mentioned are related to peroxidative damage. It is likely that human senile cataracts will be found to be caused in most cases by a combination of factors, including peroxide damage, and adequate protection against peroxides may play a significant role in the prevention of cataract.

VI. GLUTATHIONE PEROXIDASE IN HUMAN DISEASES

A. Hemolysis

1. Clinical Cases in Adults

Several clinical cases of hemolytic anemia attributed to GSH-Px deficiency have been reported in the literature. Necheles et al. (1967, 1969) described an 18-year-old Puerto Rican male who suffered a hemo-lytic episode following autotransfusion after surgery. During the hemo-lytic crisis, his blood contained numerous red cells with Heinz bodies, but these disappeared within a few weeks. Incubation with acetylphenyl-hydrazine continued to produce five or more Heinz bodies in 53% of his red cells, however. Following recovery from the hemolytic episode, about 3 months later, his reticulocyte count remained at 2.8–5%, suggesting a compensated hemolysis. His erythrocyte GSH-Px activity was approximately one-third of normal, and hemolyzates of his red cells did not show the characteristic stimulation of the hexose monophosphate shunt pathway upon incubation with hydrogen peroxide in the presence of glucose. Both of his parents and one of three siblings had GSH-Px activities slightly lower than normal, which the authors interpreted as indicative of heterozygous genetic deficiency.

Necheles *et al.* (1970) have summarized data on infants with neonatal jaundice as well as six adults with drug-induced hemolytic anemia where GSH-Px activities ranged from 47 to 78% of normal (mean equal 66%) and nine others without hemolysis whose GSH-Px activities averaged 69% of normal, all of whom were classified as heterozygous on the basis of family studies. In addition, one adult (described in the previous paragraph) with low GSH-Px activities (34% of normal) was classified as homozygous deficient. No other cause for hemolysis could be found in those who suffered from it. Drug-induced hemolytic episodes were precipitated by high doses of acetylsalicylic acid, sulfisoxazole, or nitrofurantoin.

Steinberg *et al.* (1970) and Steinberg and Necheles (1971) described the case of a woman who developed hemolytic anemia following infection and treatment with sulfisoxazole and nitrofurantoin. Her erythrocyte GSH-Px activity was found to be about 53% of normal and the characteristic stimulation of hexose monophosphate shunt activity was not seen with ascorbate, which produced hydrogen peroxide, but was seen with methylene blue, which oxidizes NADPH directly.

Gharib *et al.* (1969) reported low GSH-Px activity associated with hepatic failure and acanthocytosis in a woman who had suffered jaundice for 3 years. This woman had been consuming large quantities of alcohol for 10 years, and the relationship of the low GSH-Px activity to the symptoms described is unclear. Boivin *et al.* (1969) described the case of a 67-year-old man with chronic hemolytic anemia, methemoglobinemia, Heinz bodies, and drug sensitivity. His erythrocyte GSH-Px activity was 30% of that of subjects with comparable reticulocytosis. The activities of fourteen enzymes of the glycolytic pathway and hexose monophosphate shunt were normal or slightly elevated.

Nishimura *et al.* (1972) described a 9-month-old girl suffering from severe anemia first noticed at 4 months of age. All blood tests and the activity of several glycolytic and hexose monophosphate shunt enzymes as well as catalase activity were found to be normal. Glutathione content and hemoglobin electrophoretic patterns were also normal. The patient's erythrocyte GSH-Px activity was about 17% of normal children of the same age group, and those of the mother and father were 52 and 66%, respectively. GSH-Px was not determined on other family members. The patient also had markedly lower levels of GSH-Px in cultured leukocytes.

Although all of these investigators attribute the GSH-Px deficiency to genetic causes, dietary selenium deficiency may play a significant role in GSH-Px deficiency. It is also known that the activity of GSH-Px is greatly decreased in cases of iron-deficiency anemia (see Section IV,B,4). It is evident from these studies that GSH-Px activity is important in preventing damage to human red cells, even in the presence of normal catalase activity.

2. Hemolytic Anemia of the Newborn

The increased susceptibility of the erythrocytes of newborn infants and especially premature infants to oxidative stress is well known and has been attributed to various causes, including greater susceptibility of fetal hemoglobin to oxidation and vitamin E deficiency (Cornblath and Hartman, 1948; Gasser, 1953; Allison, 1955; Betke et al., 1956; Kravitz et al., 1956; Gross and Schroeder, 1963; Hassan et al., 1966; Oski and Barness, 1967; Ritchie et al., 1968; Bracci et al., 1970b; Melhorn and Gross, 1971a,b; Flohe, 1971; Abrams et al., 1973; Lo, 1973). Recent work, however, has focused on a reduced activity of GSH-Px in erythrocytes from newborns as a possible explanation.

Most investigators have found reduced GSH-Px activity in the erythrocytes of premature and full-term newborn infants (Gross et al., 1967; Necheles et al., 1968; Swierczewski et al., 1969; Whaun and Oski, 1970; Emerson et al., 1972; Glader and Conrad, 1972; Konrad et al., 1972; Lie-Injo et al., 1973), but two groups from Germany did not (Vetrella et al., 1970; Butenandt, 1971; Vetrella and Barthelmai, 1971). The original report by Gross et al. (1967) showed that erythrocyte GSH-Px activity (units per gram of hemoglobin) in premature and full-term infants averaged approximately two-thirds that of adults, and they suggested an important role of GSH-Px in the resistance to oxidative stress. Necheles et al. (1968) confirmed this finding. Necheles et al. (1970) studied eleven infants in whom neonatal jaundice was associated with a "moderately severe" decrease in erythrocyte GSH-Px, and in whom no other cause for hyperbilirubinemia was evident. Eight showed signs of mild hemolysis with reticulocytosis (some also had increased Heinz body formation after incubation with acetylphenylhydrazine); in these infants they postulated an inherited partial deficiency of GSH-Px. In addition one infant with very low erythrocyte GSH-Px (15% of normal) was described that was classified as homozygous-deficient. In a survey of one hundred consecutive full-term newborns, two cases of apparent hereditary deficiency of GSH-Px were uncovered. Emerson *et al.* (1972), commenting on the studies of Necheles *et al.* (1970), thought that "This incidence of a genetically transmitted defect would appear to be exceedingly high when compared with most other congenital enzyme deficiency states. . . ." Whaun and Oski (1970) also found that the average GSH-Px activity was decreased in infants. Although infants classified as GSH-Px-deficient did not become more jaundiced as a group than those infants classified as sufficient, there was a lower GSH-Px activity in those infants having the highest bilirubin levels compared to those with the lowest bilirubin values. Lie-Injo *et al.* (1974), however, found no significant difference in GSH-Px in infants with highest and lowest bilirubin levels. Emerson *et al.* (1972) also were unable to correlate decreased GSH-Px activity with increased hemolysis in newborn infants having an erythrocyte GSH-Px activity (per cell number) equal to 55% of adult controls. In some cases, the GSH-Px in newborn infants apparently is not decreased if activity is expressed per cell number, but may be slightly decreased if the activity is expressed in relation to hemoglobin, which is somewhat higher in neonatal erythrocytes (Vetrella *et al.*, 1970; Butenandt, 1971; Lie-Injo *et al.*, 1973).

Nevertheless, it is clear that GSH-Px activity is frequently lower in the newborn even when expressed per cell number (Emerson *et al.*, 1972). The work of Konrad *et al.* (1972) confirms this and is especially informative in that they measured nineteen other enzyme activities as well as glutathione and GSH-Px levels in erythrocytes of newborn and compared them to older normal subjects as well as to a group of subjects having reticulocytosis comparable to newborn infants. They found higher glutathione levels and lower GSH-Px levels in newborn subjects, with the difference being accentuated by comparison to reticulocyte-rich blood because of the higher GSH-Px activity in reticulocytosis. Higher GSH-Px activity was also associated with reticulocytosis in two other studies (Gross *et al.*, 1967; Whaun and Oski, 1970), but not in the study by Necheles *et al.* (1970). (The paper by Hopkins and Tudhope (1973) also is pertinent in regard to GSH-Px activity and alterations in blood cell populations.)

There is a good possibility that some of the variations in the degree of GSH-Px deficiency in newborns as a group, as well as the apparent existence of genetically related deficiencies of GSH-Px in individual cases, are related to the dietary selenium intake. The situation is quite analogous to that for glutathione reductase, in which many cases initially thought to be genetic deficiencies of the enzyme proved to have a nutritional origin, namely riboflavin deficiency. It is interesting that most of the reports of low GSH-Px activity in the United States were from areas where the selenium content of the forages is known to be low (Kubota et al., 1967). Although the dietary histories of the mothers of these infants were not investigated, the selenium content in human blood tends to vary with the selenium content of plants (Allaway et al., 1968). The geographic differences in blood are less pronounced, however, than the variation in locally produced foods such as milk. The relation of GSH-Px activity in the newborn to selenium status needs to be investigated.

Some investigators have reported increased sensitivity to oxidative stress of erythrocytes with low GSH-Px activity from newborn infants (Gross et al., 1967; Lubia and Oski, 1972) but the deficiency is not usually severe enough to cause spontaneous hemolysis and hyperbilirubinemia (Emerson et al., 1972; Whaun and Oski, 1970; Lie-Injo et al., 1974). The cases of four infants with especially low GSH-Px activity and spontaneous hemolysis were reported by Necheles et al. (1968). One report has appeared recently in which no difference was found between erythrocytes from adults and newborns in their response to oxidative challenge in spite of differences in GSH-Px activity (Glader and Conrad, 1972). In this study the GSH-Px in newborn erythrocytes, expressed per gram of hemoglobin, averaged 59% of adult controls and glutathione levels were slightly higher. Glutathione oxidation and the response of the hexose monophosphate shunt to a peroxide stimulus were comparable for newborn and adult controls. This finding implies that even the decreased level of GSH-Px found in newborn erythrocytes is not necessarily rate-limiting.

B. Platelet Disorders

1. Glanzmann's Thrombasthenia

Disorders of platelet function resulting in recurring bleeding episodes occur in certain individuals who are normal with respect to platelet count and the plasma coagulation factors. Platelets are involved in a number of processes in hemostasis; consequently, a number of different abnormalities in platelet function are known. The aggregation of platelets, important in temporary hemostasis at the site of injury, occurs in response to minute quantities of adenosine diphosphate or to various agents that stimulate adenosine diphosphate release. Glanzmann's thrombasthenia is a serious bleeding disorder inherited as an autosomal recessive trait and characterized by defective adenosine diphosphate-induced platelet aggregation and deficient clot retraction. The enzymatic basis of this disease has been investigated for some time.

A study by Karpatkin and Weiss (1972) of a number of enzymes in platelet extracts of three unrelated patients with Glanzmann's thrombasthenia revealed a markedly decreased level of GSH-Px in all three patients and a twofold increase in acid-soluble thiol concentration in two of the three cases. These results indicate that enzymatic pathways for maintaining glutathione were normal, but utilization of glutathione for destruction was impaired, making the platelet more susceptible to oxidative damage. The authors point out that GSH-Px and glutathione are present in platelets in relatively large amounts and suggest that lipid peroxidation of the platelet membrane or oxidation of sulfhydryl groups in other proteins may be the cause of altered platelet function associated with GSH-Px deficiency. The platelet contractile protein, thrombasthenin, implicated in platelet contraction and aggregation, is sensitive to sulfhydryl reagents. The authors also point out that the moderate decreases in platelet activities of the sulfhydryl enzymes enolase and glutathione reductase that were noted might be indirect effects of oxidative stress on sensitive enzymes. Some additional comments on the possible relation of GSH-Px to platelet function can be found in Section V,A,3.

2. Hermansky–Pudlak Syndrome

A triad of symptoms consisting of oculocutaneous albinism, mild hemorrhagic symptoms, and accumulation of ceroid pigment in reticuloendothelial cells was first described by Hermansky and Pudlak (1959). Witkop et al. (1973) have stated that many patients with this disorder have had spontaneous gingival hemorrhage and prolonged bleeding following tooth extraction, child birth, or surgery, and that aspirin may enhance these tendencies. The authors postulate that a hereditary deficiency of GSH-Px is the cause of Hermansky–Pudlak syndrome, but unfortunately no measurements of GSH-Px activity in such patients have yet been made.

C. Chronic Infection

The avoidance of chronic and recurrent bacterial or fungal infection depends upon the abundance and functional integrity of the phagocytic cells of the peripheral blood and bone marrow (Baehner, 1972). There are a few patients having a particularly severe syndrome first described by Holmes et al. (1966) called chronic granulomatous disease (CGD). Such patients respond normally to infection in terms of an appropriate leukocytosis, and particle ingestion is normal. They are almost always found to be immunologically competent. The cellular defect in CGD patients is a diminished microbicidal capacity of the PMN's, associated with one or more enzyme defects in the pathways known to be involved in the bactericidal process. A summary of the metabolic abnormalities in CGD patients as well as in less severe chronic infectious states is given in Table III. Deficiencies of glucose-6-phosphate dehydrogenase, NADH- or NADPH-dependent primary oxidases, or myeloperoxidase in human leukocytes have been extensively reviewed (Johnston and Baehner, 1971). GSH-Px is of possible importance here for the reasons discussed in Section V,A,2, but has received little attention; only one study of GSH-Px activities in cases of diminished microbicidal capacity has been carried out.

Leukocyte GSH-Px deficiency was found by Holmes *et al.* (1970) to be associated with CGD of childhood in two female patients (Table IV). This deficiency distinguishes their disease from that of male patients with the more common X-linked defect. There were no demonstrable heterozygotes in the families of the female patients. Consanguinity was established in one family. Leukocytes from the male patients were found to possess normal levels of GSH-Px. Erythrocyte GSH-Px activity was normal in patients of both sexes. Leukocytes of both male and female patients were not deficient in glutathione reductase or glucose-6-phosphate dehydrogenase activity when compared to controls.

Metabolic studies on leukocytes from these patients (Quie *et al.*, 1968) demonstrated that the increases in oxygen consumption and hexose monophosphate shunt activity characteristic of normal leukocytes undergoing phagocytosis were lacking in both the male and female patients. However, hydrogen peroxide production, myeloperoxidase, and primary oxidase activities in these patients were not reported. It is therefore impossible to ascertain whether the GSH-Px deficiency was the primary determinant of CGD in the female patients or a secondary result of some other deficiency.

GSH-Px activities have not been reported in other studies of CGD in female patients, but it would be a mistake to assume that all female CGD patients are deficient in GSH-Px. Several cases of CGD in females have been reported (Baehner and Nathan, 1968; Azimi *et al.*, 1968), where it is likely that functional deficiencies of an NADH or NADPH oxidase are responsible for the defects. On the other hand, there exist cases in which the defect could be in any one of the previously mentioned enzymes (glucose-6-phosphate dehydrogenase, glutathione reductase, myeloperoxidase, GSH-Px) other than the primary oxidase (Davis *et al.*, 1968).

TABLE III Some Studies of Microbicidal Capacity in Human Leukocytes

Condition	Microbicidal capacity	Phagocytic hexose monophosphate shunt activity	Phagocytic hydrogen peroxide ([^{14}C] formate oxidation)	Enzyme deficiency	Reference
Normal	Adequate	7–10-fold increase	3–5-fold increase	None	Baehner (1972)
Caucasian G6PD[a] deficiency (complete)	Inadequate	No increase	None	G6PD[a] (leukocyte, erythrocyte)	Gray et al. (1973)
Partial Caucasian G6PD[a] deficiency (20–50%)	Adequate	Normal increase	Normal increase	G6PD[a] (leukocyte, erythrocyte)	Baehner et al. (1972)
Chronic granulomatous disease	Inadequate	No increase	No increase	Primary oxidase (leukocyte)	Holmes et al. (1967)
Chronic granulomatous disease	Inadequate	No increase	Not reported (postulated greater than normal)	Glutathione peroxidase (leukocyte only)	Holmes et al. (1970)
Myeloperoxidase deficiency	Inadequate	Increase greater than normal	Increase greater than normal	Myeloperoxidase (neutrophil only)	Lehrer and Cline (1969)

[a] G6PD = Glucose-6-phosphate dehydrogenase.

TABLE IV Chronic Granulomatous Disease in Females with
Leukocyte Glutathione Peroxidase Deficiency[a]

Subject	GSH-Px activity (nmoles NADPH/min/mg protein)
Females with CGD	
Patient 1	12
Patient 2	20
Parents of patient 1	45, 46
Parents of patient 2	70, 90
Males with CGD (7 patients)	59 ± 14
Controls	64 (40–110)

[a] Holmes et al. (1970). Reproduced with approval of the publisher.

Leukocytic deficiency of GSH-Px in an infant has been reported without any apparent evidence of susceptibility to infection (Nishimura et al., 1972). In this case, the erythrocytes GSH-Px was also low, and hemolytic anemia was the presenting symptom (see Section VI,A,1).

If it is true that GSH-Px is present to protect the phagocyte rather than being involved in the killing process per se, it might be expected that patients with no defect other than leukocyte GSH-Px deficiency would experience milder abnormalities than the CGD cases referred to. There are syndromes that have been described in which the metabolic abnormalities are similar to CGD, but the clinical signs are not as marked and the infections are milder (Rodey et al., 1970; Shmerling et al., 1969; Bannatyne et al., 1969). It is interesting that lipopigments, which may represent end products of lipid peroxidation, are observed in patients susceptible to chronic infection (Rodey et al., 1970) and in Batten's disease, a form of cerebral degeneration with an associated deficiency of leukocyte peroxidase (Armstrong et al., 1974). GSH-Px activities in such cases would be interesting to determine.

Experimental studies with animals indicate that a lack of phagocytic GSH-Px brought about by nutritional deficiency of selenium may not be detrimental unless coupled to other factors (Serfass, 1975). Other observations, such as the reported immunoadjuvant characteristics of dietary or parenterally-administered selenium compounds (Spallholz et al., 1973, 1974) must also be considered when seeking to determine the effects of selenium status on resistance to infection. Clearly there are a number of alternatives that preclude making a direct association between GSH-Px deficiency and susceptibility to infection on the basis of data available at this time.

D. Other Diseases

The possible relationship of selenium deficiency to kwashiorkor, sudden infant death syndrome, and cancer has been briefly reviewed elsewhere in this monograph by Burk. Investigations of GSH-Px in relationship to these conditions are generally lacking. Hopkins and Tudhope (1973) assayed erythrocyte GSH-Px in 163 patients with various diseases. In fifty-five patients with carcinoma, there was a wide variation in red cell GSH-Px, but the mean value was significantly lower compared to sixty-two normal subjects. GSH-Px was also decreased in hepatomatous livers of rats treated with diethylnitrosamine (Pinto and Bartley, 1973). Abnormally high values for erythrocyte GSH-Px were found in acute myeloblastic leukemia and in myelofibrosis, whereas the enzyme activity tended to be low in chronic lymphocytic and myeloid leukemia (Hopkins and Tudhope, 1973). With respect to the apparent anticarcinogenic effects of selenium, it should be mentioned that certain carcinogenic substances are metabolized to electrophilic derivatives such as epoxides that may be the actual carcinogenic agents. Since many of these are detoxified by glutathione-linked conjugation reactions, it is possible that selenium derivatives of glutathione such as the selenopersulfides (GSSeH), with their greater nucleophilic character compared to glutathione, might help detoxify carcinogenic metabolites.

The possible relationship of GSH-Px to the aging process has received little investigation. Smith *et al.* (1973) found that GSH-Px was present at low levels in pig and human aortas. They observed that the cholesteryl hydroperoxyoctadecadienoates, which occur in human atherosclerotic plaques, were reduced to the hydroxy esters by aortic GSH-Px but at a relatively low rate.

VII. RESEARCH NEEDS

The primary importance of dietary selenium intake as a factor determining GSH-Px levels in many tissues is now well established. This relationship is so strong, that an assay for GSH-Px may be useful in assessing the selenium status of individuals. Almost without exception, GSH-Px deficiency in humans has been attributed to a genetic defect. This explanation, particularly where familial studies are lacking and a high apparent rate of incidence in a population is claimed, must be viewed with skepticism. Hereditary GSH-Px deficiency is on no firmer ground than hereditary glutathione reductase deficiency was a few years ago. There may indeed be hereditary deficiencies of GSH-Px in humans, but many other cases may prove to have a nutritional origin, as for glutathione reductase. The selenium status has to be considered before attributing an apparent deficiency of GSH-Px to genetic causes. As Burk has pointed out elsewhere in this volume, methods for the assessment of selenium status in humans are not well established; this is an area of research needing development in its own right. Unlike glutathione reductase, where the degree of stimulation of erythrocyte glutathione reductase by the flavin cofactor added *in vitro* can be used as a measure of riboflavin status, attempts to activate erythrocyte GSH-Px from selenium-deficient animals by adding selenium *in vitro* have been unsuccessful. Indeed, it is not even known whether GSH-Px has a dissociable selenium cofactor and, if so, what its chemical nature is.

When the chemical nature of selenium in GSH-Px is established, studies on the biosynthetic pathway by which the selenium is introduced into GSH-Px will be interesting. It is possible that some cases of decreased GSH-Px may be secondary effects resulting from a primary inability to utilize dietary selenium for GSH-Px synthesis as a result of hereditary, environmental, or nutritional conditions. The ability of silver and tri-*o*-cresyl phosphate to bring about a marked decrease in GSH-Px in animals fed diets adequate in selenium may involve such an effect, and the decrease in GSH-Px observed with iron deficiency might have a similar origin. Thus, even in individuals with an apparently normal selenium status, it is possible that GSH-Px deficiency could result from causes other than a direct genetic defect involving the biosynthesis of the enzyme per se.

Although GSH-Px is a multisubunit protein, little is known about possible isoenzyme forms. It would be desirable to compare the properties of GSH-Px isolated from different tissues under similar conditions. The same could be said for the enzyme from different subcellular fractions. Also, the isolation of GSH-Px from plasma would be a useful contribution, in order to verify that the apparent high levels of activity reported in some cases are not artifacts. The origin of plasma GSH-Px and the cause of the elevated GSH-Px in many tissues when high levels of dietary selenium are fed remains unknown. In the case of the apparent adaptive increase in tissue GSH-Px produced by oxidative stress, can this be a secondary result of tissue destruction followed by invasion of the tissue with phagocytic cells rich in GSH-Px?

To what extent the pathological changes in selenium deficiency can be explained by decreased GSH-Px activity, as opposed to other biological functions of selenium that many believe are yet to be discovered, is not known. Certainly the presence of selenium in GSH-Px provides a reasonable basis for explaining disorders responsive to selenium in terms of oxidative damage. A great deal of carefully planned research is needed to elucidate the relationships between pathological changes, the sites and magnitude of oxidant stress generation in various tissues and within cellular components, in relation to the distribution of vitamin E, GSH-Px, and related enzymes that function in oxidative damage. Specific suggestions along these lines have been made elsewhere (Hoekstra, 1974).

The fact that dietary selenium strongly affects GSH-Px activity does complicate the interpretation of individual cases where GSH-Px deficiency is found in association with this or that disorder, making it even more difficult to establish cause and effect relationships out of observed correlations. However, the ability to experimentally induce GSH-Px deficiency by nutritional means also provides a way of investigating whether the postulated cause and effect relationship is soundly based. One can induce GSH-Px deficiency at will, at least in experimental animals, rather than being dependent on the availability of rare individuals with the presenting symptom. This approach can be criticized because selenium deficiency might produce other changes besides GSH-Px deficiency. But it seems likely that GSH-Px is very rapidly lost from many tissues, and might be preferentially lost before other biologically active forms of selenium. At least, the attempt should be made to reproduce in selenium-deficient animals the disorders attributed to hereditary GSH-Px peroxidase deficiency in humans. It is surprising how little overlap exists between the recognized signs of selenium deficiency in animals and the symptoms recognized in humans with low GSH-Px activity. The opportunity now exists to explore selenium and GSH-Px together instead of independently, as has been the case from the time they first attracted the attention of investigators.

REFERENCES

Abrams, B. A., Gutteridge. J. M. C., Stocks, J., Friedman, M., and Dormandy, T. L. (1973) Vitamin E in neonatal hyperbilirubinaemia. *Arch. Dis. Childhood* 48, 721–724.

Aebi, H., and Suter, H. (1966). Peroxide sensitivity of acatalatic erythrocytes. *Humangenetik* 2, 328–343.

Aebi, H., Baggiolini, M., Dewald, B., Lauber, E., Suter, H., Micheli, A., and Frei, J. (1964a). Observations on two Swiss families with acatalasia II. *Enzymol. Biol. Clin.* 4, 121–151.

Aebi, H., Heiniger, J. T., and Lauber, E. (1964b). Methemoglobin formation in erythrocytes due to peroxide action. Experiments on the evaluation of the protective function of catalase and glutathione peroxidase. *Helv. Chim. Acta* 47, 1428–1440.

Albanese, A. A., and Buschke, W. (1942). On cataract and certain other manifestations of tryptophan deficiency in rats. *Science* 95, 584–586.

Allaway, W. H., Kubota, J., Losee, F., and Roth, M. (1968). Selenium, molybdenum, and vanadium in human blood. *Arch. Environ. Health* 16, 342–348.

Allen, R. C., Stjerholm, R. L., and Steele, R. H. (1972). Evidence for the generation of an electronic excitation state(s) in human polymorphonuclear leukocytes and its participation in bactericidal activity. *Biochem. Biophys. Res. Commun.* 47, 679–684.

Allison, A. C. (1955). Danger of vitamin K to the newborn. *Lancet* 1, 669.

Anderson, E. E., and Spector, A. (1971). Oxidation reduction reactions involving ascorbic acid and the hexose monophosphate shunt in corneal epithelium. *Invest. Ophthalmol.* 10, 41–53.

Armstrong, D., Dimmitt, S., and VanWormer, D. E. (1974). Studies in Batten disease. I. Peroxidase deficiency in granulocytes. *Arch. Neurol. (Chicago)* 30, 144–152.

Arstila, A. U., Smith, M. A., and Trump, B. F. (1972). Microsomal lipid peroxidation: Morphological characterization. *Science* 175, 530–532.

Azimi, P. H., Bodenbender, J. G., Hintz, R. L., and Kontras, S. B. (1968). Chronic granulomatous disease in three female siblings. *J. Amer. Med. Ass.* 206, 2865–2871.

Babior, B. M., Kipnes, R. S., and Curnutte, J. T. (1973). Biological defense mechanisms. The production by leukocytes of superoxide, a potential bactericidal agent. *J. Clin. Invest.* 52, 741–744.

Baehner, R. L. (1972). Disorders of leukocytes leading to recurrent infection. *Pediat. Clin. N. Amer.* 19, 935–956.

Baehner, R. L., and Nathan, D. G. (1968). Quantitative nitroblue tetrazolium test in chronic granulomatous disease. *N. Engl. J. Med.* 278, 971–978.

Baehner, R. L., Gilman, N., and Karnovsky, M. L. (1970). Respiration and glucose oxidation in human and guinea pig leukocytes: Comparative studies. *J. Clin. Invest.* 49, 692–700.

Baehner, R. L., Johnston, R. B., Jr., and Nathan, D. G. (1972). Comparative study of the metabolic and bactericidal characteristics of severe glucose-6-phosphate dehydrogenase deficient polymorphonuclear leukocytes and leukocytes from children with chronic granulomatous disease. *J. Reticuloendothel. Soc.* 12, 150–157.

Bagchi, K. (1959). The effects of methionine-sulfoximine induced methionine deficiency on the crystalline lens of albino rats. *Indian J. Med. Res.* 47, 437–447.

Bannatyne, R. M., Skowron, P. N., and Weber, J. L. (1969). Job's syndrome—a variant of chronic granulomatous disease. *J. Pediat.* 75, 236–242.

Barber, G. W. (1973). Human cataractogenesis: A review. *Exp. Eye Res.* 16, 85–94.

Beck, W. S. (1958). Occurrence and control of the phosphogluconate oxidation pathway in normal and leukemic leukocytes. *J. Biol. Chem.* 232, 271–287.

Bernstein, H. N. (1967). Chloroquine ocular toxicity. *Surv. Ophthalmol.* 12, 415–447.

Betke, K., Kleinhauer, E., and Lipps, M. (1956). Vergleichende untersuchungen über die spontan oxydation von Nableschnar and Erwachsenenhamoglobin. *Z. Kinderheilk.* 77, 549–553.

Beutler, E. (1965). Glucose-6-phosphate dehydrogenase deficiency and nonspherocytic congenital hemolytic anemia. *Semin. Hematol.* 2, 91–138.

Beutler, E. (1969a). Drug-induced hemolytic anemia. *Pharmacol. Rev.* 21, 73–103.

Beutler, E. (1969b). Effect of flavin compounds on GSSG-R activity: *In vivo* and *in vitro* studies. *J. Clin. Invest.* 48, 1957–1966.

220 GANTHER, HAFEMAN, LAWRENCE, SERFASS, AND HOEKSTRA

Beutler, E. (1972a). Drug-induced anemia. *Fed. Proc., Fed. Amer. Soc. Exp. Biol.* **31,** 141–146.
Beutler, E. (1972b). Disorders due to enzyme defects in the red blood cell. *Advan. Metab. Disord.* **6,** 131–160.
Beutler, E. (1972c). Glanzmann's thrombasthenia and reduced glutathione. *N. Engl. J. Med.* **287,** 1094–1095.
Beutler, E., and Srivastava, S. K. (1970). Relationship between glutathione reductase activity and drug-induced haemolytic anemia. *Nature (London)* **226,** 759–760.
Beutler, E., and West, C. (1974). Red cell glutathione peroxidase polymorphism in Afro-Americans. *Amer. J. Hum. Genet.* **26,** 255–258.
Bhuyan, K. C., and Bhuyan, D. K. (1970). Catalase in ocular tissue and its intracellular distribution in corneal epithelium. *Amer. J. Ophthalmol.* **69,** 147–153.
Bhuyan, K. C., Bhuyan, D. K., and Katzin, H. M. (1973). Amizol-induced cataract and inhibition of lens catalase in rabbit. *Ophthalmol. Res.* **5,** 236–247.
Boguslawska-Jaworska, J., and Kaplan, J. C. (1969). A simple screening test for glutathione peroxidase activity in red cells. *Clin. Chim. Acta* **26,** 459–463.
Boivin, P., Galand, C., André, R., and Debray, J. (1966). Anémies hémolytiques congénitales avec déficit isolé en glutathion réduit par déficit en glutathion synthétase. *Nouv. Rev. Fr. Hematol.* **6,** 859–866.
Boivin, P., Galand, C., Hakim, J., Rogé, J., and Guéroult, N. (1969). Anémie hémolytique avec déficit en glutathion peroxydase chez un adulte. *Enzymol. Biol. Clin.* **10,** 68–80.
Bourne, M. C., and Pyke, M. A. (1935). The occurrence of cataract in rats fed on diets deficient in vitamin B₂. *Biochem. J.* **29,** 1865–1871.
Bracci, R., Calabri, G., Bettini, F., and Princi, P. (1970a). Glutathione peroxidase in human leukocytes. *Clin. Chim. Acta* **29,** 345–348.
Bracci, R., Benedetti, P. A., and Ciambellotti, V. (1970b). Hydrogen peroxide generation in erythrocytes of newborn infants. *Biol. Neonate* **15,** 135–141.
Brewer, G. J. (1969). 6-phosphogluconate dehydrogenase and glutathione reductase. *In* "Biochemical Methods in Red Cell Genetics" (G. J. Yunis, ed.), pp. 139–165. Academic Press, New York.
Brown, D. G., and Burk, R. F. (1973). Selenium retention in tissues and sperm of rats fed a Torula yeast diet. *J. Nutr.* **103,** 102–108.
Bunce, G. E., Caasi, P., Hall, B., and Chavez, N. (1972). Prevention of cataracts in the progeny of rats fed a maternal diet based on vegetable proteins. *Proc. Soc. Exp. Biol. Med.* **140,** 1103–1107.
Bunyan, J., Diplock, A. T., Cawthorne, M. A., and Green, J. (1968). Vitamin E and stress. 8. Nutritional effects of dietary stress with silver in vitamin E-deficient chicks and rats. *Brit. J. Nutr.* **22,** 165–182.
Butenandt, O. (1971). Glutathione, glutathione peroxidase, glutathione reductase, glucose-6-phosphate dehydrogenase, lactic dehydrogenase, and catalase in erythrocytes of newborns, infants, and children and their relation to the formation of Heinz bodies. *Z. Kinderheilk.* **111,** 149–161.
Carson, P. E., and Frischer, H. (1966). Glucose-6-phosphate dehydrogenase deficiency and related disorders of the pentose phosphate pathway. *Amer. J. Med.* **41,** 744–761.
Carson, P. E., Brewer, G. J., and Ickes, C. (1961). Decreased glutathione reductase with susceptibility to hemolysis. *J. Lab. Clin. Med.* **58,** 804 (abstr.).
Cartwright, G. E., Wintrobe, M. M., Buschke, W., Follis, R. H., Jr., Suksta, A., and Humphries, S. (1945). Anemia, hypoproteinemia and cataracts in swine

fed casein hydrolyzates or Zein. Comparison with pyridoxine deficiency anemia. *J. Clin. Invest.* **24,** 268–279.

Chernick, S. S., Moe, J. G., Rodman, G. P., and Schwarz, K. (1955). A metabolic lesion in dietary necrotic liver degeneration. *J. Biol. Chem.* **217,** 829–843.

Chow, C. K., and Tappel, A. L. (1972). An enzymatic protective mechanism against lipid peroxidation damage to lungs of ozone exposed rats. *Lipids* **7,** 518–524.

Chow, C. K., and Tappel, A. L. (1973). Activities of pentose shunt and glycolytic enzymes in lungs of ozone exposed rats. *Arch. Environ. Health* **26,** 205–208.

Chow, C. K., and Tappel, A. L. (1974). Response of glutathione peroxidase to dietary selenium in rats. *J. Nutr.* **104,** 444–451.

Chow, C. K., Reddy, K., and Tappel, A. L. (1973). Effect of dietary vitamin E on the activities of the glutathione peroxidase system in rat tissues. *J. Nutr.* **104,** 618–624.

Christophersen, B. O. (1968). Formation of monohydroxypolyenic fatty acids from lipid peroxides by a glutathione peroxidase. *Biochim. Biophys.* Acta **164,** 35–46.

Christophersen, B. O. (1969). Reduction of x-ray-induced DNA and thymine hydroperoxides by rat liver glutathione peroxidase. *Biochim. Biophys.* Acta **186,** 387–389.

Cibis, P. A., Constant, M., Pribye, A., and Becker, B. (1957). Ocular lesions produced by iodoacetate acid. *AMA Arch. Ophthalmol.* **57,** [N.S.] 508–519.

Cohen, G., and Hochstein, P. (1963). Glutathione peroxidase: The primary agent for the elimination of hydrogen peroxide in erythrocytes. *Biochemistry* **2,** 1420–1428.

Cohen, G., and Hochstein, P. (1964). Generation of hydrogen peroxide in erythrocytes by hemolytic agents. *Biochemistry* **3,** 895–900.

Comporti, M., and Benedetti, A. (1972). Carbon tetrachloride-induced peroxidation of liver lipids in vitamin E pretreated rats. *Biochem. Pharmacol.* **21,** 418–420.

Cornblath, M., and Hartman, A. F. (1948). Methemoglobinemia in young infants. *J. Pediat.* **33,** 421–425.

Curnutte, J., and Babior, B. M. (1974). The effect of bacteria and serum on superoxide production by granulocytes. *J. Clin. Invest.* **53,** 1662–1672.

Curtis, P. B., Hague, S. M., and Kraybill, H. R. (1932). The nutritive value of certain animal protein concentrates. *J. Nutr.* **5,** 503–517.

Dam, H., and Glavind, J. (1940). Vitamin E and capillary permeability. *Naturwissenschaften* **28,** 207.

Davis, W. C., Douglas, S. D., and Fudenberg, H. H. (1968). Impaired neutrophil function and "granulomatous diseases." *Fed. Proc., Fed. Amer. Soc. Exp. Biol.* **27,** 671A.

Day, P. L., and Darby, W. J. (1936). The inverse relation between growth and incidence of cataract in rats given graded amounts of vitamin G containing foods. *J. Nutr.* **12,** 387–394.

Day, P. L., Langston, W. C., and O'Brien, C. S. (1931). Cataract and other ocular changes in vitamin G deficiency. *Amer. J. Ophthalmol.* **14,** 1005–1009.

DeChatelet, L. R., Cooper, M. R., and McCall, C. E. (1971). Dissociation by colchicine of the hexose monophosphate shunt activation from the bactericidal activity of the leukocyte, *Infec. Immunity* **3,** 66–71.

deDuve, C., and Baudhuin, P. (1966). Peroxisomes (microbodies and related particles). *Physiol. Rev.* **46,** 323–357.

Demus-Oole, A., Swierczewski, E. (1969a). Glutathione peroxidase in rat liver during development. I. Localization and characterization of the enzyme in the subcellular liver fractions of newborn and adult rat. *Biol. Neonate* **14,** 211–210.

Demus-Oole, A., and Swierczewski, E. (1969b). Glutathione peroxidase in rat liver during development. II. Changes in glutathione peroxidase during postnatal development of normal and hypotropic rats. *Biol. Neonate* **14**, 219–225.

Demus-Oole, A., Swierczewski, E., and Minkowski, A. (1969). Glutathione peroxidase in rat liver during development. *Z. Klin. Chem.* **7**, 209.

DeWitt, W. B. (1957). Experimental *Schistosomiasis mansoni* in mice maintained on nutritionally deficient diets. I. Effects of a Torula yeast ration deficient in Factor 3, vitamin E, and cystine. *J. Parasitol.* **43**, 119–128.

Dickson, R. C., and Tomlinson, R. H. (1967). Selenium in blood and human tissues. *Clin. Chim. Acta* **16**, 311–321.

DiLuzio, N. R. (1968). Letter to the editor. The role of lipid peroxidation and antioxidants in ethanol-induced lipid alterations. *Exp. Mol. Pathol.* **8**, 394–402.

Duchon, G., and Collier, H. B. (1971). Enzyme activities of human erythrocyte ghosts: Effect of various treatments. *J. Membrane Biol.* **6**,138–157.

Emerson, P. M., Mason, D. Y., and Cuthbert, J. E. (1972). Erythrocyte glutathione peroxidase content and serum tocopherol levels in newborn infants. *Brit. J. Haematol.* **22**, 667–680.

Ernster, L., and Nordenbrand, K. (1967). Microsomal lipid peroxidation. In "Methods in Enzymology" (R. W. Estabrook and M. E. Pullman, eds.), Vol. 10, pp. 574–580. Academic Press, New York.

Fairbanks, V. F., and Fernandez, M. N. (1969). The identification of metabolic errors associated with hemolytic anemia. *J. Amer. Med. Ass.* **208**, 316–320.

Ferguson, T. M., Atkinson, R. L., and Couch, J. R. (1954). Relationship of vitamin E to embryonic development of avian eye. *Proc. Soc. Exp. Biol. Med.* **86**, 868–871.

Ferguson, T. M., Rigdon, R. H., and Couch, J. R. (1956). Cataracts in vitamin E deficiency: An experimental study in the turkey embryo. *AMA Arch. Ophthalmol.* **55**, [N.S.] 346–355.

Flohe, L. (1969). Spezifischer nachweis der glutathion-peroxydase auf cellogel-elektrophoresestreifen und bestimmung des isoelektrischen punktes. *Hoppe-Zeyler's Z. Physiol. Chem.* **350**, 856–858.

Flohe, L. (1971). Die glutathionperoxidase: Enzymologie und biologische aspekte. *Klin. Wochenschr.* **49**, 669–683.

Flohe, L., and Brand, I. (1969). Kinetics of glutathione peroxidase. *Biochim. Biophys. Acta* **191**, 541–549.

Flohe, L., and Brand, I. (1970). Some hints to avoid pitfalls in quantitative determination of glutathione peroxidase (EC 1,11,1,9). *Z. Klin. Chem. Klin. Biochem.* **8**, 156–161.

Flohe, L., and Schlegel, W. (1971). Glutathione-peroxidase. IV. Intrazellulaire verteilung des glutathion-peroxidase-systems in der rattenleber. *Hoppe-Zeyler's Z. Physiol. Chem.* **352**, 1401–1410.

Flohe, L., Schlegel, W., and Schaich, E. (1970). Zur frage der identitat von gluta-thion peroxidase aus erythrocyten und leber ("contraction Factor I") der ratte. *Z. Klin. Chem. Klin. Biochem.* **8**, 149–155.

Flohe, L., Eisele, B., and Wendel, A. (1971a). Glutathion-peroxidase. I. Reindarstellung und molekulargewichts-bestimmungen. *Hoppe-Zeyler's Z. Physiol. Chem.* **352**, 151–158.

Flohe, L., Gunzler, W., Schaich, E., and Schneider, F. (1971b). Glutathionperoxidase. II. Substratspezifitat und hemmbarkeit durch substratanaloge. *Hoppe-Zeyler's Z. Physiol. Chem.* **352**, 159–169.

Flohe, L., Schaich, E., Voelter, W., and Wendel, A. (1971c). Glutathionperoxidase. III. Spektrale charakteristika und versuche zum reacktions mechanismus. *Hoppe-Zeyler's Z. Physiol. Chem.* 352, 170–180.

Flohe, L., Loschen, G., Gunzler, W. A., and Eichele, E. (1972). Glutathione peroxidase. V. The kinetic mechanism. *Hoppe-Zeyler's Z. Physiol. Chem.* 353, 987–999.

Flohe, L., Gunzler, W. A., and Schock, H. H. (1973). Glutathione peroxidase: A selenoenzyme. *FEBS (Fed. Eur. Biochem. Soc.) Lett.* 32, 132–134.

Fodor, G., and Kemény, G. L. (1965). On the hepato-protective effect of selenium in carbon tetrachloride poisoning in albino rats. *Experientia* 21, 666–667.

Fridovich, I. (1974). Superoxide radical and the bactericidal action of phagocytes. *N. Engl. J. Med.* 290, 624–625.

Froseth, J. A., Piper, R. C., and Carlson, J. R. (1974). Relationship of dietary selenium and oral methyl mercury to blood and tissue selenium and mercury concentrations and deficiency-toxicity signs in swine. *Fed. Proc., Fed. Amer. Soc. Exp. Biol.* 33, 660.

Gallagher, C. H. (1962). The effect of antioxidants on poisoning by carbon tetrachloride. *Aust. J. Exp. Biol. Med. Sci.* 40, 241–253.

Ganther, H. E. (1971). Reduction of the selenotrisulfide derivative of glutathione to a persulfide analogue by glutathione reductase. *Biochemistry* 10, 4089–4098.

Ganther, H. E. (1974). Biochemistry of selenium. In "Selenium" (R. A. Zingaro and W. C. Cooper, eds.) pp. 546–614. Van Nostrand-Reinhold, Princeton, New Jersey.

Ganther, H. E., and Corcoran, C. (1969). Selenotrisulfides. II. Cross-linking of reduced pancreatic ribonuclease with selenium. *Biochemistry* 7, 2557–2563.

Ganther, H. E., and Hsieh, H. (1974). Mechanisms for the conversion of selenite to selenides in mammalian tissues. In "Trace Element Metabolism in Animals" (W. G. Hoekstra et al., eds.), pp. 339–353. Univ. Park Press, Baltimore, Maryland.

Ganther, H. E., Goudie, C., Sunde, M. L., Kopecky, M. J., Wagner, P., Oh, S. H., and Hoekstra, W. G. (1972). Selenium: Relation to decreased toxicity of methylmercury added to diets containing tuna. *Science* 175, 1122–1124.

Ganther, H. E., Oh, S. H., Chitharanjan, D., and Hoekstra, W. G. (1974). Studies on selenium in glutathione peroxidase *Fed. Proc., Fed. Amer. Soc. Exp. Biol.* 33, 694.

Gasser, C. (1953). The hemolytic anemia of premature infants with spontaneous Heinz-body formation, a new syndrome observed in 14 cases. *Helv. Paediat. Acta* 8, 491–529.

Gharib, H., Fairbanks, V. F., and Bartholomew, L. G. (1969). Hepatic failure with acanthocytosis associated with hemolytic anemia and deficiency of glutathione peroxidase. *Proc. Staff Meet. Mayo Clin.* 44, 96–101.

Glader, B. E., and Conrad, M. E. (1972). Decreased glutathione peroxidase in neonatal erythrocytes: Lack of relation to hydrogen peroxide metabolism. *Pediat. Res.* 6, 900–904.

Glatzle, D., Weber, F., and Wiss, O. (1968). Enzymatic test for detection of a riboflavin deficiency. NADPH-dependent glutathione reductase of red blood cells and its activation by FAD in vitro. *Experientia* 24, 1122.

Gooley, C. M., Keyzer, H., and Setchell, F. (1969). Free radical drug enhancement. *Nature (London)* 223, 80–81.

Gram, T. E., and Fouts, J. R. (1966). Effect of α-tocopherol upon lipid peroxidation and drug metabolism in hepatic microsomes. *Arch. Biochem. Biophys.* 114, 331–335.

Gray, G. R., Stamatoyannopoulos, G., Naiman, S. C., Kliman, M. R., Klebanoff, S. J., Austin, T., Yoshida, A., and Robinson, G. C. F. (1973). Neutrophil dysfunction, chronic granulomatous disease, and non-spherocytic haemolytic anaemia caused by complete deficiency of glucose-6-phosphate dehydrogenase. *Lancet* 2, 530–534.

Green, R. C., and O'Brien, P. J. (1970). The cellular localization of glutathione peroxidase and its release from mitochondria during swelling. *Biochim. Biophys. Acta* 197, 31–39.

Grosch W., Senser, F., and Fischer, K. (1972). Einfluss von auf heringen wachsenden mikroorganismen auf die fettoxidation. III. Glutation-peroxidase-aktivitat in einer candida lipolytica-rat. *Chem. Mikrobiol. Technol. Lebensm.* 1, 214–218.

Gross, R. T., and Schroeder, E. A. R. (1963). The relationship of TPNH content to abnormalities in the erythrocytes of premature infants. *J. Pediat.* 63, 823–825.

Gross, R. T., Bracci, R., Rudolph, N. Schroeder, E., and Kochen, J. A. (1967). Hydrogen peroxide toxicity and detoxification in erythrocytes of newborn infants. *Blood* 29, 481–493.

Gunzler, W. A., Vergin, H., Muller, I., and Flohe, L. (1972). Glutathion-peroxidase. VI. Die reaktion der glutathion-peroxidase mit verschiedenen hydroperoxiden. *Hoppe-Zeyler's Z. Physiol. Chem.* 353, 1001–1004.

Hafeman, D. G., Sunde, R. A., and Hoekstra, W. G. (1974). Effect of dietary selenium on erythrocyte and liver glutathione peroxidase in the rat. *J. Nutr.* 104, 580–586.

Hall, W. K., Bowles, L. L., Sydenstricker, V. P., and Schmidt, H L., Jr. (1948). Cataracts due to deficiencies of phenylalanine and of histidine in the rat. A comparison with other types of cataracts. *J. Nutr.* 36, 277–295.

Hamberg, H., Svensson, J., Wakabayashi, T., and Samuelsson, B. (1974). Isolation and structure of two prostaglandin endoperoxides that cause platelet aggregation. *Proc. Nat. Acad. Sci. U.S.* 71, 345–349.

Harley, J. D., Robin, H., Meuser, M. A., and Hertzberg, R. (1966). Cataracts in glucose-6-phosphate dehydrogenase deficiency. *Brit. Med. J.* 1, 421.

Hassan, H. A., Hashim, S. A., Van Itallie, T., and Sebrell, W. H. (1966). Syndrome in premature infants associated with low plasma vitamin E levels and high polyunsaturated fatty acids in the diet. *Amer. J. Clin. Nutr.* 19, 147–157.

Helge, H., and Barness, K. (1966). Congenital hemolytic anemia, cataract, and glucose-6-phosphate dehydrogenase deficiency. *Deut. Med. Wochenschr.* 91, 1584–1590.

Hermansky, F., and Pudlak, P. (1959). Albinism associated with hemorrhagic diathesis and unusual pigmented reticular cells in the bone marrow: Report of two cases with histochemical studies. *Blood* 14, 162–169.

Hinman, J. W. (1972). Prostaglandins. *Annu. Rev. Biochem.* 41, 161–178.

Hochstein, P., and Ernster, L. (1963). ADP-activated lipid peroxidation coupled to the TPNH oxidase system of microsomes. *Biochem. Biophys. Res. Commun.* 12, 388–394.

Hochstein, P., and Utley, H. (1968). Hydrogen peroxide detoxification by glutathione peroxidase and catalase in rat liver homogenates. *Mol. Pharmacol.* 4, 574–579.

Hochstein, P., Nordenbrand, K., and Ernster, L. (1964). Evidence for the involvement of iron in the ADP-activated peroxidation of lipids in microsomes and mitochondria. *Biochem. Biophys. Res. Commun.* 14, 323–328.

Hoekstra, W. G. (1974). Biochemical role of selenium. In "Trace Element Metabolism in Animals" (W. G. Hoekstra et al., eds.), pp. 61–76. Univ. Park Press, Baltimore, Maryland.

Hoekstra, W. G. (1975). Biochemical function of selenium and its relation to vitamin E. Fed. Proc., Fed. Amer. Soc. Exp. Biol. 34, 2083–2089.

Hoekstra, W. G., Hafeman, O., Oh, S. H., Sunde, R. A., and Ganther, H. E. (1973). Effect of dietary selenium on liver and erythrocyte glutathione peroxidase in the rat. Fed. Proc., Fed. Amer. Soc. Exp. Biol. 32, 885.

Hogberg, J., Bergstrand, A., and Jakobsson, S. V. (1973). Lipid peroxidation of rat-liver microsomes. Its effect on the microsomal membrane and some membrane-bound microsomal enzymes. Eur. J. Biochem. 37, 51–59.

Holmberg, N. J. (1968). Purification and properties of glutathione peroxidase from bovine lens. Exp. Eye Res. 7, 570–580.

Holmes, B., Quie, P. G., Windhorst, D. B., and Good, R. A. (1966). Fatal granulomatous disease of childhood. An inborn abnormality of phagocytic function. Lancet 1, 1225.

Holmes, B., Page, A. R., and Good, R. A. (1967). Studies of the metabolic activity of leukocytes from patients with a genetic abnormality of phagocytic function. J. Clin. Invest. 46, 1422–1431.

Holmes, B., Park, B. H., Malawista, S. E., Quie, P. G., Nelson, D. L., and Good, R. A. (1970). Chronic granulomatous disease in females. N. Engl. J. Med. 283, 217–221.

Hopkins, J., and Tudhope, G. R. (1973). Glutathione peroxidase in human red cells in health and disease. Brit. J. Haematol. 25, 563–575.

Hove, E. L. (1948). Interrelation between α-tocopherol and protein metabolism. III. The protective effect of vitamin E and certain nitrogenous compounds against CCl₄ poisoning in rats. Arch. Biochem. 17, 467–474.

Jacob, H. S. (1971). Mechanism of hemoglobin precipitation into Heinz bodies: Possible relevance to cataract formation. Exp. Eye Res. 11, 356–364.

Jacob, H. S., Ingbar, S. H., and Jandl, J. H. (1965). Oxidative hemolysis and erythrocyte metabolism in hereditary acatalasia. J. Clin. Invest. 44, 1187–1199.

Jaffe, E. R. (1970). Hereditary hemolytic disorders and enzymatic deficiencies of human erythrocytes. Blood 35, 116–134.

Jaffe, E. R., Rieber, E. E., Anderson, H. M., Kosower, N. S., and Penny, J. L. (1968). Glutathione reductase activity and hemolysis in hemoglobin C disease. J. Clin. Invest. 47, 51a.

Jenkins, K., and Hidiroglou, M. (1972). Comparative metabolism of ⁷⁵Se-selenite, ⁷⁵Se-selenate, and ⁷⁵Se-selenomethionine in bovine erythrocytes. Can. J. Physiol. Pharmacol. 50, 927–935.

Johnston, R. B., Jr., and Baehner, R. L. (1971). Chronic granulomatous disease: Correlation between pathogenesis and clinical findings. Pediatrics 48, 730–748.

Kagan, V. E., Shvedova, A. A., Novikov, K. N., and Kozlov, Y. P. (1973). Light-induced free radical oxidation of membrane lipids in photoreceptors of frog retina. Biochim. Biophys. Acta 330, 76–79.

Kaplan, J. C. (1971). Defects of glutathione reducing and synthesizing reactions in the red cells. Rev. Eur. Etud. Clin. Biol. 16, 523–528.

Karpatkin, S., and Weiss, H. J. (1972). Deficiency of glutathione peroxidase associated with high levels of reduced glutathione in Glanzmann's thrombasthenia. N. Engl. J. Med. 287, 1062–1066.

Karremann, G., Isenberg, I., and Szent-Györgi, A. (1959). On the mechanism of action of chlorpromazine. *Science* 130, 1191–1192.

Keitt, A. S. (1971). Enzymes deficient hemolytic anemias—mechanisms, diagnosis, and treatment. *Mod. Treat.* 8, 402–418.

Khandwala, A., and Gee, J. B. L. (1973). Linoleic acid hydroperoxide: Impaired bacterial uptake by alveolar macrophages, a mechanism of oxidant lung injury. *Science* 182, 1364–1365.

Kinoshita, J. H. (1955). Carbohydrate metabolism of the lens. *AMA Arch. Ophthalmol.* 54, [N.S.] 360–368.

Kinoshita, J. H. (1964). Selected topics in ophthalmic biochemistry. *Arch. Ophthalmol.* 72, 554–572.

Klayman, D. L. (1973). Selenols and their derivatives (excluding selenides). *In* "Organic Selenium Compounds: Their Chemistry and Biology" (D. L. Klayman and H. H. Gunther, eds.), pp. 157–171. Wiley (Interscience), New York.

Klebanoff, S. (1971). Intraleukocytic microbicidal defects. *Annu. Rev. Med.* 22, 39–62.

Konrad, P. N., Valentine, W. N., and Paglia, D. E. (1972). Enzymatic activities and glutathione content of erythrocytes in the newborn. Comparison with red cells of older normal subjects and those with comparable reticulocytosis. *Acta Haematol.* 48, 193–201.

Kravitz, H., Elegant, L. D., Kaiser, E., and Kagan, B. M. (1956). Methemoglobin values in premature and mature infants and children. *Amer. J. Dis. Child.* 91, 1–5.

Kubota, J., Allaway, W. H., Carter, D. L., Cary, E. E., and Lazar, V. A. (1967). Selenium in crops in the United States in relation to the selenium-responsive diseases of livestock, *J. Agr. Food. Chem.* 15, 448–453.

Kuck, J. F. R., Jr. (1970). The lens. *In* "Biochemistry of the Eye" (C. N. Graymore, ed.), pp. 319–371. Pergamon, Oxford.

Lausecker, C., Heidt, P., Fischer, D., Hartleyb, H., and Lohr, G. W. (1965). Anémie hémolytique constitutionnelle avec déficit in 6-phospho-gluconate-déshydrogénase. *Arch. Fr. Pediat.* 22, 789–797.

Lawrence, R. A. (1975). Ph.D. Thesis, University of Wisconsin.

Lawrence, R. A., Sunde, R. A., Schwartz, G. L., and Hoekstra, W. G. (1974). Glutathione peroxidase activity in rat lens and other tissues in relation to dietary selenium intake. *Exp. Eye Res.* 18, 563–569.

Lee, M., Dong, A., and Yano, J. (1969). Metabolism of ⁷⁵Se-selenite by human whole blood *in vitro*. *Can. J. Biochem.* 47, 791–797.

Lehrer, R. I., and Cline, M. J. (1969). Leukocyte myeloperoxidase deficiency and disseminated candidiasis. *J. Clin. Invest.* 48, 1478–1488.

Lerman, S. (1959). Enzymatic factors in experimental galactose cataract. *Science* 130, 1473–1474.

Lerman, S. (1965). Metabolic pathways in experimental sugar and radiation cataract. *Physiol. Rev.* 45, 98–122.

Levander, O. A., Morris, V. C., and Higgs, D. J. (1974). Characterization of the selenium in rat liver mitochondria as glutathione peroxidase. *Biochem. Biophys. Res. Commun.* 58, 1047–1052.

Lie-Injo, L. E., Wong, W. P., and Ng, T. (1973). Reduced glutathione, glutathione reductase, glutathione peroxidase, and pyruvate kinase in the erythrocytes of human newborns and adults in Malaysia. *Brit. J. Haematol.* 25, 577–584.

Lie-Injo, L. E., Ng, T., and Balakrishnan, S. (1974). Red cell enzymes in cord blood and plasma bilirubin levels in the first week of life. *Clin. Chim. Acta* **50**, 77–83.

Linden, O., and Work, E. (1953). Experimental liver necrosis in rats. I. Changes in liver, blood, and spleen glutathione and ascorbic acid levels in dietetic liver necrosis. *Biochem. J.* **55**, 554–562.

Little, C. (1972). Steroid hydroperoxides as substrates for glutathione peroxidase. *Biochim. Biophys. Acta* **284**, 375–381.

Little, C., and O'Brien, P. J. (1968). An intracellular GSH-peroxidase with a lipid peroxidase substrate. *Biochem. Biophys. Res. Commun.* **31**, 145–150.

Little, C., Olinescu, R., Reid, K. G., and O'Brien, P. J. (1970a). Properties and regulation of glutathione peroxidase. *J. Biol. Chem.* **245**, 3632–3636.

Little, C., Olinescu, R. M., and O'Brien, P. J. (1970b). Inhibition of glutathione peroxidase by coenzyme A. *Biochem. Biophys. Res. Commun.* **41**, 287–293.

Lo, S. S. (1973). Vitamin E and hemolytic anemia in premature infants. *Arch. Dis. Childhood* **48**, 360–365.

Lubia, B., and Oski, F. A. (1972). Red cell metabolism in the newborn infant. VI. Irreversible oxidant-induced injury. *J. Pediat.* **81**, 698–704.

McCay, P. B., Poyer, J. L., Pfeifer, P. M., May, H. E., and Gilliam, J. M. (1971). A function for α-tocopherol: Stabilization of the microsomal membrane from radical attack during TPNH-dependent oxidations. *Lipids* **6**, 297–306.

MacDonald, C. M. (1973). The effects of ethanol on hepatic lipid peroxidation and on the activities of glutathione reductase and peroxidase. *FEBS (Fed. Eur. Biochem. Soc.) Lett.* **35**, 227–230.

MacDougall, L. G. (1972). Red cell metabolism in iron deficiency anemia. III. The relationship between glutathione peroxidase, catalase, serum vitamin E and susceptibility of iron-deficient red cells to oxidative hemolysis. *J. Pediat.* **80**, 775–782.

Mandell, G. L. (1972). Functional and metabolic derangements in human neutrophils induced by a glutathione antagonist. *J. Reticuloendothel. Soc.* **11**, 129–137.

Marcus, A. J. (1969). Platelet function. *N. Engl. J. Med.* **280**, 1213–1220.

Marquis, N. R., Vigdahl, R. L., and Tavormina, P. A. (1969). Platelet aggregation. I. Regulation by cyclic AMP and prostaglandin E_1. *Biochem. Biophys. Res. Commun.* **36**, 965–972.

May, H. E., and McCay, P. B. (1968). Reduced triphosphopyridine nucleotide oxidase-catalyzed alterations of membrane phospholipids. I. Nature of lipid alterations. *J. Biol. Chem.* **243**, 2288–2295.

Melhorn, D. K., and Gross, R. T. (1971a). Vitamin E-dependent anemia in the premature infant. I. Effect of large doses of medicinal iron. *J. Pediat.* **79**, 569–580.

Melhorn, D. K., and Gross, R. T. (1971b). Vitamin E-dependent anemia in the premature infant. II. Relationships between gestational age and absorption of vitamin E. *J. Pediat.* **79**, 581–588.

Meyers, L. S., Jr. (1973). Free radical damage of nucleic acids and their components by ionizing radiation. *Fed. Proc., Fed. Amer. Soc. Exp. Biol.* **32**, 1882–1884.

Mills, G. C. (1957). Hemoglobin catabolism. I. Glutathione peroxidase, an erythrocyte enzyme which protects hemoglobin from oxidative breakdown. *J. Biol. Chem.* **229**, 189–197.

Mills, G. C. (1959). The purification and properties of glutathione peroxidase of erythrocytes. *J. Biol. Chem.* **234**, 502–506.

Mills, G. C. (1960). Glutathione peroxidase and the destruction of hydrogen peroxide in animal tissues. *Arch. Biochem. Biophys.* **86**, 1–5.

228 GANTHER, HAFEMAN, LAWRENCE, SERFASS, AND HOEKSTRA

Mills, G. C., and Randall, H. P. (1958). Hemoglobin catabolism. II. The protection of hemoglobin from oxidative breakdown in the intact erythrocyte. *J. Biol. Chem.* 232, 589–598.

Muth, O. H. (1960). Carbon tetrachloride poisoning of ewes on a low selenium ration. *Amer. J. Vet. Res.* 21, 86–87.

Nakamura, W., Hosoda, S., and Hayashi, K. (1974). Purification and properties of rat liver glutathione peroxidase. *Biochim. Biophys. Acta* 358, 251–261.

Necheles, T. F., Maldonado, N., Barquet-Chediak, A, and Allen, D. M. (1967). Homozygous erythrocyte glutathione peroxidase deficiency. *Blood* 30, 880–881 (abstract).

Necheles, T. F., Boles, T. A., and Allen, D. M. (1968). Erythrocyte glutathione peroxidase deficiency and hemolytic disease of the newborn infant. *J. Pediat.* 72, 319–324.

Necheles, T. F., Maldonado, N., Barquet-Chediak, A., and Allen, D. M. (1969). Homozygous erythrocyte glutathione peroxidase deficiency: Clinical and biochemical studies. *Blood* 33, 164–169.

Necheles, T. F., Stimberg, M. H., and Cameron, D. (1970). Erythrocyte glutathione peroxidase deficiency. *Brit. J. Haematol.* 19, 605-612.

Neely, C. L., and Kraus, A. P. (1972). Mechanism of drug-induced hemolytic anemia. *Advan. Intern. Med.* 18, 59-76.

Nicholls, P. (1965). Activity of catalase in the red cell. *Biochim. Biophys. Acta* 99, 286-297.

Nicholls, P. (1972). Contributions of catalase and glutathione peroxidase to red blood cell peroxide removal. *Biochim. Biophys. Acta* 279, 306–309.

Nicholls, P., and Schonbaum, G. R. (1963). Catalases. In "The Enzymes" (P. D. Boyer, H. Lardy, and K. Myrbäck, eds.), 2nd ed., Vol. 8, pp. 147–225. Academic Press, New York.

Nishimura, Y., Chida, N., Hayashi, T., and Arakawa, T. (1972). Homozygous glutathione-peroxidase deficiency of erythrocytes and leukocytes. *Tohoku J. Exp. Med.* 108, 207–217.

Noguchi, T., Cantor, A. H., and Scott, M. L. (1973). Mode of action of selenium and vitamin E in prevention of exudative diathesis in chicks. *J. Nutr.* 103, 1502–1511.

Noseworthy, J., Jr., and Karnovsky, M. L. (1972). Role of peroxide in the stimulation of the hexose monophosphate shunt during phagocytosis by polymorphonuclear leukocytes. *Enzyme* 13, 110–131.

O'Brien, P. J. (1969). Intracellular mechanisms for the decomposition of a lipid peroxide. I. Decomposition of a lipid peroxide by metal ions, heme compounds, and nucleophiles. *Can. J. Biochem.* 47, 485–492.

O'Brien, P. J., and Little, C. (1969). Intracellular mechanisms for the decomposition of a lipid peroxide. II. Decomposition of a lipid peroxide by subcellular fractions. *Can. J. Biochem.* 47, 493–499.

Oh, S-H. (1975). Ph.D. Thesis, University of Wisconsin.

Oh, S. H., Ganther, H. E., and Hoekstra, W. G. (1974a). Selenium as a component of glutathione peroxidase isolated from ovine erythrocytes. *Biochemistry* 13, 1825–1829.

Oh, S. H., Sunde, R. A., Pope, A. L., and Hoekstra, W. G. (1974b). Glutathione peroxidase response to Se intake in lambs. *J. Anim. Sci.* 39, 247.

Omaye, S. T., and Tappel, A. L. (1974a). Effect of dietary selenium on glutathione peroxidase in the chick. *J. Nutr.* 104, 747–753.

Omaye, S. T., and Tappel, A. L. (1974b). Glutathione peroxidase, glutathione reductase, and thiobarbituric acid reactive products in muscles of chickens and mice with genetic muscular dystrophy. *Life Sci.* 15, 137–145.

Oski, F. A., and Barness, L. A. (1967). Vitamin E deficiency: A previously unrecognized cause of hemolytic anemia in the premature infant. *J. Pediat.* 70, 211–220.

Paglia, D. E., and Valentine, W. N. (1967). Studies on the quantitative and qualitative characterization of erythrocyte glutathione peroxidase. *J. Lab. Clin. Med.* 70, 158–169.

Paniker, N. V., and Iyer, G. Y. N. (1965). Erythrocyte catalase and detoxification of hydrogen peroxide. *Can. J. Biochem.* 43, 1029–1039.

Paniker, N. V., and Iyer, G. Y. N. (1969). Protective factors in the detoxication of hydrogen peroxide in the red blood cell. *Can. J. Biochem.* 47, 405–410.

Paniker, N. V., and Iyer, G. Y. N. (1972). Role of red blood cell catalase in the protection of hemoglobin against hydrogen peroxide. *Indian J. Biochem. Biophys.* 9, 176–178.

Paniker, N. V., Srivastava, S. K., and Beutler, E. (1970). Glutathione metabolism of the red cells. Effect of glutathione reductase deficiency on the stimulation of hexose monophosphate shunt under oxidative stress. *Biochim. Biophys. Acta* 215, 456–460.

Paterson, C. A. (1971). Effects of drugs on the lens. *Int. Ophthalmol. Clin.* 11(2), 63–97.

Patterson, E. L., Milstrey, R., and Stokstad, E. L. R. (1957). Effect of selenium in preventing exudative diathesis in chicks. *Proc. Soc. Exp. Biol. Med.* 95, 617–620.

Piccardo, M. G., and Schwarz, K. (1958). The electron microscopy of dietary necrotic liver degeneration. *In* "Liver Function" (R. W. Brauer, ed.), pp. 528–540. Amer. Inst. Biol. Sci., Washington, D.C.

Pike, R. L. (1951). Congenital cataract in albino rats fed different amounts of tryptophan and niacin. *J. Nutr.* 44, 191.

Pinto, R. E., and Bartley, W. (1969a). The effect of age and sex on glutathione reductase and glutathione peroxidase activities and on aerobic glutathione oxidation in rat liver homogenates. *Biochem. J.* 112, 109–115.

Pinto, R. E., and Bartley, W. (1969b). The nature of the sex-linked differences in glutathione peroxidase activity and aerobic oxidation of glutathione in male and female rat liver. *Biochem. J.* 115, 449–455.

Pinto, R. E., and Bartley, W. (1973). Glutathione reductase and glutathione peroxidase activities in hepatomatous livers of rats treated with diethylnitrosamine. *FEBS (Fed. Eur. Biochem. Soc.) Lett.* 32, 307–309.

Piper, P., and Vane, J. (1971). The release of prostaglandins from lung and other tissues. *Ann. N. Y. Acad. Sci.* 180, 363–385.

Pirie, A. (1965a). A light catalyzed reaction in the aqueous humor of the eye. *Nature (London)* 205, 500–501.

Pirie, A. (1965b). Glutathione peroxidase in lens and a source of H_2O_2 in aqueous humor. *Biochem. J.* 96, 244–253.

Pirie, A., Rees, J. R., and Holmberg, N. J. (1970). Diquat cataract: Formation of the free radical and its reaction with constituents of the eye. *Exp. Eye Res.* 9, 204–218.

Popov, K., Jordanov, I., and Nikiforova, M. (1970). Influence of ATP, riboflavin, succinate, and glutamate *in vitro* on the hemolytic action of chlorpromazine. *Dokl. Bolg. Acad. Nauk* 23, 221; *Chem. Abstr.* 73, Abstract No. 2266 (1970).

Poyer, J. L., and McCay, P. B. (1971). Reduced triphosphopyridine nucleotide oxidase-catalyzed alterations of membrane phospholipids. IV. Dependence on Fe^{+3}. *J. Biol. Chem.* 246, 263–269.

Prins, H. K., Oort, M., Loos, J. A., Zurcher, C., and Beckers, T. (1966). Congenital nonspherocytic hemolytic anemia associated with glutathione deficiency of the erythrocytes: Hematological and biochemical studies. *Blood* 27, 145–166.

Pryor, W. A. (1973). Free radical reactions and their importance in biochemical systems. *Fed. Proc., Fed. Amer. Soc. Exp. Biol.* 32, 1862–1869.

Quie, P. G., Kaplan, E. L., Page, A. R., Gruskay, F. L, and Malawista, S. E. (1968). Defective polymorphonuclear leukocyte function and chronic granulomatous disease in two female children. *N. Engl. J. Med.* 278, 976–979.

Recknagel, R. O.(1967). Carbon tetrachloride hepatotoxicity. *Pharmacol. Rev.* 19, 145–208.

Recknagel, R. O., and Ghoshal, A. K. (1966). Lipoperoxidation as a vector in carbon tetrachloride hepatotoxicity. *Lab. Invest.* 15, 132–148.

Reddy, K., and Tappel, A. L. (1974). Effect of dietary selenium and autoxidized lipids on the glutathione peroxidase system of gastrointestinal tract and other tissues in the rat. *J. Nutr.* 104, 1069–1078.

Reed, P. W. (1969). Glutathione and the hexose monophosphate shunt in phagocytizing and hydrogen peroxide-treated rat leukocytes. *J. Biol. Chem.* 244, 2459–2464.

Rees, J. R., and Pirie, A. (1967). Possible reactions of 1,2-naphthoquinone in the eye. *Biochem. J.* 102, 853–863.

Reim, M., Henrels, B., and Cattepoel, H. (1974). Glutathione peroxidase in some ocular tissues. *Ophthalmol. Res.* 6, 228–234.

Ritchie, J. H., Mathews, B. F., McMasters, V., and Grossman, M. (1968). Edema and hemolytic anemia in premature infants: A vitamin E deficiency syndrome. *N. Engl. J. Med.* 270, 1185–1190.

Rodey, G. E., Park, B. H., Ford, D. K., Gray, B. H., and Good, R. A. (1970). Defective bactericidal activity of peripheral blood leukocytes in lipochrome histiocytosis. *Amer. J. Med.* 49, 322–327.

Rodvien, R., Gillum, A., and Weintraub, L. R. (1974). Decreased glutathione peroxidase activity secondary to severe iron deficiency: A possible mechanism responsible for the shortened life span of the iron-deficient cell. *Blood* 43, 281–289.

Rotruck, J. T., Hoekstra, W. G., and Pope, A. L. (1971). Glucose-dependent protection by dietary selenium against hemolysis of rat erythrocytes *in vitro*. *Nature* (*London*), *New Biol.* 231, 223–224.

Rotruck, J. T., Pope, A. L., Ganther, H. E., and Hoekstra, W. G. (1972). Prevention of oxidative damage to rat erythrocytes by dietary selenium. *J. Nutr.* 102, 689–696.

Rotruck, J. T., Pope, A. L., Ganther, H. E., Swanson, A. B., Hafeman, D., and Hoekstra, W. G. (1973). Selenium: Biochemical role as a component of glutathione peroxidase. *Science* 179, 588–590.

Schaeffer, A. J., and Murray, J. P. (1950). Tryptophan determination in cataracts due to deficiency or delayed supplementation of tryptophan. *Arch. Ophthalmol.* 43, 202–216.

Schneider, F., and Flohe, L. (1967). Untersuchungen uber die glutathion: H_2O_2-oxydoreducktase (glutathion-peroxydase). *Hoppe-Zeyler's Z. Physiol. Chem.* 348, 540–552.

Schrauzer, G. N., Rhead, W. J., and Evans, G. A. (1973). Selenium and cancer: Chemical interpretation of a plasma "cancer test." *Bioinorgan. Chem.* 2, 329–340.

Schwartz, J. P., Cooperberg, A. A., and Rosenberg, A. (1974). Platelet-function studies in patients with glucose-6-phosphate dehydrogenase deficiency. *Brit. J. Haematol.* **27,** 273–280.

Schwarz, K. (1961). Development and status of experimental work on Factor 3-selenium. *Fed. Proc., Fed. Amer. Soc. Exp. Biol.* **20,** 666–673.

Schwarz, K. (1962). Vitamin E, trace elements, and sulfhydryl groups in respiratory decline. *Vitam. Horm.* (*New York*) **20,** 463–484.

Schwarz, K. (1965). Role of vitamin E, selenium, and related factors in experimental nutritional liver disease. *Fed. Proc., Fed. Amer. Soc. Exp. Biol.* **24,** 58–67.

Schwarz, K., and Foltz, C. M. (1957). Selenium as an integral part of Factor 3 against dietary necrotic liver degeneration. *J. Amer. Chem. Soc.* **79,** 3292–3293.

Scialom, C., Najeau, Y., and Bernard, J. (1966). Anémie hémolytique congénitale non-sphérocytoire avec déficit incomplet en 6-phosphogluconate déshydrogénase. *Nouv. Rev. Fr. Hematol.* **6,** 452–457.

Scott, M. L. (1973). Nutritional importance of selenium. *In* "Organic Selenium Compounds: Their Chemistry and Biology" (D. L. Kayman and W. H. H. Gunther, eds.), pp. 629–661. Wiley (Interscience), New York.

Serfass, R. E. (1975). Ph.D. Thesis, University of Wisconsin.

Serfass, R. E., and Ganther, H. E. (1975). Defective microbicidal activity in glutathione peroxidase-deficient neutrophils of selenium-deficient rats. *Nature* **155,** 640–641.

Serfass, R. E., Hinsdill, R. D., and Ganther, H. E. (1974). Protective effect of dietary selenium on Salmonella infection: Relation to glutathione peroxidase and superoxide dismutase activities of phagocytes. *Fed. Proc., Fed. Amer. Soc. Exp. Biol.* **33,** 694.

Seward, C. R., Vaughan, G., and Hove, E. L. (1966). Effect of selenium on incisor depigmentation and carbon tetrachloride poisoning in vitamin E-deficient rats. *Proc. Soc. Exp. Biol. Med.* **121,** 850–852.

Shmerling, D. H., Prader, A., Hitzig, W. H., Giedion, A., Hadorn, B., and Kuhni, M. (1969). The syndrome of exocrine pancreatic insufficiency, neutropenia, metaphyseal dysostosis and dwarfism. *Helv. Paediat. Acta* **24,** 547–553.

Shull, L. R., and Cheeke, P. R. (1973). Antiselenium activity of tri-O cresyl phosphate in rats and Japanese quail. *J. Nutr.* **103,** 560–568.

Sies, H., Gerstenecker, C., Menzel, H., and Flohe, L. (1972). Oxidation in the NADP system and release of GSSG from hemoglobin-free perfused rat liver during peroxidation of glutathione by hydroperoxides. *FEBS* (*Fed. Eur. Biochem. Soc.*) *Lett.* **27,** 171–175.

Silver, M. J., Hoch, W., Kocsis, J. J., Ingerman, C. M., and Smith, J. B. (1974). Arachidonic acid causes sudden death in rabbits. *Science* **183,** 1085–1087.

Slater, T. F. (1972). "Free Radical Mechanisms in Tissue Injury." Pion, London.

Smith, A. G., Harland, W. A., and Brooks, C. J. W. (1973). Glutathione peroxidase in human and animal aortas. *Steroids Lipids Res.* **4,** 122–128.

Smith, J. B., Ingerman, C., Kocsis, J. J., and Silver, M. J. (1974). Formation of an intermediate in prostaglandin biosynthesis and its association with the platelet release reaction. *J. Clin. Invest.* **53,** 1468–1472.

Smith, P. J., Tappel, A. L., and Chow, C. K. (1974). Glutathione peroxidase activity as a function of dietary selenomethionine. *Nature* (*London*) **247,** 392–393.

Sondegaard, E. (1967). Selenium and vitamin E interrelationships. *In* "Selenium in Biomedecine" (O. H. Muth, ed.), pp. 365–381. Avi Publ., Westport, Connecticut.

Spallholz, J. E., Martin, J. L., Gerlach, M. L., and Heinzerling, R. H. (1973). Enhanced immunoglobulin M and immunoglobulin G antibody titers in mice fed selenium. *Infec. Immunity* **8**, 841–843.

Spallholz, J. E., Heinzerling, R. H., Gerlach, M. L., and Martin, J. L. (1974). The effect of selenite, tocopheryl acetate and selenite:tocopheryl acetate on the primary and secondary immune responses of mice administered tetanus toxoid or sheep red blood cell antigen. *Fed. Proc., Fed. Amer. Soc. Exp. Biol.* **33**, 696.

Sprinker, L. H., Harr, J. R., Newberne, P. M., Whanger, P. D., and Weswig, P. H. (1971). Selenium deficiency lesions in rats fed vitamin E supplemented rations. *Nutr. Rep. Int.* **4**, 335–339.

Srivastava, S. K., and Beutler, E. (1969). The transport of oxidized glutathione from human erythrocytes. *J. Biol. Chem.* **244**, 9–16.

Srivastava, S. K., and Beutler, E. (1970). Increased susceptibility of riboflavin deficient rats to galactose cataract. *Experientia* **26**, 250.

Srivastava, S. K., and Beutler, E. (1972). Galactose cataract in riboflavin deficient rats. *Biochem. Med.* **6**, 372–379.

Stadtman, T. C. (1974). Selenium biochemistry. *Science* **183**, 915–922.

Steinberg, M. H., and Necheles, T. F. (1971). Erythrocyte glutathione peroxidase deficiency. Biochemical studies on the mechanisms of drug-induced hemolysis. *Amer. J. Med.* **50**, 542–546.

Steinberg, M. H., Brauer, M. J., and Necheles, T. F. (1970). Acute hemolytic anemia associated with glutathione-peroxidase deficiency. *Arch. Intern. Med.* **125**, 302–303.

Strauss, R. R., Paul, B. B., and Sbarra, A. J. (1968). Effect of phenylbutazone on phagocytosis and intracellular killing by guinea pig polymorphonuclear leukocytes. *J. Bacteriol.* **96**, 1982–1988.

Strauss, R. R., Paul, B. B., Jacobs, A. A., and Sbarra, A. J. (1969). The role of the phagocyte in host-parasite interactions. XIX. Leukocytic glutathione reductase and its involvement in phagocytosis. *Arch. Biochem. Biophys.* **135**, 265–271.

Swanson, A. A., and Truesdale, A. W. (1971). Elemental analysis in normal and cataractous human lens tissue. *Biochem. Biophys. Res. Commun.* **45**, 1488–1496.

Swanson, A. B. (1975). Ph.D. Thesis, University of Wisconsin.

Swanson, A. B., Wagner, P. A., Ganther, H. E., and Hoekstra, W. G. (1974). Antagonistic effects of silver and tri-o-cresyl phosphate on selenium and glutathione peroxidase in rat liver and erythrocytes. *Fed. Proc., Fed. Amer. Soc. Exp. Biol.* **33**, 693.

Swanson, M. (1973). Drugs, chemicals, and hemolysis. *Drug Intel. and Clin. Pharm.* **7**, 6–24.

Swierczewski, E., Demus-Oole, A. M., and Minkowski, A. (1969). Glutathione peroxidase and catalase in the erythrocytes of premature, full term, and hypotrophic infants. *Z. Klin. Chem.* **7**, 208–209.

Tam, B. K., and McCay, P. B. (1970). Reduced triphosphopyridine nucleotide oxidase-catalyzed alterations of membrane phospholipids. III. Transient formation of phospholipid peroxides. *J. Biol. Chem.* **245**, 2295–2300.

Thompson, J. N., and Scott, M. L. (1969). Role of selenium in the nutrition of the chick. *J. Nutr.* **97**, 335–342.

Tieri, O., and Vecchione, L. (1963). Monolateral cataract provoked with iodoacetic acid. *Acta Ophthalmol.* **41**, 205–212.

Totter, L. R., and Day, P. L. (1942). Cataract and other ocular changes resulting from tryptophan deficiency. *J. Nutr.* **24,** 159–166.

Tudhope, G. R., and Leece, S. P. (1971). Red cell catalase and the production of methemoglobin, Heinz bodies, and changes in osmotic fragility due to drugs. *Acta Haematol.* **45,** 290–302.

Ugazio, G., Koch, R. R., and Recknagel, R. O. (1973). Reversibility of liver damage in rats rendered resistant to carbon tetrachloride by prior carbon tetrachloride administration: Bearing on the lipoperoxidation hypothesis. *Exp. Mol. Pathol.* **18,** 281–289.

Valentine, W. N. (1972). Red cell enzyme deficiencies as a cause of hemolytic disorders. *Annu. Rev. Med.* **23,** 93–100.

van Heyningen, R. (1969). The lens: Metabolism and cataract. *In* "The Eye" (H. Davson, ed.), 2nd ed., Vol. 1, pp. 381–388. Academic Press, New York.

van Heyningen, R., and Pirie, A. (1953). Reduction of glutathione coupled with oxidative decarboxylation of malate in cattle lenses. *Biochem. J.* **53,** 436–444.

van Heyningen, R., and Pirie, A. (1967). The metabolism of naphthalene and its toxic effect on the eye. *Biochem. J.* **102,** 842–858.

Vargaftig, B. B., and Zirinis, P. (1973). Platelet aggregation induced by arachidonic acid is accompanied by release of potential inflammatory mediators distinct from PGE$_2$ and PGF$_{2\alpha}$. *Nature (London), New Biol.* **244,** 114–116.

Vetrella, M., and Barthelmai, W. (1971). Erythrocyten·Enzyme bei menschlichen Feten. *Monatsschr. Kinderheilk.* **119,** 265–267.

Vetrella, M., and Barthelmai, W. (1972). Studies on drug-induced hemolysis: Effects of menadione and its water soluble preparations on the glutathione peroxidase of human erythrocytes. *Klin. Wochenschr.*. **50,** 234–238.

Vetrella, M., Barthelmai, W., and Reitkolter, J. (1970). Erythrocyte glutathione peroxidase activity from fetal to adult ages. *Klin. Wochenschr.* **48,** 85–88.

Vogt, M. T., Thomas, C., Vassallo, C. L., Basford, R. E., and Gee, J. B. L. (1971). Glutathione-dependent peroxidative metabolism in the alveolar macrophage. *J. Clin. Invest.* **50,** 401–410.

von Sallman, L., Reid, M. E., Grimes, P. A., and Collins, E. M. (1959). Tryptophan-deficiency cataract in guinea pigs. *AMA Arch. Ophthalmol.* [N.S.] **62,** 662–672.

Wagner, P. A. (1975). Ph.D. Thesis, University of Wisconsin.

Wagner, P. A., Hoekstra, W. G., and Ganther, H. E. (1975). Alleviation of silver toxicity by selenite in the rat in relation to tissue glutathione peroxidase. *Proc. Soc. Exp. Biol. Med.* **148,** 1106–1110.

Waller, H. D. (1968). Glutathione reductase deficiency. *In* "Hereditary Disorders of Erythrocyte Metabolism" (E. Beutler, ed.), pp. 185–208. Grune & Stratton, New York.

Waller, H. D., and Gerok, W. (1964). Schwere strahleninduzierte hamolyse bei hereditarem mangel an reduziertem glutathion in blutzellen. *Klin Wochenschr.* **47,** 948–954.

Walter, R., Schlesinger, D. H., and Schwartz, I. L. (1969). Chromatographic separation of isologous sulfur- and selenium-containing amino acids: Reductive scission of the selenium-selenium bond by mercaptans and selenols. *Anal. Biochem.* **27,** 231–243.

Westring, D. W., and Pisciotta, A. V. (1966). Anemia, cataract, and seizures in a patient with glucose-6-phosphate dehydrogenase deficiency. *Arch. Intern. Med.* **118,** 385–390.

Whaun, J. M., and Oski, F. A. (1970). Relation of red cell glutathione peroxidase to neonatal jaundice. *J. Pediat.* **76,** 555–560.

Wills, E. D. (1971). Effects of lipid peroxidation on membrane-bound enzymes of the endoplasmic reticulum. *Biochem. J.* **123,** 983–991.

Witkop, C. J., Jr., White, J. G., Gerritsen, S. M., Townsend, D., and King, R. A. (1973). Hermansky-Pudlak syndrome (HPS): A proposed block in glutathione peroxidase. *Oral Surg., Oral Med. Oral. Pathol.* **35,** 790–806.

Wu, C. (1965). Glutamine synthetase. VI. Mechanism of the dithiol-dependent inhibition by arsenite. *Biochim. Biophys. Acta* **96,** 134–147.

Zeller, E. A. (1953). Contribution to the enzymology of the normal and cataractous lens. III. On the catalase of the crystalline lens. *Amer. J. Ophthalmol.* **38,** [3] 51–53.

33
Metabolism and Function
of Manganese

R. M. Leach, Jr.

I. INTRODUCTION

Manganese was shown to be essential in 1931, when this element was found to be necessary for growth and reproduction in rats and mice (Kemmerer *et al.*, 1931; Orent and McCollum, 1931). Several years later, Wilgus *et al.* (1936) demonstrated that manganese prevented a skeletal abnormality called "perosis" in chickens. Although manganese has been shown to be essential for many species of animals, there are as yet no well-defined occurrences of manganese deficiency in man.

II. METABOLISM OF MANGANESE

A. Absorption

Little is known concerning the mechanism of manganese absorption. Thomson *et al.* (1971) found this element to be absorbed equally well throughout the length of the small intestine. There are several dietary substances that interfere with manganese availability in the intestinal tract. Prior to the discovery that manganese was the nutrient essential for perosis prevention, it was recognized that excessive mineral supplements aggravated this leg abnormality. In fact, the identification of the contaminants in a phosphate supplement that alleviated rather than aggravated the condition lead to the discovery that manganese was the nutrient that prevented this condition. The chemical explanation for the adverse effect of calcium and phosphorus was presented later by Schaible and Bandemer (1942). In addition, Davis et al. (1962) have reported that isolated soy protein also interferes with manganese utilization.

Considerable effort has been expended on the possible relationship between iron and manganese. Wilgus and Patton (1939) noted that addition of ferric citrate to the diet accentuated the severity of perosis. The reciprocal observation was made by Hartman et al. (1955) and Matrone et al. (1959). In these studies, the addition of manganese to diets of several species of animals depleted of iron resulted in depressed hemoglobin levels. Addition of iron to the diets prevented the antagonistic effects of manganese. The authors postulated that manganese was interfering with iron absorption rather than hematopoiesis. Forth and Rummel (1973) have recently reviewed the knowledge relating to iron absorption and concluded that a mutual inhibition of absorption could be demonstrated for iron and manganese.

B. Manganese Homeostasis

Extensive research has been conducted on the metabolism of manganese (Maynard and Cotzias, 1955; Cotzias and Greenough, 1958; Borg and Cotzias, 1958a; Britton and Cotzias, 1966; Hughes et al., 1966; Papavasiliou et al., 1966; Bertinchamps et al., 1966). Manganese homeostasis appears to be regulated at the excretory level rather than at the site of absorption. The liver is the key tissue in this regulation, with the bile serving as an important route of excretion. Biliary excretion is particularly important in adjusting to a manganese load. However, the bile is not the exclusive route of manganese excretion, since it was found that biliary ligation did not abolish manganese excretion by the intestinal tract.

In contrast to intestinal absorption, where there appears to be some interaction between iron and manganese, the pathway of manganese within the body appears to be very specific. It was found that only manganese would accelerate the exit of radiomanganese from the body.

Administration of a variety of other elements did not increase excretion, indicating that there was not an interaction between manganese and other elements of similar chemical properties as is observed with many other trace elements.

In spite of this apparent lack of interaction, there are several substitutions between manganese and other elements that have been reported. Several investigators (Borg and Cotzias, 1958b; Hancock and Fritze, 1973) have reported the isolation of manganese-containing porphyrins. Also, Scrutton et al. (1972) found magnesium to substitute for manganese in pyruvate carboxylase, a manganese metalloprotein.

The status of a specific blood carrier for manganese is unclear at the present time. Although Cotzias and Bertinchamps (1960) proposed the existence of a specific manganese-carrying protein called transmanganin, there is not widespread agreement that manganese is associated with a specific protein in blood (Nandedkar et al., 1973; Chapman et al., 1973).

Within the cell, much of the manganese is found in the mitochondria. The significance of this observation will become apparent in subsequent discussion of the physiological and biochemical aspects of manganese function.

C. Genetic Interaction with Manganese Metabolism

Several genetic interrelationships with manganese metabolism have been discovered. Most extensively studied has been the relationship between the *pallid* gene in mice and manganese metabolism (Erway et al., 1966, 1971). A mutant gene affecting coat color in mice, *pallid*, also produces a congenital ataxia very similar to that observed with manganese-deficient normal mice. Supplement of the mutant diet with high levels of manganese during pregnancy prevents the occurrence of the congenital ataxia. The mutant gene itself and the effects of this gene on pigmentation are unaltered by the manganese treatment. It should be noted that the high levels (1500–2000 ppm) of manganese needed to prevent this condition in mutant mice is greatly in excess of the amount of manganese needed to prevent congenital ataxia in normal mice. Cotzias et al. (1972) demonstrated that mice with the *pallid* gene differed from normal mice in the metabolism of radiomanganese. The manganese concentration of certain tissues, such as bone and brain, was also decreased in the mutant mice.

Erway and Mitchell (1973) have reported similar findings in pastel mink. The occurrence of screw neck, a postural defect, can be reduced through supplementation with 1000 ppm manganese.

In addition to the specific relationship between the above genes and manganese metabolism, Hurley and Bell (1974) have reported substantial individual and strain differences in response to feeding low or borderline levels of manganese to mice. These observations are similar to those of Gallup and Norris (1939), who reported breed and strain differences in the amount of manganese required to prevent perosis in the chick.

D. Manganese Metabolism and Biogenic Amines

The similarity between the symptoms of chronic manganese poisoning and Parkinson's disease led to the study of the possible relationship between manganese and biogenic amines. Mena *et al.* (1970) have reported that the administration of L-dopa (dihydroxyphenylalanine) to patients with chronic manganese toxicity resulted in a disappearance of rigidity and hypokinesia as well as improvement of postural reflexes and restitution of balance. This compound (L-dopa) has also been shown to be of some benefit in alleviating some of the symptoms of Parkinson's disease (Cotzias *et al.*, 1971).

Papavasiliou *et al.* (1968) have proposed that cyclic AMP is the link between biogenic amines and manganese metabolism. In these studies, substances that altered cyclic AMP also altered manganese metabolism, as evidenced by increased liver retention accompanied by decreased biliary excretion. Cotzias *et al.* (1972) have extended these studies to mice with the *pallid* gene, where it was found that mice with this mutant gene differed from normal mice in the metabolism of L-dopa and tryptophan as well as manganese.

III. BIOCHEMICAL AND PHYSIOLOGICAL CHANGES ASSOCIATED WITH MANGANESE DEFICIENCY

As might be expected, the changes associated with manganese deficiency vary according to species of animal and degree of deficiency. However, there are several symptoms common to several species of animals, i.e., skeletal abnormalities and postural defects (ataxia). As discussed earlier, manganese was shown to prevent a skeletal defect called perosis in chickens (Wilgus *et al.*, 1936). Since that time, it has been found to prevent skeletal abnormalities in other species of animals, such as the rat (Amdur *et al.*, 1945), guinea pig (Everson *et al.*, 1959), swine (Plumlee *et al.*, 1956), and cattle (Rojads *et al.*, 1965). The initial observations concerning manganese and perosis prevention led to the search for a role for manganese in the calcification process. Much of the evidence obtained did not support such a hypothesis (Caskey *et al.*, 1939; Parker *et al.*, 1955). This led to the suggestion of the possibility that manganese was playing a role in chondrogenesis rather than osteogenesis (Wolbach and Hegsted, 1953). Evidence has been obtained in several laboratories that supports such a hypothesis. Leach and Muenster (1962) reported that there was severe reduction in cartilage mucopolysaccharide content associated with manganese deficiency. These findings plus subsequent histological studies (Leach, 1968) support the view that manganese affects skeletal formation through chondrogenesis rather than osteogenesis.

Further studies on other species of animals lend support to the above conclusion. Tsai and Everson (1967) have shown that manganese deficiency had similar effects upon the mucopolysaccharide content of guinea pig cartilage. Alteration in ^{35}S metabolism is also observed in manganese-deficient rats (Hurley, 1968). In addition to the effect on skeletal development, Longstaff and Hill (1972) have reported similar compositional changes in eggshell matrix. These results help to explain the earlier effects on eggshell formation described by Lyons (1939).

There is a substantial amount of evidence that indicates that the effect of manganese on mucopolysaccharide metabolism is also responsible for the congenital ataxia that many investigators have observed with a deficiency of this element (Norris and Caskey, 1939; Hill *et al.*, 1950; Hurley *et al.*, 1958). The postural defects (ataxia) associated with both manganese deficiency and the *pallid* gene in mice appear to be due to defective development of the otoliths, structures found in the inner ear that are thought to be involved in equilibrium (Erway *et al.*, 1966, 1970). Extensive studies have demonstrated that there are alterations in mucopolysaccharide metabolism associated with abnormal otolith development (Shrader and Everson, 1967; Hurley, 1968; Shrader *et al.*, 1973). Both histochemical and radiosulfate metabolism studies were used in reaching this conclusion.

Although a defect in mucopolysaccharide metabolism explains many of the symptoms associated with manganese deficiency, there are other changes that cannot be explained in this manner. Liver mitochondria isolated from deficient mice exhibit normal phosphate esterified to oxygen consumption ratio (P.O) but have a reduced oxygen uptake (Hurley *et al.*, 1970). Examination of the ultrastructure reveals abnormalities including elongation and reorientation of cristae. Further studies by Bell and Hurley (1973) report that the ultrastructural changes associated with manganese deficiency occur in other tissues as well. All tissues examined showed alterations in integrity of their cell membranes as well as changes in the endoplasmic reticulum. It was thought that the morphological changes observed in the mitochondria might explain the lowered oxidation rate noted in their previous study. The lipid accumulation noted in these studies is interesting in view of the earlier report by Amdur *et al.* (1946) on the lipotropic effect of manganese. It is interesting to note that Maynard and Cotzias (1955) found the mitochondria to be where much of the manganese was localized within the cell.

Other defects in carbohydrate metabolism have been observed with manganese deficiency. Many of the guinea pigs with a congenital deficiency have short survival times and exhibit aplasia or hypoplasia of pancreatic tissue. Furthermore, these studies indicated that those animals that survive to adult age exhibit abnormal tolerance to intravenously administered glucose (Shrader and Everson, 1968; Everson and Shrader, 1968). Subsequent studies in the same laboratory (Everson, 1968) revealed differences in urinary myoinositol content.

Another interrelationship between manganese and carbohydrate metabolism has been proposed by Doisy (1972). Presumptive evidence was presented for coincident deficiencies of vitamin K and manganese in man. The patient exhibited an inability to elevate clotting proteins in response to vitamin K. Hypocholesterolemia was also observed with this patient. The effect upon blood clotting was confirmed with chicks deficient in manganese and vitamin K. These animals had a reduced ability to respond to vitamin K. It was suggested that manganese was necessary for prothrombin biosynthesis in response to vitamin K. We have been unable to obtain similar effects of manganese on blood clotting in our laboratory (R. M. Leach, unpublished data, 1973).

The reported hypocholesterolemia is also of interest in view of the reported effects of manganese and vanadium on cholesterol metabolism (for a review, see Underwood, 1971). Recently, it has been found that manganese deficiency does not influence the cholesterol content of the hen's egg (R. M. Leach, unpublished data, 1973).

IV. BIOCHEMICAL FUNCTION
OF MANGANESE

A. General Considerations

Extensive information is available on the interaction between manganese and proteins such as enzymes. As with most of the other essential transition elements, the relationship between manganese and enzymes can be classified into two categories—metalloenzymes and metal–enzyme complexes. This type of categorization is based upon affinity of the metal for the enzyme rather than on a functional basis. For a detailed discussion of the role of manganese and other metals in enzyme catalysis, an excellent review by Mildvan (1970) may be examined.

Unlike other essential transition elements, the number of manganese metalloenzymes is very limited, while the enzymes that can be activated (metal–enzyme complexes) are numerous. These enzymes include hydrolases, kinases, decarboxylases, and transferases (Vallee and Coleman, 1964). Usually this type of enzymatic activation is relatively nonspecific, making it difficult to correlate pathological defects with biochemical function. However, a group of transferases called glycosyl transferases offers such a possibility.

B. Manganese and Glycosyl Transferases

Glycosyl transferases are enzymes involved in the transfer of sugar from sugar nucleotides to a variety of acceptors. The enzymes are important in the synthesis of polysaccharides and glycoproteins. A survey of the metal requirements of these enzymes indicated that most of the glycosyl transferases require manganese or some other metal ion for activity (Leach, 1971).

Thus, the need for manganese for the activation of enzymes involved in polysaccharide synthesis can be related to the impairment in mucopolysaccharide metabolism that is associated with the symptoms of manganese deficiency. Leach (1971) presented data that supports such a relationship. First of all, the glycosyl transferases involved in mucopolysaccharide synthesis required metal ions for optimum activity. In most instances, manganese was the most effective ion.

The enzymatic activity of tissues from manganese-deficient and control animals was studied by Leach et al. (1969). When the enzymes necessary for chondroitin sulfate synthesis in the 105,000 g particulate fraction from deficient and control tissues were compared, the preparations from the deficient tissues incorporated more radioactive substrate. The incorporation of more substrate by the deficient tissues was interpreted as an indication of more acceptor sites reflecting suboptimum *in vivo* synthetic activity. Carbohydrate analysis of this particulate fraction supported such a hypothesis.

Studies on the possible mechanism of action of manganese on the above glycosyl transferases are difficult because both the enzyme and the acceptor are present in the same insoluble particle. An alternate approach to a study of the mechanism of action of manganese would be to choose a soluble glycosyl transferase as a model system. This was done by Morrison and Ebner (1971a,b) who investigated the galactosyl transferase found in bovine milk. It was concluded that the reaction had an ordered mechanism, with the reactants adding in the order Mn^{2+}, UDP–sugar, and acceptor. The manganese and the enzyme formed a metal–enzyme complex that did not dissociate after each catalytic cycle.

C. Manganese Metalloenzymes

As mentioned previously, the number of manganese metalloenzymes that have been isolated and identified is limited (see Table I). It is interesting that several have been isolated from mitochondria, an organelle rich in manganese.

The most extensively studied manganese metalloenzyme is pyruvate carboxylase, which was isolated from chick liver mitochondria by Scrutton et al. (1966). This enzyme contains 4 moles of tightly bound manganese and 4 moles of biotin and catalyzes the conversion of pyruvate to oxaloacetate. The enzyme also requires a divalent ion not related to the tightly bound metal component of the enzyme for activation. Studies on the tightly bound manganese by Mildvan et al. (1966) resulted in the proposal that the electrophilic character of the bound manganese facilitates the proton departure from the methyl group of pyruvate and the carboxyl transfer from the carboxybiotin residue to pyruvate.

Scrutton et al. (1972) also studied the metal content of pryuvate carboxylase under conditions of manganese deficiency. Magnesium was found to replace manganese as the bound metal in pyruvate carboxylase

TABLE I Some Characteristics of Manganese-Containing Metalloproteins

Protein	M.W.	Mn/mole (oxidation state)	Source	Reference
Pyruvate carboxylase	500,000	4(II)	Avian liver	Scrutton et al. (1966)
Superoxide dismutase	39,500	2(III)	Escherichia coli	Keele et al. (1970)
	40,000	2(III)	S. mutans	Vance et al. (1972)
Avimanganin	89,000	1(III)	Avian liver	Scrutton (1971)
Manganin	56,000	1	Peanuts	Dickert and Rozacky (1969)
Concanavalin A	190,000	1(II)	Jackbean	Agrawal and Goldstein (1968)

isolated from manganese deficient chicks. This substitution caused only minor alterations in the catalytic properties of the enzyme.

In contrast to the above observation with pyruvate carboxylase, manganese deficiency resulted in a depletion of manganese from avimanganin as well as a reduction in the amount of this metalloprotein (Scrutton, 1971). Avimanganin is a protein of unknown function that contains 1 mole of bound manganese(III) per 89,000 mole weight.

Thus, two manganese metalloproteins are affected differently by manganese deficiency. With pyruvate carboxylase, magnesium is substituted for manganese under conditions of dietary deficiency, while the amount of avimanganin is reduced under similar conditions.

V. SUMMARY AND CONCLUSIONS

Manganese is essential for growth, reproduction, and skeletal development in all species of animals that have been investigated. However, with the exception of the chicken, normal diets for most species contain sufficient manganese to prevent deficiency symptoms. This applies to man as well, since there is little evidence for manganese deficiency in the human population. The quantitative needs for manganese can be altered by substances that interfere with manganese metabolism.

Manganese homeostasis is controlled through variable excretion via the bile and intestinal tract rather than at the site of absorption. Although the pathway of manganese metabolism within the body is fairly specific, genetics and biogenic amines are two factors that can influence the metabolism of this element. Within the cell, much of the manganese is localized in mitochondria, which have served as starting material for the isolation of several manganese-containing metalloenzymes. Further evidence of the important relationship between manganese and mitochondria is illustrated by the discovery that manganese deficiency results in alterations in the structure and metabolism of these cellular organelles.

The need for manganese for the prevention of skeletal and postural (ataxia) abnormalities, as well as normal egg shell formation, can be related to the need for this element in mucopolysaccharide synthesis. This appears to be related to the observation that manganese is the preferred metal cofactor for many glycosyl transferases, which are important enzymes in polysaccharide and glycoprotein synthesis. The role of manganese in the prevention of other aberrations in carbohydrate metabolism remains obscure at the present time.

Many aspects of manganese metabolism and function warrant further clarification. Some examples of fruitful areas of research include: (1) mechanism of absorption, (2) role in the metabolism and function of mitochondria, (3) relationship to biogenic amines, and (4) relationship to blood clotting and vitamin K.

REFERENCES

Agrawal, B. B. L., and Goldstein, I. J. (1968). Protein carbohydrate interaction. VII. Physical and chemical studies on concanavalin A, the hemogglutinin of the Jackbean. *Arch. Biochem. Biophys.* 124, 218–229.

Amdur, M. O., Norris, L. C., and Heuser, G. F. (1945). The need for manganese in bone development by the rat. *Proc. Soc. Exp. Biol. Med.* 59, 254–255.

Amdur, M. O., Norris, L. C., and Heuser, G. F. (1946). The lipotropic action of manganese. *J. Biol. Chem.* 164, 783–784.

Bell, L. T., and Hurley, L. S. (1973). Ultrastructural effects of manganese deficiency in liver, heart, kidney and pancreas of mice. *Lab. Invest.* 29, 723–736.

Bertinchamps, A. J., Miller, S. T., and Cotzias, G. C. (1966). Interdependence of routes of excreting manganese. *Amer. J. Physiol.* 211, 217–224.

Borg, D. C., and Cotzias, G. C. (1958a). Manganese metabolism in man: Rapid exchange of Mn^{56} with tissue as demonstrated by blood clearance and liver uptake. *J. Clin. Invest.* 37, 1269–1278.

Borg, D. C., and Cotzias, G. C. (1958b). Incorporation of manganese into erythrocytes as evidence for a manganese porphyrin in man. *Nature (London)* 182, 1677–1678.

Britton, A. A., and Cotzias, G. C. (1966). Dependence of manganese turnover on intake. *Amer. J. Physiol.* 211, 203–206.

Caskey, C. D., Gallup, W. D., and Norris, L. C. (1939). The need for manganese in the bone development of the chick. *J. Nutr.* 17, 407–417.

Chapman, B. E., MacDermott, T. E., and O'Sullivan, W. J. (1973). Studies on manganese complexes of human serum albumin. *Bioinorg. Chem.* 3, 27–38.

Cotzias, G. C., and Bertinchamps, J. (1960). Transmanganin, the specific manganese-carrying protein of human plasma. *J. Clin. Invest.* 39, 979.

Cotzias, G. C., and Greenough, J. J. (1958). The high specificity of the manganese pathway through the body. *J. Clin. Invest.* 37, 1298–1305.

Cotzias, G. C., Papavasiliou, P. S., Ginos, J., Streck, A., and Düby, S. (1971). Metabolic modification of Parkinson's Disease and of chronic manganese poisoning. *Annu. Rev. Med.* 22, 305–326.

Cotzias, G. C., Tang, L. C., Miller, S. T., Sladic-Simic, D., and Hurley, L. S. (1972). A mutation influencing the transportation of manganese, L-Dopa, and L-Tryptophan. *Science* 176, 410–412.

Davis, P. N., Norris, L. C., and Kratzer, F. H. (1962). Interference of soybean meal with the utilization of trace minerals. *J. Nutr.* 77, 217–223.

Dickert, J. W., and Rozacky, E. (1969). Isolation and partial characterization of manganin, a new manganoprotein from peanut seeds. *Arch. Biochem. Biophys.* 134, 473–477.

Doisy, E. A., Jr. (1972). Micronutrient controls on biosynthesis of clotting proteins and cholesterol. *In* "Trace Substances in Environmental Health" (D. D. Hemphill, ed.), Vol. VI, p. 193. University of Missouri, Columbia.

Erway, L., Hurley, L. S., and Fraser, A. (1966). Neurological defect: Manganese in phenocopy and prevention of a genetic abnormality of inner ear. *Science* **152**, 1766–1768.

Erway, L., Hurley, L. S., and Fraser, A. S. (1970). Congenital ataxia and otolith defects due to manganese deficiency in mice. *J. Nutr.* **100**, 643–654.

Erway, L., Fraser, A., and Hurley, L. S. (1971). Prevention of congenital otolith defect in *Pallid* mutant mice by manganese supplementation. *Genetics* **67**, 97–108.

Erway, L. C., and Mitchell, S. E. (1973). Prevention of otolith defect in pastel mink by manganese supplementation. *J. Hered.* **64**, 111–119.

Everson, G. J. (1968). Preliminary study of carbohydrates in the urine of mangansedeficient guinea pigs at birth. *J. Nutr.* **96**, 283–288.

Everson, G. J., and Shrader, R. E. (1968). Abnormal glucose tolerance in manganesedeficient guinea pigs. *J. Nutr.* **94**, 89–94.

Everson, G. J., Hurley, L. S., and Geiger, J. F. (1959). Manganese deficiency in the guinea pig. *J. Nutr.* **68**, 49–56.

Forth, W., and Rummel, W. (1973). Iron absorption. *Physiol. Rev.* **53**, 724–792.

Gallup, W. D., and Norris, L. C. (1939). The amount of manganese required to prevent perosis in the chick. *Poultry Sci.* **18**, 76–82.

Hancock, R. G. V., and Fritze, K. (1973). Chromatographic evidence for the existence of a manganese porphryin in erythrocytes. *Bioinorg. Chem.* **3**, 77–87.

Hartman, R. H., Matrone, G., and Wise, G. H. (1955). Effect of high dietary manganese on hemoglobin formation. *J. Nutr.* **57**, 429–439.

Hill, R. M., Holtkamp, D. E., Buchanan, A. R., and Rutledge, E. K. (1950). Manganese deficiency in rats with relation to ataxia and loss of equilibrium. *J. Nutr.* **41**, 359–371.

Hughes, E. R., Miller, S. T., and Cotzias, G. C. (1966). Tissue concentrations of manganese and adrenal function. *Amer. J. Physiol.* **211**, 207–210.

Hurley, L. S. (1968). Genetic-nutritional interactions concerning manganese. *In* "Trace Substances in Environmental Health" (D. Hemphill, ed.), Vol. II, pp. 41–51. University of Missouri, Columbia.

Hurley, L. S., and Bell, L. T. (1974). Genetic influence on response to dietary manganese deficiency in mice. *J. Nutr.* **104**, 133–137.

Hurley, L. S., Everson, G. J., and Geiger, J. F. (1958). Manganese deficiency in rats: Congenital nature of ataxia. *J. Nutr.* **66**, 309–319.

Hurley, L. S., Theriault, L. L., and Dreosti, I. E. (1970). Liver mitochondria from manganese-deficient and pallid mice: Function and ultrastructure. *Science* **170**, 1316–1318.

Keele, B. B., McCord, J. M., and Fridovich, I. (1970). Superoxide dismutase from *Escherichia coli* B. *J. Biol. Chem.* **245**, 6176–6181.

Kemmerer, A. R., Elvehjem, C. A., and Hart, E. B. (1931). Studies on the relation of manganese to the nutrition of the mouse. *J. Biol. Chem.* **92**, 623–630.

Leach, R. M., Jr. (1968). Effect of manganese upon the epiphyseal growth plate in the young chick. *Poultry Sci.* **47**, 828–830.

Leach, R. M., Jr. (1971). Role of manganese in mucopolysaccharide metabolism. *Fed. Proc., Fed. Amer. Soc. Exp. Biol.* **30**, 991–994.

Leach, R. M., Jr., and Muenster, A. M. (1962). Studies on the role of manganese in bone formation. I. Effect upon mucopolysaccharide content of chick bone. *J. Nutr.* **78**, 51–56.

Leach, R. M., Jr., Muenster, A. M., and Wein, E. M. (1969). Studies on the role of manganese in bone formation. II. Effect upon chondroitin sulfate synthesis in chick epiphyseal cartilage. *Arch. Biochem. Biophys.* **133**, 22–28.

Longstaff, M., and Hill, R. (1972). The hexosamine and uronic acid contents of the matrix of shells of eggs from pullets fed on diets of different manganese content. *Brit. Poultry Sci.* 13, 377–385.

Lyons, M. (1939). Some effects of manganese on eggshell quality. *Arkansas Agr. Exp. Sta. Bull.* 374, 1.

Matrone, G., Hartman, R. H., and Clawson, A. J. (1959). Manganese-iron antagonism in the nutrition of rabbits and baby pigs. *J. Nutr.* 67, 309–317.

Maynard, L. S., and Cotzias, G. C. (1955). The partition of manganese among organs and intracellular organelles of the rat. *J. Biol. Chem.* 214, 489–495.

Mena, I., Court, J., Fuenzalida, S., Papavasiliou, P. S., and Cotzias, G. C. (1970). Modification of chronic manganese poisoning. *N. Engl. J. Med.* 282, 5.

Mildvan, A. S. (1970). In "The Enzymes" (P. D. Boyer, ed.), 3rd ed., Vol. 2, pp. 445–536. Academic Press, New York.

Mildvan, A. S., Scrutton, M. C., and Utter, M. F. (1966). Pyruvate carboxylase. VII. A possible role for tightly bound manganese. *J. Biol. Chem.* 241, 3488–3498.

Morrison, J. F., and Ebner, K. E. (1971a). Studies on galactosyltransferase: Kinetic investigations with n-acetylglucosamine as the galactosyl group acceptor. *J. Biol. Chem.* 246, 3977–3984.

Morrison, J. F., and Ebner, K. E. (1971b). Studies on galactosyltransferase: Kinetic investigations with glucose as the galactosyl group acceptor. *J. Biol. Chem.* 246, 3985–3998.

Nandedkar, A. K. N., Nurse, C. E., and Friedberg, F. (1973). Mn^{++} binding by plasma proteins. *Int. J. Peptide and Protein Res.* 5, 279–281.

Norris, L. C., and Caskey, C. D. (1939). A chronic congenital ataxia and osteodystrophy in chicks due to manganese deficiency. *J. Nutr.* 17, Suppl., 16–17.

Orent, E. R., and McCollum, E. V. (1931). Effects of deprivation of manganese in the rat. *J. Biol. Chem.* 92, 651–678.

Papavasiliou, P. S., Miller, S. T., and Cotzias, G. C. (1966). Role of liver in regulating distribution and excretion of manganese. *Amer. J. Physiol.* 211, 211–216.

Papavasiliou, P. S., Miller, S. T., and Cotzias, G. C. (1968). Functional interaction between biogenic amines, 3'-5'-cyclic AMP and manganese. *Nature (London)* 220, 74–75.

Parker, H. E., Andrew, F. N., Carrick, C. W., Creek, R. D., and Hauge, S. M. (1955). Effect of manganese on bone formation studied with radioactive isotopes. *Poultry Sci.* 34, 1154–1158.

Plumlee, M. P., Thrasher, D. M., Beesen, W. M., Andrews, F. N., and Parker, H. E. (1956). The effects of a manganese deficiency upon the growth, development and reproduction of swine. *J. Anim. Sci.* 15, 352–367.

Rojas, M. A., Dyer, I. A., and Cassatt, W. A. (1965). Manganese deficiency in the bovine. *J. Anim. Sci.* 24, 664–667.

Schaible, P. J., and Bandemer, S. A. (1942). The effect of mineral supplements on the availability of manganese. *Poultry Sci.* 21, 8–14.

Scrutton, M. C. (1971). Purification and some properties of a protein containing bound manganese (avimanganin). *Biochemistry* 10, 3897–3905.

Scrutton, M. C., Utter, M. F., and Mildvan, A. S. (1966). Pyruvate carboxylase. VI. The presence of tightly bound manganese. *J. Biol. Chem.* 241, 3480–3487.

Scrutton, M. C., Griminger, P., and Wallace, J. C. (1972). Pyruvate carboxylase: Bound metal content of the vertebrate liver enzyme as a function of diet. *J. Biol. Chem.* 247, 3305–3313.

Shrader, R. E., and Everson, G. J. (1967). Anomalous development of otoliths associated with postural defects in manganese-deficient guinea pigs. *J. Nutr.* **91,** 453–460.

Shrader, R. E., and Everson, G. J. (1968). Pancreatic pathology in manganese-deficient guinea pigs. *J. Nutr.* **94,** 269–281.

Shrader, R. E., Erway, L. C., and Hurley, L. S. (1973). Mucopolysaccharide synthesis in the developing inner ear of manganese-deficient and pallid mutant mice. *Teratology* **8,** 257–266.

Thomson, A. B. R., Olatunbosun, D., and Valberg, L. S. (1971). Interrelation of intestinal transport system of manganese and iron. *J. Lab. Clin. Med.* **78,** 642–655.

Tsai, H. C. C., and Everson, G. J. (1967). Effect of manganese deficiency on the acid mucopolysaccharides in cartilage of guinea pigs. *J. Nutr.* **91,** 447–452.

Underwood, E. J. (1971). "Trace Elements in Human and Animal Nutrition," 3rd ed., pp. 419–420. Academic Press, New York.

Vallee, B. L., and Coleman, J. E. (1964). Metal coordination and enzyme action. *Compr. Biochem.* **12,** 165–235.

Vance, P. G., Keele, B. B., Jr., and Rajagopalan, K. V. (1972). Superoxide dismutase from *Streptococcus mutans. J. Biol. Chem.* **247,** 4782–4786.

Wilgus, H. S., and Patton, A. R. (1939). Factors affecting manganese utilization in the chicken. *J. Nutr.* **18,** 35–45.

Wilgus, H. S., Norris, L. C., and Heuser, G. F. (1936). The role of certain inorganic elements in the cause and prevention of perosis. *Science* **84,** 252–253.

Wolbach, S. B., and Hegsted, D. M. (1953) Perosis: Epiphyseal cartilage in choline and manganese deficiencies in the chick. *AMA Arch. Pathol.* **56,** 437–453.

34

Fluoride Metabolism—Effect of Pre-eruptive or Posteruptive Fluoride Administration on Rat Caries Susceptibility

J. M. Navia, C. E. Hunt, F. B. First, and
A. J. Narkates

I. INTRODUCTION

Fluoride has been shown to be a safe and effective cariostatic agent, and thus beneficial to oral health, when provided at a level of 1 ppm in drinking water or in various topical applications (Marthaler, 1967; Caldwell and Thomas, 1970). However, its mode of action, optimal time–dose relationship, and interactions with other elements have not been sufficiently clarified. While some trace elements have been reported to have cariostatic properties (Navia, 1970), fluoride is without question

249

the most effective. It has also been suggested as a possible factor in the control of metabolic bone diseases (Rich et al., 1964), and therefore it is important to understand its metabolism in order to improve the effectiveness of its use.

Fluoride metabolism has been reviewed in monographs published by WHO (1970), the National Academy of Sciences (1971), and in publications by Hodge and Smith (1970), Jenkins et al. (1970), and Underwood (1971). Fluoride from inorganic sources is rapidly absorbed and distributed throughout the body. Some fluoride crosses the gastric mucosa, but most is quickly absorbed from the small intestine. Probably as much as 95% of the total body fluoride is incorporated into skeletal and dental tissues. The distribution of fluoride within the bone varies; it is higher in cancellous than in compact bone. Growing bones are more biologically active and seem to incorporate fluoride more readily (Weidmann and Weatherell, 1970) and in proportion to the levels found in the extracellular compartment at the time of mineralization. If ectopic calcification develops in soft tissues, then fluoride will tend to accumulate in these tissues also (Smith et al., 1960; Call et al., 1965).

Fluoride is found in bone and tooth apatite (Eanes and Posner, 1970), substituting for hydroxyl groups at selected sites in the apatite lattice. Pure fluoroapatite is rarely found, for if all the hydroxyl positions in the apatite were exchanged for fluoride, its concentration in the fluoroapatite formed would be 3.8%, and most bone and enamel do not approach such a value except for shark enamel (Glas, 1962), which seems to contain fluoroapatite. No evidence has been reported that CaF_2 is present in the skeleton, but it has been found in enamel topically treated with fluoride. This molecule is easily lost from the surface, but the fluoride associated with apatite structures remains in the enamel (Baud and Bang, 1970).

The level of fluoride in drinking water and consequently its concentration in bone has been associated with the incidence of osteoporosis (Leone et al., 1954, 1955, 1960). The hypothesis was formulated (Rich et al., 1964) that bone resorptive diseases such as osteoporosis and Paget's disease might be controlled by administration of doses as high as 100 mg of fluoride ion per day. Studies in rats (Lane and Steinberg, 1973) in which fluoride was compared to diphosphonates in its ability to inhibit osteoporosis of disuse showed no beneficial effect for fluoride. Results of studies in which pigs were used as animal models (Spencer et al., 1971) indicated that there were no intrinsic differences in strength of cortical bone from femurs of swine on rations with or without fluoride.

Hodge and Smith (1968) reviewed results from several human studies and concluded that the beneficial effects of fluoride were not clearly established, although a reduction of bone pain and urinary calcium excretion in multiple myeloma had been documented. Recent studies (Riggs et al., 1972) have suggested that combination treatments of sodium fluoride together with calcium supplements may stimulate formation of normal bone. Further work is necessary to elucidate the timing and dosage level as well as the tissue fluoride concentrations necessary to control these metabolic bone diseases.

Body fluids such as saliva, bile, and blood contain fluoride concentrations ranging from 0.1 to 0.2 ppm. These levels again vary proportionally to fluoride intake in the diet and the drinking water. Dietary fluoride is highly dependent on whether the region is fluoridated or not; in fluoridated areas, the dietary fluoride content exclusive of the drinking water has been reported (Kramer et al., 1974) to range from 1.7 to 3.4 mg/day, and in nonfluoridated areas, the fluoride intake was found to be approximately 1 mg/day.

In general, the mammary gland and the placenta seem to act as barriers that interfere with fluoride transfer to the milk or the fetus (Zipkin and Babeaux, 1965), although Armstrong et al. (1970) have questioned the existence of such a placental barrier. Fluoride is usually excreted through the kidneys, although up to 10% may be eliminated in the feces. Some fluoride may be excreted through sweat glands, though this amount is difficult to ascertain and depends on factors such as temperature and activity of the individual. It is important to stress that excretion of fluoride is rapid and that a large percentage of an orally or parenterally administered dose is excreted within a few hours (Muhler et al., 1966).

The cariostatic effect of fluoride for humans has been demonstrated clearly in epidemiological studies (Arnold et al., 1962; Ast et al., 1956) of individuals consuming water that contained an optimal level of 1 or 2 ppm of fluoride. While water fluoridation is an effective public health measure that should be "the cornerstone of any national program of dental caries prevention" (Horowitz, 1973), there are other approaches to the use of this valuable element in caries control.

Fluoride could be made available during fetal life when the deciduous teeth are actively mineralizing. Carlos et al. (1962) and Horowitz and Heifetz (1967) studied several cohorts of children who had different patterns of prenatal exposure followed by continuous exposure to fluoridated water. They found no meaningful additional benefits from the maternal ingestion of fluoridated water if the offspring also ingested fluoridated water from birth. The placenta seemed to act as a barrier that limited the availability of maternal fluoride to the fetal tissues (Babeaux and Zipkin, 1966). In view of these and other studies, the U.S. Food and Drug Administration (1966) banned from the market those products that contained fluoride and for which claims were made that they would prevent caries in the offspring of mothers consuming such products.

Fluoride also might be made available to the suckling infant if the mother has a sufficiently high intake of fluoride. Zipkin and Babeaux (1965) have reviewed the subject of maternal transfer of fluoride and concluded that human milk contains a low concentration of fluoride (0.1–0.2 ppm fluoride), which is not significantly increased even with a dietary intake of fluoride as high at 5 mg/day.

Distinct systemic effects of fluoride have been difficult to evaluate in most human studies due to availability of fluoride during both pre- and posteruptive stages of tooth development. Animal studies (Stookey et al., 1962; König et al., 1960; Shaw and Sognnaes, 1954) that were directed to evaluate the systemic effects of fluoride on caries have also been inconclusive because more than one developmental period was examined.

Kruger (1964) conducted a study to evaluate the combined effect of pre-eruptive and posteruptive administration of fluoride on rat molars and caries, but used the parenteral rather than the oral route to administer the fluoride. Therefore, studies were necessary in which the caries effect of orally administered fluoride, provided at different stages of tooth development, could be clearly identified and understood. It would also be of great advantage in implementing the use of fluoride as a cariostatic agent to know its mechanism of action. Some of the mechanisms that have been suggested to explain its cariostatic properties are: (1) alteration of tooth crown morphology; (2) formation of large, perfect crystals of apatite; (3) stimulation of remineralization processes at the enamel surface; (4) decreased solubility of enamel; and (5) decreased bacterial enzymatic activity. Probably all of these mechanisms are in some measure responsible for the cariostatic effect of fluorides, but it would be extremely useful to understand which ones are most important, as this would suggest the time during tooth development when fluoride administration and what dosage would bring about its best cariostatic effect.

It is our hypothesis that to obtain the most beneficial cariostatic effect of fluoride a critical dose and period of fluoride administration should be identified. Departure from these optimal conditions may increase rather than decrease the susceptibility to caries. Our objective in this investigation was to study such time–dose relationships in the rat model to evaluate fluoride incorporation into molars, as well as its cariostatic effect. In these studies, the fluoride doses were given either by gavage strictly during tooth formation, prior to eruption, or in the drinking water after eruption of the tooth. The caries challenge was uniformly administered after tooth eruption to measure the susceptibility of the treated rat molars to caries.

II. MATERIALS AND METHODS

A. Animals

Either 1-day-old pups with a lactating dam or 15 days timed-pregnant rats (COBS-CR) were obtained from Charles River Laboratories, Wilmington, Massachusetts. Pups were randomized, weighed, and the number per litter adjusted to nine. Rats were housed in polycarbonate cages with stainless steel tops and hardwood sterilized bedding (Ab-sorb-dri). Animals were kept in a room with controlled lighting (12 hours light, 12 hours darkness), temperature (70°–72°F), and humidity (50%). Dams in experiments designed to study pre-eruptive effects of fluorides were fed *ad libitum* the nutritionally adequate, purified diet MIT #200 (Navia *et al.*, 1969) in a gel form (2% agar). At 17 days of age, the pups were provided distilled water and a caries-promoting powdered diet, #305, which is identical to diet #200 except that 62% of the sucrose is replaced with cornstarch. The final composition of diet #305 has therefore 62% cornstarch and 5% sucrose and when fed to these young rats it induces carious lesions on the buccal, sulcal, and interproximal molar areas. All rats were weighed at the beginning of the experiment, at weaning time, and weekly thereafter, as well as at sacrifice time.

B. Experimental Design—Posteruptive Effects of Fluoride

Six rat dams with their litters were maintained on diet #305 from day 1 until 18 days of age, when the pups were weaned and assigned to either of two groups—one receiving distilled water and the other receiving water containing 25 ppm fluorine as sodium fluoride. Twenty-six animals were assigned to the control group and twenty-six to the group receiving fluoride. At day 37, the animals were sacrificed, the first maxillary molar extracted for fluoride analysis, and the mandibles set aside for caries scoring.

C. Experimental Design—Pre-eruptive Effects of Fluoride

1. Experiment #1

Twenty-four litters of 1-day-old male pups were used, from which eighteen litters were selected so that body weight of pups ranged from 11.5 to 12.5 gm. The rat dams were rotated among the litters during lactation to randomize the effect of possible differences in milk production among dams.

All treatments were blocked within the litters and started when the pups were 5 days old. Nine groups of rats received by gavage daily doses of a sodium fluoride solution in distilled water. Fluoride dosage for the different groups was as follows:

Group:	A	B	C	D	E	F	G	H
F⁻ dosage (μg/10 gm body weight):	0	15	30	45	60	75	90	105

The pups within each litter were marked and assigned to one of the eight groups; the ninth pup was a repeat of one of the groups and provided a measure of internal variability within the litters. Intubations were continued through day 17, at which time tooth eruption begins under the described experimental conditions (Menaker and Navia, 1973). A plastic 1 ml tuberculin syringe with intravenous tubing was used to deliver the daily doses of fluoride into the stomach.

Starting on day 17, the pups were fed diet #305 and distilled water, and the oral cavity of all pups was swabbed with a fecal solution to equalize the oral flora. Fresh fecal pellets from the dams were suspended in physiological saline solution and used to swab the pups on the seventeenth, eighteenth, and nineteenth days of age. All pups were weaned on the eighteenth day and sacrificed on the thirty-fifth day.

2. Experiment #2

This study was designed to evaluate fluoride incorporation into the molar teeth of rats administered a fluoride dose for various lengths of time and starting at different developmental stages of the teeth. In this experiment, the level of fluoride given the rat pups by gavage was kept constant at 45 μg/10 gm of body weight, and only the initial time and length of administration was varied. Eighteen timed-pregnant rats (COBS, Sprague-Dawley) were received in our laboratories and fed diet #200 in gel form and water *ad libitum*.

At birth, the litters were weighed and adjusted to nine pups per litter. The treatments were blocked within litters. Each pup in the litter was identified and assigned to one of the nine groups shown in the tabulation below.

Group	Fluoride treatment period (days of age)	Total no. of fluoride doses
1	4–7	4
2	4–10	7
3	4–13	10
4	4–16	13
5	7–16	10
6	10–16	7
7	13–16	4
8	8–11	4
9 (controls)	0	0

Rats in group 9 received no fluoride during the experimental period (4–16 days of age) and served as controls, while those in group 4 were dosed daily with the fluoride solution throughout this period. The caries promoting diet #305 was fed from 17 days of age until sacrifice at 35 days of age. The first maxillary molars were then extracted and analyzed to determine incorporation of fluoride under these experimental conditions.

D. Caries Scores

The rat heads were lightly steamed in the autoclave, the mandibles were dissected, cleaned of soft tissue, dried, and stained with a solution of murexide (0.04% ammonium purpurate in 70% aqueous ethanol). The molars were scored for caries on buccal, sulcal, and interproximal surfaces using the method of Keyes (1958).

E. Fluoride Analysis

Maxillary first molars were extracted and dried. The roots were removed, and the pulp cavity exposed and cleaned by means of a sharp instrument and a blast of pressurized air. The crowns were pulverized in a glass mortar, weighed, and dissolved in 0.5 M perchloric acid. Citrate buffer (0.5 M, pH 5.8) was added, and the concentration of fluoride in the tooth crown was measured with a fluoride electrode (Orion Instrument Co., Cambridge, Massachusetts) and an expanded-scale potentiometer (McCann, 1968). The sample readings were compared with those obtained from standard solutions of sodium fluoride. All molar crown samples were treated in exactly the same manner.

F. Statistical Analysis

All the data was analyzed at the University of Alabama in Birmingham computer facilities using analysis of variance and Duncan's multiple mean comparisons to test the significance of the results.

III. RESULTS

Caries scores of rats administered fluoride (25 ppm) in the drinking water posteruptively from day 18 to 37 are tabulated in Table I. Administration of fluoride in this manner reduced enamel lesions (E) on the buccal surface of molars 24.8% and deep dentinal lesions 54.4%. This posteruptive effect has been demonstrated repeatedly both in animal and human studies (Hodge and Smith, 1970). The effect of fluoride on the sulcal areas is also clear. Fluoride-treated rats had a 19.7% reduction in enamel lesions (E) on the sulcal surfaces and a somewhat higher reduction (38.2%) in lesions that involved deep dentinal areas of the sulci. The response of smooth tooth surface areas in humans to the cariostatic effect of fluoride has also been found to be better than the caries protection observed in the pit and fissure areas.

No significant differences in body weights were observed between the two groups of rats (Table II). However, the fluoride levels in maxil-

TABLE I   Caries Scores of Molars from Rats Offered Either Distilled Water or Water Containing Fluoride[a]

| | | Caries scores (mean ± SD) | | | |
| | | Buccal | | Sulcal | |
Treatment	No. of rats	E^b	$D_m{}^c$	E^b	$D_m{}^c$
Control	26	12.1 ± 1.0	7.8 ± 1.1	13.7 ± 0.4	8.1 ± 0.7
Fluoride	26	9.1 ± 0.8	3.6 ± 0.6	11.0 ± 0.5	5.0 ± 0.6
Caries reductions		24.8%	54.4%	19.7%	38.1%

[a] 25 ppm posteruptively from day 18 to day 37.
[b] E = Scores for carious surfaces that involve the enamel.
[c] D_m = Scores for carious surfaces that extend into the dentin.

TABLE II Mean Body Weights and Fluoride Content of First
Maxillary Crowns from Rats Offered Either
Distilled Water or Water Containing Fluoride[a]

Treat- ment	No. of rats	Mean body weight (gm)	Fluoride (μg/mg)
Control	15	189 ± 6	0.013 ± 0.001
Fluoride	15	194 ± 6	0.160 ± 0.008

[a] Mean ± SD; 25 ppm fluoride administered posteruptively
from day 18 to 37 of age.

lary teeth were significantly different (0.013 versus 0.160 μg F$^-$/mg molar
crown), indicating that fluoride offered posteruptively can accumulate
in the rat molar in spite of the rapid enamel maturation that takes
place immediately after eruption.

Pre-eruptive administration of fluoride from day 5 to 17, the period
when molars are undergoing active mineralization, was not found to
be cariostatic under these experimental conditions (Table III and Fig.
1). Administration of a daily dose of fluoride at a level of 15 μg F$^-$/10

TABLE III Caries Scores of Molars from Rats Administered Various Daily Doses of
Fluoride During Tooth Mineralization Prior to Eruption[a]

Group	Treat- ment[b]	No. of animals	Caries scores		
			Buccal (E)[c]	Sulcal (D$_s$)[d]	Proximal (E)[c]
A	0	17	8.0 ± 0.9	9.8 ± 0.6	2.0 ± 0.4
B	15	19	7.6 ± 0.9	8.7 ± 0.5	1.4 ± 0.4
C	30	17	9.6 ± 1.1	9.1 ± 0.6	2.8 ± 0.4
D	45	12	9.3 ± 1.5	9.3 ± 0.9	3.2 ± 0.5
E	60	17	9.6 ± 1.2	7.8 ± 0.7	3.3 ± 0.4
F	75	17	12.4 ± 1.1	10.4 ± 0.7	4.4 ± 0.3
G	90	18	13.2 ± 1.1	9.2 ± 0.8	4.8 ± 0.3
H	105	20	15.4 ± 1.0	11.9 ± 0.8	4.8 ± 0.3

[a] All rats were challenged with a caries-promoting diet #305 from day 17 to termination
of the experiment on day 35.
[b] Fluoride dose μg/10 gm body weight.
[c] E = scores for carious surfaces that involve the enamel.
[d] D$_s$ = scores for carious surfaces that extend into the dentin.

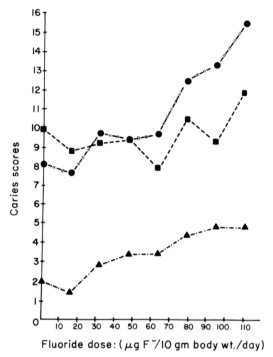

Fluoride dose: (μg F⁻/10 gm body wt./day)

FIG. 1.   Buccal (E) (●), sulcal (D$_s$) (■), and proximal (E) (▲) caries scores for rats administered different levels of fluoride pre-eruptively (4 to 17 days of age).

gm body weight had a tendency to lower caries scores on all molar surfaces, but these effects were not statistically significant. As the fluoride dose level was increased beyond the lowest dose, there was a parallel increase in the caries scores of the buccal and interproximal surfaces. However, the response of the sulcal caries (D_s) was not similar to that of buccal and proximal surfaces, for caries scores of groups receiving the lower levels of fluorine fluctuated around the control level of 9.8. Both when the dose was raised to 75 μg F⁻/10 gm of body weight and at higher doses, the caries scores were found to be significantly higher (Table IV).

In general, pre-eruptive administration of fluoride to young rats had no significant effect on body weight at termination of the study (Table V). At 17 days of age, there were slightly lower body weights for the rats receiving the higher fluoride doses, but this effect was not large or significant. Gross examination of the animals indicated no differences between the rats in the control group and those receiving fluoride.

As indicated previously, the fluoride content of maxillary molars from

TABLE IV   Duncan's Evaluation of Ranked Comparisons of Caries Scores Means from Rats Administered Different Levels of Fluoride[a]

Buccal (E) scores

Group:	H	G	F	E	C	D	A	B
Treatment:	105	90	75	60	30	45	0	15
$\bar{X}$:	15.4	13.2	12.4	9.6	9.6	9.3	8.0	7.6

Sulcal (D_s) scores

Group:	H	F	A	D	G	C	B	E
Treatment:	105	75	0	45	90	30	15	60
$\bar{X}$:	11.9	10.4	9.8	9.3	9.2	9.1	8.7	7.8

Proximal (E) scores

Group:	G	H	F	E	D	C	A	B
Treatment:	90	105	75	45	60	30	0	15
$\bar{X}$:	4.8	4.8	4.4	3.3	3.2	2.8	2.0	1.4

[a] All means underscored by the same line are not statistically significant at $p < 0.05$. Treatment expressed as ppm F.

rats receiving fluoride in the drinking water (posteruptively) was found to be 0.160 μg F$^-$/mg of tooth (Table II). This level of fluoride was within the range of fluoride concentrations found in molars of rats given fluoride pre-eruptively. Administration of a dose containing 15 μg F$^-$/10 gm of body weight increased the fluoride levels of tooth crowns from

TABLE V   Mean Body Weights of Rat Pups Administered Different Fluoride Doses during Tooth Development (4–17 Days)

Group	Treatment (μgF/10 gm body wt.)	Mean body weight (gm)			
		5 days	10 days	17 days	33 days
A	0	13.3	24.2	42.6	111.2
B	15	13.3	24.0	41.1	112.7
C	30	13.7	24.0	41.3	113.7
D	45	13.3	23.6	37.3	112.3
E	60	13.4	23.0	39.9	113.8
F	75	13.6	22.9	39.2	114.0
G	90	13.6	22.6	39.2	115.5
H	105	13.3	21.7	38.4	107.7

0.027 in controls to 0.099 μg/mg. At this level, a tendency to lower caries values was found (Fig. 1). Increasing the fluoride dosage gave a linear increase in fluoride content of molar crowns up to a dose of 60 μg F$^-$/10 gm body weight. The fluoride values seem to plateau at 0.77 μg/mg, when the highest dose level of 105 μg F$^-$/10 gm was given pre-eruptively (Fig. 2). The increase in fluoride level of tooth crowns from rats administered fluoride pre-eruptively paralleled the increase in severity of carious lesions observed on the buccal, sulcal, and proximal molar surfaces of the fluoride-treated rats.

In general, pre-eruptive administration of fluorine levels above 15 μg/10 gm body weight, which corresponds to 1.5 mg/kg body weight, were found to be deleterious in terms of dental caries. Interestingly, rats given fluoride in the drinking water posteruptively at a level of 25 ppm fluoride consume approximately 3.8 mg of fluoride per kg of body weight without any deleterious effects and with a significant protection against caries.

Incorporation of fluoride into molars was not found to be the same throughout the pre-eruptive period (Fig. 3). In the second experiment,

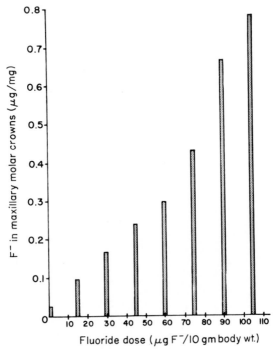

FIG. 2. Fluoride concentration (μg/mg of tooth) in maxillary first molar crowns from rats administered different fluoride doses pre-eruptively (4 to 17 days of age).

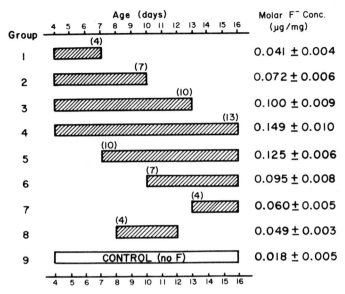

FIG. 3. Experimental design and fluoride concentration (μg/mg of tooth) in maxillary first molar crowns from rats administered pre-eruptively a single level of fluoride (45 μg F$^-$/10 gm body weight) for different lengths of time and during different stages of molar mineralization. The total number of fluoride doses in each case is given in parentheses.

where fluoride solutions were intubated daily for different lengths of time at various stages of tooth development, it was shown that incorporation of fluoride was greatest at the later stages immediately prior to eruption into the oral cavity. Molars from rats in group 7 had 0.060 μg F$^-$/mg, while those from groups 8 and 1 had approximately 30% less (0.049 and 0.041) even though the rats had received an equal number of fluoride doses. The same pattern was observed when groups 6 and 5 are compared respectively to groups 2 and 3. The former presented higher fluoride concentrations than the latter group, which received fluoride at earlier stages of development.

The level of fluoride in the maxillary crowns of rats in group 4, which received fluoride supplements throughout the experimental period, was lower than the one found in group D in Experiment #1. It should be noted that the rat dams in Experiment #2 were fed the gel diet containing less than 2 ppm fluoride during pregnancy, while the dams in Experiment #1 were suckling 1-day-old pups when the experiment started. It should also be pointed out that the experimental period in Experiment #1 was 14 days, while Experiment #2 was 1 day shorter (13 days). Whether one day at this critical time prior to eruption could account for the difference in fluoride concentration is not known and is being investigated.

IV. DISCUSSION

Results of studies of the effects of fluoride on caries in humans have not enabled investigators to distinguish clearly between pre-eruptive and posteruptive effects of this element. For this reason, it is essential to use a controlled experimental approach to try to understand the levels at which fluoride will reduce the incidence and severity of caries, as well as the time during tooth development when it should be administered to obtain the greatest cariostatic effect without danger of a negative effect on the teeth or the host.

In a recent paper, Aasenden and Peebles (1974) studied a group of children from nonfluoridated communities who had ingested a 0.5 mg fluoride supplement per day from 1 week to 4 months after birth until 3 years of age and then continued on a 1 mg/day supplement until 10 years of age, when oral examinations were done. This group was compared with children from the same communities who had not received fluoride and with group of children with a lifetime exposure to fluoridated water. Comparison of mean scores of decayed and filled surfaces per child for all teeth and for first molars showed that the group supplemented with fluoride had lower scores than the other two groups in a ratio of 1:2:5, with the nonfluoridated group having the highest scores. These authors also evaluated the incidence and severity of fluorosis and found the mean fluorosis index to be twice as high in the group supplemented with fluoride (0.88) as in those that received fluoridated water throughout life (0.40). Fourteen percent had moderate lesions in the supplemented group, while only 2.2% had these lesions in the group drinking fluoridated water.

This human study shows the combined pre- and posteruptive effects of fluoride and does not attempt to separate them. The net reduction in caries, therefore, is the result of the addition of these two effects of fluoride. In view of the reported higher incidence of enamel fluorosis in the human study, it is possible that an even greater beneficial effect may have been seen had the fluoride administration started immediately before eruption and continued thereafter rather than earlier. Our results, obtained with experimental animal models, suggest a definite advantage in providing the element immediately before eruption, when fluoride uptake is greatest, and including the early posteruptive maturation period

in the oral cavity. This approach would avoid possible deleterious alteration during the period of greatest ameloblast activity, and yet would
increase fluoride concentration in the outer enamel surface. It would
make fluoride available to strengthen the resistance of the tooth (Navia,
1973) by influencing the maturation process of enamel, pellicle formation, and bacterial plaque metabolism (Bowen and Hewitt, 1974) on
the enamel surface.

Posteruptive administration of fluoride in the drinking water offered
to weanling rats decreased the severity of carious lesions, particularly
on the buccal surfaces. Molars of these rats were found to have a substantial level of fluoride (0.160 $\mu g/mg$) when compared to those of control
rats (0.013 μg F/mg). Fluoride given pre-eruptively during the time
of tooth mineralization also increased the fluoride level of the tooth
but did not make the molars caries resistant. Actually, the caries susceptibility was increased at the higher doses of fluoride. These data suggest
that fluoride content of molars is not the sole factor responsible for
the cariostatic effect. Results obtained in this investigation support the
concept that posteruptive administration of fluorides is most beneficial,
especially if it includes the time when the tooth is actually emerging
into the oral cavity. At this time even a short exposure of the molars
to fluoride is capable of confering a lasting protection against caries.
Madsen and Edmonds (1964) fed a diet supplemented with sodium
fluoride to weanling cotton rats for only 2 days (12 and 13 days of
age) when first molars of this strain of rats start to erupt. At 40 days
of age, they found a significant reduction in molar caries scores between
treated rats and untreated controls. Only the newly erupted first molars
were protected significantly by early fluoride treatment. A similar response to another cariostatic agent, sodium trimetaphosphate, was observed when it was offered immediately after tooth eruption (Navia
et al., 1968).

The experiments involving the posteruptive administration of fluoride
differed from the pre-eruptive studies because (a) they included a different period in tooth development, and (b) they had an increased frequency of exposure. Fluoride in the drinking water comes in contact
with the tooth surface as often as the rat drinks. Exposure therefore
is fairly frequent, and the fluoride comes in contact with enamel and
with the film of bacteria that covers it several times during a 24 hour
period. Thus, the fluoride has an opportunity to act on the maturing
enamel surface as well as the bacterial plaque. This plaque, as suggested
by Charlton *et al.* (1974), may prepare the enamel surface for fluoride
uptake in a manner similar to that of acidulated phosphate solutions,
which prepare the enamel surface prior to a topical fluoride application.

Frequent exposure to fluoride may then facilitate the incorporation of fluoride into the outer enamel–plaque interface and stimulate its subsequent cariostatic action.

When different dosages of fluoride were given pre-eruptively to study the caries effect of such treatments, no gross toxicity signs were detected in the rats. Mean body weights for rats in the different groups did not show significant differences. Fluoride levels in the crowns were increased significantly as the intubated dosage of fluoride was raised, and caries scores were found to be directly correlated with the increased level of fluoride in the molars. No benefit was obtained, therefore, from such systemic treatment, and in fact a definite detriment resulted. Several investigators (Allan, 1963; Kruger, 1967, 1968, 1969; Walton and Eisenmann, 1974) have studied and described the detrimental effects of parenteral high doses of fluoride on the ameloblast, amelogenesis, and enamel structure.

In studies reported here the approach was to use the oral route of administration and a series of dose levels ranging from low to moderately high. It should be stressed that none of these treatments induced gross pathosis in the rats. It may be that intermediate levels between the control (0 fluoride) and the second dose level (30 μg/10 gm of body weight) might bring about an increased protection against the caries challenge instituted at weaning. However, it seems improbable that the level of fluoride incorporation obtained in this manner might be protective, since the fluoride level obtained when the element was given posteruptively, and found to be cariostatic, was approximately equal compared with that obtained at the level of 30 μg F/10 gm body weight.

The difference between the two approaches to fluoride administration might be even greater than is apparent, since the pattern of distribution of fluoride in these teeth is quite different. The fluoride concentration in surface enamel of the molars from rats offered fluoride posteruptively was probably much higher than in surface enamel from rats receiving fluoride pre-eruptively. To achieve pre-eruptively a level of fluoride in the outer layers of enamel similar to those obtained by posteruptive administration of fluoride might require a toxic dose that would be detrimental rather than beneficial to the developing tissues.

V. CONCLUSION

Results of these investigations suggest that administration of supplemental fluoride should be considered and evaluated at times when the tooth is erupting or has recently erupted. It is at these times that the cariostatic effects are found to be most dramatic. Administration of supplemental fluoride before tooth eruption under our experimental conditions is noneffective and possibly even detrimental, especially when other trace elements are given concomitantly. Hunt and Navia (1973, 1975) have shown repeatedly that when elements previously supposed to have cariostatic properties are administered together with fluoride during tooth formation, there is an enhancement of enamel hypoplasia, which makes the molars highly susceptible to caries. The interaction shown to exist between trace elements and fluoride (Buttner, 1963) is important and should be investigated further.

The local administration of frequent doses of fluoride to the erupted tooth seems to be an ideal approach to insure the maximum effectiveness of this highly beneficial element to oral health.

VI. SUMMARY

Fluoride was administered either pre-eruptively, by gavage of a solution of sodium fluoride, or posteruptively in the drinking water. Several levels of fluoride, ranging from 0 to 105 μg/10 gm body weight, and different time periods were tested in the preeruptive experiments, and a single level of 25 ppm was evaluated in the posteruptive studies.

Administration of a level of 15 μg/10 gm body weight throughout the pre-eruptive period was found to decrease caries scores, although this effect was not significant. Increasing caries scores were observed with all other fluoride treatments from 30 to 105 μg/10 gm body weight. The level of fluoride in crowns of maxillary first molars increased in proportion to the amount of systemically administered fluoride. Higher incorporation of fluoride was obtained when the fluoride was administered at a time close to eruption of the molar. Pre-eruptive administration of fluoride did not affect body weight gain or produce signs of pathosis in the rats.

When the fluoride was offered posteruptively, there was also an increase in fluoride level in the crowns and a significant decrease in caries scores in all surfaces ranging from 20 to 54% reduction.

The data obtained in these studies support the concept that supplemental fluoride is most effective when it is given at and following the time of eruption, and that little benefit is gained from pre-eruptive administration, which could be even deleterious if the dose level and the presence of other interfering elements is not kept under control.

Water fluoridation and topical administration of frequent doses of fluoride to the erupted tooth seem to be ideal approaches to insure the maximum effectiveness of this highly beneficial element to oral health.

ACKNOWLEDGMENTS

We wish to express our deep appreciation to Dr. E. Bradley, who gave us expert advice on the design of experiments and the statistical analysis. These investigations were supported with NIDR Grants No. DE-03230 and DE-02670 of the National Institutes of Health, Washington, D.C.

REFERENCES

Aasenden, R., and Peebles, T. C. (1974). Effect of fluoride supplementation from birth on human deciduous and permanent teeth. *Arch. Oral Biol.* **19**, 321–326.

Allan, J. H. (1963). Observations on the development of dental enamel in acute experimental fluorosis. *O.R.C.A.* (Suppl. to *Arch. Oral Biol.*) pp. 41–51.

Armstrong, W. D., Singer, L., and Makowski, E. L. (1970). Placental transfer of fluoride and calcium. *Amer. J. Obstet. Gynecol.* **107**, 432–434.

Arnold, F. A., Likins, R. C., Russell, A. L., and Scott, D. B. (1962). Fifteenth year of Grand Rapids fluoridation study. *J. Amer. Dent. Ass.* **65**, 780–785.

Ast, D. B., Smith, D. J., Wachs, B., and Cantwell, K. T. (1956). Newburgh-Kingston caries-fluorine study. XIV. Combined clinical and roentgenographic dental findings after 10 years of fluoride experience. *J. Amer. Dent. Ass.* **52**, 314–325.

Babeaux, W. L., and Zipkin, I. (1966). Dental aspects of the prenatal administration of fluoride. *J.Oral Ther. Pharmacol.* **3**, 124–135.

Baud, C. A., and Bang, S. (1970). Electron probe and x-ray diffraction microanalyses of human enamel treated *in vitro* by fluoride solutions. *Caries Res.* **4**, 1–13.

Bowen, W. H., and Hewitt, M. J. (1974). Effect of fluoride on extracellular polysaccharide production by *Streptococcus mutans*. *J. Dent. Res.* **53**, 627–629.

Buttner, W. (1963). Action of trace elements on the metabolism of fluoride. *J. Dent. Res.* **42**, 453–460.

Caldwell, R., and Thomas, J. (1970). Application of chemical agents for the control of dental caries. *Advan. Chem. Ser.* **94**, 161–180.

Call, R. A., Greenwood, D. A., LeCheminant, W. H., Shupe, J. L., Nielsen, H. M., Olson, L. E., Lamborn, R. E., Mangelson, F. L., and Davis, R. V. (1965). Histological and chemical studies in man on effects of fluoride. *Pub. Health Rep.* **80**, 529–538.

Carlos, J. P., Gittelsohn, A. M., and Haddon, W. (1962). Caries in deciduous teeth in relation to maternal ingestion of fluoride. *Pub. Health Rep.* **77**, 658–660.

Charlton, G., Blainey, B., and Schamschula, R. G. (1974). Associations between dental plaque and fluoride in human surface enamel. *Arch. Oral Biol.* **19**, 139–143.

Eanes, E. D., and Posner, A. S. (1970). Structure and chemistry of bone mineral. *In* "Biological Calcification: Cellular and Molecular Aspects" (H. Schraer, ed.), pp. 1–26. Appleton, New York.

Glas, J. E. (1962). Studies on the ultrastructure of dental enamel. VI. *Odontol. Rev.* **13**, 315–326.

Hodge, H. C., and Smith, F. A. (1968). Fluorides and man. *Annu. Rev. Pharmacol.* **8**, 395.

Hodge, H. C., and Smith, F. A. (1970). Minerals: Fluorine and dental caries. *Advan. Chem. Ser.* **94**, 93–115.

Horowitz, H. S. (1973). Fluoride: Research on clinical and public health applications. *J. Amer. Dent. Ass.* **87**, 1013–1018.

Horowitz, H. S., and Heifetz, S. B. (1967). Effects of prenatal exposure to fluoridation on dental caries. *Pub. Health Rep.* **82**, 297–304.

Hunt, C. E., and Navia, J. M. (1973). Effects of Sr, Mo, Li, and B on developing teeth and other tissues of neonatal rats. *In* "Trace Substances in Environmental Health" (D. D. Hemphill, ed.), Vol. VI, pp. 159–168. University of Missouri, Columbia.

Hunt, C. E., and Navia, J. M. (1975). Preeruptive effects of Mo, B, Sr, and F on caries in the rat. *Arch. Oral Biol.* **20**, 497–501.

Jenkins, G. N., Venkateswarlu, P., and Zipkin, I. (1970). Physiological effects of small doses of fluoride. Chapter 6. *World Health Organ. Monogr.* No. 59 163–223.

Keyes, P. H. (1958). Dental caries in the molar teeth of rats. II. A method for diagnosis and scoring several types of lesions simultaneously. *J. Dent. Res.* **37**, 1088–1099.

König, von K. G., Marthaler, T. M., Schait, A., and Mühlemann, H. R. (1960). Karies-hemmung durch Fluor in Wasser, Milch und Futter und Skelettfluorspeicherung im Rattenversuch bei Verabreichung wahrend und nach abschluss der Zahventurcklung. *Schweiz. Monatsschr. Zahnheilk.* **70**, 279.

Kramer, L., Osis, D., Wiatrawski, E., and Spencer, H. (1974). Dietary fluoride in different areas in the United States. *Amer. J. Clin. Nutr.* **27**, 590–594.

Kruger, B. J. (1964). Preeruptive and posteruptive effect of fluoride on rat molars. *Aust. Dent. J.* **9**, 90–93.

Kruger, B. J. (1967). Histologic effects of fluoride and molybdenum on developing dental tissues. *Aust. Dent. J.* **12**, 54–60.

Kruger, B. J. (1968). Ultrastructural changes in ameloblasts from fluoride treated rats. *Arch. Oral Biol.* **13**, 969–977.

Kruger, B. J. (1969). Electron microscopy of enamel formed in the presence of fluoride and molybdenum. *J. Dent. Res.* **48**, 1303–1307.

Lane, J. M., and Steinberg, M. E. (1973). The role of diphosphonates in osteoporosis of disuse. *J. Trauma* **13**, 863–869.

Leone, N. C., Shimkin, M. B., Arnold, F. A., Stevenson, C. A., Zimmerman, E. R., Geiser, P. A., and Lieberman, J. E. (1954). Medical aspects of excessive fluoride in a water supply. *Pub. Health Rep.* **69**, 925–936.

Leone, N. C., Stevenson, C. A., Hilbish, T. F., and Sosman, M. C. (1955). A roentgenologic study of a human population exposed to high-fluoride domestic water. *Amer. J. Roentgenol., Radium Ther. Nucl. Med.* **74**, 874–885.

Leone, N. C., Stevenson, C. A., Besse, B., Harves, L. E., Dauber, T. A., and Claffey, W. J. (1960). Effects of absorption of fluoride. II. A radiological investigation of 546 human residents of an area in which the drinking water contained only a minute trace of fluoride. *Arch. Environ. Health* **21**, 326–327.

McCann, H. G. (1968). Determination of fluoride in mineralized tissues using the fluoride ion electrode. *Arch. Oral Biol.* **13**, 475–477.

Madsen, K. O., and Edmonds, E. J. (1964). Prolonged effect on caries of short term fluoride treatment. I. Sensitivity of newly erupted cotton rat molars to dietary fluoride. *Arch. Oral Biol.* **9**, 209–217.

Marthaler, T. M. (1967). The value in caries prevention of other methods of increasing fluoride ingestion, apart from fluoridated water. *Int. Dent. J.* **17**, 606–618.

Menaker, L., and Navia, J. M. (1973). Effect of undernutrition during the perinatal period on caries development in the rat. IV. Effects of differential tooth incidence. *J. Dent. Res.* **52**, 692–697.

Muhler, J. C., Stookey, G. K., Spear, L. B., and Bixler, D. (1966). Blood and urinary fluoride studies following the ingestion of single doses of fluoride. *J. Oral Ther. Pharmacol.* **2**, 241–260.

National Academy of Sciences. (1971). "Biological Effects of Atmospheric Pollutants: Fluoride." Div. Med. Sci., Nat. Res. Counc., Washington, D.C.

Navia, J. M. (1970). Effects of minerals on dental caries. *Advan. Chem. Ser.* **94**, 123–160.

Navia, J. M. (1973). Prevention of dental caries: Agents which increase tooth resistance to dental caries. *Int. Dent. J.* **22**, 427–440.

Navia, J. M., Lopez, H., and Harris, R. S. (1968). Cariostatic effects of sodium trimetaphosphate when fed to rats during different stages of tooth development. *Arch. Oral Biol.* **13**, 779–786.

Navia, J. M., Lopez, H., and Harris, R. S. (1969). Purified diet for dental caries research with rats. *J. Nutr.* **97**, 133–140.

Rich, C., Ensick, J., and Ivanovich, P. (1964). The effects of sodium fluoride on calcium metabolism of subjects with metabolic bone diseases. *J. Clin. Invest.* **43**, 545–556.

Riggs, B. L., Jowsey, J., Kelly, P. J., and Hoffman, D. L. (1972). Treatment for postmenopausal and senile osteoporosis. *Med. Clin. N. Amer.* **56**, 989–997.

Shaw, J. H., and Sognnaes, R. F. (1954). Experimental rat caries. V. Effect of fluorine on the caries-conduciveness of a purified ration. *J. Nutr.* **53**, 207–214.

Smith, F. A., Leone, N. C., and Hodge, H. C. (1960). The effects of absorption of fluoride. V. Chemical determination of fluoride in human soft tissues following prolonged ingestion of fluoride at various levels. *AMA Arch. Ind. Health* **21**, 330–337.

Spencer, G. R., El-Sayed, F. I., Kroening, G. H., Pell, K. L., Shoup, N., Adams, D. F., Franke, M., and Alexander, J. E. (1971). Effects of fluoride, calcium, and phosphorus on porcine bone. *Amer. J. Vet. Res.* **32**, 1751–1774.

Stookey, G. K., Osborne, J., and Muhler, J. C. (1962). Effects of pre- and postnatal fluoride on caries. *Dent. Progr.* **2**, 137.

Underwood, E. J. (1971). "Trace Elements in Human and Animal Nutrition," 3rd ed. Academic Press, New York.

U.S. Food and Drug Administration. (1966). Statements of general policy or interpretation, Oral prenatal drugs containing fluorides for human use. *Fed. Regist.* Washington, D.C.

Walton, R. E., and Eisenmann, D. R. (1974). Ultrastructural examination of various stages of amelogenesis in the rat following parenteral fluoride administration. *Arch. Oral Biol.* **19**, 171–182.

Weidmann, S. M., and Weatherell, J. A. (1970). Fluorides and human health. *World Health Organ., Monogr. Ser.* **59**, 104–128.

Zipkin, I., and Babeaux, W. L. (1965). Maternal transfer of fluoride. *J. Oral Ther. Pharmacol.* **1**, 652–665.

35
Methodology of Trace Element Research

E. J. Underwood

I. INTRODUCTION

As one of the pioneer workers in the trace element field, I have had considerable opportunity to appraise and even to participate in many of the various methods used in trace element research. I have come to appreciate the special and demanding characteristics of these methods, both with respect to facilities and to the knowledge and skills required of the investigator. I propose to look first at some of the particular characteristics of trace elements that make their investigation so demanding and at the same time so challenging. Consideration will then be given to the two main methods that have been used in arriving at our present state of knowledge of the nutritional physiology of the trace elements. These are (1) the studies of naturally occurring "area" problems, and (2) the purified diet and protected environment investigations. These types of investigation overlap in time and in some aspects of their methodology, especially in their dependence on analytical methods of great accuracy and refinement.

II. TRACE ELEMENT DIVERSITY AND CHARACTERISTICS

The only characteristic that the trace elements have in common is that they normally occur or function in living tissues in low concentra-

269

tions relative to the major elements. They vary markedly in their physico-chemical properties, as well as in their biological properties, so that there is no common chemical denominator to aid the investigator. One has only to think of the fourteen trace elements now known to be essential for animal life, ranging from the halogens iodine and fluorine, through the transition metals, to silicon and vanadium, which have only recently been added to the essential list. This chemical diversity, which is increased by the inclusion of potentially toxic elements like lead, mercury, and cadmium, with which the essential elements interact, poses special analytical challenges. The analytical challenges to the investigator are compounded by (1) the very low concentrations usually involved, (2) problems of contamination from the environment and from the reagents and instruments used in obtaining and processing the samples, and (3) the forms or chemical combinations in which the trace elements occur in foods and tissues. Many of the trace elements are linked by coordination or covalent bonds to organic compounds of varying size, lability, and biological potency. The investigator has therefore to be concerned with more than total concentrations in his investigations; he may have to consider also the proportions of much more complex compounds. Even the valence of the element, as with chromium, can be important.

A further complicating factor in trace element research, to add to the difficulties of the investigator, is that of interaction. The nutritional physiology of the trace elements is rarely confined to a single element in isolation from others because of the frequency of interactions at the absorptive and the cellular level, which can affect minimum requirements and influence maximum tolerances. Indeed, the trace elements interact with each other and with other nutrients to such an extent that the margin between the levels at which the effects on the organism are beneficial and those that are toxic may be quite small or even overlap. This is particularly striking in studies with copper and molybdenum and also with zinc and cadmium and with selenium and mercury. The inevitability of significant interactions among other elements and nutrients should increasingly be taken into account in the methodology of trace element research.

III. THE ESSENTIAL ELEMENTS

On present evidence, twenty-six or the ninety naturally occurring elements are essential to life. These consist of eleven major elements—carbon, hydrogen, oxygen, nitrogen, sulfur, calcium, phosphorus, potassium, sodium, chlorine, and magnesium—and fifteen elements generally accepted as trace elements. These are iron, iodine, copper, zinc, manganese, cobalt, nickel, molybdenum, boron, selenium, chromium, fluorine, tin, silicon, and vanadium. Boron is included, but so far it has only been shown to be essential for plant life. A further twenty to thirty elements occur in usually low and variable concentrations in living tissues, and for these, no essential functions have yet been found. It is very likely that some of them will be found to perform some vital functions, but at the present state of knowledge, they seem merely to reflect the contact of the organism with its environment.*

It appears from the foregoing that evolution has selected certain elements for the essential functioning of living organisms and has rejected or ignored others for this purpose. No rationale exists for explaining why or how certain elements have been found uniquely suitable to perform various vital functions and others have not. However, there are certain facts that may give pointers to the existence of other potentially useful elements. For example, if we look at the periodic table we see that only three of the twenty-six elements known to be essential to life have an atomic number above 34. These are iodine, tin, and molybdenum. Furthermore, of the fourteen known essential trace elements, no less than nine occupy positions between atomic numbers 23 and 34. The significance of this interesting fact is unknown, but it does suggest that we ought to be paying special attention to other elements similarly placed in the periodic table.

The atomic number interval 23–34 includes three elements—gallium, germanium, and arsenic†—for which no vital roles are known. Surely these three elements should logically be considered prime targets for the trace element investigator interested in delineating the full range of essential elements in nutrition. By the same reasoning, the nutritional potential of bromine deserves further critical attention. With an atomic number of 35, bromine is next on this apparently critical atomic number sequence of 23 to 34. We have already been given some tantalizing hints that bromine may have some nutritional significance. Bromide can completely replace chloride in the growth medium of several species of halophytic algae (McClachlan and Craigie, 1967) and can substitute for part of the chloride requirement of chicks (Leach and Nesheim, 1963). Nearly twenty years ago, it was shown that chicks fed a semisynthetic diet exhibited a significant growth response to trace additions

---

* Author's note: Recent evidence indicates that arsenic must now be considered an essential element for the rat (Nielsen et al., 1975).

† See previous footnote.

of bromine (Huff *et al.*, 1956) and that mice fed the same diet containing iodinated casein to produce a hyperthyroid-induced growth retardation responded similarly to supplemental bromine (Bosshardt *et al.*, 1956). These investigations were conducted prior to the advent of the plastic isolator technique and the demonstration of the need to control atmospheric contamination. Bromine is so ubiquitous in nature, that the application of this technique seems to provide the best if not the only hope of confirming or otherwise the earlier indications of an essential role for this element.

The methods and tools in the armamentarium of the physical chemist and the molecular biologist are beginning to unfold other possibilities of biological potentiality among the trace elements. For example, Vallee (1971) has shown that cobalt and cadmium can be substituted *in vitro* for the native zinc atoms in several zinc metalloenzymes and the enzyme remains active, and Stiefel (1973) has studied the five known molybdenum metalloenzymes—nitrogenase, xanthine oxidase, nitrate reductase, aldehyde oxidase, and sulfite oxidase. A simple molecular mechanism, embodying coupled electron–proton transfer to and from the substrate and compatible with the coordination chemistry of molybdenum, is presented and discussed for each of the enzymes and the reactions they catalyze. The particular suitability of molybdenum, as distinct from most other metals, for these physiological uses is thus revealed in physicochemical terms. Using the same reasoning, Stiefel makes the interesting point that vanadium, but not tungsten or chromium, has many of the significant attributes of molybdenum and may display some activity, and that rhenium is a further likely candidate to replace molybdenum with retention of enzyme activity. Comparable studies of the molecular biology of other metalloenzymes will no doubt provide equally revealing insights into the physiological potential of the trace elements.

IV. NATURALLY OCCURRING "AREA" PROBLEMS WITH TRACE ELEMENTS

In certain restricted areas in many parts of the world, animals and man have suffered from various debilitating diseases with well-marked clinical and pathological manifestations that have been shown to be caused by naturally occurring trace element deficiencies, toxicities, and imbalances. The solution of these "area" problems has provided some of the most scientifically stimulating and economically rewarding activities in the whole field of trace element research.

The most remarkable area study involving a trace element is undoubt-

edly that of Chatin (1852), the French botanist who published his pioneer observations on the iodine content of soils, waters, and foods in
Europe over 120 years ago and who concluded from these observations
that the occurrence of endemic goiter in man was associated with a
deficiency of environmental iodine. This association had been suggested
in 1830 by Prévost (Towery, 1953), but Chatin (1852) was the first
to provide convincing analytical data. This can be seen as an extraordi-
nary achievement for that time when it is realized that the iodine concentrations had to be measured in micrograms per gram long before the
development of the sophisticated and refined physical methods of analysis now available to the trace element worker. Chatin's achievement
is made even more remarkable by the fact that a further forty years
elapsed before the German chemist Baumann (1896) showed that iodine
is concentrated in the thyroid gland and that this concentration is diminished in endemic goiter.

   The most significant methodological development in the subsequent
investigation of a wide range of trace element area problems was the
emergence in the 1920s of the technique of emission spectrography.
This technique had limited quantitative accuracy in its earlier stages,
but it permitted the simultaneous detection of some twenty to thirty
elements in low concentrations, thus allowing comparisons of the mineral
composition of soils and plants and animal tissues from affected and
nonaffected areas. The outstanding usefulness of emission spectrography
in the methodology of trace element research in the 1930s can be gauged
from the fact that the use of this technique gave the all-important initial
leads to the solution and control of three major area problems. I refer
to the demonstration that excessive intakes of molybdenum from herbage
is the cause of the scouring disease of cattle known as "teart" occurring
in certain parts of England (Ferguson et al., 1938), to the finding that
enzootic neonatal ataxia of lambs in parts of Western Australia is a
manifestation of copper deficiency in the ewe (Bennetts and Chapman,
1937), and to the important demonstration that molybdenum intakes
can have a profound effect upon copper metabolism in herbivorous animals (Dick and Bull, 1945). The disease of poultry known as "slipped
tendon" is not an area problem, but the lead to its discovery as a manifestation of manganese deficiency also came from a spectrographic study
of a calcium phosphate supplement observed surprisingly to prevent
rather than exacerbate the condition (Wilgus et al., 1936, 1937).

   Emission spectrography played no part in the discovery of cobalt
deficiency in sheep and cattle as an important area problem, a discovery
in which I was personally involved, but the investigations did provide
other methodological challenges, particularly in respect to inorganic and

analytical chemistry, which deserve to be mentioned in the present context.

Workers in New Zealand had shown that a wasting disease of cattle known as "bush sickness" in parts of that country was not due to either a toxic or an infectious agent. Since the affected animals were anemic, the administration of iron compounds was tried and found to be highly effective in preventing and curing the disease. Iron deficiency then became accepted as the cause of this and similar diseases (Underwood, 1971). In our investigation in Western Australia of a similar wasting disease of cattle, correctly named enzootic marasmus, we (1) became suspicious of the very large doses of iron salts and compounds required to cure the disease, (2) could find little relation between the effectiveness of a given dose and the amount of iron it supplied, (3) found considerable stores of iron in the liver, spleen, and bone marrow of affected animals, and (4) most significantly of all, discovered that whole liver was curative in oral doses that supplied insignificant amounts of iron. We then removed the iron from the potent iron compounds limonite ($Fe_2O_3 \cdot H_2O$) by exploiting the specific solubility of ferric chloride in ethyl ether. The limonite had to be dissolved in concentrated hydrocholoric acid and then extracted in a huge Soxhlet type apparatus in large enough quantities to feed to affected lambs and calves. When this was done, the iron fraction was found to be completely noncurative and the potency to reside in the "iron-free" fraction.

These findings disproved the iron-deficiency theory and led us to the hypothesis that the disease was due to an environmental deficiency of an element present in trace amounts as a contaminant in the curative iron compounds. The iron-free extract of limonite was then fractionated into groups of elements by the classic group separation methods used by analytical chemists at the time. Large amounts had to be prepared, because each separation had to be fed for 2–4 weeks or more to lambs or calves. Potency was found to reside in the so-called zinc group containing zinc, manganese, nickel, and cobalt. After some misleading tests with a contaminated nickel oxide, the curative element was shown to be cobalt, and extremely small amounts of this element, as low as 0.1 mg/day, were found to prevent and cure the disease in lambs, and the same was true for slightly larger amounts in calves.

The formidable practical and chemical difficulties inherent in this research program continued when it came to estimating the levels of cobalt in animal tissues, pastures, and soils. We had to develop analytical procedures capable of estimating accurately concentrations below 0.1 ppm cobalt, the only physical device then available being simple optical colorimetry. This meant using very large samples requiring large quantities of reagents, all of which had to be specially purified for the purpose. Some idea of the magnitude of the task can be gained from the fact that it took me about five days to analyze a single sample in duplicate. At the present time, ten times this number of samples can be analyzed for cobalt in one-tenth the time by atomic absorption spectrometry.

Before leaving this outline of the methodology employed in the early demonstration of cobalt as an essential element in ruminant nutrition, I would like to refer briefly again to our dicovery that whole liver administered orally was curative of wasting disease. Liver was tested in this way because it had just been shown to control pernicious anemia in man, and anemia was evident in our affected animals. Subsequently, we found liver ash to be ineffective when administered orally in comparable doses to whole liver. This led us to the hypothesis, put forward as early as 1937, that the potency of liver may be due to the presence of a stored factor and that cobalt may function through the production of this factor within the body (Filmer and Underwood, 1937). Eleven years were to pass before this "stored factor" was shown by others to be the cobalt-containing vitamin B_{12} and a further three years before it was established that cobalt deficiency in ruminants is actually a vitamin B_{12} deficiency brought about by the inability of the rumen microorganisms, in the presence of inadequate dietary cobalt, to synthesize sufficient vitamin B_{12} to meet the needs of the host animal's tissues (see Underwood, 1971).

V. METHODOLOGICAL PROBLEMS WITH PURIFIED AND SPECIAL DIETS

Trace element research with purified diets began in the early part of this century with the pioneer studies of Gabriel Bertrand in Paris and of J. S. McHargue in Missouri. The nature and importance of vitamins were little understood at that time. In these circumstances, the investigators were faced with the problem of either including in the semipurified diets some crude vitamin-rich materials such as yeast or liver extract, which incidentally supplied some trace elements, or of feeding these diets supplemented only with the trace element under study. In the first case, the experimental animals usually grew and remained healthy whether supplemented with the trace element under study or not, and in the second case they usually failed to grow or thrive, also whether the trace element in question was added or not. It is hardly surprising, therefore, that their results were inconclusive.

The Wisconsin group, led by E. B. Hart, was not faced with the vitamin problem just described, because, initially at least, they were using cows' milk as a basal diet. In a series of studies with iron that served to invalidate the old concept that organic forms of iron were nutritionally superior to inorganic iron salts, certain anomalies in the results were noticed. This led the investigators to suspect that another element in addition to iron was necessary to prevent milk anemia in young rats. This suspicion was confirmed, and in 1928, copper was shown to be essential for growth and hemoglobin formation in the rat (Hart *et al.*, 1928). Within three years, the same group showed that rats and mice fed a milk diet supplemented with both iron and copper required supplements of a further element, which turned out to be manganese, if their fertility was to be maintained (Kemmerer *et al.*, 1931). The Wisconsin workers had cleverly exploited the fact that cows' milk, kept free of contact with metal, is inherently deficient in iron, copper, and manganese, relative to the requirements of the young rat, while being at the same time rich in other essential nutrients.

This experimental technique was no longer possible for the next trace element shown to be essential for mammalian nutrition by the Wisconsin group—zinc—because milk is a relatively good source of this element. They were therefore obliged to develop a semipurified solid diet resulting in poor growth and skin lesions in rats, preventable and curable by supplemental zinc (Todd *et al.*, 1934).

Although a great deal was learned about trace elements and other branches of nutrition and great strides were made in analytical methods, no further additions to the list of essential trace elements came from studies with purified diets for more than twenty years after the initial demonstration of the essentiality of zinc in 1934. Then came molybdenum in 1956 (Higgins *et al.*, 1956), selenium in 1957 (Schwarz and Foltz, 1957), and chromium in 1959 (Schwarz and Mertz, 1959). Vitamin research had progressed to the point where pure crystalline vitamins had become available, thus eliminating one important source of trace element contamination. Later, the essential amino acids became available in pure crystalline form, so that whole protein dietary components, with their considerable opportunities for trace element contamination, were no longer necessary. The use of such a highly purified diet, containing less than 0.005 ppm selenium but otherwise adequate for chicks, provided the first clear and unequivocal evidence that selenium is a dietary essential for growth, independent of or additional to its function as a substitute for vitamin E (Thompson and Scott, 1969). This beautiful experiment strikingly illustrates the demanding nature of trace element research at this level of sophistication. The investigators had to develop an otherwise nutritionally adequate diet containing less than 5 parts per *billion* of selenium and to evolve and use a physical analytical methodology capable of measuring selenium concentrations of this minute magnitude. The next step forward in the methodology of trace element research was the development of a controlled environment system for experiments with rats and chicks used in conjunction with the highly purified types of diets mentioned earlier (Smith and Schwarz, 1967). The animals are isolated in a system in which plastics are used for all components, and there is no metal, glass, or rubber. An air lock facilitates passage of articles in and out of the so-called trace-element-sterile environment, and two air filters remove all dust down to a particle size of 0.35 μm. The virtual exclusion of atmospheric contamination of the animals and their food, water, and utensils is the crucial final step, because deficiency signs appear in rats after 1–3 weeks on the purified diets in the closed environment, whereas animals fed the same diets under conventional conditions remain normal (Schwarz, 1972). These facts highlight the ever-present problems of contamination that face the trace element investigator. The plastic isolator technique has been so successful in minimizing environmental contamination, that no less than five new essential trace elements—tin, fluorine, silicon, nickel, and vanadium—have emerged through its use by Schwarz and others over the last few years (Schwarz, 1972).

The discoveries of new trace elements, some of which, notably chromium, nickel, and vanadium, are present and function in living tissues in parts per billion rather than parts per million, not only pose formidable problems in minimizing environmental contamination of samples and reagents, but also present special analytical difficulties.

The analytical challenge facing trace element investigators has been, and to some extent still is, particularly severe with chromium. The concentrations of chromium in blood and urine are normally so low that conventional atomic absorption spectrometry is inadequate to the task. In the well known review article by Mertz (1969), a wide range of values for blood chromium concentrations was reported, with the majority lying between 20 and 30 ppb. The use of the graphite furnace with flameless atomic absorption produced very much lower values. Direct analysis of serum, i.e., no digestion other than the ashing within the furnace, is reported to yield values of around 1 ppb, whereas a wet predigestion prior to injection into the furnace results in concentrations close to 4 ppb (W. Mertz, private communication). The disagreement among reported chromium concentrations is as great or greater with other biological materials such as liver. It seems that chromium exists in such materials in a number of forms, some of which are highly volatile and can escape detection by existing methods. The proportions of the different forms present could vary not only among different tissues, but presumably also from sample to sample of the same tissue. Furthermore, if this is the complex and difficult position with chromium it would be surprising if similar problems did not exist with some of the other trace elements. This possibility certainly needs to be taken into consideration in future research with these elements. The development of more accurate and sensitive analytical techniques, combined with assessments of physiological activity, thus emerges increasingly as the most difficult and certainly among the most challenging problems in the methodology of trace element research.

REFERENCES

Baumann, E. J. (1896). Ueber das normale vorkommen von jod im thierkorper. *Hoppe-Zeyler's Z. Physiol. Chem.* 21, 319–330.

Bennetts, H. W., and Chapman, F. E. (1937). Copper deficiency of sheep in Western Australia. *Aust. Vet. J.* 13, 138–149.

Bosshardt, D. K., Huff, J. W., and Barnes, R. H. (1956). Effect of bromine on chick growth. *Proc. Soc. Exp. Biol. Med.* 92, 219–226.

Chatin, A. (1852). Recherche de l'iode dan l'air, les eaux, le sol, et les produits alimentoures des Alpes de la France et du Piedmont. *C. R. Acad. Sci.* 34, 14–18 and 51–54.

Dick, A. T., and Bull, L. B. (1945). Some preliminary observations on the effect of molybdenum on copper metabolism in herbivorous animals. *Aust. Vet. J.* 21, 70–72.

Ferguson, W. S., Lewis, A. H., and Watson, S. J. (1938). Action of molybdenum in nutrition of milking cattle. *Nature (London)* 141, 553.

Filmer, J. F., and Underwood, E. J. (1937). Enzootic Marasmus: Further data concerning the potency of cobalt as a curative and prophylactic agent. *Aust. Vet. J.* 13, 57–64.

Hart, E. B., Steenbock, H., Waddell, J., and Elvehjem, C. A. (1928). Iron in nutrition. VII. Copper as a supplement to iron for hemoglobin building in the rat. *J. Biol. Chem.* 77, 797–812.

Higgins, E. S., Richert, D. A., and Westerfeld, W. W. (1956). Molybdenum deficiency and tungstate inhibition studies. *J. Nutr.* 59, 539–559.

Huff, J. W., Bosshardt, D. K., Miller, O. P., and Barnes, R. H. (1956). A nutritional requirement for bromine. *Proc. Soc. Exp. Biol. Med.* 92, 216–219.

Kemmerer, A. R., Elvehjem, C. A., and Hart, E. B. (1931). Studies on the relation of manganese to the nutrition of the mouse. *J. Biol. Chem.* 92, 623–630.

Leach, R. M., and Nesheim, M. C. (1963). Studies on chloride deficiency in chicks. *J. Nutr.* 81, 193–199.

McClachlan, J., and Craigie, J. S. (1967). Bromide, a substitute for chloride in a marine algal medium. *Nature (London)* 214, 604–605.

Mertz, W. (1969). Chromium: Occurrence and function in biological systems. *Physiol. Rev.* 49, 163–239.

Nielsen, F. H., Givand, S. H., and Myron, D. R. (1975). *Fed. Proc.* 34, 923 (abstract).

Schwarz, K. (1972). Elements newly identified as essential for animals. In "Nuclear Activation Techniques in the Life Sciences." IAEA Vienna (unpublished).

Schwarz, K., and Foltz, C. M. (1957). Selenium as an integral part of Factor 3 against dietary necrotic liver degeneration. J. Amer. Chem. Soc. 79, 3293–3294.

Schwarz, K., and Mertz, W. (1959). Chromium (111) and the glucose tolerance factor. Arch. Biochem. Biophys. 85, 292–295.

Smith, J. C., and Schwarz, K. (1967). A controlled environment system for new trace element deficiencies. J. Nutr. 93, 182–188.

Stiefel, E. J. (1973). Proposed molecular mechanism for the action of molybdenum in enzymes: Coupled proton and electron transfers. Proc. Nat. Acad. Sci. U.S. 70, 988–992.

Thompson, J. N., and Scott, M. L. (1969). Role of selenium in the nutrition of the chick. J. Nutr. 97, 335–342.

Todd, W. R., Elvehjem, C. A., and Hart, E. B. (1934). Zinc in the nutrition of the rat. Amer. J. Physiol. 107, 146–156.

Towery, B. T. (1953). The physiology of iodine. Bull. W.H.O. 9, 175–182.

Underwood, E. J. (1971). "Trace Elements in Human and Animal Nutrition," 3rd ed. Academic Press, New York.

Vallee, B. L. (1971). Spectral characteristics of metals in metalloenzymes In "Newer Trace Elements in Nutrition" (W. Mertz and W. E. Cornatzer, eds.). Dekker, New York.

Wilgus, H. S., Jr., Norris, L. C., and Heuser, G. F. (1936). The role of certain inorganic elements in the cause and prevention of perosis. Science 84, 252–253.

Wilgus, H. S., Jr., Norris, L. C., and Heuser, G. F. (1937). The role of manganese and certain other trace elements in the prevention of perosis. J. Nutr. 14, 155–167.

36

Mineral Interrelationships

C. H. Hill

I. INTRODUCTION

As the science of nutrition has progressed through stages of identification, quantification of requirements, and studies of physiological function of nutrients, it has been apparent that there are certain interactions between nutrients that complicate interpretation of the results of experiments. An instance of the latter interaction was the controversy over the requirement of animals for zinc which was found to be lower when determined with a casein diet than when determined with a soybean protein-based diet. This has been resolved as being a result of zinc interacting with a phytate–protein complex in the soybean protein that reduces the availability of zinc. An instance of the former interaction is that of copper, molybdenum, and sulfate. Pastures high in molybdenum can precipitate copper deficiency in cattle if the sulfate level is high enough. This interaction is under investigation in a number of laboratories around the world at this time.

These known interactions, particularly among the elements, have led some nutritionists, myself among them, to set out deliberately to uncover interactions that might occur and be important. In the field of mineral nutrition, there are approximately fifteen elements that are or may be essential, excluding carbon, nitrogen, oxygen, and hydrogen and some eighty-three others for which no such claim has as yet been made. The sheer number of elements prohibits an all-encompassing approach to mineral interaction studies, nor is such an approach necessary.

II. INTERACTION OF TRACE ELEMENTS

The biological interaction of elements must be based on the physicochemical properties of their ions. This concept has led us to propose

281

that ions whose valence shell electronic structures were similar would be antagonistic to each other biologically (Hill and Matrone, 1970). There are, however, antagonistic relationships between the ions of certain elements whose electronic structures are not at all similar. The evidence to date suggests that these interactions may be the result of a chemical combination of the ions. These two kinds of interactions are illustrated below.

Let us examine possible interrelationships between iron and other elements. Iron in the ferric state has a d^5 electronic configuration. That is, in the third electronic shell there are five electrons in the d orbitals, while the ferrous ion has six d electrons. Divalent manganese also is a d^5 ion, while trivalent cobalt is a d^6 ion. Based on the similarity between the electronic structures of these ions, an antagonistic relationship between manganese and iron as well as cobalt and iron could be predicted. Experimental work has shown that these antagonisms exist. Hartman et al. (1955) reported that the feeding of as little as 45 ppm manganese to lambs being fed a milk diet lowered hemoglobin levels from 10.2 gm/100 ml of blood in the controls to 6.9 at 8 weeks of age. In subsequent work, Matrone et al. (1959) measured the regeneration of hemoglobin levels of pigs that had been made anemic by feeding a milk diet in the presence of high levels of manganese. The initial level of hemoglobin was 5 gm/100 ml, and after 27 days, the change in hemoglobin levels was as is presented in Table I. These effects could be prevented by the addition of more iron to the diet. Thomson et al. (1971a) presented evidence indicating that in iron deficiency manganese as well as iron was absorbed more rapidly in both rats and man. In further work to this point, Pollack et al. (1965) reported that manganese, cobalt, and iron were absorbed more rapidly by iron-deficient rats. Some of their results are presented in Table II. These data taken together strongly indicate that manganese does act as an antagonist of iron, particularly at the level of absorption, and that the presence of iron reduces the absorption of manganese.

The data in Table II indicate that more cobalt is absorbed in iron deficiency than in control animals. Forth and Rummel (1971), using isolated segments of rat intestine in situ, found a mutual antagonism between cobalt and iron in absorption as illustrated in Table III. Thomson et al. (1971b) reported that the interaction of these two elements results from the competition for intestinal transport mechanisms. To add another species of animal to this kind of investigation, we have found that the addition of cobalt to an iron-deficient diet resulted in a greater degree of anemia when the chicks were fed equal amounts of feed (Table IV) (Chetty, 1972). These data indicate that cobalt also acts as an iron antagonist, and so two elements that could be predicted to act antagonistically to iron based on the similarity of their electronic structures have been found to do so.

Our interest in the study of interactions arose from our interest in copper metabolism, particularly in relation to anemia caused by simple copper deficiency. We had found that chicks did not always become anemic when fed a dried skim milk diet containing as little as 1 ppm copper. In an attempt to accentuate the deficiency, we investigated possible copper antagonists. The electronic structure of the cuprous ion is d^{10}, while that of the cupric ion is d^8p^1. These structures are not unique in that Zn^{2+}, Cd^{2+}, and Hg^{2+} all have the same structure of the valence shell as the cuprous ion, while Ag^{2+} has the same structure as the cupric ion. If the thesis that similar electronic structure of the ions would result in biological antagonisms was correct, all of these elements should be antagonistic to copper. In a study to determine if zinc would act as an antagonist to copper, the results presented in Table V were obtained. Two hundred parts per million of zinc did increase the anemia of the copper-deficient but not the copper-supplemented chicks. Mortality was increased in the presence of 100 ppm zinc in the deficient chicks, but not in the supplemented group. As little as 50 ppm zinc decreased growth in the absence but not the presence of copper. These data then indicate that zinc could act as a copper antagonist.

The studies with cadmium were somewhat more complex, because the cadmium ion is not only isoelectronic with the cuprous ion, but also with the zinc ion, and zinc is also an essential element. In order to investigate these possible interactions, a factorial experiment was carried out with the results shown in Table VI. There was a significant interaction of cadmium and zinc as far as growth was concerned, and a significant interaction between copper and cadmium as far as mortality was concerned. The results of study on the interaction of silver and copper are presented in Table VII. In the absence of copper, silver reduced growth, increased mortality, reduced hemoglobin levels, and reduced aortic elastin. All of these effects were prevented by the addition of copper to the diet, so that silver, too, can act as a copper antagonist.

The studies of the possible mercury–copper interaction were approached by using a four-way factorial experiment in which cadmium and zinc as well as mercury and copper were varied. The results are presented in Table VIII and simplified in Table IX. Statistical analysis revealed that there was a significant mercury–copper interaction, but it was not the same kind of interaction seen in the studies referred to above. In this case, mercury depressed the weight of chicks fed the copper-supplemented diet but not the copper-deficient diet, in contrast to the effect of zinc in this same experiment and in those experiments referred to before. These data indicate that mercury does not act as a copper antagonist. The reason for the different effect of mercury may be related to the fact that the 6s electrons of mercury are much less reactive than the 4s orbitals of copper and the fact that mercury tends to coordinate with two ligands linearly and form polymeric structures in contrast to the favored coordination number of four for copper and the formation of tetrahedral complexes by the cuprous ion and square planar complexes by the cupric ion. At any rate, zinc, cadmium, and silver are antagonistic to copper, cadmium is antagonistic to zinc, and in these particular instances as well as those of cobalt and manganese with iron, the thesis that ions whose electronic structures are similar will act antagonistically to each other is supported.

This concept is also apparently valid when anions are considered. Our interest in this aspect of mineral metabolism stemmed from a series of studies with vanadate. While at low levels vanadium has been proposed as an essential element, at higher levels it has been found to be extremely toxic. At levels of 25 ppm or less, it has been found to uncouple oxidative phosphorylation both *in vivo* and *in vitro* (Hathcock *et al.*, 1966). Because of this property of vanadate, we compared the orbital structure of vanadate with phosphate as well as with arsenate, another known uncoupler. In addition, we examined the orbital structures of chromate and selenate (Fig. 1). In all five anions the oxygens are attached to the central atom in an sp^3 arrangement and thus form tetrahedral structures. While in the phosphate anion the 3s and 3p orbitals are used, in the other four it is the 4s and 4p. Chromate and selenate have two π bonds instead of the one in the other three anions. In order to determine whether or not chromium would interact with vanadate, Wright (1968) fed these two ions to chicks with the results on growth and mortality shown in Table X. Chromium was effective in overcoming the growth depression and mortality associated with feeding 20 ppm vanadate. In another study on the effect of these ions on oxidative phosphorylation *in vivo* (Table XI), it was shown that chromium partially overcame the effect of vanadate in uncoupling oxidative phosphorylation. In an *in vitro* test using chicken liver mitochondria, the results presented in Table XII were obtained. Chromate partially prevented the uncoupling by vanadate. Thus, *in vivo* and *in vitro* chromate is antagonistic to vanadate. It should be pointed out that the *in vivo* studies were conducted using $CrCl_3$. It is possible that the large amounts of chromium required to counteract a given amount of vanadate in this situation were the result of an inefficient oxidation of the Cr^{3+} to Cr^{6+}. The *in vitro* experiments were conducted with both vanadate and chromate. In further experiments on the mechanism of this interaction, it was found that vanadate inhibited the uptake of chromate by respiring mito-

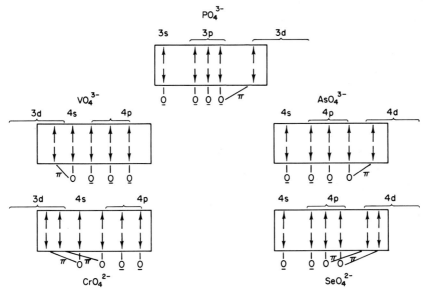

FIG. 1. Molecular orbitals of PO_4^{3-}, VO_4^{3-}, AsO_4^{2-}, CrO_4^{2-}, and SeO_4^{2-} anions.

chondria and that chromate inhibited the uptake of vanadate (Table XIII), again indicating a mutual antagonism between these two anions.

The interaction between selenate and arsenate has been known for many years. Moxon (1938) reported that arsenic would counteract the toxicity of seleniferous grain. This interaction has been found to occur in dogs (Rhian and Moxon, 1943), pigs (Moxon, 1941a), cows (Moxon et al., 1944), and chicks (Moxon, 1941b). In studies conducted by C. H. Hill (unpublished), it was found that the inclusion of 5 or 10 ppm selenite in the drinking water resulted in decreased growth of chicks unless an equal amount of arsenate was also present (Table XIV). When the arsenate was less than half the concentration of selenate, the interaction was much less apparent. In studies on the physiological basis for this interaction, Ganther and Baumann (1962a) reported that the injection of arsenite with selenium in rats shifted the elimination of selenium from the lungs to the GI tract (Table XV). In following up this work, Levander and Baumann (1966) reported that the presence of arsenic led to an increased selenium excretion in the bile; conversely, the presence of selenium led to an increased biliary excretion of arsenic (Tables XVI, XVII). In our studies on the interaction of these two elements, the effect of selenate on the uncoupling of oxidative phosphorylation was examined (Wright, 1968). The results (Table XVIII) indicate that selenate is effective in counteracting the uncoupling effect of arsenate.

We believe the basis for this interaction is the reciprocal inhibition of uptake of these two ions by respiring mitochondria as is indicated in Table XIX.

The sulfate anion is analogous to selenate, and studies have shown that sulfate is to some degree capable of preventing the toxic effects of selenate. As an example, Halverson and Monty (1960) reported that feeding sulfate improved the growth of selenium-fed rats (Table XX). In a further study, Halverson et al. (1962) reported that sulfate would counteract the effect of selenate much more effectively than selenite, as is indicated in Table XXI. Ganther and Baumann (1962b), on the other hand, reported that sulfate counteracted the growth-depressing effect of both selenite and selenate but that sulfite was not effective in counteracting the toxicity of selenite (Table XXII). While the details of the mechanisms underlying this interaction remain to be worked out, it is clear that there is an antagonistic relationship between sulfate and selenium.

The data presented on the studies of the interaction of the various oxyanions of the vanadium–chromium, arsenic–selenium, and sulfate–selenium pairs indicate that the pairs whose orbital structures are closely related will act antagonistically to each other. These findings reinforce the concept that the similar electronic structures of the ions of elements may be a basis for their antagonistic relationship.

There are, however, antagonistic relationships between elements whose electronic structures are not similar. Ganther et al. (1972) reported that dietary selenium would counteract the toxicity of methylmercury added to the drinking water of rats. At this time we were conducting experiments on the effects of elements on selenium toxicity and were particularly concerned with mercury. The results of one such experiment is presented in Table XXIII. Selenium, fed as SeO_2 at a level of 40 ppm, was quite toxic in the absence of mercury but not in its presence. In an experiment to determine if the effect of mercury could be duplicated by other metals, zinc, copper, and iron were examined (Table XXIV). While zinc and iron were without effect, copper alleviated the growth depression somewhat and had a striking effect on the mortality associated with feeding this level of selenium. In another experiment, in which copper and cadmium were included in the diet in equimolar amounts to selenium, the results presented in Table XXV were obtained. Again, copper alleviated the mortality associated with feeding selenium. While cadmium did not appear to alleviate either the growth depression or mortality, a statistical analysis revealed that there was a significant cadmium–selenium interaction in that there was less of an increase in mortality than would be expected based on the data obtained when either were fed alone. While the mechanism underlying these interactions is unknown, it seemed likely to us that a compound of selenium with these other elements might be formed that was less toxic than selenium alone. In order to test this hypothesis, products of selenium with mercury, cadmium, and copper were prepared and fed to chicks. On the basis of selenium analysis, these products were probably the mercuric, cupric, and cadmium selenites. The results of feeding the mercuric–selenium compound are presented in Table XXVI. The growth data reveal that the compound is relatively innocuous. The results of feeding the copper and cadmium compounds are presented in Table XXVII. These compounds, too, are less toxic than selenium alone. The ease with which these compounds are formed makes tenable the hypothesis that the interaction observed when mercury, copper, or cadmium are fed with selenium is the result of the formation of these compounds. Why these compounds should be less toxic than the selenium contained in them is still unknown. Ganther and Baumann (1962a) reported that the injection of cadmium, unlike the injection of arsenic, tended to increase retention of selenium in rat carcasses. Johnson and Pond (1974) have reported that both organic and inorganic mercuric compounds tended to increase the kidney levels of selenium, and that methylmercury increased the selenium content of the brain of rats while selenium reduced the toxicity of $HgCl_2$ as well as phenylmercuriacetate and methylmercury. A similar finding was reported by Parizek et al. (1971), who injected pregnant rats with radioactive selenium in the presence and absence of mercury. An example of their results is presented in Table XXVIII. As the level of mercury was increased, the level of selenium in the blood and liver increased. In contrast, it was found that as the mercury levels were increased in the dams, the fetuses contained less selenium, indicating a decreased placental transfer. Gunn et al. (1968) reported that selenium would protect mouse testes from vascular injury caused by cadmium, but in those groups receiving both selenium and cadmium, higher concentrations of those elements were found in the testes than in the tests of animals receiving either element alone.

III. RESEARCH NEEDS

The data presented in this report indicate that between elements there exist striking interrelationships of such a magnitude that a toxic level may be rendered innocuous, and a marginal level of an essential element may be rendered frankly deficient. As more of these interrelationships are uncovered and as the mechanisms underlying the interactions are better understood, we will be better able to predict the consequences of aberrations of the mineral components of our environment.

It follows from this reasoning that future research in this area should be directed toward searches for biological interrelationships between essential and nonessential elements. With the approaches referred to above this can be done in a systematic way. Other types of interactions may be uncovered, synergistic instead of antagonistic, for instance, which may be useful in reaching an understanding of mineral metabolism. Concomitant with such searches, studies should be carried out to determine the exact biochemical bases of the interactions. Are the effects observed a reflection of interactions at the absorptive sites, or do they reflect changes in the excretory patterns? Do metals closely related chemically substitute for each other in enzyme structures *in vivo* and thereby change enzymatic activity? Questions such as these remain to be answered.

TABLE I   Effect of Manganese
on Regeneration of
Hemoglobin in Pigs[a]

Mn (ppm)	Hb gain (gm/100 ml)
0	6.09
125	3.38
500	3.18
2000	1.40

[a] From Matrone et al. (1959).

TABLE II   Effect of Iron Deficiency on
Absorption of Copper,
Manganese, Cobalt, and
Iron[a]

Metal	Amount absorbed (% of 5 μmoles)	
	Control	Iron deficient
Cu	6.2	5.8
Mn	3.5	5.7
Co	18.4	34.8
Fe	9.2	27.8

[a] From Pollack et al. (1965).

TABLE III   Mutual Antagonism between Cobalt and Iron on Absorption[a]

Co (μM)	Fe absorbed (%)	Fe (μM)	Co absorbed (%)
0	38	0	60
0.05	32	0.05	42
0.5	13	0.5	27
5.0	2	5.0	10

[a] From Forth and Rummel (1971).

TABLE IV   Cobalt–Iron Interactions in Chicks[a]

Treatment (ppm)		Body weight (gm)	Hemoglobin (gm/100 ml)
Fe	Co		
0	0	107	5.81
0	100	101	3.31
100	0	89	9.32
100	100	91	8.75

[a] From Chetty (1972).

TABLE V   Interaction of Zinc and Copper on Hemoglobin

Zinc (ppm)	Hemoglobin (gm/100 ml)	
	0 ppm Cu	10 ppm Cu
0	6.5	8.5
50	5.9	8.0
100	6.0	8.8
200	4.8	8.0
300	4.1	6.6

TABLE VI   Interaction of Cadmium With Zinc and Copper

Cd (ppm)	Zn (ppm)	Body weight (gm)		Mortality[a]		Significant effects
		Cu, 0 ppm	Cu, 10 ppm	Cu, 0 ppm	Cu, 10 ppm	
0	0	214	246	4	1	Cu[b], Cd[b]
100	0	131	163	17	1	(Cd×Cu)[b]
0	200	174	222	13	0	
100	200	149	187	19	1	

[a] Number out of 20 chicks at 19 days.
[b] $P < 0.01$.

TABLE VII   *In Vivo* Interaction between Silver and Copper

Ag (ppm)	Cu (ppm)	3-week body weight (gm)[a]			Mortality— 4 weeks[a]			Hemoglobin (gm/100 cm³)[b]			Aortic elastin (% wet weight)[c]		
		0	10	25	0	10	25	0	10	25	0	10	25
0		145	196	232	5	2	3	7.45	7.17	7.72	7.58	11.63	12.12
10		125	190	229	5	1	0	6.37	7.32	9.00	5.39	11.68	10.46
25		139	199	244	3	0	2	6.05	7.35	8.22	4.92	14.58	12.45
50		126	240	243	10	2	0	5.02	7.40	7.30	6.67	12.05	11.15
100		110	174	240	12	1	4	4.62	7.00	7.60	5.26	11.03	11.33
200		96	187	207	13	0	0	3.52	7.75	8.32	4.78	11.59	12.46

[a] 20 chicks started in each treatment.
[b] Mean of 4 determinations in each treatment.
[c] Mean of 5 determinations in each treatment.

TABLE VIII   Interactions between Copper, Mercury, Zinc and Cadmium[a]

		Average weight at 2 weeks of age (gm)			
		Cu, 0 ppm		Cu, 25 ppm	
		Hg, 0 ppm	Hg, 400 ppm	Hg, 0 ppm	Hg, 400 ppm
Cd, 0 ppm	Zn, 0 ppm	144	123	160	138
	Zn, 400 ppm	87	108	147	138
Cd, 100 ppm	Zn, 0 ppm	82	81	100	78
	Zn, 400 ppm	87	100	115	91

[a] 20 chicks per treatment.

TABLE IX Interactions of Copper with Mercury and Zinc

	Body weight at 2 weeks (gm)	
	Cu, 0 ppm	Cu, 25 ppm
Hg		
0 ppm	100	130
400 ppm	104	111
Zn		
0 ppm	107	119
400 ppm	95	123

TABLE X Effects of Dietary Vanadium and Chromium on Growth and Mortality of Chicks[a]

Cr (ppm)	Body weight at 3 weeks[b] (gm)		Mortality at 3 weeks (%)	
	V, 0 ppm	V, 20 ppm	V, 0 ppm	V, 20 ppm
0	238	98	6.7	86.6
500	256	125	6.7	66.7
1000	232	158	10.0	40.0
2000	182	193	6.7	13.3

Duncan's multiple range tests[c]:
Body weight:

98   125   138   182   193   232   238   256

Mortality:

6.7 6.7 6.7 10.0 13.3   40.0 66.7 86.6

[a] From Wright (1968). Chicks were fed the dried skim milk diet supplemented as indicated with NH_4VO_3 and/or $CrCl_3$.
[b] Averages of 5–15 chicks.
[c] Any two values underscored by the same line are not significantly different; any two not underscored by the same line are significantly different; $P = 0.05$.

TABLE XI   Effect of Dietary Vanadium and Chromium on
the P/O Ratio in Chicken Liver Mitochondria[a]

	P/O		
Vanadium, ppm	Cr, 0 ppm	Cr, 100 ppm	Cr, 400 ppm
0	1.80	1.78	1.75
10	1.09	1.29	1.59
20	0.65	1.03	1.30

Duncan's multiple range test[b]:
0.65   1.03   1.09   1.29   1.30   1.59   1.75   1.78   1.80

[a] From Wright (1968). Reaction medium and conditions for P/O measurements were as follows: 40 mM succinate, 20 mM phosphate, 5 mM ADP, 4 mM KF, 10–15 mg mitochondrial protein/ml; pH 7.4; room temperature 24°–28°C. Each reported P/O ratio is the average of 6 individual determinations.
[b] Any two values underscored by the same line are not significantly different; any two not underscored by the same line are significantly different; $P = 0.05$.

TABLE XII   Interaction of Vanadate and Chromate on
Oxidative Phosphorylation[a]

	P/O[b]	
Chromate (mM)	Vanadate, 0 mM	Vanadate, 1 mM
0	1.85	0.75
0.1	1.62	0.98
1.0	1.75	1.38
10	1.81	1.30

[a] Reaction conditions and media were the same as in Table XI. From Wright (1968).
[b] Each reported P/O ratio is the average of 6 determinations.

TABLE XIII   Effect of Vanadate and
Chromate on the Uptake of
$^{51}CrO_4$ and $^{48}VO_4$ by Respiring
Mitochondria[a]

$^{51}CrO_4$ versus VO_4 (1 mM CrO_4 and VO_4 as indicated)		$^{48}VO_4$ versus CrO_4 (1 mM VO_4 and CrO_4 as indicated)	
VO_4 mM	cpm	CrO_4 mM	cpm
0	15,559	0	7,979
1	9,803[b]	1	3,880[b]

[a] From Wright (1968).
[b] $P < 0.05$.

TABLE XIV   Interaction of Selenium
and Arsenic in Drinking
Water on the Growth of
Chicks[a]

Se (ppm)	As (ppm)	2-week gain (gm)
0	0	185
2.5	0	207
2.5	2.5	199
5.0	0	142
5.0	5.0	196
10.0	0	37
10.0	10.0	175
10.0	5.0	181
10.0	2.5	100

[a] C. H. Hill (unpublished).

TABLE XV Effect of Injected Arsenite on
the Metabolism of Injected
Selenium[a]

| | Se conc. (% of dose)[b] | |
	Control	Arsenite injected
Volatile compounds	21.6	9.8
G.I. Tract	7.1	32.0
Urine	12.0	12.9
Blood	1.33	0.69
Liver	18.8	10.5
Kidney	1.6	6.4
Carcass	30.2	22.7

[a] From Ganther and Baumann (1962a).
[b] 2.0 mg/kg Se as Na_2SeO_3 injected subcutaneously and 2.9 mg/kg As as $NaAsO_2$ injected intraperitoneally.

TABLE XVI Effect of Arsenite on the Biliary Excretion and Tissue
Distribution of Selenite[a]

| | Selenium concentration (% of dose)[b] | |
	Saline injected only[c]	Arsenite injected[c]
Bile	4.0 ± 0.4	40.8 ± 7.2
Liver	51.3 ± 3.0	20.9 ± 3.0
Gastrointestinal contents	1.7 ± 0.3	1.5 ± 0.3
Carcass[d]	33.5 ± 1.2	29.7 ± 2.8
Kidneys	2.8 ± 0.3	7.4 ± 1.2
Blood (1 ml)	0.29 ± 0.02	0.84 ± 0.15
Bile volume (ml)	3.0 ± 0.2	3.8 ± 0.5

[a] From Levander and Baumann (1966).
[b] Distribution of radioactivity 3 hr after subcutaneous injection of 0.5 mg Se/kg body weight as $Na_2^{75}SeO_3$ containing approximately 0.5 μCi ^{75}Se as $H_2^{75}SeO_3$; weight of animals 274–290 gm, average 281; recovery of isotope 90.9–101.8% of the dose, average 97.4%; mean of 3 animals ± SE.
[c] Subcutaneous injection of saline or 1 mg As per kilogram as $NaAsO_2$ followed the selenite injection by 10 min.
[d] Includes all organs and tissues of animal except liver, kidneys, and 1 ml of blood.

TABLE XVII   Effect of Selenite on the Biliary Excretion of Arsenic[a]

	Arsenic concentration (% of dose)[b]	
	Saline injected only[c]	Selenite infected[c]
Bile	9.2 ± 1.2	18.3 ± 1.7
Liver	19.0 ± 1.5	11.0 ± 0.6
Gastrointestinal contents	1.6 ± 0.2	1.7 ± 0.2
Carcass	54.0 ± 1.5	52.7 ± 1.3
Kidneys	4.5 ± 0.0	5.2 ± 0.1
Blood (1 ml)	0.57 ± 0.08	1.56 ± 0.06

[a] From Levander and Baumann (1966).

[b] Distribution of radioactivity 50 min after subcutaneous injection of 1.0 mg As/kg body weight as $Na^{76}AsO_2$ containing approximately 0.5 μCi ^{76}As as $H^{76}AsO_2$; mean of 4 rats ± SE; weight of animals 240–264 gm; average 253 gm; recovery of isotope 84.2–95.0% of the dose, average 89.9%.

[c] Subcutaneous injection of saline or 0.5 mg Se per kilogram preceded the arsenite injection by 10 min; bile was collected for 1 hr.

TABLE XVIII   Effects of Various Concentrations of Selenate on the Arsenate Uncoupling of Oxidative Phosphorylation[a]

Selenate (mM)	P/O[b]	
	Arsenate 0 mM	Arsenate 20 mM
0	1.72	0.59
2	1.68	1.26
.20	1.56	1.46
50	1.58	1.30

Duncan's multiple range test[c]:

0.59 1.26 1.30 1.46 1.56 1.58 1.68 1.72

[a] Reaction media and conditions were the same as in Table XI, except that each contained 1 mM inorganic phosphate. From Wright (1968).

[b] Each reported P/O ratio is the average of 4 individual determinations.

[c] Any two values underscored by the same line are not significantly different; any two not underscored by the same line are significantly different; $P = 0.05$.

TABLE XIX   Effect of Arsenate and Selenate on
the Uptake of ^{75}Se and [76]As,
respectively, by Respiring
Mitochondria[a]

[75]SeO$_4$ versus AsO$_4$ (2 mM P$_i$, 40 mM SeO$_4$)		[76]AsO$_4$ versus SeO$_4$ (2 mM P$_i$, 40 mM AsO$_4$)	
AsO$_4$ (mM)	cpm[b]	SeO$_4$ (mM)	cpm[b]
0	449,070	0	12,221
40	215,080	40	5,556
$M^c = 0.536^d$		$M^c = 0.675^d$	

[a] From Wright (1968). Reaction media contained
5 mM ADP, 4 mM KF, 10–15 mg mitochondrial pro-
tein/ml; pH 7.4, 24°–28°C, 1 µCi of isotope/sample.
[b] Averages of 6 observations.
[c] M is the substitute τ value for comparing 2
means.
[d] P < .01.

TABLE XX   Interaction of Selenium
and Sulfate in Rats[a]

	Weight gain (gm)	
K$_2$SO$_4$	Se, 0 ppm	Se, 10 ppm
0	141	56
0.29	137	69
0.58	136	89
0.67	119	94

[a] From Halverson and Monty (1960).

TABLE XXI   Interaction of Sulfate with Selenate
and Selenite in Rats[a]

	Daily weight gain (gm)	
	Sulfate, 0%	Sulfate, 2%
Control	7.4	
Selenate, 10 ppm	1.0	3.4
Selenite, 10 ppm	1.0	1.7

[a] From Halverson et al. (1962).

TABLE XXII Interaction of Sulfur and Selenium on Rat Growth[a]

	Weight gain (gm)		
	Control	Sulfate, 1%	Sulfite, 89%
Control	154		
Selenite, 10 ppm	80	103	83
Selenate, 10 ppm	67	92	92

[a] From Ganther and Baumann (1962b).

TABLE XXIII Interaction of Selenium and Mercury on Growth of Chicks[a]

	2-week gain (gm)
Control	213
Selenium, 40 ppm	16
Mercury, 500 ppm	167
Selenium, 40 ppm + mercury, 500 ppm	183

[a] Selenium fed as SeO_2, mercury as $HgCl_2$.

TABLE XXIV Effect of Mercury, Zinc, Copper, and Iron on Selenium Toxicity in Chicks

Diet	3-week weight gain (gm)		3-week mortality (%)	
	Se, 0 ppm	Se, 40 ppm	Se, 0 ppm	Se, 40 ppm
Control	367	67	12.1	48.5
Hg, 500 ppm	279	295	42.4	53.6
Zn, 500 ppm	398	22	9.1	50.9
Cu, 500 ppm	319	92	6.1	6.1
Fe, 500 ppm	395	25	6.1	53.0

TABLE XXV   Effect of Copper and Cadmium on Selenium Toxicity in Chicks

Diet	2-week weight gain (gm)		2-week mortality (%)	
	Se, 0 ppm	Se, 40 ppm	Se, 0 ppm	Se, 40 ppm
Control	224	19	2.5	20.0
Cu, 32 ppm	227	19	2.5	6.2
Cd, 57 ppm	123	23	15.0	21.2

TABLE XXVI   Effect of Selenium and Mercury and Their Reaction Product on Growth of Chicks

Treatment	3-week weight gain (gm)
Control	373
Se, 10 ppm	276
Se, 20 ppm	100
Hg, 50 ppm	364
Se, 10 ppm + Hg, 25 ppm	354
Se, 20 ppm + Hg, 50 ppm	336
[HgSeX] = 8 ppm Se	360
[HgSeX] = 16 ppm Se	366

TABLE XXVII   Effect of Cadmium and Copper Reaction Products with Selenium on Growth of Chicks

Treatment	2-week weight gain (gm)
Control	222
Cd, 14.6 ppm	216
Cu, 8.3 ppm	219
Se, 10 ppm	152
[CdSeX] = 10 ppm Se	187
[CuSeX] = 10 ppm Se	196

TABLE XXVIII Mercury–Selenium Interaction
in Pregnant Mice[a]

| HgCl₂ (μmole/kg body weight) | Selenium content (% of dose) | |
	Blood (1 ml)	Liver (whole organ)
0	0.26	5.93
2.5	0.63	9.01
5.0	0.82	13.37
10.0	0.94	15.22
20.0	1.18	16.73

[a] From Parizek et al. (1971).

ACKNOWLEDGMENTS

These studies were supported in past by grant no. 9 ROI HE 14719-10 NTN from the National Science Foundation and by grant No. 10 HEW S ROI HL 14719-11 NTN from the National Institutes of Health.

REFERENCES

Chetty, K. N. (1972). Interactions of cobalt and iron in chicks. Ph.D. Thesis, North Carolina State University, Raleigh.

Forth, W., and Rummel, W. (1971). Absorption of iron and chemically related metals in vitro and in vivo. In "Intestinal Absorption of Metal Ions, Trace Elements and Radionuclides" (S. C. Skoryna and D. Waldron-Edward, eds.), pp. 173–191. Pergamon, Oxford.

Ganther, H. E., and Baumann, C. A. (1962a). Selenium metabolism. I. Effects of diet, arsenic and cadmium. J. Nutr. 77, 210–216.

Ganther, H. E., and Baumann, C. A. (1962b). Selenium metabolism. II. Modifying effects of sulfate. J. Nutr. 77, 408–414.

Ganther, H. E., Goudie, C., Sunde, M. L., Kopecky, M. J., Wagner, P., Oh, S. H., and Hoekstra, W. G. (1972). Selenium: Relation to decreased toxicity of methylmercury added to diets containing tuna. Science 175, 1122–1124.

Gunn, S. A., Gould, T. C., and Anderson, W. A. D. (1968). Mechanisms of zinc, cysteine, and selenium protection against cadmium-induced vascular injury to mouse tests. J. Reprod. Fert. 15, 65–70.

Halverson, A. W., and Monty, K. J. (1960). An effect of dietary sulfate on selenium poisoning in the rat. J. Nutr. 70, 100–102.

Halverson, A. W., Guss, P. L., and Olson, O. E. (1962). Effect of sulfur salts on selenium poisoning in the rat. J. Nutr. 77, 459–464.

300 C. H. HILL

Hartman, R. H., Matrone, G., and Wise, G. H. (1955). Effect of high dietary manganese on hemoglobin formation. *J. Nutr.* **57**, 429–439.

Hathcock, J. N., Hill, C. H., and Tove, S. B. (1966). Uncoupling of oxidative phosphorylation by vanadate. *Can. J. Biochem.* **44**, 983–988.

Hill, C. H., and Matrone, G. (1970). Chemical parameters in the study of *in vivo* and *in vitro* interactions of transition elements. *Fed. Proc., Fed. Amer. Soc. Exp. Biol.* **29**, 1474–1481.

Johnson, S. L., and Pond, W. G. (1974). Inorganic vs organic Hg toxicity in growing rats: Protection by dietary Se but not Zn. *Nutr. Rep. Int.* **9**, 135–147.

Levander, O. A., and Baumann, C. A. (1966). Selenium metabolism. VI. Effect of arsenic on the excretion of selenium in the bile. *Toxicol. Appl. Pharmacol.* **9**, 106–115.

Matrone, G., Hartman, R. H., and Clawson, A. J. (1959). Studies on manganese-iron antagonism in the nutrition of rabbits and baby pigs. *J. Nutr.* **67**, 309–317.

Moxon, A. L. (1938). Effect of arsenic on the toxicity of seleniferous grains. *Science* **88**, 81.

Moxon, A. L. (1941a). Influence of arsenic on selenium poisoning in hogs. *Proc. S. Dak. Acad. Sci.* **21**, 34–36.

Moxon, A. L. (1941b). The influence of some proteins on the toxicity of selenium. Ph.D. Thesis, University of Wisconsin, Madison.

Moxon, A. L., Rhian, M. A., Anderson, H. D., and Olson, O. E. (1944). Growth of steers on seleniferous range *J. Anim. Sci.* **3**, 299–309.

Pařízek, J., Oštadalová, I., Kalousková, J., Babický, A., Pavík, L., and Bíbr, B. (1971). Effect of mercuric compounds on the maternal transmission of selenium in the pregnant and lactating rat. *J. Reprod. Fert.* **25**, 157–170.

Pollack, S., George, J. N., Reba, R. C., and Kaufman, R. M. (1965). The absorption of non-ferrous metals in iron deficiency. *J. Clin. Invest.* **4**, 1470–1473.

Rhian, M., and Moxon, A. L. (1943). Chronic selenium poisoning in dogs and its prevention by arsenic. *J. Pharmacol. Exp. Ther.* **78**, 249–263.

Thomson, A. B. R., Olatunbosun, D., and Valberg, L. S. (1971a). Interrelation of intestinal transport system for manganese and iron. *J. Lab. Clin. Med.* **78**, 642–655.

Thomson, A. B. R., Valberg, L. S., and Sinclair, D. G. (1971b). Competitive nature of the intestinal transport mechanism for cobalt and iron in the rat. *J. Clin. Invest.* **50**, 2384–2394.

Wright, W. R. (1968). Metabolic interrelationship between vanadium and chromium. Ph.D. Thesis, North Carolina State University, Raleigh.

37

Perinatal Effects of Trace Element Deficiencies

Lucille S. Hurley

I. INTRODUCTION

A relationship between trace elements and prenatal or perinatal development has been suspected for some time, but extensive investigation of the effects of trace element deficiencies during the prenatal or perinatal period has occurred only relatively recently. The earliest recognized example of such a relationship is probably that of iodine deficiency and the thyroid gland, which is associated in the adult with goiter and in the fetus with cretinism. Cretinism has been recognized since the sixteenth century, and by the beginning of the nineteenth century, its connection with goiter was realized. Soon thereafter, a relationship between iodine and goiter was postulated, and in 1846 Prévost and Maffoni proposed for the first time that endemic goiter (and by implication also endemic cretinism) was due to iodine deficiency (Langer, 1960).

It is now known that the mental and physical retardation characteristic of cretinism is brought about by insufficiency of thyroxine apparently related to iodine deficiency. Although it is not clear that cretinism results from a simple uncomplicated deficiency of iodine, it is well known that in certain areas where there was a high rate of endemic goiter and low iodine content of the soil, the incidence of cretinism was very high. After the iodization of salt was instituted, the incidence of endemic cretinism as well as of goiter fell markedly (Clements, 1960; Kelly and Snedden, 1960). In animals, there is both experimental and field evidence that iodine deficiency during pregnancy produces abnormal development of the offspring, notably hairless skin, hypertrophied thyroids, and retarded development (Underwood, 1971).

Reports on the essentiality of the trace metals for prenatal development began to appear in the 1930s with the observations by Orent and McCollum (1931) and Daniels and Everson (1935) on debility in offspring of manganese-deficient rats, Lyons and Insko (1937) on nutritional chondrodystrophy in chick embryos resulting from manganese deficiency, and Bennetts and Chapman (1937) on enzootic ataxia caused by copper deficiency in lambs. The role of trace elements in metabolism and in human and animal disease and the effects of trace element deficiencies in prenatal or perinatal life have been extensively reviewed in recent symposia and monographs (Asling and Hurley, 1963; Underwood, 1971; Hoekstra et al., 1974; Hurley, 1974b). This paper will therefore not attempt to provide comprehensive historical reviews of the literature for all of the trace elements, but will instead concentrate on summarizing more recent work on effects on development of deficiencies of copper, manganese, zinc, and magnesium. Magnesium is not usually considered to be a trace element, but in many ways it acts in a manner similar to that of the trace metals, and since it is being included in the subject matter of this treatise, it will be included in this chapter as well.

II. COPPER

Since the work of Bennetts in Australia (Bennetts and Beck, 1942) and Inness and Shearer in England (1940), it has been known that copper deficiency in pregnant ewes results in a nervous disorder of lambs. This condition is characterized by lack of coordination and paralysis of the hind quarters and is called "swayback" or "enzootic neonatal ataxia." The disorder affects brain development, apparently through interference with phospholipid synthesis and myelination. Everson and her colleagues (1967, 1968) experimentally produced similar effects in guinea pigs with a copper-deficient diet. Ataxia, retarded growth, brain abnormalities, and aneurisms were observed among the progeny. Agenesis of the cerebellum was a striking finding in the guinea pigs, as it was in sheep (Follis, 1958). In rats, Carlton and Kelly (1969) have also observed brain lesions in the offspring of pregnant females on a copper-deficient diet, although unlike the sheep, the changes were generally restricted to the cerebral cortex and corpus striatum and did not include the cerebellum.

Abnormalities in offspring of copper-deficient rats have been observed in other tissues as well as in brain. O'Dell (1968) found that the aortas

from newborn rats of copper-deficient females showed abnormal separation of the elastic lamina and less well-stained elastin than those from
normal newborns. O'Dell and co-workers (1961) also found in offspring
of copper-deficient rats that newborn animals were anemic and nonviable
and were afflicted with edema and characteristic subcutaneous hemor-
rhages. They showed a high incidence of skeletal anomalies and many
had abdominal hernias. Histological examination of the skin revealed
a paucity of hair follicles.

Recent studies concerning copper in perinatal development have been
made in our laboratory and suggest the existence of an interaction between copper metabolism and a certain mutant gene in mice called
crinkled (cr) (Hurley and Bell, 1974a). The effects of this gene resemble
in some respects those of copper deficiency. Abnormal texture of hair,
reduced number of hair follicles, thin epidermis, and increased mortality
in early life are characteristics of both conditions (Underwood, 1971;
Falconer et al., 1952). Neonatal survival of mutant offspring of females
fed high dietary copper during pregnancy and lactation was twice as
high as those of females fed a normal control diet. High dietary copper
also produced increased pigmentation, increased hair growth, and increased thickness of the skin in mutant offspring. Scanning electron
microscopy revealed the existence in crinkled mice of abnormal hairs
characteristic of Menkes' kinky hair syndrome, a genetic disease of children known to involve copper metabolism (Menkes, 1972; Danks et
al., 1972). In addition to hair changes and defective copper metabolism,
Menkes' disease is characterized by slow growth, early mortality, and
cerebral degeneration. The neonatal mortality, the abnormalities of hair
and skin that we have reported for the crinkled mutant, and its relationship to copper metabolism suggest that crinkled may be similar in some
respects to Menkes' disease (Hurley and Bell, 1975).

III. MANGANESE

The most striking effect of a deficiency of manganese during prenatal
development is ataxia in the offspring, characterized by incoordination,
lack of equilibrium, and retraction of the head. This ataxic condition
has been reported in a number of species, including the chick (Norris
and Caskey, 1939), guinea pig (Everson et al., 1959), rat (Shils and
McCollum, 1943), mouse (Erway et al., 1970), and pig (Plumlee et
al., 1956). Studies of the critical period for the production of ataxia
in manganese-deficient rats showed that it occurred between day 14
and day 18 of gestation (Hurley et al., 1958; Hurley and Everson, 1963).
This observation, in combination with studies of the development of

body-righting reflexes in these animals (Hurley and Everson, 1959) led to the finding that manganese deficiency produced abnormal development of the inner ear (Hurley et al., 1960; Asling et al., 1960).

The ataxic condition observed in manganese-deficient offspring is also seen in mice homozygous for a certain mutant gene called *pallid* (Lyon, 1953). These mice, like manganese-deficient animals, have abnormal equilibrium and abnormal body-righting reflexes, which are especially evident in water. The gene also affects pigmentation, giving the animals a pale color. When pregnant mice homozygous for the gene *pallid* are given a diet containing a high level of manganese during pregnancy, the abnormal development of their offspring is prevented. In both the manganese-deficient offspring and the mutant animals, the basic anatomical defect is an absence or abnormal development of the otoliths, the calcified structures in the vestibular portion of the inner ear that are responsible for normal body-righting reflexes (Erway et al., 1966, 1970, 1971; Shrader and Everson, 1967).

In a study in which otolith morphology was quantified, morphological development of the otoliths was only 68% of normal in pallid offspring with 1000 ppm of manganese in the maternal diet, although function (that is, ability to maintain balance in the water) was 100% of normal. Completely normal otolith morphology was not achieved until the level of manganese in the diet reached 1500 ppm (Erway et al., 1971).

In another study, the influence of the genetic background of mice on their response to manganese deficiency during prenatal development was studied with some inbred strains of mice and in comparison with pallid mutants as well. In young of hybrid animals, otolith development increased from 22% of normal with 1 ppm of manganese in the diet to 99–100% of normal with 45 ppm of manganese or the stock diet. The progeny of strain C57 black mice fed 3 ppm of manganese had otolith scores similar to those of young hybrids fed the same diet, but young of strain SEC/REJ and DBA/2J given 3 ppm of manganese showed much lower otolith scores than did the hybrids. However, when fed a diet containing 45 ppm manganese, the three inbred strains as well as the hybrids had progeny with nearly 100% normal otolith development. These results suggest that, except for mutants, what is considered to be the recommended dietary level of a trace element is probably sufficient to prevent signs of deficiencies for most individuals. However, at low or borderline levels of dietary intake, responses of individuals will vary greatly depending in part on their genetic background (Hurley and Bell, 1974b).

The implications of this hypothesis for humans are obvious. Indeed, I would like to offer the speculation that the association of cretinism with iodine deficiency, which occurred only in localized areas of goiter regions (Clements, 1960), may have been due to such an interaction of genetics and nutrition, leading to an exaggerated response to a deficiency level of iodine.

In seeking to understand the cause of the failure of otolith development resulting from manganese deficiency or the pallid gene, two possibilities were apparent. Failure of calcification can occur through abnormal metabolism of calcium or through abnormal development of the matrix upon which calcification of the otolithic crystals takes place. Studies of calcium metabolism in manganese-deficient rats showed that no abnormalities could be observed (Hurley et al., 1969). On the other hand, the large variety of abnormalities of the skeleton produced by manganese deficiency, including disproportionate growth (Hurley et al., 1961a,b), chondrodystrophy (Lyons and Insko, 1937), and epiphyseal dysplasia (Hurley and Asling, 1963), as well as both chemical and histological work of others, suggested that the major defect might lie in the synthesis of mucopolysaccharides (Asling and Hurley, 1963).

In vitro studies of fetal cartilage showed reduced and delayed uptake of ^{35}S in tibiae from manganese-deficient fetuses (Hurley et al., 1968a). This finding was consistent with the hypothesis that the skeletal abnormalities produced by manganese deficiency, both pre- and postnatally, resulted from abnormal or depressed synthesis of mucopolysaccharides. Leach and Muenster (1962; Leach et al., 1969) and Tsai and Everson (1967) have also shown that in vivo synthesis of acid mucopolysaccharides in skeletal cartilage was decreased by manganese deficiency.

However, the specific question of causation of abnormal otolith development remained. This was investigated by injecting radioactive sulfate into pregnant mice, either manganese-deficient or pallid, and examining the incorporation of radioactive material into the otolithic matrices of the fetuses. Manganese deficiency of the pallid gene caused reduced incorporation of ^{35}S in the macular cells of the inner ear with the formation of a nonmetachromatic, variably PAS-positive otolithic matrix that did not contain ^{35}S. At 16 days of gestation, in inner ears of normal and nonpallid mice, silver grains seen in autoradiography were localized in the matrix of the otolithic membrane. No such incorporation was seen in the manganese-deficient and pallid young. Otoconia and the metachromatic material of the otolithic membrane were both absent from the ears of 16 and 17 day manganese-deficient and pallid fetal mice (Shrader et al., 1973).

Recently, it has been shown by Erway and Mitchell (1973) that a mutant gene analogous to pallid occurs in mink. In this economically important species, a recessive mutation called pastel and commercially known as Royal Pastel or Autumn Haze causes the light brown color that is valued. Approximately 25% of the pastel mink exhibit an ataxic condition (called "screwneck" by the breeders) as a pleiotropic effect of the pastel gene. Erway and Mitchell have now demonstrated that this condition is also caused by reduction or absence of the otoliths and that it can be prevented entirely by manganese supplementation of the pregnant females. The discovery of analogous genes interacting with manganese in at least two species, as well as the copper-crinkled example discussed earlier, suggest that similar interactions may occur in other species, including the human.

Two other effects of manganese deficiency that may not be related to its effect during prenatal development are, however, worthy of mention. One is the role of manganese in brain function. Manganese-deficient rats, whether or not they are ataxic, are more susceptible to convulsions than are normal animals (Hurley et al., 1961c, 1963). This shows that manganese is required for normal function of the brain. Manganese is also required for the integrity of cell membranes. In ultrastructural studies of pancreas, kidney, heart, and liver, dietary deficiency of manganese was seen to cause changes in the classic ultrastructural parameters of the cell types examined. All manganese-deficient tissues observed showed alterations in the integrity of their cell membranes. In addition, the endoplasmic reticulum was swollen and irregular. Mitochondria were found with elongated stacked cristae in liver, heart, and kidney cells. In addition, microbodies occurred in greater number in liver cells from manganese-deficient animals than from controls (Bell and Hurley, 1973). These changes are consistent with the biochemical abnormalities observed in isolated liver mitochondria from manganese-deficient animals in which, although P/O ratios are normal, oxygen uptake is reduced (Hurley et al., 1970).

IV. ZINC

The importance of zinc for embryonic development was first demonstrated in chicks by Hoekstra and his colleagues (Turk et al., 1959; Keinholz et al., 1961) and by Blamberg et al. (1960). Gross malformations in embryos from zinc-deficient hens included skeletal defects, brain abnormalities, microphthalmia, and visceral herniation.

In rats, work from our laboratory has shown that high incidences of congenital malformations result from zinc deficiency in the maternal diet (Hurley and Swenerton, 1966). When female rats were given a zinc-deficient diet during pregnancy (days 0 to 21), even though they had been fed a normal stock diet until the beginning of gestation, about half of the implantation sites were resorbed, full-term young weighed about half of controls, and 90% of fetuses showed gross congenital malformations. Food intake controls had normal young (Hurley et al., 1971). The observation of teratogenic effects from zinc deficiency has since been confirmed by several laboratories in various parts of the world (Mills et al., 1969; Warkany and Petering, 1972; Dreosti et al., 1972). Shorter periods of deficiency were also teratogenic. When the zinc deficiency regime occurred from day 6 to 14 of pregnancy, about half the young were abnormal. Even when the deficiency lasted for only the first 10 days of pregnancy, 22% of the full-term fetuses were malformed (Hurley et al., 1971).

Recently, Warkany and Petering (1973) have shown that when the deficiency period of zinc was limited to 3 days, from the tenth to the twelfth, a small but significant percentage of young were abnormal and had important malformations of the brain. Malformations produced by zinc deficiency affect every organ system (Hurley et al., 1971), and anomalies of the nervous system were especially impressive (Hurley and Shrader, 1972). Zinc-deficient fetuses showed hyperplasia of the esophageal mucosa, a lesion characteristic of zinc deficiency in juvenile animals (Diamond and Hurley, 1970).

Studies were undertaken to investigate the mechanisms bringing about the abnormality of embryonic development. A number of enzymes were assayed both chemically and histochemically in severely deficient growing animals and in full-term fetuses. In most cases, no differences were seen between controls and zinc-deficient animals. There were some differences in cellular localization of enzyme reactivity, but in general it appeared that intensity of enzyme activity was a function of the cell types present and that enzyme changes were probably not causative factors in producing the congenital malformations of zinc deficiency (Hurley et al., 1968b; Swenerton and Hurley, 1968; Swenerton et al., 1972).

The evidence available at present suggests that congenital malformations in zinc-deficient embryos may be brought about by impaired synthesis of nucleic acids. DNA synthesis was studied by measuring the uptake of tritiated thymidine. The uptake of tritiated thymidine was much lower than normal in zinc-deficient embryos at 12 days of gestation, suggesting that DNA synthesis was depressed (Swenerton et al., 1969). This conclusion is consistent with work of others using different systems and indicating a requirement for zinc in DNA synthesis (Fujioka and Lieberman, 1964; Weser et al., 1969; Sandstead and Rinaldi, 1969). More recent studies have shown that thymidine kinase activity is depressed in zinc deficient embryos (Dreosti and Hurley, 1975).

An outstanding aspect of zinc deficiency is the rapidity with which it occurs (Swenerton and Hurley, 1968; Hurley *et al.*, 1971). The rapid effect of zinc deficiency arises from the need for a constant source of zinc in order to maintain plasma levels. When rats were given a zinc-deficient diet at the beginning of pregnancy, plasma zinc concentration dropped sharply. After only 24 hrs of the deficiency regime, plasma zinc fell by approximately 40% (Dreosti *et al.*, 1968). This fast change was brought about by lack of mobilization of zinc from maternal stores. After 21 days of a deficient diet, the zinc content of bone was the same in pregnant as it was in nonpregnant rats, although the zinc content of the fetuses was abnormally low and they were malformed. These results indicated that the pregnant rat cannot mobilize zinc from maternal tissues in amounts sufficient to supply the needs of normal fetal development (Hurley and Swenerton, 1971).

Because of these observations, we developed the hypothesis that zinc could be released from the skeleton only under conditions in which there is breakdown of bone itself. The hypothesis was tested by comparing the effects of a diet lacking calcium as well as zinc with the effects of a diet deficient in zinc alone. The teratogenic effects of zinc deficiency were alleviated by lack of dietary calcium. Female rats fed the diet deficient in both calcium and zinc had larger litters, fewer resorptions, and fewer malformed fetuses than did those fed the diet deficient in zinc alone. Furthermore, the ash, zinc, and calcium concentrations of bone were also reduced in rats receiving neither calcium nor zinc during pregnancy (Hurley and Tao, 1972). However, alleviation of the teratogenic effects of zinc deficiency by calcium deficiency did not occur in parathyroidectomized rats (Tao and Hurley, 1975). These results support the hypothesis that conditions bringing about resorption of bone increase the availability of skeletal zinc.

A similar effect occurred when increased breakdown of maternal tissue was brought about by giving pregnant females a diet deficient in protein as well as in zinc. In this case, with a diet containing either 8 or 5% protein, the percentage of implantation sites affected was markedly lower than in rats receiving a diet deficient only in zinc (Hurley *et al.*, 1973).

The experiments described thus far were made under extreme conditions of zinc deficiency. It was also of interest to examine the effect of milder states of zinc deficiency, which might be more relevant to human problems. One approach, therefore, was to correlate the level of zinc in the diet with the incidence of malformations and to determine the concentration of dietary zinc that would prevent such malformations. This was done by feeding pregnant rats diets containing various levels of zinc. Rats given diets containing less than 9 ppm zinc during pregnancy had a high incidence of fetal death and malformation. In addition, both total litter weight and fetal weight at term correlated with the level of dietary zinc up to 14 ppm, but there was no correlation between the fetal zinc content or maternal plasma zinc at term and the incidence of malformation. However, plasma zinc during the second trimester was so correlated. These results suggest that in seeking measures for the evaluation of zinc nutriture in pregnant women, it appears that determination of plasma zinc level during the second trimester would provide a better index than such measurements at term (Hurley and Cosens, 1974).

Another approach used in examining the results of mild rather than severe zinc deficiency was to study the effects of transitory deficiency during prenatal life. Normal pregnant rats were given a zinc-deficient diet from day 6 to day 14 of gestation. Maternal plasma zinc levels fell rapidly but returned quickly to original values after zinc was given. Young born to these females showed low birth weight, high incidence of congenital malformation, high rate of stillbirths, and very poor survival to weaning, although postnatal growth of survivors was normal. Most of the postnatal mortality occurred in the first week. None of these effects was seen in control groups, either *ad libitum*-fed or with restricted food intake. The concentration of zinc in postpartum maternal plasma and milk, as well as in plasma of the pups, was normal, suggesting that postnatal zinc nutriture of the young was adequate. The poor survival of young born to females fed a zinc-deficient diet for a short period of time may be due to congenital abnormalities or to failure to suckle because of weakness at birth. The results show that a short period of zinc deficiency during prenatal life caused an irreversible change that subsequently affected postnatal development (Hurley and Mutch, 1973).

Zinc deficiency during the suckling period also has very deleterious effects on development of the young. When females were given a zinc-deficient diet at parturition the growth of their offspring was significantly retarded. Even when the young were given a normal control diet at weaning, their growth rate improved, but they did not obtain the body weight of the normal *ad libitum*-fed controls. Their survival to weaning was also greatly reduced, and these effects were produced by insufficient intake of zinc from the mother's milk. The zinc content of the milk was significantly reduced (Mutch and Hurley, 1974). Nishimura (1953) found similar effects in suckling mice rendered zinc-deficient through deprivation of colostrum.

Zinc is also an essential element for the reproduction of monkeys. In experiments with *Macaca radiata*, the bonnet monkey, it was found that zinc-deficient females had signs of abnormal ovarian development. In mature females, no pregnancies resulted from 32 matings, as compared with 18 and 24% of pregnancies in controls (H. Swenerton and L. S. Hurley, unpublished data).

V. MAGNESIUM

Another essential metal that is similar to zinc in its rapidity of action is magnesium. With a severe deficiency of magnesium, embryonic death and malformation result (Hurley and Cosens, 1970). With a milder deficiency, some embryos survive but they are small and may be malformed. In addition, they are edematous and pale, with low plasma protein and severe anemia (Hurley and Cosens, 1971). Although packed cell volume (PCV) and hemoglobin were normal in maternal blood, in the fetuses, hemoglobin, PCV, and red blood cell count were markedly reduced in the deficient animals (Hurley, 1971). Cohlan *et al.* (1970) and Dancis *et al.* (1971) have also observed a fall in maternal plasma magnesium, decreased magnesium concentration in the fetuses, and fetal anemia in magnesium deficiency in rats during pregnancy.

VI. CONCLUSION

Wilson (1973) has estimated that 65–70% of developmental defects in man are of unknown origin. I would like to conclude with the postulation that in humans, nutritional deficiencies (even marginal or short term) superimposed upon a particularly susceptible genetic constitution, with perhaps a drug, toxin, or other environmental factor interacting, could cause aberrations of developmental processes with deleterious effects in the perinatal period (Hurley, 1968, 1969, 1974a).

REFERENCES

Asling, C. W., and Hurley, L. S. (1963). The influence of trace elements on the skeleton. *Clin. Orthop. Relat. Res.* **27**, 213–264.

Asling, C. W., Hurley, L. S., and Wooten, E. (1960). Abnormal development of the otic labyrinth in young rats following maternal dietary manganese deficiency. *Anat. Rec.* **136**, 157.

Bell, L. T., and Hurley, L. S. (1973). Ultrastructural effects of manganese deficiency in liver, heart, kidney and pancreas of mice. *Lab. Invest.* **29**, 723–736.

Bennetts, H. W, and Beck, A. B. (1942). Enzootic ataxia and copper deficiency of sheep in Western Australia. *Aust. Counc. Sci. Ind. Res., Bull.* **147**.

Bennetts, H. W., and Chapman, F. E. (1937). Copper deficiency in sheep in Western Australia: A preliminary account of the aetiology of enzootic ataxia of lambs and an anemia of ewes. *Aust. Vet. J.* **13**, 138–149.

Blamberg, D. L., Blackwood, U. B., Supplee, W. C., and Combs, G. F. (1960).

Effect of zinc deficiency in hens on hatchability and embryonic development. *Proc. Soc. Exp. Biol. Med.* **104**, 217–220.

Carlton, W. W., and Kelly, W. A. (1969). Neural lesions in the offspring of female rats fed a copper-deficient diet. *J. Nutr.* **97**, 42–52.

Clements, F. W. (1960). Health significance of endemic goitre and related conditions. *In* "Endemic Goitre." *World Health Organ., Monogr. Ser.* **44**, pp. 245–260.

Cohlan, S. Q., Jansen, V., Dancis, J., and Piomelli, S. (1970). Microcytic anemia with erythroblastosis in the offspring of magnesium deprived rats. *Blood* **36**, 500–506.

Dancis, J., Springer, D., and Cohlan, S. Q. (1971). Fetal homeostasis in maternal malnutrition. II. Magnesium deprivation. *Pediat. Res.* **5**, 131–136.

Daniels, A. L., and Everson, G. J. (1935). The relation of manganese to congenital debility. *J. Nutr.* **9**, 191–203.

Danks, D. M., Campbell, P. E., Stevens, B. J., Mayne, V., and Cartwright, E. (1972). Menkes' kinky hair syndrome. An inherited defect in copper absorption with widespread effects. *Pediatrics* **50**, 188–201.

Diamond, I., and Hurley, L. S. (1970). Histopathology of zinc-deficient fetal rats. *J. Nutr.* **100**, 325–329.

Dreosti, I. E., and Hurley, L. S. (1975). Depressed thymidine kinase activity in zinc-deficient rat embryos. *Proc. Soc. Exp. Biol. Med.* **150**, 161–165.

Dreosti, I. E., Tao, S., and Hurley, L. S. (1968). Plasma zinc and leukocyte changes in weanling and pregnant rats during zinc deficiency. *Proc. Soc. Exp. Biol. Med.* **127**, 169–174.

Dreosti, I. E., Grey, P. C., and Wilkens, P. J. (1972). Deoxyribonucleic acid synthesis, protein synthesis and teratogenesis in zinc-deficient rats. *S. Afr. Med. J.* **46**, 1585–1588.

Erway, L., and Mitchell, S. E. (1973). Prevention of otolith defect in pastel mink by manganese supplementation. *J. Hered.* **64**, 110–119.

Erway, L., Hurley, L. S., and Fraser, A. (1966). Neurological defect: Manganese in phenocopy and prevention of a genetic abnormality of inner ear. *Science* **152**, 1766–1768.

Erway, L., Hurley, L. S., and Fraser, A. (1970). Congenital ataxia and otolith defects due to manganese deficiency in mice. *J. Nutr.* **100**, 643–654.

Erway, L., Fraser, A., and Hurley, L. S. (1971). Prevention of congenital otolith defect in *Pallid* mutant mice by manganese supplementation. *Genetics* **67**, 97–108.

Everson, G. J., Hurley, L. S., and Geiger, J. F. (1959). Manganese Deficiency in the guinea pig. *J. Nutr.* **68**, 49–57.

Everson, G. J., Tsai, H. C., and Wang, T. (1967). Copper deficiency in the guinea pig. *J. Nutr.* **93**, 533–540.

Everson, G. J., Shrader, R. E., and Wang, T. (1968). Chemical and morphological changes in the brain of copper-deficient guinea pigs. *J. Nutr.* **96**, 115–125.

Falconer, D. S., Fraser, A. S., and King, J. W. B. (1952). The genetics and development of "crinkled," a new mutant in the house mouse. *J. Genet.* **50**, 324–346.

Follis, R. H., Jr. (1958). "Deficiency Disease," pp. 301–305. Thomas, Springfield, Illinois.

Fujioka, M., and Lieberman, I. (1964). A Zn^{++} requirement for synthesis of deoxyribonucleic acid by rat liver. *J. Biol. Chem.* **239**, 1164–1167.

Hoekstra, W. G., Suttie, J. W., Ganther, H. E., Mertz, W. (1974). "Trace Element Metabolism in Animals-2." *International Symposium on Trace Element Metabolism in Animals, 2nd.* University Park Press, Baltimore.

Hurley, L. S. (1968). The consequences of fetal impoverishment. *Nutr. Today* 3, 3–10.

Hurley, L. S. (1969). Nutrients and genes: Interactions in development. *Nutr. Rev.* 27, 3–6.

Hurley, L. S. (1971). Magnesium deficiency during pregnancy and its effects on the offspring. A comprehensive review. *Proc. Int. Symp. Magnesium Defic. Hum. Pathol., 1971* Imprimerie Amelot, Brionne, France, pp. 481–492.

Hurley, L. S. (1974a). Zinc deficiency, potatoes, and congenital malformations in man. *Teratology* 10, 205–206.

Hurley, L. S. (1974b). Aspects of mineral metabolism in the perinatal period. *In* "Perinatal Pharmacology: Problems and Priorities" (J. Dancis and J. C. Hwang, eds.), pp. 149–158. Raven, New York.

Hurley, L. S., and Asling, C. W. (1963). Localized epiphyseal dysplasia in offspring of manganese-deficient rats. *Anat. Rec.* 145, 25–38.

Hurley, L. S., and Bell, L. T. (1974a). Amelioration by copper supplementation of mutant gene crinkled in mice. *Teratology* 9, A22.

Hurley, L. S., and Bell, L. T. (1974b). Genetic influence on response to dietary manganese deficiency. *J. Nutr.* 104, 133–137.

Hurley, L. S., and Bell, L. T. (1975). Amelioration by copper supplementation of mutant gene effects in the crinkled mouse. *Proc. Soc. Exp. Biol. Med.* 149, 830–834.

Hurley, L. S., and Cosens, G. (1970). Teratogenic magnesium deficiency in pregnant rats. *Teratology* 3, 202.

Hurley, L. S., and Cosens, G. (1971). Congenital malformations and fetal anemia resulting from magnesium deficiency in rats. *Fed. Proc., Fed. Amer. Soc. Exp. Biol.* 30, 516.

Hurley, L. S, and Cosens, G. (1974). Reproduction and prenatal development in relation to dietary zinc level. *In* "2nd International Symposium on Trace Element Metabolism" (C. F. Mills, ed.) (in press).

Hurley, L. S., and Everson, G. J. (1959). Delayed development of righting reflexes in offspring of manganese-deficient rats. *Proc. Soc. Exp. Biol. Med.* 102, 360–362.

Hurley, L. S., and Everson, G. J. (1963). Influence of timing of short-term supplementation during gestation on congenital abnormalities of manganese-deficient rats. *J. Nutr.* 79, 23–27.

Hurley, L. S., and Mutch, P. B. (1973). Prenatal and postnatal development after transitory gestational zinc deficiency in rats. *J. Nutr.* 103, 649–656.

Hurley, L. S., and Shrader, R. E. (1972). Congenital malformations of the nervous system in zinc-deficient rats. *Int. Rev. Neurobiol., Suppl.* 1, 7–51.

Hurley, L. S., and Swenerton, H. (1966). Congenital malformations resulting from zinc deficiency in rats. *Proc. Soc. Exp. Biol. Med.* 123, 692–697.

Hurley, L. S., and Swenerton, H. (1971). Lack of mobilization of bone and liver zinc under teratogenic conditions of zinc deficiency in rats. *J. Nutr.* 101, 597–604.

Hurley, L. S., and Tao, S. H. (1972). Alleviation of teratogenic effects of zinc deficiency by simultaneous lack of calcium. *Amer. J. Physiol.* 222, 322–325.

Hurley, L. S., Everson, G. J., and Geiger, J. F. (1958). Manganese deficiency in rats: Congenital nature of ataxia. *J. Nutr.* 66, 309–320.

Hurley, L. S., Wooten, E., Everson, G. J., and Asling, C. W. (1960). Anomalous development of ossification in the inner ear of offspring of manganese-deficient rats. *J. Nutr.* 71, 15–20.

Hurley, L. S., Everson, G. J., Wooten, E., and Asling, C. W. (1961a). Disproportionate growth in offspring of manganese-deficient rats. I. The long bones *J. Nutr.* **74**, 274–281.

Hurley, L. S., Wooten, E., and Everson, G. J. (1961b). Disproportionate growth in offspring of manganese-deficient rats. II. Skull, brain, and cerebrospinal fluid pressure. *J. Nutr.* **74**, 282–288.

Hurley, L. S., Woolley, D. E., and Timiras, P. S. (1961c). Threshold and pattern of electroshock seizures in ataxic manganese-deficient rats. *Proc. Soc. Exp. Biol. Med.* **106**, 343–346.

Hurley, L. S., Woolley, D. E., Rosenthal, E., and Timiras, P. S. (1963). Influence of manganese on susceptibility of rats to convulsions. *Amer. J. Physiol.* **204**, 493–496.

Hurley, L. S., Gowan, J., and Shrader, R. (1968a). Genetic-nutritional interaction in relation to manganese and calcification. *Tissue Calcifies, Symp. Euro., 5th, 1967* (G. Milhaud, M. Owen, and H. J. J. Blackwood, eds.) pp. 101–104.

Hurley, L. S., Dreosti, I. E., and Swenerton, H. (1968b). Studies on zinc enzymes and nucleic acid synthesis in relation to congenital malformations in zinc-deficient rats. *Proc. West. Hemisphere Nutr. Congr., 2nd, 1968* p. 39.

Hurley, L. S., Gowan, J., and Milhaud, G. (1969). Calcium metabolism in manganese-deficient and zinc-deficient rats. *Proc. Soc. Exp. Biol. Med.* **130**, 856–860.

Hurley, L. S., Theriault, L., and Dreosti, I. E. (1970). Liver mitochondria from manganese-deficient and pallid mice: Function and ultrastructure. *Science* **170**, 1316–1318.

Hurley, L. S., Gowan, J., and Swenerton, H. (1971). Teratogenic effects of short-term and transistory zinc deficiency in rats. *Teratology* **4**, 199–204.

Hurley, L. S., Sucher, K., Story, D., and Cosens, G. (1973). Interaction of dietary protein and zinc in the pregnant rat. *J. Nutr.* **103**, xxv.

Innes, J. R. M., and Shearer, G. D. (1940). "Swayback": A demyelinating disease of lambs with affinities to Schilder's encephalitics in man. *J. Comp. Pathol. Ther.* **53**, 1.

Keinholz, E. W., Turk, D. E., Sunde, M. L., and Hoekstra, W. G. (1961). Effects of zinc deficiency in the diets of hens. *J. Nutr.* **75**, 211–221.

Kelly, F. C., and Snedden, W. W. (1960). Prevalence and geographical distribution of endemic goitre. In "Endemic Goitre." *World Health Organ., Monogr. Ser.* **44**, 27–233.

Langer, P. (1960). History of goitre. In "Endemic Goitre." *World Health Organ., Monogr. Ser.* **44**, 9–25.

Leach, R. M., Jr., and Muenster, A. M. (1962). Studies of the role of manganese in bone formation. I. Effect upon mucopolysaccharide content of chick bone. *J. Nutr.* **78**, 51–57.

Leach, R. M., Jr., Muenster, A. M., and Wein, E. M. (1969). Studies on the role of manganese in bone formation. II. Effect upon chondroitin sulfate synthesis in chick epiphyseal cartilage. *Arch. Biochem. Biophys.* **133**, 22–28.

Lyon, M. F. (1953). Absence of otoliths in the mouse: An effect of the pallid mutant. *J. Genet.* **51**, 638–650.

Lyons, M., and Insko, W. M., Jr. (1937). Chondrodystrophy in the chick embryo produced by manganese deficiency in the diet of the hen. *Ky. Agr. Exp. Sta. Bull.* **371**.

Menkes, J. H. (1972). Kinky hair disease. *Pediatrics* **50**, 181–183.

Mills, C. F., Quarterman, J., Chesters, J. K., Williams, R. B., and Dalgarno, A. C. (1969). Metabolic role of zinc. *Amer. J. Clin. Nutr.* **22**, 1240–1249.

Mutch, P. B., and Hurley, L. S. (1974). Effect of zinc deficiency during lactation on postnatal growth and development. *J. Nutr.* **104**, 828–842.

Nishimura, H. (1953). Zinc deficiency in suckling mice deprived of colostrum. *J. Nutr.* **49**, 79–93.

Norris, L. C., and Caskey, C. D. (1939). A chronic congenital ataxia and osteodystrophy in chicks due to manganese deficiency. *J. Nutr.* **17**, Suppl., 16–17.

O'Dell, B. L. (1968). Trace elements in embryonic development. *Fed. Proc., Fed. Amer. Soc. Exp. Biol.* **27**, 199–204.

O'Dell, B. L., Hardwick, B. C., and Reynolds, G. (1961). Mineral deficiencies of milk and congenital malformations in the rat. *J. Nutr.* **73**, 151–157.

Orent, E. R., and McCollum, E. V. (1931). Effects of deprivation of manganese in the rat. *J. Biol. Chem.* **92**, 651.

Plumlee, M. P., Thrasher, D. M., Beeson, W. M., Andrews, F. N., and Parker, H. E. (1956). The effects of a manganese deficiency upon the growth, development, and reproduction of swine. *J. Anim. Sci.* **15**, 352.

Sandstead, H., and Rinaldi, R. A. (1969). Impairment of deoxyribonucleic acid synthesis by dietary zinc deficiency in the rat. *J. Cell. Physiol.* **73**, 81–83.

Shils, M. E., and McCollum, E. V. (1943). Further studies on the symptoms of manganese deficiency in the rat and mouse. *J. Nutr.* **26**, 1–31.

Shrader, R. E., and Everson, G. J. (1967). Anomalous development of otoliths associated with postural defects in manganese-deficient guinea pigs. *J. Nutr.* **91**, 453–460.

Shrader, R. E., Erway, L., and Hurley, L. S. (1973). Mucopolysaccharide synthesis in the developing inner ear of manganese-deficient and pallid mutant mice. *Teratology* **8**, 257–266.

Swenerton, H., and Hurley, L. S. (1968). Severe zinc deficiency in male and female rats. *J. Nutr.* **95**, 8–18.

Swenerton, H., Shrader, R., and Hurley, L. S. (1969). Zinc-deficient embryos: Reduced thymidine incorporation. *Science* **166**, 1014–1015.

Swenerton, H., Shrader, R., and Hurley, L. S. (1972). Lactic and malic dehydrogenases in testes of zinc-deficient rats. *Proc. Soc. Exp. Biol. Med.* **141**, 283–286.

Tao, S. H., and Hurley, L. S. (1975). Effect of dietary calcium deficiency during pregnancy on zinc mobilization in intact and parathyroidectomized rats. *J. Nutr.* **105**, 226–232.

Tsai, H. C. C., and Everson, G. J. (1967). Effect of manganese deficiency on the acid mucopolysaccharides in cartilage of guinea pigs. *J. Nutr.* **91**, 447–453.

Turk, D. E., Sunde, M. L., and Hoekstra, W. G. (1959). Zinc deficiency experiments with poultry. *Poultry Sci.* **38**, 1256.

Underwood, E. J. (1971). "Trace Elements in Human and Animal Nutrition," 3rd ed., pp. 83–87. Academic Press, New York.

Warkany, J., and Petering, H. G. (1972). Congenital malformations of the central nervous system in rats produced by maternal zinc deficiency. *Teratology* **5**, 319–334.

Warkany, J., and Petering, H. G. (1973). Congenital malformations of the brain produced by short zinc deficiencies in rats. *Amer. J. Ment. Defic.* **77**, 645–653.

Weser, U., Seeber, S., and Warnecke, P. (1969). Reactivity of Zn^{2+} on nuclear DNA and RNA biosynthesis of regenerating rat liver. *Biochim. Biophys. Acta* **179**, 422.

Wilson, J. G. (1973). "Environment and Birth Defects," pp. 48–82. Academic Press, New York.

38

Effects of Oral Contraceptive Agents on Trace Element Metabolism—A Review

J. Cecil Smith, Jr., and Ellen D. Brown

I. INTRODUCTION

Oral contraceptive agents (OCA) have become a widely accepted means of birth control in the United States, with more than one-third of all married couples using the method in 1970, only ten years after its introduction (Westoff, 1972). Specifically, nearly six million married women were users of oral contraceptives in 1970. The increasing use of these preparations emphasizes the need for a thorough understanding of their metabolic effects. A recent report (Weindling and Henry, 1974) has summarized the effect of OCA use on general biochemical parameters. This report will review pertinent studies concerning the influence of oral contraceptives on trace element metabolism.

II. ORAL CONTRACEPTIVES AND TRACE ELEMENT METABOLISM

There are three main types of oral contraceptives currently available (Haller, 1969).

1. *Progestogen–estrogen* combinations in which each tablet contains both hormones in a fixed dose. These are taken for 20–21 days with a tablet-free interval of 7 days before the next course.

2. *Sequential or serial* preparations, consisting of a course of an estrogen alone followed by a course of progestogen plus estrogen. These also have a tablet-free interval.

3. *Progestogen-only* compounds, in which the preparation contains only one hormone in a fixed dose and is taken continuously without a break.

The effect on trace element metabolism may vary among these three types of preparations depending on the hormones and dosage present.

In addition to its hormone composition, contamination of the OCA by the trace element under investigation must be considered. However, one study indicates that trace element contamination may not be a major problem in preparations currently used. Dawson *et al.* (1973) analyzed eleven different brands of OCA for sodium, potassium, magnesium, calcium, iron, copper, zinc, cobalt, and manganese but found no significant quantities of the trace elements.

A. Copper

It has been known for many years that serum copper increases during pregnancy (Cartwright, 1950; Markowitz *et al.*, 1955). In addition, Lahey *et al.* (1953) reported that serum concentrations were significantly higher in females than in males. These studies suggested that hormones could either directly or indirectly affect serum copper concentration. Later, Russ and Raymunt (1956) investigated the influence of estrogens on total serum copper and ceruloplasmin after they observed that the blue color attributed to ceruloplasmin was always more intense after patients had received estrogen therapy. This study involved eight subjects with various diseases. After 3–4 weeks of 1 mg daily of ethinylestradiol, marked increases in both serum copper and ceruloplasmin occurred. The authors concluded that "in view of these observations and reports that serum copper concentrations are significantly higher in females than in males the possible interrelationship between . . . ceruloplasmin and estrogen metabolism is suggested." Gault *et al.* (1966) also reported that ceruloplasmin concentrations increased in four subjects taking estrogen. These early investigations indicated that estrogen therapy resulted in an increase in the concentration of the serum copper-binding protein ceruloplasmin. Since a majority of the serum copper is bound to ceruloplasmin, significant positive correlations have been found between these two parameters of copper metabolism (Underwood, 1971). Therefore, when ceruloplasmin is increased, there is a corresponding elevation in serum copper concentration.

Carruthers *et al.* (1966) reported that high serum copper concentrations occurred in OCA users in a "normal" control population of twenty-five healthy OCA users compared to a control group of twenty-three healthy females. Six different oral contraceptive preparations including one sequential preparation were being used. The serum copper concentration for the control group was 121 ± 11.4 μg/100 ml (mean ± SD), with a ceruloplasmin level of 31 ± 5.7 mg/100 ml. In contrast, the mean serum copper was 258 μg/100 ml and the ceruloplasmin 80 mg/100 ml for those subjects taking the oral contraceptives. In three subjects, serum copper and ceruloplasmin concentrations were measured before and during medication. The results indicated that more than a twofold increase in both serum copper and ceruloplasmin occurred after medication of 17–22 days. These authors found a positive correlation coefficient of 0.94 between serum copper and ceruloplasmin concentrations.

In 1968, our laboratory (Halsted *et al.*, 1968) reported plasma copper concentrations in twenty-five pregnant women and ten receiving OCA. The results are shown in Table I and indicate a highly significant increase ($p < 0.001$) both in pregnancy and after ingestion of oral contraceptives.

Schenker *et al.* (1971b) determined the serum copper concentration in 502 women who were receiving four different types of oral contraceptive preparations including two that were sequential. The serum copper level in ninety-one healthy female controls was 129 ± 7.4 μg/100 ml (mean ± SE). The mean serum copper concentration in the females taking the oral contraceptives increased strikingly to 207 μg/100 ml. There was no direct correlation between duration of the therapy and serum copper concentrations. The rise in serum copper level appeared after two cycles of treatment and remained rather constant. Nine subjects were followed for fifty-four cycles and exhibited sustained elevated serum copper levels approximating 200 μg/100 ml. Six patients who

TABLE I Plasma Copper in Pregnancy and After Oral Contraceptives

Subjects	Number	Plasma copper (μg/100 ml) (mean ± SD)	Significance levels
Controls	37	118 ± 21	—
Pregnancy	25	250 ± 38	$p < 0.001$
On oral contraceptives	10	300 ± 70	$p < 0.001$

experienced clinical side effects from the OCA had serum copper concentrations of more than 300 $\mu g/100$ ml. When the oral contraceptive was stopped, the copper level in these six patients returned to near normal range within 4–6 weeks. Other results by these authors indicated that neither the type (combined or sequential) nor the steroid composition altered the increases in serum copper with OCA use.

In another publication, Schenker et al. (1971a) reported results similar to the above study. Specifically, serum copper was determined in 342 cases, 251 subjects taking OCA and 91 controls. The results indicated that the serum copper in the control females was 129 ± 7.4 (mean $\pm$ SE) $\mu g/100$ ml, compared to 205 ± 26 $\mu g/100$ ml for the subjects taking the oral contraceptives. These authors stated disagreement with the general belief that the estrogen component alone is the factor in the oral contraceptive preparations responsible for the increased serum copper concentration. They conclude "that the rise of serum copper content in subjects taking oral contraceptives is not due to the estrogenic compound alone . . . but that the progestive agents also play a role." They support this conclusion in part by the finding that serum copper was 205 ± 25.9 $\mu g/100$ ml (mean $\pm$ SE) in four subjects receiving chlormadinone alone, a progestogen with "no estrogenic activity." The control level for serum copper was 129 ± 7.4 (mean $\pm$ SE) $\mu g/100$ ml.

Serum protein alterations, including ceruloplasmin, produced in women receiving synthetic estrogens was studied by Musa et al. (1967). Five subjects received 0.5 mg of ethinylestradiol and six received 0.25 mg of ethinylestradiol plus one tablet of Enovid-E, which contains 0.1 mg ethinylestradiol-3 methyl ether and 2.5 mg norethynodrel. Using several methods of quantitation, ceruloplasmin was significantly increased after the steroid treatment, confirming the earlier results of Russ and Raymunt (1956). No differences in the response to ethinylestradiol with or without the synthetic progestational agent were apparent. Serum copper was not reported.

Laurell et al. (1967) also reported ceruloplasmin levels for thirty women before and 6 months after a regular regime of a combined contraceptive. Ceruloplasmin increased significantly and was similar in magnitude to the level occurring during late pregnancy. Serum copper was not determined.

Briggs and co-workers have published a series of papers regarding oral contraceptives and copper metabolism. Briggs et al. (1970) noted the development of the technique of daily administration of a continuous small dose of a synthetic progestogen alone without estrogen. This was an effort to prevent side effects generally considered to be associated with the estrogen component of the combined oral contraceptives. (They state, without reference, that "chronic increases of ceruloplasmin have been suspected as being implicated in the etiology of certain side-effects of oral contraceptives—notably, migraine and chloasma. . . .") They therefore investigated the effects on copper metabolism of a progestogen-only oral contraceptive. In their study, six normal healthy young women received 0.3 mg daily of the progestogen (norethisterone acetate). As a control, two other women received a combined estrogen–progestogen product (Minovlar, 50 μg ethinylestradiol plus 1.0 mg norethisterone acetate). The results of this study indicated that the progestogen alone did not affect serum copper or ceruloplasmin, whereas the product containing estrogen produced a marked increase in serum copper and ceruloplasmin.

Briggs and Briggs (1973) reported the dose-related changes on serum proteins, including ceruloplasmin of an estrogen (mestranol) given alone or in combination with a progestogen. In addition, the effect of two progestogen agents alone was studied. Oral daily doses of mestranol ranging from 25 to 120 μg were given to groups of ten to twelve healthy women, 19–36 years of age, for a period of 21 days. A dose-dependent increase was observed in ceruloplasmin ranging from 41 ± 11 mg/100 ml (mean $\pm$ SD) for the lowest mestranol dose (25 μg) to 71 ± 15 mg/100 ml for the highest dose (120 μg). The pretreatment ceruloplasmin concentration was 39 ± 8 mg/100 ml. Similar increases in ceruloplasmin had been noted previously by these same workers (Briggs and Briggs, 1971a) when the levels of a different estrogen (ethinylestradiol) were increased from 10 to 75 μg per day. The minimum daily oral dose of estrogen required to induce a statistical increase in ceruloplasmin was 10 μg for ethinylestradiol and 60 μg for mestranol. The ceruloplasmin concentration remained unchanged when 1.0 mg norethisterone was added to the daily doses of either 50 μg or 100 μg mestranol or 50 μg ethinylestradiol. In contrast, the serum ceruloplasmin level was significantly increased when either 1.0 mg ($p < 0.05$) or 10 mg ($p < 0.02$) of norethisterone was given daily without any estrogen to five women for 21 consecutive days. However, when another progestogen (megestrol acetate) was given alone to a different group of five women for 21 days in similar daily doses (1.0 or 10 mg) there was no effect upon ceruloplasmin levels. The authors conclude that the progestogens used in this study ". . . had little action on serum proteins when given alone at the dose used in the oral contraceptives, though larger amounts produced significant changes." (The dose used in the contraceptives is usually 1 mg). However, their data indicate a "slightly increased" ($p < 0.05$) ceruloplasmin concentration after a 1 mg daily dose of the progestogen norethisterone, a dose similar to that used in the combined pill. It is possible that the increase could be due to the reported production of estrogenic metabolites from the metabolism of norethisterone (Brown and Blair, 1960; Breuer, 1964; Paulsen, 1965). In fact an earlier publication by Briggs and Briggs (1970) recognized that norethisterone produced metabolites with estrogenic activity and reported that slightly increased serum copper levels occurred when 1 mg of norethisterone acetate was given to ten to twelve healthy young women. Specifically, the controls had a copper concentration of 125 ± 8 μg/100 ml (mean $\pm$ SD), whereas those receiving the progestogen norethisterone acetate (1 mg) had copper levels of 152 ± 11 μg/100 ml.

O'Leary and Spellacy (1968) reported increased serum copper values after fourteen healthy females ingested "10 mg. of norethynodrel with mestranol daily for 21 days." In a subsequent report by O'Leary and Spellacy (1969) plasma copper concentrations were determined in three groups of women: twenty-seven controls, thirty pregnant, and sixteen receiving an oral contraceptive containing 9.85 mg of norethynodrel and 0.15 mg mestranol. The mean plasma copper concentrations were increased from 142 μg/100 ml for the controls to 231 μg/100 ml for those pregnant and 241 μg/100 ml for those receiving the oral contraceptive.

More recently, the effect of oral contraceptives on serum copper levels in 224 Nigerian women has been reported by Olatunbosun et al. (1973). Eighty-seven of the women had been fitted with an intrauterine contraceptive device (IUCD), twenty-eight were receiving Ovral 28,* and sixty-five Norlestrin Fe.* (Both contraceptives contain 50 μg of ethynylestradiol.) In addition, forty-four women served as controls. The results indicated no significant difference in the serum copper concentrations between the control or IUCD group—110 $\pm$ 20 μg/100 ml (mean $\pm$ SD) and 102 $\pm$ 21 μg/100 ml, respectively. In contrast, those receiving either oral contraceptive had significantly higher serum copper concentrations—144 $\pm$ 26 μg/100 ml for Ovral 28 or 142 $\pm$ 25 μg/100 ml for Norlestrin Fe. The authors note that the increase in copper concentration in women taking the oral contraceptive, although significant, was only 30% in contrast to increases of 60–200% of control values reported by others (Carruthers et al., 1966; O'Leary and Spellacy, 1969; Halsted et al., 1968; Schenker et al., 1971a). They suggest the possibility that the "concentration of the plasma proteins responsible for copper transport is lower in Nigerian women than elsewhere and that there is also a reduction in their ability to synthesize increased amounts of these proteins. . . ." They further speculate "that the increase in plasma globulin levels . . . in Nigerians is responsible for the relative reduction in the

* Total steroid composition of these commercial products was not given.

concentration of the proteins responsible for the binding and transport of copper and steroids."

A concept based on the pharmacological action of copper to prevent pregnancy has recently been advanced. Zipper *et al.* (1969a) reported that a small piece of copper wire placed in the uterus of rabbits prevented implantation of the blastocyst. Subsequently, this group (Zipper *et al.*, 1969b, 1971) has further studied and developed this concept. As a result copper is now incorporated into several IUCDs and clinical evaluations have been conducted (Bernstein *et al.*, 1972; Oster, 1972). A clinical study with a limited number of subjects (Daunter and Elstein, 1973) indicated lower serum and ceruloplasmin concentrations in users of copper-containing IUDCs compared to those taking combined oral contraceptives.

Hagenfeldt (1972) also studied the effect of copper-containing IUCDs upon trace elements including copper, in the endometrium, cervical mucus, and plasma. Sixteen women were involved in the study. Samples were taken before insertion, during 1 year's use, and after removal of the device. The data indicated that no changes occurred in plasma copper as a result of the release of copper from the device. The amount of copper released from the device was estimated to be 10.3 mg per year, an amount considered to be nonharmful.

In summary, there is unanimous agreement that serum copper and ceruloplasmin are consistently elevated in users of OCA, as summarized in Table II. There is also general agreement that the increase in serum copper concentration is a result of an increase in the copper-binding protein ceruloplasmin. The magnitude of the increase approximates that found during pregnancy. The majority of the studies indicate that the estrogen component of the oral contraceptive is responsible for the increase. Recently a copper-containing IUCD has been proposed. In a limited number of studies, there have been no apparent alterations in regard to copper metabolism.

B. Zinc

Johnson (1961) reported that plasma zinc was depressed during pregnancy. However, while analyzing blood samples in our laboratory from healthy nonpregnant female volunteers to establish a normal range for plasma zinc concentrations, we noted occasional low values. It was later determined that these low values could be related to those females ingesting oral contraceptives and was of similar magnitude to the decrease found during the third trimester of pregnancy (Halsted *et al.*, 1968).

TABLE II Selected References Concerning Serum Copper and Ceruloplasmin Concentrations in Oral Contraceptive Steroid Users

Investigator	Length of treatment	Ceruloplasmin (mg/100 ml)[a]		Copper (μg/100 ml)[a]		OCA brand name	Estrogen component (μg)	Progestogen component (mg)
		Control	Steroid	Control	Steroid			
Carruthers et al. (1966)	1–47 months	31 ± 5.7 (23)	87 ± 11[b] (12)	121 ± 11.4 (23)	275 ± 43[b] (12)	Feminor[c]	Mestranol[c] (100/75)	Norethynodrel[c] (5)
	2–18 months	31 ± 5.7 (23)	63 ± 9[b] (5)	121 ± 11.4 (23)	229 ± 49[b] (5)	Norlestrin	Ethinylestradiol (50)	Norethisterone acetate (2.5)
	1–48 months	31 ± 5.7 (23)	83 ± 22[b] (4)	121 ± 11.4 (23)	256 ± 28[b] (4)	Ovulen	Mestranol (100)	Ethynodiol diacetate (1)
Schenker et al. (1971b)	1–60 cycles	—	—	129 ± 7.4 (91)	203 ± 47.5 (108)	Metrulen-M	Mestranol (100)	Ethynodiol diacetate (1)
		—	—	129 ± 7.4 (91)	208 ± 73.5 (163)	Gynovlar	Ethinylestradiol (50)	Norethisterone (3)
		—	—	129 ± 7.4 (91)	198 ± 49.5 (141)	Nogest-S[d]	Ethinylestradiol[d] (75)	Metroxyprogesterone[d] (5)
Briggs and Briggs (1970)	3–4 weeks	—	—	129 ± 7.4 (91)	218 ± 50.3 (90)	Sequelan[e]	Mestranol[e] (100/75)	Norethyprogesterone[e] (5)
		—	—	125 ± 8 (10–12)[f]	235 ± 25 (10–12)	—	Ethinylestradiol (50)	Norethisterone acetate (1)
		—	—	125 ± 8 (10–12)	130 ± 8 (10–12)	—	—	Norethisterone acetate (0.3)
		—	—	125 ± 8 (10–12)	152 ± 11 (10–12)	—	—	Norethisterone acetate (1)
		—	—	125 ± 8 (10–12)	136 ± 10 (10–12)	—	Ethinylestradiol (10)	—
		—	—	125 ± 8 (10–12)	181 ± 16 (10–12)	—	Ethinylestradiol (20)	—
		—	—	125 ± 8 (10–12)	227 ± 18 (10–12)	—	Ethinylestradiol (50)	—
		—	—	125 ± 8 (10–12)	128 ± 10 (10–12)	—	—	—
Briggs and Briggs (1973)	3 weeks	39 ± 8 (45)	41 ± 11 (12)	—	—	—	Mestranol (25)	d(l)-Norgestrel (1)
		39 ± 8 (45)	45 ± 13 (12)	—	—	—	Mestranol (50)	—
		39 ± 8 (45)	53 ± 10 (10)	—	—	—	Mestranol (75)	—
		39 ± 8 (45)	65 ± 13 (12)	—	—	—	Mestranol (100)	—
		39 ± 8 (45)	48 ± 5 (10)	—	—	—	Ethinylestradiol (10)	—
		39 ± 8 (45)	76 ± 8 (11)	—	—	—	Ethinylestradiol (50)	—
		39 ± 8 (45)	78 ± 10 (10)	—	—	—	Ethinylestradiol (75)	—
	3 weeks	37 ± 9 (20)	49 ± 18 (5)	—	—	—	—	Norethisterone (1)
		37 ± 9 (20)	54 ± 15 (5)	—	—	—	—	Norethisterone (10)
		37 ± 9 (20)	39 ± 12 (5)	—	—	—	—	Megestrol acetate (1)
		37 ± 9 (20)	41 ± 14 (5)	—	—	—	—	Megestrol acetate (10)

[a] All analyses data of copper and ceruloplasmin presented as mean ± S.D.; number of subjects in parentheses.
[b] Calculated from data provided.
[c] Sequential oral contraceptive; 100 μg of mestranol given on days 5–19 of the cycle, then 75 μg of mestranol and 5 mg norethynodrel on days 20–24.
[d] Sequential oral contraceptive; 75 μg of ethinylestradiol given on days 5–19 of cycle, then 75 μg of ethinylestradiol plus 5.0 mg of metroxyprogesterone given on days 20–24.
[e] Sequential oral contraceptive; 100 μg of mestranol given on days 5–19 of cycle, then 75 μg mestranol plus 5.0 mg of norethyprogesterone given on days 20–24.
[f] Each patient served as her own control.

A subsequent study from our laboratory (Halsted and Smith, 1970) involving a greater number of subjects also demonstrated a decreased plasma zinc concentration during pregnancy and while taking the oral contraceptive. These findings are shown in Table III.

As seen in Table III both pregnancy and oral contraceptives resulted in depressed plasma zinc concentrations. However, this study revealed that plasma zinc concentration was not depressed to as great an extent by the oral contraceptive as by pregnancy. Specifically, the mean difference between the controls and pregnant females was 34 μg/100 ml, compared to 16 μg/100 ml for the comparison of controls with those ingesting oral contraceptives ($p < 0.001$).

O'Leary and Spellacy (1969) noted in a preliminary report that plasma zinc was not significantly altered in sixteen subjects ingesting the oral contraceptive Enovid 10. Likewise, although the mean plasma zinc levels tended to be lower in thirty pregnant women, the differences were not statistically significant. However, Halsted et al. (1969) questioned the technique in respect to collection and preparation of samples and suggested a "strong probability of contamination," since the control values as well as those for pregnancy and women taking oral contraceptives were "much higher than is reasonable to expect."

Briggs et al. (1971b) also reported the effects of contraceptive steroids on plasma zinc. Twenty-five subjects were investigated, twenty women and five men, ranging in age from 18 to 38 years. Selected results from that study are shown in Table IV. The results indicate that a daily dose of 0.05 mg of the estrogen ethinylestradiol given alone or in combination with the progestogens norethisterone acetate or $d(l)$-norgestrel produced a significant decrease in plasma zinc.

Likewise, Schenker et al. (1971a) reported serum zinc levels in a large number of subjects taking various preparations of oral contraceptives, both combined and sequential. Specifically, serum zinc was determined in 342 cases, 251 subjects taking OCA and 91 controls. The results

TABLE III Plasma Zinc Concentrations in Pregnancy and After Oral Contraceptives

Subjects	Number	Zinc (μg/100 ml) (mean ± SD)	Significance level
Control	27	97 ± 11	—
Pregnant	107	63 ± 12	$p < 0.001$
On oral contraceptives	30	81 ± 14	$p < 0.001$

TABLE IV   Effect of Oral Contraceptive Steroids on Plasma Zinc Concentration[a]

Steroid	Daily oral dose (mg)	Plasma zinc (μg/100 ml) (mean ± SD)	Significance level
None	—	99 ± 14	—
Ethinylestradiol	0.05	83 ± 16	$p < 0.01$
Norethisterone acetate	1.0	99 ± 15	NS[b]
d(1)Norgestrel	0.25	100 ± 15	NS
Ethinylestradiol plus norethisterone acetate	0.05 + 1.0	82 ± 15	$p < 0.01$
Ethinylestradiol plus d(1)norgestrel	0.05 + 0.25	84 ± 12	$p < 0.01$

[a] Data from Briggs and Briggs, 1971b.
[b] Not significant.

indicated a significant decrease ($p < 0.001$) in plasma zinc concentration as a result of OCA use. The zinc concentration of the control group approximated 115 μg/100 ml (actual level not given), whereas the OCA users exhibited a mean of 97 μg/100 ml. In a subsequent paper, Schenker et al. (1972) presented data indicating a significant increase in erythrocyte carbonic anhydrase B during the use of oral contraceptives as well as during pregnancy. They speculated that the decrease in the concentration of zinc in the plasma of subjects taking oral contraceptives may result from a "shift of zinc from plasma to the red cells where it is incorporated mainly as carbonic anhydrase." However, analysis in our Laboratory, of erythrocytes from seventeen females who had been ingesting oral contraceptives from 2 months to 6 years revealed no significant increase in the zinc concentration.[*]

In addition, Briggs et al. (1971b) noted that a relatively high dosage (5 mg) of the progestogen norethisterone acetate also produced a "small decrease" in plasma zinc, 89 ± 15 μg/100 ml, compared to 99 ± 14 for the controls. They speculate that this could be due to the action of estrogenic metabolites of this progestogen.

The above results are similar to the findings of an investigation in our Laboratory (McBean et al., 1971) that studied the effect of oral contraceptive hormones on zinc metabolism in the rat. The design of the study included four groups of rats fed the following diets: (1)

[*] Smith, J. C., and McBean, L. D. (1975) Unpublished data. Veterans Administration Hospital, Washington, D.C.

TABLE V   Effect of OCA Hormones on Plasma Zinc Concentration in Female Rats

Hormone	Plasma zinc (μg/100 ml)	Significance level
None	181 ± 23	—
Norethindrone	169 ± 19	NS[a]
Mestranol	149 ± 7.5	$p < 0.02$
Norethindrone plus mestranol	157 ± 21	NS

[a] N.S., not significant.

control diet, (2) control diet containing norethindrone, (3) control diet containing mestranol, and (4) control diet containing norethindrone and mestranol. On a comparative body weight basis, the quantity of norethindrone and mestranol consumed by the rats was maintained at approximately ten times the amount in a daily dose of the oral contraceptive Ortho-Novum.* The duration of the experiment was 110 days. The results concerning the plasma zinc concentration are shown in Table V. The data indicate that the estrogen mestranol significantly lowered plasma zinc concentration, whereas the progestational agent (norethindrone) had little effect.

Aitken *et al.* (1973) reported the effect of the long-term administration of mestranol on plasma zinc concentration using a total of 231 subjects. The individuals studied included three groups: (1) 53 estrogen-treated oophorectomized women, (2) 128† oophorectomized without treatment, and (3) 50 women with hysterectomy alone. The estrogen-treated oophorectomized women received 20–40 μg of mestranol daily for at least 1 year prior to study. None of the other subjects were receiving hormone treatment. The results indicated that the estrogen-treated group had a significantly lower ($p < 0.001$) plasma zinc concentration than either control group. Specifically, the estrogen treated oophorectomized women had a plasma zinc concentration of 96.8 ± 10.6 μg/100 ml (mean ± SD), compared to 108.9 ± 11.5 or 106.8 ± 11.1 μg/100 ml for the oophorectomized or hysterectomized, respectively.

In contrast, a preliminary report by McKenzie (1974) involving eleven

* Ortho-Novum, Ortho Pharmaceutical Division, Raritan, New Jersey, contains 2 mg of norethindrone and 0.10 mg of mestranol.
† Calculated from information provided.

women aged 22–25 years noted that plasma zinc was unchanged after administration of the oral contraceptive. The initial serum zinc concentration before taking the oral contraceptive was (mean ± SD) 103 ± 19 μg/100 ml, compared to 108 ± 19 μg/100 ml after 3–10 months of ingesting the oral contraceptive.

In summary, there is some conflict in the literature in regard to the effect of oral contraceptive steroids on zinc metabolism as indicated by changes in plasma or serum zinc concentrations. Although the majority of reports indicate a significant decrease in plasma or serum zinc concentration after ingestion of the oral contraceptives or its estrogenic steroid two preliminary reports find no significant changes. One animal study reported depressed plasma zinc concentration in animals after ingestion of an estrogen alone. The levels fed were approximately ten times that in a daily human dose of oral contraceptive, on a comparative body weight. No human studies have reported the effect of the oral contraceptives on parameters of zinc metabolism other than plasma or serum concentrations. Since plasma copper and ceruloplasmin concentrations are often inversely related to plasma zinc concentration future studies should elucidate the significance of the increased levels of plasma copper and ceruloplasmin observed in the oral contraceptive users in respect to zinc metabolism. Specifically, depressed serum zinc concentrations in OCA users may be a result of increased serum copper and ceruloplasmin concentrations.

C. Iron

Iron-deficiency anemia is a common disorder among fertile women. Menstrual blood loss, pregnancy, or a marginal diet are frequently implicated in this problem. When early reports (Pincus et al., 1958; Rice-Wray et al., 1962; Larsson-Cohn, 1966; Nilsson and Solvell, 1967) concerning the effects of OCA noted decreased blood loss, investigators began to examine the effects of OCA on iron status.

Burton (1967) found that OCA users had significantly ($p < 0.001$) elevated levels of serum iron and total iron-binding capacity (TIBC), while hemoglobin levels remained normal. He compared thirty women using various combination type OCA to a group of thirty control women. The serum iron concentration for the control group was 89.3 ± 45.4 μg/100 ml (mean ± SD), while TIBC was 361.3 ± 49.0 μg/100 ml. In contrast, the OCA users had a mean serum iron concentration of 157.3 ± 78.6 μg/100 ml and a TIBC of 504.3 ± 87.7. After 12 months of OCA use, serum iron and TIBC remained elevated. Mardell and Zilva (1967) confirmed the findings of elevated serum iron and TIBC after examining eight OCA users. The women had used a variety of combination type OCA for periods ranging from 1 week to 4 years. Serum iron (126.4 ± 24.9 μg/100 ml versus 87.9 ± 31.0 μg/100 ml) and TIBC (449 ± 67.4 μg/100 ml versus 370 ± 32.2 μg/100 ml) were higher for the group of OCA users, regardless of length of treatment. Hemoglobin levels were not measured. Both groups of investigators (Burton, 1967; Mardell and Zilva, 1967) suggested that the circulating estrogens and/or progestogen was the key factor in the alterations in iron metabolism.

In regard to hemoglobin, it is generally agreed that pregnancy results in a decrease in hemoglobin concentration (McFee, 1973; Fisch and Freedman, 1973). However, there are conflicting results regarding the effect of OCA on hemoglobin. For example, Burton (1967) reported that hemoglobin remained unchanged in OCA users. However, Zadeh *et al.* (1967) presented data suggesting that "the steroid contraceptive pill of 'combined' formulation leads to an increase in the concentration of hemoglobin." However, their data do not clearly support such a broad statement. They tested ninety-four women receiving six different types of combined OCA. These users were compared to fifty-three control women. The mean hemoglobin level of the OCA users (13.7 ± 0.10 gm/100 ml, mean ± SE) did not differ significantly from the mean value of the controls (13.4 ± 0.11 gm/100 ml). Only when the proportion of women with a high hemoglobin concentration (greater than 14 gm/100 ml) was considered did the authors see a significant ($p < 0.01$) increase with OCA use after 1–12 months. Longer periods of use did not result in an increased proportion of women with high hemoglobin.

For sequential type OCA, Powell *et al.* (1970) found a significant increase in hemoglobin levels in twelve women subjects when compared to a group of controls (13.7 ± 0.46 gm/100 ml, mean ± SD versus 12.7 ± 0.7 gm/100 ml, respectively). The length of treatment was not indicated.

Likewise, a recent study (Fisch and Freedman, 1973) involving 1083 OCA [type or composition of OCA not given] users showed a slight but statistically significant decrease in hemoglobin level. However, the decrease was not nearly as marked as for 316 pregnant subjects.

Additional studies regarding hemoglobin levels are summarized in Table VI. It is evident that the majority of studies indicate no alteration due to OCA use. However, the number of subjects is often small.

Several reports have investigated transferrin concentration in order to explain the elevation of TIBC found in OCA users. Using polyacrylamide electrophoresis, Musa *et al.* (1967) found no change in transferrin concentration in eleven women receiving 0.5 mg ethinylestradiol

TABLE VI   Selected References Concerning Hemoglobin, Serum Iron, and TIBC in OCA Users[a]

Investigator	Length of treatment	Hemoglobin (%)(mean ± SD)			Serum Iron (μg/100 ml)(mean ± SD)		
		Control	OCA users	Significance level	Control	OCA users	Significance level
Burton (1967)	>6 months	13.2 ± 0.46 (30)	13.4 ± 0.96 (30)	NS	89.3 ± 45.4 (30)	157.3 ± 78.6 (30)	$p < 0.001$
Mardell and Zilva (1967)	1 week– 4 years	—	—	—	87.9 ± 31.0 (NG)	126.4 ± 24.9 (8)	—[b]
Zadeh et al. (1967)	1–24+ months[c]	13.4 ± 0.11[c] (53)	13.7 ± 0.10[c] (94)	NS	—	—	—
Thein et al. (1969)	2 months– 9 years	14.1 ± 1.2 (9)	13.9 ± 1.0 (9)	NS	90 ± 29[e] (9)	173 ± 55[e] (9)	$p < 0.01$
Mardell et al. (1969)	2 weeks– 4 years	14.3 ± 0.6 (21)	14.6 ± 1.1 (76)	NS	94 ± 43 (21)	116 ± 29 (76)	$p < 0.01$
Briggs and Staniford (1969)	2–4 cycles	13.4 ± 0.6 (3)	13.3 ± 0.7 (2)	NT	89 ± 25 (3)	112 ± 28 (2)	NT
	1–2 cycles	13.4 ± 0.6 (3)	13.2 ± 0.5 (6)	NT	89 ± 25 (3)	115 ± 21 (6)	NT
Jacobi et al. (1969)	3 months– 7 years	—	—	—	102 ± 38.1 (11)	175 ± 41.2 (37)	$p < 0.001$
		—	—	—	102 ± 38.1 (11)	159 ± 25.9 (8)	$p < 0.005$
Powell et al. (1970)	NG	12.7 ± 0.7 (10)	13.7 ± 0.46 (12)	$p < 0.01$	102 ± 38.1 (11)	133 ± 37.43 (11)	$p < 0.05$
Briggs and Briggs (1970)	3–4 weeks	—	—	—	93 ± 25 (10–12)	122 ± 28 (10–12)	NT
Briggs and Briggs (1972)	3 months	—	—	—	89 ± 25 (NG)	115 ± 21 (5)	NT
Norrby et al. (1972)	3 cycles	12.7 ± 1.3[h] (6)[i]	12.4 ± 1.3[h] (6)	NT	116 ± 65[e,h] (6)[i]	152 ± 58[e,h] (6)	NT

[a] Symbols: NG = not given, NS = not significant, NT = not tested. Number in each group given in ( ).
[b] The OCA users were considered to be "very significantly higher" than the controls by the authors, but the level of significance was not given.
[c] Standard error.
[d] Composition not reported by authors.
[e] Plasma iron.

| TIBC (μg/100 ml)(mean ± SD) | | | | | | |
Control	OCA users	Significance level	OCA brand name	Type	Estrogen component (μg)	Progestogen component (mg)
1.3 ± 49.0 (30)	504.3 ± 87.7 (30)	$p < 0.001$	Ovulen	Combination	Mestranol (100)	Ethynodiol diacetate (1)
			Lyndiol	Combination	Mestranol (150)	Lynestrenol (5)
			Lyndiol 2.5	Combination	Mestranol (75)	Lynestrenol (2.5)
			Gynovlar	Combination	Ethinylestradiol (50)	Norethisterone acetate (3)
0 ± 32.2 (NG)	449 ± 67.4 (8)	NT	Orthonovin (3)	Combination	Mestranol (100)	Norethisterone (2)
			Ovulen (2)	Combination	Mestranol (100)	Ethynodiol diacetate (1)
			Anovlar (1)	Combination	Ethinylestradiol (50)	Norethisterone acetate (4)
			Lyndiol (1)	Combination	Mestranol (150)	Lynestrenol (5)
			Volidan (1)	Combination	Ethinylestradiol (50)	Megestrol acetate (4)
—	—	—	Anovlar[d]	Combination	Ethinylestradiol (50)	Norethisterone acetate (4)
			Gynovlar[d]	Combination	Ethinylestradiol (50)	Norethisterone acetate (3)
			Lyndiol[d]	Combination	Mestranol (150)	Lynestrenol (5)
			Ortho-Novin[d]	Combination	Mestranol (100)	Norethisterone (2)
			Ovulen[d]	Combination	Mestranol (100)	Ethynodiol diacetate (1)
			Ovran[d]	Combination	Ethinylestradiol (50)	Norgestrel (0.5)
0 ± 33 (9)	359 ± 61 (9)	$p < 0.01$	Lyndiol[d]	Combination	Mestranol (150)	Lynestrenol (5)
			Orthonovum 1[d]	Combination	Mestranol (50)	Norethindrone (1)
			Orthonovum 2[d]	Combination	Mestranol (100)	Norethindrone (2)
			Ovulen[d]	Combination	Mestranol (100)	Ethynodiol diacetate (1)
8 ± 31 (21)	445 ± 54 (76)	$p < 0.001$	Ovulen (21)	Combination	Mestranol (100)	Ethynodiol diacetate (1)
			Gynovlar (13)	Combination	Ethinylestradiol (50)	Norethisterone acetate (3)
			Ortho-Novin (12)	Combination	Mestranol (100)	Norethisterone (2)
			Lyndiol 2.5 (10)	Combination	Mestranol (75)	Lynestrenol (2.5)
			Lyndiol (8)	Combination	Mestranol (150)	Lynestrenol (5)
			Volidan (5)	Combination	Ethinylestradiol (50)	Megestrol acetate (4)
			Anovlar (4)	Combination	Ethinylestradiol (50)	Norethisterone acetate (4)
			Norinyl (1)	Combination	Mestranol (50)	Norethisterone (1)
			Sequens[f] (2)	Sequential	Mestranol[f]	Chlormadione acetate[f] (2)
58 ± 38 (3)	465 ± 65 (2)	NT	Minovlar (2)	Combination	Ethinylestradiol (50)	Norethisterone acetate (1)
58 ± 38 (3)	428 ± 59 (6)	NT	SH 420 C (6)	Progestogen only	—	Norethisterone acetate (0.3)
37 ± 49.4 (11)	512 ± 66.4 (36)	$p < 0.001$	NG	Combination	—	—
37 ± 49.4 (11)	511 ± 101.0 (8)	$p < 0.005$	NG	Sequential	—	—
37 ± 49.4 (11)	554 ± 89.87 (11)	$p < 0.001$	Neonovum[g]	Sequential	Mestranol[g] (100)	Anagestone[g] (0.125/0.25)
			ORF 1658[g]	Sequential	Mestranol[g] (100)	Anagestone[g] (1/2)
			SQI III[g]	Sequential	Mestranol[g] (100)	Anagestone[g] 0.25/0.50
51 ± 35 (10–12)	465 ± 65 (10–12)	NT	Minovlar	Combination	Ethinylestradiol (50)	Norethisterone acetate(1)
58 ± 38 (NG)	428 ± 59 (5)	NT	NG	Progestogen only	—	Norethisterone acetate (0.3)
08 ± 62[h] (6)	383 ± 44[h] (6)	NT	Conlunett (6)	Combination	Mestranol (100)	Norethisterone (1)

[f] Sequential type preparation—mestranol for 15 days of cycle and mestranol and chlormadione for 5 days of cycle.
[g] Sequential type preparation—mestranol for days 5–25 of a cycle, anagestone taken at the first level for days 12–18 and at the second levels for days 19–25. Each patient acted as her own control.
[h] Standard deviations calculated from data provided.
[i] Each patient acted as her own control.

or 0.25 mg ethinylestradiol plus one tablet of Enovid-E (0.1 mg ethinyl-estradiol-3 methyl ether and 2.5 mg norethynodrel). The women served as their own controls, contributing a blood sample before treatment and one after only 20 days of treatment. The authors concluded that transferrin levels failed to respond to "estrogen treatment."

Mardell *et al.* (1969) also treated patients for 20 days and used poly-acrylamide electrophoresis to estimate transferrin concentration. Two volunteers received Volidan (4 mg megestrol acetate and 0.05 mg ethinylestradiol) or Orthonovin (2 mg norethisterone and 0.1 mg mestra-nol). As illustrated in Fig. 1, the rise with TIBC during OCA treatment was paralleled with an increase in transferrin concentration. Both levels decreased with the removal of hormone treatment.

Jacobi *et al.* (1969) used a direct immunochemical technique to mea-sure transferrin levels in forty women receiving a combined OCA and nine taking a sequential type. Transferrin as well as TIBC were signifi-cantly ($p < 0.001$) elevated in both types of OCA when compared to a group of twenty-two control women. The mean immunochemical trans-ferrin level (mg/100 ml) for the control group was 279 ± 58.5 (mean $\pm$ SD), while the combined type OCA group mean was 464 ± 81.7 and the sequential type OCA group was 444 ± 97.0. TIBC

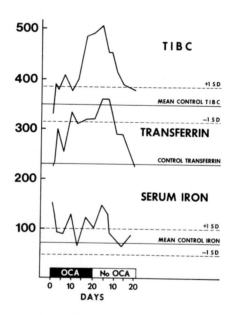

FIG. 1. Effect of oral contraceptive agents (OCA) on the concentration of serum iron (µg/100 ml), transferrin (mg/100 ml), and total iron-binding capacity (TIBC) (µg/100 ml) in one volunteer. Modified from Mardell *et al.* (1969).

(μg/100 ml) values were 387 ± 49.4 for the control group, 512 ± 66.4 for the combined OCA users, and 511 ± 101.0 for the sequential OCA users. SGOT values were normal in all groups. Thus, the authors suggest that the increase in transferrin with OCA use is not due to liver damage but perhaps to increased protein synthesis.

Horne et al. (1970) also used an immunoassay to confirm that transferrin levels are increased with OCA use. Seven women received Ovulen (1 mg ethynodiol diacetate and 0.1 mg mestranol) and two received Norinyl-1 (1 mg norethisterone with 0.05 mg mestranol). Transferrin levels measured after 2–6 weeks of treatment were significantly higher. Transferrin concentration was 278 ± 68 mg/100 ml (mean ± SD) before treatment and 375 ± 84 mg/100 ml after treatment for the nine women.

There has been considerable controversy concerning which specific hormone from OCA affects transferrin levels. As noted previously, Musa et al. (1967) concluded that transferrin levels did not respond to "estrogen treatment." However, Briggs and Staniford (1969) investigated two women receiving Minovlar, a combination type OCA (1 mg norethisterone acetate and 0.05 mg ethinylestradiol) for two to four cycles and six receiving SH 420 C, a progestogen-only preparation (0.3 mg norethisterone acetate) for one to two cycles. These OCA users were compared to three control women. Serum iron and TIBC increased in both groups of OCA users when compared with the control group. Serum iron (μg/100 ml) was 89 ± 25 (mean ± SD) for the control group, 112 ± 28 for the Minovlar users, and 115 ± 21 for the SH 420 C users, while TIBC (μg/100 ml) was 358 ± 38 for the controls, 465 ± 65 for the Minovlar users, and 428 ± 59 for the SH 420 C users. The authors concluded that these changes were induced by norethisterone acetate and not estrogen. A later study (Briggs and Briggs, 1972) on five women using the same dose of norethindrone acetate (0.3 mg) supported this conclusion. Progesten treatment increased both serum iron (115 ± 21 μg/100 ml, mean ± SD versus 89 ± 25 μg/100 ml) and TIBC (428 ± 59 mg/100 ml versus 358 ± 38 mg/100 ml) when compared to a control group.

Powell et al. (1970) challenged the conclusion that progestogen therapy influences iron metabolism in OCA use. They claimed that the progestogen norethisterone acetate used by Briggs and Staniford has estrogenic metabolites. Powell et al. administered medroxyprogesterone acetate, a pure progestational agent that has no estrogenic properties, to eighteen women who had previously taken an OCA of the sequential type. During OCA treatment (sequential), seum iron, TIBC, and transferrin concentrations were elevated. Specifically, serum iron, TIBC, and transferrin concentrations during the treatment period were 133 ± 37.43

$\mu g/100$ ml (mean $\pm$ SD), 554 ± 89.87 $\mu g/100$ ml, and 455 ± 98.89 $\mu g/100$ ml, in contrast to the control values of 102 ± 32.1, 387 ± 49.4, and 279 ± 58.5, respectively. However, these levels decreased significantly after treatment was stopped and 300 mg medroxyprogesterone acetate was given by injection. The authors conclude that the data indicate that alterations in serum iron, TIBC, and transferrin resulting from the administration of OCA are due to the estrogen rather than the progestogen component.

Briggs and Briggs (1970) responded to Powell et al. (1970) by noting that medroxyprogesterone acetate has considerable glucocorticoid activity, and the effect of corticoid–sex hormone interactions on iron metabolism is unknown. They presented data in which various doses of oral estrogen and progesterone were given separately and in combination to groups of ten to twelve healthy young women for 3–4 weeks. The results are shown in Table VII. Ethinylestradiol and norethisterone acetate together produced an increase in serum iron and TIBC. The estrogen component alone in doses up to 50 μg daily did not have an effect on these parameters. In contrast both norethisterone acetate and $d(l)$-norgestrel, a progestogen virtually free of estrogenic metabolites, increased serum iron, and TIBC.

Another area of controversy concerns the relationship of changes in serum iron to TIBC and transferrin. Briggs and Staniford (1969) maintain that increases in serum transferrin cause the elevated serum iron levels in OCA users, since both parameters increase with OCA treatment. Zilva (1969) and Mardell et al. (1969) contend that the changes in

TABLE VII   Effect of Varying Levels of Contraceptive Steroids on Serum Iron and TIBC[a]

Steroid	Daily dose[b]	Serum iron ($\mu g/100$ ml) (mean $\pm$ SD)	TIBC ($\mu g/100$ ml) (mean $\pm$ SD)
None	—	93 ± 25	361 ± 35
Ethinylestradiol	10	95 ± 28	355 ± 38
	20	96 ± 31	359 ± 32
	50	90 ± 30	365 ± 40
Norethisterone acetate	300	118 ± 21	428 ± 49
	1000	119 ± 30	425 ± 51
Ethinylestradiol + norethisterone acetate	50 } +1000 }	122 ± 28	465 ± 65
$d(1)$-Norgestrel	1000	118 ± 25	432 ± 42

[a] Data from Briggs and Briggs (1970).
[b] 10–12 women in each treatment group.

levels are independent of each other. They note that serum iron levels change during the menstrual cycle and in early stages of pregnancy, and this change cannot be accounted for by changes in TIBC. Furthermore, they cite one individual case (Mardell *et al.*, 1969) where serum iron did not increase while TIBC did. However, neither group has presented definitive evidence for either viewpoint.

Thein *et al.* (1969) examined the question of blood loss and iron metabolism in OCA users. Only women with a measured menstrual iron loss of less than 0.2 mg. per day were included in their study. This level of iron loss was well below the mean of 0.51 mg iron lost for sixty-four untreated women volunteers. There were nine subjects in a control group and nine in a group taking a combination type of OCA. None of the subjects was taking iron supplements. Even with comparable menstrual loss, OCA were associated with significant elevations of plasma iron and TIBC. The OCA group had a mean plasma iron (μg/100 ml) of 173 ± 55, while the control group mean was 90 ± 29. The mean TIBC (μg/100 ml) was 359 ± 61 in the OCA group and 270 ± 33 in the control group.

Recently, Norrby *et al.* (1972) completed a detailed study on the influence of OCA on iron absorption and metabolism. The absorption of iron and blood parameters were measured by a whole body counter after a dose of $^{59}Fe^{2+}$ as ferrous sulfate at four different time periods in six healthy women. Two study periods occurred before OCA administration. The first study was under basal conditions and the second after a phlebotomy of 400 ml of blood. Then the blood was reinfused to reestablish basal conditions. After three cycles of receiving Conlunett (1 mg norethisterone and 0.1 mg mestranol), the two study periods were repeated. All menstrual losses were measured and an additional phlebotomy during OCA treatment compensated for diminished menstrual losses. Table VIII summarizes the author's observations. No statistical analyses were reported, but trends are evident. A statistical analysis by us from the data provided generally verified these trends, though large variations prevented acceptable confidence levels ($p < 0.05$) for some comparisons. Mean hemoglobin and hematocrit were similar before and during OCA therapy, while phlebotomy had no significant effect on either parameter. Contraceptive therapy tended to raise the plasma iron from the basal period and after phlebotomy, though individual variations were large. After both phlebotomies, plasma iron was markedly lowered. TIBC significantly increased with contraceptive therapy and also was raised after phlebotomy. In all subjects, phlebotomy induced an increased iron absorption; however, OCA treatment had no apparent effect.

TABLE VIII   Effect of OCA Use and Blood Loss on Various Parameters of Iron Metabolism[a]

	Before OCA		During OCA	
Parameter	Basal	After phlebotomy	Basal	After phlebotomy
Hemoglobin (gm/100 ml)	12.7 ± 1.3	12.0 ± 1.0	12.4 ± 1.3	11.7 ± 1.0
Hematocrit (%)	38.6 ± 2.6	36.1 ± 1.7	38.6 ± 2.6	36.5 ± 1.8
Plasma iron (μg/100 ml)	116 ± 65	55 ± 24	152 ± 58	72 ± 46
TIBC (μg/100 ml)	308 ± 62	332 ± 57	383 ± 44	436 ± 57
Iron absorption (%)	52.8 ± 16.7	82.2 ± 17.4	51.8 ± 29.4	80.2 ± 12.1

[a] Data from Norrby et al. (1972). Mean ± SD; $N = 6$ for all parameters; SD calculated from data provided.

Norrby *et al.* (1972) suggested four possible causes for increased plasma iron during OCA use:

1. *Increased iron absorption.* Their study found no influence by OCA on iron absorption.

2. *Decreased blood loss due to decreased menstrual losses.* Elevated plasma iron levels occurred during OCA therapy in spite of unchanged blood loss.

3. *Decreased erythropoiesis.* Hemoglobin and hematocrit were unchanged with OCA and the response to phlebotomy was similar to untreated controls.

4. *Increased mobilization from stores.* By eliminating the other three possibilities the authors conclude that increased plasma iron during OCA use is due to increased mobilization from iron stores. Although bone marrow hemosiderin was examined, no change after OCA treatment was observed. However, marked increases in plasma iron would decrease stores by only a few milligrams of iron; thus, it would be unlikely for bone marrow smears to reflect the change.

These conclusions have important implications and need to be confirmed. Also, this particular study was concerned only with the response to OCA after three cycles. After a longer period of time, iron absorption and mobilization may change in response to OCA.

After reviewing the effect of OCA on iron metabolism, Theuer (1972) has suggested that the dietary needs of women taking OCA may be slightly less than normal women. However, no reported balance studies have been performed to test this hypothesis.

In summary, OCA appear to have a significant effect on iron metabolism. Serum iron and TIBC are consistently elevated in OCA users. Hemoglobin is usually reported to be unchanged or only slightly altered. OCA treatment seems to result in an increase in transferrin, which in turn causes the elevated TIBC. A controversy exists concerning which component, estrogen or progestin, is responsible for the rise in transferrin. Also, it is unclear if serum iron and TIBC rise independently with OCA treatment or if serum iron rises as a result of an increased TIBC.

Apparently, decreased menstrual losses cannot account for the altered iron metabolism in OCA users. Comparing OCA users and controls with similar menstrual losses or adjusting decreased menstrual losses with a phlebotomy did not eliminate the association between OCA treatment and elevated serum iron and TIBC. Furthermore, no difference was found in iron absorption after three cycles of OCA treatment.

It is clearly established that OCA use elevates serum iron and TIBC. Additional experiments, including iron turnover and balance studies, are required to elucidate the mechanisms of these changes and their effect on iron metabolism and status.

D. Magnesium

Magnesium, although not a trace element by usual definitions, has been included in our review because this element has been demonstrated to be involved in numerous metabolic reactions, including the blood clotting mechanism. In addition, recent reports have implicated magnesium in various thrombotic syndromes (Allanby et al., 1966; Durlach, 1967). In view of the involvement of magnesium in the clotting mechanism (Szelenyi, 1973), and the apparent link between OCA and thromboembolism (Sartwell et al., 1969), the magnesium status in OCA users should receive serious consideration. However, the effect of OCA on magnesium status, including serum or plasma magnesium, has not been clearly established.

In regard to the reports implicating magnesium as an important factor in various thrombotic syndromes, Allanby et al. (1966) successfully treated a patient with thrombotic microangiopathy with heparin and magnesium. They felt magnesium was an important part of the recovery of their patient. Durlach (1967) observed one patient with magnesium-deficiency phlebothrombosing disease. Plasma, erythrocyte, and platelet levels; urinary magnesium ratios; and magnesium balance confirmed the deficiency and "oral magnesium therapy with physiological doses controlled the whole clinical pattern." Thus, it appears that magnesium deficiency may result in thrombosis.

Inman et al. (1970) noted a positive correlation between the dose of estrogen in OCA and thromboembolic disease. No significant differences could be detected between sequential and combined OCA containing the same doses of estrogen, nor between the two estrogens ethinylestradiol and mestranol.

Goldsmith and Goldsmith (1966) reported lowered serum magnesium concentrations in users of Enovid-5, a combination type OCA (5 mg norethynodrel and 0.075 mg mestranol) after 3–33 months of treatment. Forty-six samples from four OCA users differed significantly ($p < 0.001$) from 175 samples from ten normally ovulating women. The OCA users had a mean serum magnesium (mEq/liter) of 1.53 ± 0.09 (mean $\pm$ SD) in contrast to the control group mean of 1.82 ± 0.11. When urinary magnesium was determined for four OCA users and four controls, the authors found a significant decrease among the OCA users (2.6 ± 0.5 μEq/min for OCA users versus 4.6 ± 0.8 μEq/min for the control group). Thus, they concluded that the decrease in serum magnesium content was not due to increased excretion. Rather, they suggest that the data indicate an alteration in magnesium metabolism. A subsequent study (Goldsmith et al., 1970) comparing four Enovid users to five normal ovulating women demonstrated a decrease in serum magnesium at the time of ovulation in normal women (about 0.15 mEq/liter) and a significant decline (0.15 mEq/liter) during the first 8 days of Enovid usage. The authors advance the theory that increased estrogen levels at ovulation and during contraceptive therapy may cause the observed decrease in serum magnesium. They speculate that serum magnesium may decline due to estrogen inhibition of bone resorption. Alternatively, increased intracellular binding may occur due to increased protein synthesis.

In contrast, Thin (1971) found no detectable effect of OCA treatment on levels of magnesium in the plasma, platelets, and red-blood cells in ten users of Gynovlar (0.05 mg ethinylestradiol and 3 mg norethisterone acetate). Mean values (standard deviation not given) before treatment (1.98 mg/100 ml, 0.34 mg/gm dry weight, and 4.42 mg/gm cells, respectively) were compared at 3 months (1.98 mg/100 ml, 0.47 mg/gm dry weight, and 4.09 mg/gm cells), and 6 months (1.92 mg/100 ml, 0.47 mg/gm dry weight, and 4.41 mg/gm cells). A second group of Gynovlar users had no significant change in all of the blood magnesium parameters after 1–4 years of treatment when compared to the before treatment group.

Dale and Simpson (1972) used a large sample of women [131 controls and 96 users of a combination OCA (100 μg mestranol and 1 mg ethynodiol diacetate)] to investigate serum magnesium in OCA users. There were no significant differences between the two groups (2.12 ± 0.31 mg/100 ml, mean $\pm$ SD for the controls versus 2.09 ± 0.38 mg/100 ml for the OCA users). Furthermore, no differences were noted when serum magnesium levels were arranged by known cycle day. When the data was examined in regard to length of treatment (0–3 months, 7–12 months, and >12 months), no significant differences were found.

Dale and Simpson (1972) also reported that ninety-eight women receiving a long-acting injectable progestin, depomedroxyprogesterone acetate (DMPA), had serum magnesium concentrations significantly higher than the control group (2.29 ± 0.21 mg/100 ml, mean ± SD, for the DMPA group versus 2.12 ± 0.31 mg/100 ml for the controls). The dose of DMPA injected and the length of treatment were not given. Using an oral progestogen, Briggs and Briggs (1972) did not find a significant alteration in serum magnesium. Five women receiving norethisterone acetate (0.3 mg daily) for 3 months had a mean magnesium concentration of 2.3 ± 0.2 mg/100 ml (mean ± SD), while a control group had a mean of 2.5 ± 0.2 mg/100 ml.

The different results among investigations may be due to the composition of the contraceptive preparations used. Table IX summarizes the type of OCA used and the reported effects on serum or plasma magnesium. Thin (1971) notes that the higher dose of estrogen in Enovid, such as used by Goldsmith and Goldsmith (1966) in their investigations, may affect serum magnesium, while a lower dose may fail to elicit a response. Also, Dale and Simpson (1972) speculate that a possible counterbalancing effect exists between some progestational steroids and the estrogen component in the combination type of OCA.

In summary, the effect of OCA on magnesium metabolism has not been clearly delineated. Only a few studies have been conducted and often with too few subjects. Blood magnesium may be dependent on the dosage of the steroids, particularly the estrogen component. Additional studies with a larger number of women receiving various levels of estrogens are needed to establish the effect of OCA on magnesium metabolism, particularly in view of the reported complications of estrogen related thromboembolism.

E. Iodine

The parameters of iodine metabolism that have received the most investigational attention have not been concerned directly with iodine per se but rather with thyroid function. These parameters have included the concentration of protein bound iodine (PBI) and thyroxine binding globulin (TBG) in the plasma or serum, the uptake of ^{131}I by the thyroid, and the uptake of $[^{131}I]$triiodothyronine (T_3) by red blood cells and resin (Starup and Friis, 1967). It has been shown previously that in-

TABLE IX   Plasma or Serum Magnesium Concentrations in OCA Users

Reference	Length of treatment	OCA users[a] (mean ± SD) (mg%)	Number of Patients	Controls[a] (mean ± SD) (mg%)	Number of Patients	Level of significance	OCA brand name	Type	Estrogen component (μg)	Progestogen component (mg)
Goldsmith and Goldsmith (1966)	3–33 months	1.53 ± 0.09 (S)	4	1.82 ± 0.11 (S)	10	$p < 0.001$	Enovid[b]	Combination	Mestranol[b] (75)	Norethynodrel[b] (5)
Thin (1971)	6 months	1.92[c] (P)	10	1.98[c,d] (P)	10	N.S.	Gynovlar	Combination	Ethinylestradiol (50)	Norethisterone acetate (3)
Dale and Simpson (1972)	1–4 years	1.93[c] (P)	10	1.98[c,d] (P)	10	N.S.	—[e]	Combination	Mestranol (100)	Ethynodiol diacetate (1)
		2.09 ± 0.38 (S)	96	2.12 ± 0.31 (S)	131	N.S.	—[e]	Progestogen only[f]	—	Depomedroxy-progesterone acetate[f] (—[e])
		2.29 ± 0.21 (S)	98	2.12 ± 0.31 (S)	131	$p < 0.001$	—[e]	Progestogen only	—	Norethisterone acetate (0.3)
Briggs and Briggs (1972)	3 months	2.3 ± 0.2 (S)	5	2.5 ± 0.2 (S)	—[e]	N.S.	—[e]	Progestogen only	—	Norethisterone acetate (0.3)

[a] S = serum; P = plasma; N.S., not significant; meq/liter reported by Goldsmith and Goldsmith; all other references used mg %.
[b] Composition not reported by authors.
[c] No standard deviation given.
[d] The control group represents the pretreatment mean for the patients receiving OCA for 6 months.
[e] Not reported.
[f] Injected.

creased PBI values and decreased levels of red-cell or resin uptake of triiodothyronine are characteristically associated with normal pregnancy (Sterling and Tabachnick, 1961; Goolden *et al.*, 1967; Hamolsky *et al.*, 1959). For reviews concerning thyroid function in pregnancy, see Man (1972); for thyroid function during OCA use, see Weindling and Henry (1974). In addition, several studies have indicated that an increase of TBG and PBI occurs after the administration of estrogens to human subjects (Alexander and Mormorston, 1961; Engbring and Engstrom, 1959; Ingbar and Freinkel, 1960). Likewise, it was reported earlier that the red-cell uptake of T_3 was decreased during treatment with estrogens (Hamolsky *et al.*, 1959). Thus, Winikoff and Taylor (1966) suggested that the concentration of PBI and parameters related to binding capacity will be altered in proportion to the amount of estrogen present in the OCA.

In regard to the effect of progestogens alone on thyroid function, Hollander *et al.* (1963) reported an increase in PBI and a reduced red-cell uptake for triiodothyronine in thirty-eight euthyroid women who received 5 mg of norethynodrel for 20 days. The mean concentration of protein-bound iodine was 7.9 μg/100 ml, compared to 5.5 μg/100 ml for normal females. In contrast, three males who received 5.0 mg of the progestogen medroxyprogesterone acetate for 20 days showed no significant change in PBI.

Several investigators have found no significant change in the uptake of ^{131}I by the thyroid after treatment with a combination of estrogens and progestogens (Irizarry *et al.*, 1966; Winikoff and Taylor, 1966; Starup and Friis, 1967). However, Fisher *et al.* (1966) and Williams *et al.* (1966) reported significant decreases in the resin uptake of T_3 during treatment with norethynodrel plus mestranol. In addition, Winikoff and Taylor (1966) and Starup and Friis (1967) observed significant decreases in the resin or red blood cell uptake of T_3 during treatment with several different oral contraceptives.

The majority of studies have reported significant increases in protein-bound iodine during oral contraception (Florsheim and Faircloth, 1964; Larsson-Cohn, 1965, 1969). However, Walser *et al.* (1964) found no significant change in protein-bound iodine during treatment with norethisterone acetate plus ethinylestradiol. Starup and Friis (1967) reported "a definite, but not significant, increase in protein-bound iodine" in eighty-one euthyroid women treated cyclically with a daily dose of 5 mg of megestrol acetate plus 0.1 mg of mestranol for an average of 16 months.

In a comprehensive study of the effects of different types of oral contraceptives on thyroid metabolism, Larsson-Cohn (1969) reported that protein-bound iodine was increased and the resin uptake of $[^{125}I]T_3$

was decreased in women taking combined or sequential OCA. Specifically, a total of 277 women aged 16–42 years (mean 26.0 years) and taking various types of oral contraceptives were studied. A group consisting of forty-seven women with a similar mean age served as controls. The results indicated that the protein-bound iodine of the control group was 5.1 ± 1.2 $\mu g/ml$ of plasma (mean $\pm$ SD) and the $[^{125}I]T_3$ resin uptake was $98 \pm 10\%$. For 119 subjects receiving four types of combined oral contraceptives, the protein-bound iodine increased to 7.3 ± 1.5 $\mu g/ml$ of plasma, whereas the $[^{125}I]T_3$ uptake was decreased to $70 \pm 9\%$. In contrast, neither the PBI nor the $[^{125}I]T_3$ uptake was altered in 116 subjects receiving "low doses" of progestogens administered daily. These data suggested that progestogens had no effect on protein-bound iodine and T_3 uptake, indicating that the estrogen component was responsible for the changes observed.

In summary, the majority of investigations report that protein-bound iodine is increased and T_3 uptake is decreased with OCA treatment. The estrogen component appears to be the causative agent.

III. FUTURE RESEARCH NEEDS

More than six million United States women are routinely ingesting exogenous steroids for a nonclinical reason, i.e., to prevent contraception. Some of these individuals have been using this method of contraception for more than a decade. We feel that one of the most pressing research needs regards the heretofore uninvestigated effect of long-term alterations in trace element metabolism. For example, does the sustained elevation of serum copper and ceruloplasmin with the probable depression of serum zinc represent a clinical hazard? Presumably, during pregnancy, changes such as the increased serum copper and ceruloplasmin levels are in response to a biochemical or physiological need that subsides after termination of pregnancy, resulting in a return to normal range for these biochemical entities. However, in the case of OCA users, the changes in serum copper, ceruloplasmin, and other trace element levels result from exogenous synthetic steroids. These long-term effects of sustained alterations in trace element concentrations in nonpregnant females remain unknown and may represent a hazard.

Metabolic balance studies are also needed. Although cumbersome, they would add valuable information as to whether the dietary requirements of trace elements are altered by OCA usage. It should be noted that an alteration in the plasma level of a trace element does not necessarily reflect changes in dietary requirements.

As methods become available to quantitate the "newer" essential trace elements (e.g., chromium and nickel), investigations concerning the effect of oral contraceptive steroids on the metabolism of these elements should be initiated. Lastly, since OCA usage may result in alterations in the metabolism of other nutrients, such as vitamins A and B_6, it is important to study the interrelationships between trace elements and other nutrients. It is conceivable that the change in metabolism of a particular vitamin is a result of a primary effect on the metabolism of a specific trace element.

In summary, additional studies with a greater number of subjects are needed concerning the specific effects of OCA on trace element metabolism. The majority of studies simply have surveyed the trace element status in OCA users, usually noting that blood levels of certain trace elements are altered.

Now that alterations in trace element metabolism have become apparent, it is imperative to determine why such changes occur and to delineate more carefully the mechanisms involved. In addition, the clinical consequences of these prolonged alterations now deserve serious and definitive study.

ACKNOWLEDGMENTS

We gratefully acknowledge Dr. J. A. Halsted, Clinical Professor of Medicine, Albany Medical College, Albany, New York; Dr. U. S. Seal, Director of VACURG Reference Laboratory, Veteran's Administration Hospital, Minneapolis, Minnesota; Dr. G. P. Schechter, Chief, Hematology Research, Veteran's Administration Hospital, Washington, D.C., for review of the manuscript and helpful suggestions. In addition, we thank Mary Netzow, Chief Librarian, and her staff for assistance with the references.

This research has been supported in part by NIH NICHD Contract No. 1-HD-2-2783.

REFERENCES

Aitken, J. M., Lindsay, R., and Hart, D. M. (1973). Plasma zinc in pre- and post-menopausal women: Its relationship to oestrogen therapy. *Clin. Sci.* **44**, 91–94.

Alexander, R. W., and Mormorston, J. (1961). Effect of two synthetic estrogens on the level of serum protein-bound iodine in men and women with atherosclerotic heart disease. *J. Clin. Endocrinol. Metab.* **21**, 243–251.

Allanby, K. D., Huntsman, R. G., and Sacker, L. S. (1966). Thrombotic microangiopathy. Recovery of a case of heparin and magnesium therapy. *Lancet* **1**, 237–239.

Bernstein, G. S., Israel, R., Seward, P., and Mishell, D. R. (1972). Clinical experience with Cu-7 intrauterine device. *Contraception* **6**, 99–107.

Breuer, H. (1964). Studies on the metabolism of 17-ethinyl-19-nortestosterone. *Int. J. Fert.* **9**, 181–187.

Briggs, M., and Briggs, M. (1973). Effects of some contraceptive steroids on serum proteins of women. *Biochem. Pharmacol.* **22**, 2277–2281.

Briggs, M., and Staniford, M. (1969). Oral contraceptives and blood iron. *Lancet* **2**, 742.

Briggs, M., Austin, J., and Staniford, M. (1970). Oral contraceptives and copper metabolism. *Nature (London)* **225**, 81.

Briggs, M. H., and Briggs, M. (1970). Contraceptives and serum proteins. *Brit. Med. J.* **3**, 521–522.

Briggs, M. H., and Briggs, M. (1971a). Effects of oral ethinylestradiol on serum proteins in normal women. *Contraception* **3**, 381–386.

Briggs, M. H., Briggs, M., and Austin, J. (1971b). Effects of steroid pharmaceuticals on plasma zinc. *Nature (London)* **232**, 480–481.

Briggs, M. H., and Briggs, M. (1972). Preliminary studies on metabolic effects of a continuous-dose, progestogen-only, oral contraceptive. *Afr. J. Med. Sci.* **3**, 105–115.

Brown, J. B., and Blair, H. A. F. (1960). Urinary estrogen metabolites of 19-norethisterone and its esters. (Summary.) *Proc. Roy. Soc. Med.* **53**, 433.

Burton, J. L. (1967). Effect of oral contraceptives on haemoglobin, packed cell volume, serum-iron, and total iron-binding capacity in healthy women. *Lancet* **1**, 978–980.

Carruthers, M. E., Hobbs, C. B, and Warren, R. L. (1966). Raised serum copper and caeruloplasmin levels in subjects taking oral contraceptives. *J. Clin. Pathol.* **19**, 498–500.

Cartwright, G. E. (1950). In "Copper Metabolism; A Symposium on Animal, Plant, and Soil Relationships" (W. D. McElroy and B. Glass, eds.), p. 274. Johns Hopkins Press, Baltimore, Maryland.

Dale, E., and Simpson, G. (1972). Serum magnesium levels of women taking an oral or long-term injectable progestational contraceptive. *Obstet. Gynecol.* **39**, 115–119.

Daunter, B., and Elstein, M. (1973). Serum levels of copper, caeruloplasmin and caeruloplasmin oxidase activity in women using copper-containing intrauterine devices and in women taking combined oral contraceptives. *J. Obstet. Gynaecol. Brit. Commonw.* **80**, 644–647.

Dawson, E. B., Frey, M. J., Monistere, N., and McGanity, W. J. (1973). Essential metals in oral contraceptive tablets. *Amer. J. Obstet. Gynecol.* **116**, 412–414.

Durlach, L. (1967). Magnesium-deficiency thrombosis. *Lancet* **1**, 1382.

Engbring, N. H., and Engstrom, W. W. (1959). Effects of estrogen and testosterone on circulating thyroid hormone. *J. Clin. Endocrinol. Metab.* **19**, 783–796.

Fisch, I. R., and Freedman, S. H. (1973). Oral contraceptives and the red blood cell. *Clin. Pharmacol. Ther.* **14**, 245–249.

Fisher, D. A., Oddie, T. H., and Epperson, D. (1966). Norethynodrel-mestranol and thyroid function. *J. Clin. Endocrinol. Metab.* **26**, 878–884.

Florsheim, W. H., and Faircloth, M. A. (1964). Effects of oral ovulation inhibitors on serum protein-bound iodine and thyroxine binding proteins. *Proc. Soc. Exp. Biol. Med.* **117**, 56–58.

Gault, M. H., Stein, J., and Aronoff, A. (1966). Serum ceruloplasmin in hepatobiliary and other disorders: Significance of abnormal values. *Gastroenterology* **50**, 8–18.

Goldsmith, N. F., and Goldsmith, J. R. (1966). Epidemiological aspects of magnesium and calcium metabolism. *Arch. Environ. Health* **12**, 607–619.

Goldsmith, N. F., Pace, N., Baumberger, J. P., and Ury, H. (1970). Magnesium and citrate during the menstrual cycle: Effect of an oral contraceptive on serum magnesium. *Fert. Steril.* **21**, 292–300.

Goolden, A. W. G., Gartside, J. M., and Sanderson, C. (1967). Thyroid status in pregnancy and in women taking oral contraceptives. Lancet 1, 12–15.

Hagenfeldt, K. (1972). Intrauterine contraception with the copper-T device. I. Effect on trace elements in the endometrium, cervical mucus and plasma. Contraception 6, 37–54.

Haller, J. (1969). "Hormonal Contraception." Geron X, Inc., Los Altos, California.

Halsted, J. A., and Smith, J. C., Jr. (1970). Plasma-zinc in health and disease. Lancet 1, 322–324.

Halsted, J. A., Hackley, B. M., and Smith, J. C., Jr. (1968). Plasma-zinc and copper in pregnancy and after oral contraceptives. Lancet 2, 278.

Halsted, J. A., Smith, J. C., Jr., Hackley, B. M., and McBean, L. (1969). Plasma zinc and copper levels. Amer. J. Obstet. Gynecol. 105, 645–646.

Hamolsky, M. W., Golodetz, A., and Freedberg, A. S. (1959). The plasma protein-thyroid hormone complex in man. III. Further studies on the use of the in vitro red blood cell uptake of ^{131}I-tri-iodothyronine as a diagnostic test of thyroid function. J. Clin. Endocrinol. Metab. 19, 103–116.

Hollander, C. S., Garcia, A. M., Stugis, S. H., and Selenkow, H. A. (1963). The effect of an ovulatory suppressant on the serum protein-bound iodine and the red-cell uptake of radioactive tri-iodothyronine. N. Engl. J. Med. 269, 501–504.

Horne, C. H. W., Howie, P. W., Weir, R. J., and Goudie, R. B. (1970). Effect of combined oestrogen-progestogen oral contraceptives on serum levels of α_2-macroglobulin, transferrin, albumin, and IgG. Lancet 1, 49–51.

Ingbar, S. H., and Freinkel, M. L. (1960). Regulation of the peripheral metabolism of the thyroid hormones. Recent Progr. Horm. Res. 16, 353–403.

Inman, W. H. W., Vessey, M. P., Westerholm, B., and Engelund, A. (1970). Thromboembolic disease and the steroidal content of oral contraceptives. A report to the Committee on Safety of Drugs. Brit. Med. J. 2, 203–209.

Irizarry, S., Paniagua, M., Pincus, G., Janer, J. L., and Friaz, Z. (1966). Effect of cyclic administration of certain progestin-estrogen combinations on the 24-hour radioiodine thyroid uptake. J. Clin. Endocrinol. Metab. 26, 6–10.

Jacobi, J. M., Powell, L. W., and Gaffney, T. J. (1969). Immunochemical quantitation of human transferrin in pregnancy and during the administration of oral contraceptives. Brit. J. Haematol. 17, 503–509.

Johnson, N. C. (1961). Study of copper and zinc metabolism during pregnancy. Proc. Soc. Exp. Biol. Med. 108, 518–519.

Lahey, M. E., Gubler, C. J., Cartwright, G. E., and Wintrobe, M. M. (1953). Studies on copper metabolism. VI. Blood copper in normal human subjects. J. Clin. Invest. 32, 322–328.

Larsson-Cohn, U. (1965). Oral contraception and serum protein-bound iodine. Lancet 1, 317.

Larsson-Cohn, U. (1966). An appraisal of the clinical effect of three different oral contraceptive agents and their influence on transaminase activity. Acta Obstet. Gynecol. Scand. 45, 499–514.

Larsson-Cohn, U. (1969). Effects of different types of oral contraceptives on the protein-bound iodine and the ^{125}I-triiodothyronine uptake on Sephadex. Scand. J. Clin. Lab. Invest. 23, 373–378.

Laurell, C. B., Kullander, S., and Thorell, J. (1967). Effect of administration of a combined estrogen-progestin contraceptive on the level of individual plasma proteins. Scand. J. Clin. Lab. Invest. 21, 337–343.

McBean, L. D., Smith, J. C., Jr., and Halsted, J. A. (1971). Effect of oral contraceptive hormones on zinc metabolism in the rat. *Proc. Soc. Exp. Biol. Med.* **137**, 543–547.

McFee, J. G .(1973). Anemia: A high risk complication in pregnancy. *Clin. Obstet. Gynecol.* **16**, 153–171.

McKenzie, J. M. (1974). Influence of oral contraceptives on serum zinc and copper concentrations. *Fed. Proc., Fed. Amer. Soc. Exp. Biol.* **33**, 2724 (abstr.).

Man, E. B. (1972). Thyroid function in pregnancy and infancy. *CRC Crit. Rev. Clin. Lab. Sci.* **3**, 203–225.

Mardell, M., and Zilva, J. (1967). Effect of oral contraceptives on the variations in serum-iron during the menstrual cycle. *Lancet* **2**, 1323–1325.

Mardell, M., Symmons, C., and Zilva, J. F. (1969). A comparison of the effect of oral contraceptives, pregnancy and sex on iron metabolism. *J. Clin. Endocrinol. Metab.* **29**, 1489–1495.

Markowitz, H., Gubler, C. J., Mahoney, J. P., Cartwright, G. E., and Wintrobe, M. M. (1955). Studies on copper metabolism. XIV. Copper, ceruloplasmin and oxidase activity in sera of normal human subjects, pregnant women. *J. Clin. Invest.* **34**, 1498–1508.

Musa, B. U., Doe, R. P., and Seal, U. S. (1967). Serum protein alterations produced in women by synthetic estrogens. *J. Clin. Endocrinol. Metab.* **27**, 1463–1469.

Nilsson, L., and Solvell, L. (1967). Clinical studies on oral contraceptives—a randomized, doubleblind, crossover study of 4 different preparations (Anovlar[R] mite, Lyndiol[R] mite, Ovulen[R], and Volidan[R]). *Acta Obstet. Gynecol. Scand., Suppl.* **46**, 1–31.

Norrby, A., Rybo, G., and Solvell, L. (1972). The influence of a combined oral contraceptive on the absorption of iron. *Scand. J. Haematol.* **9**, 43–51.

Olatunbosun, D. A., Adeniyi, F. A., and Adadevoh, B. K. (1973). The effect of oral contraceptives on serum copper levels in Nigerian women. *J. Obstet. Gynaecol. Brit. Commonw.* **80**, 937–939.

O'Leary, J. A., and Spellacy, W. N. (1968). Serum copper alteration after ingestion of an oral contraceptive. *Science* **162**, 682.

O'Leary, J. A. and Spellacy, W. N. (1969). Zinc and copper levels in pregnant women and those taking oral contraceptives. *Amer. J. Obstet. Gynecol.* **103**, 131–132.

Oster, G. K. (1972). Chemical reactions of the copper intrauterine devices. *Fert. Steril.* **23**, 18–23.

Paulsen, C. A. (1965). Progestin metabolism: Special reference to estrogenic pathways. *Metab., Clin. Exp.* **14**, 313–319.

Pincus, G., Rock, J., Garcia, C., Rice-Wray, E., Paniagua, M., and Rodriquez, I. (1958). Fertility control with oral medication. *Amer. J. Obstet. Gynecol.* **75**, 1333–1346.

Powell, L. W., Jacobi, J. M., Gaffney, T. J., and Adam, R. (1970). Failure of a pure progestogen contraceptive to affect serum levels of iron, transferrin, protein-bound iodine, and transaminase. *Brit. Med. J.* **3**, 194–195.

Rice-Wray, E., Schulz-Contreras, M., Guerrero, I., and Aranda-Rossell, A. (1962). Long-term administration of norethindrone in fertility control. *J. Amer. Med. Ass.* **180**, 355–358.

Russ, E. M., and Raymunt, J. (1956). Influence of estrogens on total serum copper and caeruloplasmin. *Proc. Soc. Exp. Biol. Med.* **92**, 465–466.

Sartwell, P. E., Masi, A. T., Arthes, F. G., Greene, G. R., and Smith, H. E. (1969).

Thromboembolism and oral contraceptives: An epidemiological case-control study. *Amer. J. Epidemiol.* **90**, 366–380.

Schenker, J. G., Hellerstein, S., Jungreis, E., and Polishuk, W. Z. (1971a). Serum copper and zinc levels in patients taking oral contraceptives. *Fert. Steril.* **22**, 229–234.

Schenker, J. G., Jungreis, E., and Polishuk, W. Z. (1971b). Oral contraceptives and serum copper concentration. *Obstet. Gynecol.* **37**, 233–234.

Schenker, J. G., Ben-Yoseph, Y., and Shapira, E. (1972). Erythrocyte carbonic anhydrase B levels during pregnancy and use of oral contraceptives. *Obstet. Gynecol.* **39**, 237–240.

Starup, J., and Friis, T. (1967). Thyroid function in oral contraception. *Acta Endocrinol.* (*Copenhagen*) **56**, 525–532.

Sterling, K., and Tabachnick, M. (1961). Resin uptake of I-131 triiodothyronine as a test of thyroid function. *J. Clin. Endocrinol. Metab.* **21**, 456–464.

Szelenyi, I. (1973). Magnesium and its significance in cardiovascular and gastrointestinal disorders. *World Rev. Nutr. Diet.* **17**, 189–224.

Thein, M., Beaton, G. H., Milne, H., and Veen, M. J. (1969). Oral contraceptive drugs: Some observations on their effect on menstrual loss and haematological indices. *Can. Med. Ass. J.* **101**, 678–679.

Theuer, R. (1972). Effect of oral contraceptive agents on vitamin and mineral needs: A review. *J. Reprod. Med.* **8**, 13–19.

Thin, C. G. (1971). The effect of an oral contraceptive agent on the concentrations of calcium and magnesium in plasma, erythrocytes and platelets in women. *Ann. Clin. Res.* **3**, 103–106.

Underwood, E. J. (1971). "Trace Elements in Human and Animal Nutrition," 3rd ed., p. 67. Academic Press, New York.

Walser, H. C., Margulis, R. R., and Ladd, J. E. (1964). Effects of prolonged administration of progestins on the endometrium and the function of the pituitary, thyroid and adrenal agents. *Int. J. Fert.* **9**, 189–195.

Weindling, H., and Henry, J. B. (1974). Laboratory test results altered by "the pill." *J. Amer. Med. Ass.* **229**, 1762–1768.

Westoff, C. F. (1972). The modernization of U.S. contraceptive practice. *Contraception* **4**, 9–12.

Williams, D. W., Denardo, J. S., and Zelenik, J. S. (1966). Thyroid function and Enovid, *Obstet. Gynecol.* **27**, 232–237.

Winikoff, D., and Taylor, K. (1966). Oral contraceptives and thyroid function tests. *Med. J. Aust.* **2**, 108–112.

Zadeh, J. A., Karabus, C. D., and Fielding, J. (1967). Haemoglobin concentration and other values in women using an intrauterine device or taking corticosteroid contraceptive pills. *Brit. Med. J.* **4**, 708–711.

Zilva, J. F. (1969). Oral contraceptives and blood-iron. *Lancet* **2**, 847.

Zipper, J. A., Medel, M., and Prager, R. (1969a). Suppression of fertility by intrauterine copper and zinc in rabbits. A new approach to intrauterine contraception. *Amer. J. Obstet. Gynecol.* **105**, 529–534.

Zipper, J. A., Tatum, H. J., Pastene, L., Medel, M., and Rivera, M. (1969b). Metallic copper as an intrauterine contraceptive adjunct to the "T" device. *Amer. J. Obstet. Gynecol.* **105**, 1274–1278.

Zipper, J. A., Tatum, H. J., Medel, M., Pastene, L., and Rivera, M. (1971). Contraception through the use of intrauterine metals. I. Copper as an adjunct to the "T" device. The endouterine copper "T." *Amer. J. Obstet. Gynecol.* **109**, 771–774.

39

Human Intake of Trace Elements

Carol I. Waslien

I. INTRODUCTION

Deficiencies in man of several trace elements have been reported from countries in the Middle East. Zinc deficiency appearing as growth retardation and delayed sexual maturity was observed by Prasad and co-workers (1961, 1963) in both Iran and Egypt. Iron deficiency is common throughout the region and is particularly prevalent at all ages and in both sexes in Egypt (Patwardhan and Darby, 1972). Possible selenium and chromium deficiencies were suggested by Hopkins and Majaj (1966) as occurring in Jordanian children with protein–calorie malnutrition. And lastly, endemic goiter is seen in the oases of Egypt (Coble et al., 1968), the mountains of Lebanon (ICNND, 1962a), and in Iraq (Caughey and Follis, 1965) and Iran (Caughey et al., 1970).

II. DIET IN THE TRACE ELEMENT DEFICIENCY OF EGYPTIANS

Many causative agents interplay to influence this deficiency of trace elements. Febrile diseases, which are endemic in most of the countries, have been shown in other chapters of this treatise to alter significantly serum and urinary levels of iron and zinc. Blood losses associated with the parasitic diseases hookworm and schistosomiasis are known to cause iron deficiency, but they may also result in significant losses of other trace elements. Some of the secondary lesions of the liver or kidney

347

associated with schistosomiasis, amebiasis, and other parasitic diseases may also contribute to these trace element deficiencies. In Egypt, nearly every resident of a village has one or more parasites, and a significant percentage of these villagers are also typhoid or hepatitis carriers. In addition, other characteristics of Middle Eastern diets, such as the high phytate content of bread, which constitutes 50–80% of the rural village diet (Waslien et al., 1972), may greatly influence trace element status.

Until recently, it was not possible to evaluate the role of diet in the etiology of these deficiencies, since no information was available on trace element content of local foodstuffs. Samples of ninety-eight different foods commonly consumed by the lower socioeconomic segment of the Egyptian population have recently been analyzed for iron and zinc by X-ray fluorescence and for selenium and chromium by neutron activation. These estimates were used to make an approximation of the nutrient intake by families likely to have trace element deficiencies. Composites of additional diets were directly analyzed for their content of these elements. These approximations have been compared with similar reports from other countries. The reports of intakes of other trace elements that may be important either as essential nutrients or toxic dietary contaminants have also been reviewed in light of their potential importance in the Middle East.

The composites were made from the hospital diet of eleven Egyptian children, ranging in age from 10 to 39 months, who had recovered from the acute stage of kwashiorkor and who no longer exhibited edema (Table I). The diets consisted of milk, bread, rice, beans, and small amounts of cooked vegetables and meat. A duplicate of one day's food for each child was collected. Each days composite was blended, lyophilized, and the protein, energy, selenium, and chromium contents of the dried samples were determined.

The median energy intake, 1940 kcal/day, exceeded that of healthy children but was not unusual for children recovering from kwashiorkor, particularly in light of the marked depression in body weight that was observed. The median body weight of these children was only 70% of normal for children of this age, and all children were more than 15% underweight. Those children with the most marked body weight deficits tended to have the highest calorie intakes. Protein intake was also high, 53 gm/day, probably reflecting the high food intake. There was a wide spread in selenium intakes, 3.3–371 μg/day, but ten of the eleven values were closely clustered around the median of 29.4 μg/day and showed a twentyfold difference from 3 to 66 μg. There was also a wide range in the chromium values, which varied from 76.8 to 1057 μg/day, or a fifteenfold difference, with a median value of 129 μg. This wide disper-

TABLE I   Trace Element Content of Diet of Children Recovering from Kwashiorkor

Patient no.	Age (months)	Weight (kg)	Wt./age % Normal[a]	Calorie		Protein		Diet composition					
								Selenium			Chromium		
				kcal/ day	kcal/ kg body wt	gm/ day	gm/ kg body wt	µg/ day	µg/ kg	µg/ 1000 kcal	µg/ day	µg/ kg	g/ 1000 kcal
88	23	7.9	65	1970	250	55	7.0	65.6	8.4	33.3	92.5	11.7	47.0
91	18	9.3	82	2580	277	76	8.2	4.2	0.4	1.6	77.9	8.4	30.2
92	17	7.0	64	1940	277	51	7.3	33.4	4.8	17.2	98.7	14.1	50.8
93	27	9.3	72	1770	191	27	2.9	3.3	0.4	1.9	76.8	8.3	43.3
94	39	10.1	67	2620	259	84	8.3	51.3	5.1	19.6	1057.2	106.6	403
96	20	7.0	60	1530	219	45	6.4	370.9	53.0	197	108.2	15.4	70.6
97	10	5.5	59	1740	316	47	8.5	6.3	1.1	3.6	250.2	45.5	143.6
98	22	8.4	70	1680	173	45	5.4	5.7	0.7	3.4	493.8	58.7	294
99	22	9.8	81	1890	224	67	6.8	29.4	3.0	15.5	139.8	14.3	74.1
100	24	9.3	75	1940	208	73	7.8	25.4	2.7	13.1	557.1	60.0	287
104	24	9.1	73	1970	217	—	—	30.5	3.3	15.5	—	—	—
Median	22	9.1	70	1940	224	53	7.2	29.4	3.0	15.5	129.0	14.8	72.3

[a] Jelliffe (1966).

sion in both selenium and chromium values may reflect variation in the heat treatment of the foods included in the composites, in addition to reflecting inclusion of different proportions of the foodstuffs and their individual contamination with selenium or chromium. Losses in both nutrients have been observed when food samples are subjected to high temperatures. Recent studies in this laboratory on unprocessed fruits and vegetables indicate that chromium values are two to ten times greater in lyophilized samples than in samples of the same foods dried at 100°C. Some selenium values were also higher in lyophilized food. There is a great deal of variation in the difference between oven-dried and lyophilized values for different foods that possibly reflects varying proportions of the several organic compounds that bind selenium or chromium.

The levels of selenium and chromium in the hospital diets were not related to the total amount of food eaten, nor were selenium and chromium levels correlated with each other. In addition, there was no correlation between energy intake and levels of either nutrients. There was a significant correlation ($p < 0.05$) between chromium contents of the diets and their protein level.

Information was collected on the home diet from fifty mothers of a similar group of Egyptian children who were being treated for protein–calorie malnutrition (Table II) (Waslien et al., 1972). An estimate was made of food intake from the response of the women to an oral questionnaire regarding the frequency of purchasing items from a list of commonly consumed foods. A 24-hour dietary recall was also made to cross check the composition of the day's meals, and recipes were collected. The calorie and protein content of the typical day's diet was calculated from tables of food composition for middle eastern foods and iron, zinc, selinium, and chromium contents were estimated from determinations made on individual foodstuffs.

The home diet of the families of these malnourished children was apparently inadequate in energy content, but not when corrected for the age and size of the family members. The average family had two adults and three children less than 10 years of age, and thus the recommended average calorie intake for the family should be between 1400 and 1500 kcal. The protein content of the diet was also adequate. Bread made from a mixture of high-extraction wheat flour and stone-ground corn meal provided the majority of protein, calories, and each of the trace elements with the exception of selenium.

The dietary intake of iron observed in this study, 15 mg, was lower than that found by chemical analysis of food composites for Egyptian school boys, 27 mg, reported by Carter et al. (1969). This lower intake

TABLE II   Home Diet of Families with Malnourished Children

Food	Median values for foods						Calculated intakes						
	Energy (kcal)[c]	Protein (gm)	Fe[a]	Zn[a]	Se[a]	Cr[a]	Dry wt (gm)	Energy (kcal)	Protein (gm)	Fe[b]	Zn[b]	Se[b]	Cr[b]
Bread	361	11.4	4.9	2.3	0.002	0.007	225	812	25.6	11.6	6.2	0.004	0.016
Cereal products	354	7.2	1.3	1.0	0.019	0.010	71	252	5.1	0.9	0.7	0.013	0.007
Broad beans	354	25.0	4.2	3.1	0.003	0.004	19	67	4.7	0.8	0.6	<0.001	0.009
Other beans	349	22.6	5.9	3.1	0.004	0.035	18	63	4.1	1.1	0.6	0.001	0.006
Meat, fish, poultry	630	20.8	2.4	9.3	0.014	0.012	6	38	1.2	0.1	0.5	0.001	<0.001
Eggs	612	20.3	3.8	6.5	0.021	0.006	0.6	4	0.1	<0.1	<0.1	<0.001	<0.001
Vegetables	365	12.9	6.7	2.1	0.004	0.015	17	62	2.2	1.1	0.4	0.001	0.002
Fruits	408	6.7	1.1	0.8	0.003	0.009	4	16	0.3	<0.1	<0.1	<0.001	<0.001
Milk, cheese	500	25.5	Trace	Trace	0.001	Trace	9	45	2.3	Trace	Trace	0.001	0.008
Sugar	400	0	0	0	0	0	24	96	0	0	0	0	0
Total								1455	45.6	15.0	8.0	0.021	0.048
Percent from bread								56	56	73	65	19	33
Percent from bread and cereal products								73	67	79	71	81	48
Trace element intake/1000 kcal								—	—	10.3	5.5	0.014	0.033

[a] In mg/100 gm dry weight.
[b] In mg/person/day.
[c] In units/100g dry weight.

TABLE III Iron in Diets

Group	Country	Type of study	Diet iron mg/day	Diet iron mg/1000 kcal	Diet iron mg/day body wt	References
Infants (months)						
0-6	USA	Cow's milk	5.4[a]	—	—	Murthy et al. (1972)
0-6	USSR	Breast-fed	—	—	0.20-0.25	Reshetkina (1968)
0-6	USSR	Bottle-fed	—	—	0.30	Reshetkina (1968)
<12	Guatemala	Calculated	4.9	5.7	—	Flores et al. (1966)
1	USA	Calculated	14.5	—	—	R. A. Stewart (personal communication, 1974)
3	USA	Calculated	12.5	—	—	R. A. Stewart (personal communication, 1974)
6	USA	Calculated	11.5	—	—	R. A. Stewart (personal communication, 1974)
Children (years)						
1-<3	Uruguay (urban)	Calculated	9.8	6.7	—	Valassi and Reynolds (1966)
1-<3	Uruguay (rural)	Calculated	8.3	5.7	—	Valassi and Reynolds (1966)
1-<2	Guatemala	Calculated	4.4	9.2	0.51	Flores et al. (1966)
1-4	USSR	Children's home	6.8	4.3	—	Vorob'eva and Bol'sanina (1964)
2-<3	Guatemala	Calculated	8.3	10.1	0.85	Flores et al. (1966)
3-<4	Guatemala	Calculated	9.7	10.1	0.86	Flores et al. (1966)
3-<5	Uruguay (urban)	Calculated	13.8	8.3	—	Valassi and Reynolds (1966)
3-<5	Uruguay (rural)	Calculated	9.0	6.1	—	Valassi and Reynolds (1966)
3-6	USA	Calculated	8-14	—	0.6	Monier-Williams (1950)
3-7	USSR	Children's home	16.1	6.3	—	Vorob'eva and Bot'sanina (1964)
4-5	Guatemala	Calculated	11.0	9.8	0.81	Flores et al. (1966)
7-16	USSR	Children's home	30	9.5	—	Voreb'eva and Bol'sanina (1964)
10-13	USA	Balance study	8.5-11.2	—	—	Schlaphoff and Johnson (1949)
13-15M	USA	Calculated	14.2	5.6	—	Wharton (1963)
13-15F	USA	Calculated	10.4	4.8	—	Wharton (1963)
13-19M	USA	Calculated	14.1	5.0	—	Hampton et al. (1967)
13-19F	USA	Calculated	9.7	4.9	—	Hampton et al. (1967)
14-17M	Egypt	Self-selected	27.2	12.2	—	Carter et al. (1969)
16-18M	USA	Calculated	14.8	5.3	—	Wharton (1963)
16-18F	USA	Calculated	11.0	5.4	—	Wharton (1963)
16-19M	USA	Representative	35.6	8.4	—	Zook and Lehmann (1965)

School children	Holland	Calculated	12.8	5.7	—	Wretlind (1970)
	Holland	Calculated	13.4	5.8	—	Wretlind (1970)
	Nigeria	Calculated	13.0	5.2	—	Hauck (1961)
16–25M	Alaska	Calculated	12.1	6.4	—	Mann (1962)
Adults						
M	USA	Balance studies	15–28	—	—	Tipton et al. (1969)
M	USA	Balance study	12–15	—	—	Tipton et al. (1966)
W	USA	Balance study	6.5–7	—	—	Johnson et al. (1951)
M–F	USA	Hospital (winter)	9.2	—	—	Gormican (1970)
M–F	USA	Hospital (summer)	7.6	—	—	Gormican (1970)
M–F	USSR	Hospital	19–39	—	—	Soroka (1970)
M–F	USSR	Hospital	24–38	11–13	—	Soroka (1967)
M–F	UK	Self-selected	12.0	—	—	Soman et al. (1969)
M–F	Japan	Self-selected	19.0	—	—	Soman et al. (1969)
M–F	India	Self-selected	39.4	—	—	Soman et al. (1969)
F	USA	Representative	10–12	—	—	Underwood (1971)
M–F	India	Representative	9	—	—	Underwood (1971)
M–F	Holland	Representative	14.5	5.2	—	Wretlind (1970)
M–F	Australia	Representative	20–22	—	—	Underwood (1971)
Households	Bolivia	Self-selected	41.4	22.4	—	ICNND (1964b)
	Columbia	Self-selected	17.0	11.4	—	ICNND (1960b)
	Ecuador	Self-selected	19.7	12.0	—	ICNND (1960a)
	Ethiopia	Self-selected	390	156	—	ICNND (1959)
	Malaya	Self-selected	29	10.6	—	ICCND (1964a)
	Nigeria	Self-selected	59	23.4	—	ICNND (1967a)
	Paraguay	Self-selected	17.8	8.0	—	ICNND (1967a)
	Thailand	Self-selected	23.2	7.6	—	ICNND (1961)
	Trinidad and Tobago	Self-selected	11.0	8.0	—	ICNND (1962a)
	Uruguay (urban)	Self-selected	23	9.1	—	Valassi and Reynolds (1966)
	Venezuela	Self-selected	34	14.9	—	ICNND (1963)
	Alaska	Calculated	10.5	5.7	—	Mann (1962)
	Finland	Calculated	13.0	4.8	—	Wretlind (1970)
	Italy	Calculated	11.2	3.0	—	Wretlind (1970)
	Pakistan (urban)	Calculated	8.7	4.9	—	ICNND (1966)
	Pakistan (rural)	Calculated	9.7	4.3	—	ICNND (1966)
	Egypt	Calculated	15.0	10.3	—	Unpublished analysis

[a] Calculated on the basis of an average milk consumption of 850 ml/day.

TABLE IV Zinc in Diets

Group	Country	Type of study	Diet zinc			References
			mg/day	mg/1000 kcal	mg/kg body wt	
Infants						
6–8 days	UK	Human milk	0.7–5.0	—	0.2–1.2	Schlage and Wortberg (1972)
1–5 week	Sweden	Human and cow's milk	1.0–1.5	—	—	Schlage and Wortberg (1972)
1 month	USA	Calculated	1.8	—	—	R. A. Stewart (personal communication, 1974)
3 months	USA	Calculated	1.7	—	—	R. A. Stewart (personal communication, 1974)
6 months	USA	Calculated	4.1	—	—	R. A. Stewart (personal communication, 1974)
9 months	USA	Calculated	2.7	—	—	Sandstead (1973)
0–1 year	USSR	Self-selected	—	—	0.51	Reshetkina (1969)
0–1 year	Australia	Human or cow's milk	2.6–4.2[a]	—	—	Underwood (1971)
Children (years)						
1–4	USSR	Children's home	4.6	2.9	0.54	Vorob'eva and Bol'sanina (1964)
2	USSR	Balance study	4.3	—	—	Vorob'eva (1967)
3–5	Germany	Institution	6.4	4.2	0.36	Schlage and Wortberg (1972)
3–6	USA	Balance study	3.8–5.9	—	0.22–0.31	Schlage and Wortberg (1972)
3–7	USSR	Children's home	7.1	2.8	0.54	Vorob'eva and Bol'sanina (1964)
3–7	USSR	Children's home (winter)	6.7	—	—	Kerimova (1968)
		Children's home (summer)	7.3	—	—	Kerimova (1968)
6–10 F	USA	Balance study	4.6–9.3	—	—	Engel et al. (1966)
7–9 F	USA	Balance study	4.7–6.9	—	—	Price et al. (1970)
7–9 F	USA	Balance study	4.5	2.2	—	Price and Bunce (1972)
7–16	USSR	Children's home	13.6	4.3	0.54	Vorob'eva and Bol'sanina (1964)
8–10	USSR	Balance study	10.9	—	—	Vorob'eva (1967)

8–12	USA	Balance study	16	—	0.5	Schlage and Wortberg (1972)
9–12	USA	Children's homes	9.1	—	—	Murthy et al. (1971)
10–13	Germany	Children's home	10.2	4.8	0.28	Schlage and Wortberg (1972)
10–12	USA	School lunches	12.3[b]	5.3	—	Murphy et al. (1971)
14–17 M	Egypt	Self-selected	11.5	5.0	—	Carter et al. (1969)
14–30 F	USA	Self-selected	13.2	9.0	—	White (1969)
Adults						
M–F	USA	Balance study	12.4	—	—	Sandstead (1973)
F	USA	Balance study	10–14	—	—	Schlage and Wortberg (1972)
M	Iran (urban)	Balance study	27–32	12–14	—	Reinhold et al. (1973)
M	Iran (rural)	Balance study	26–36	11–16	—	Reinhold et al. (1973)
M–F	UK	Balance study	5.6–22.0	—	—	Schlage and Wortberg (1972)
M	USA	Institution	15.5	—	—	Schroeder et al. (1967)
M–F	USA	Hospital diet	8.5	3.5	—	Schroeder et al. (1967)
M–F	USA	Hospital (winter)	14.5	—	—	Gormican (1970)
M–F	USA	Hospital (summer)	13.3	—	—	Gormican (1970)
M–F	USSR	Hospital diet	10.2–15.9	4.6–5.2	—	Soroka (1967)
M–F	USA	Hospital diet	8.7–15.9	—	—	Soroka (1970)
M–F	USA	Self-selected	10–15	—	0.2	Schlage and Wortberg (1972)
M–F	USA	Self-selected	14.4	—	—	Schlage and Wortberg (1972)
M–F	USA	Self-selected	5.0–22.5	—	—	Allen and Pierce (1968)
M–F	Germany	Self-selected	6–40	—	—	Schlage and Wortberg (1972)
M–F	UK	Self-selected	12.0	—	—	Soman et al. (1969)
M–F	Japan	Self-selected	14.0	—	—	Soman et al. (1969)
M–F	India	Self-selected	16.1	—	—	Soman et al. (1969)
F	New Zealand	Self-selected	11.5	—	—	Gutherie (1973)
Households	USA	Calculated	8–13	—	—	Schroeder et al. (1967)
	USA	Calculated	12	—	—	Eggleton (1939)
	China	Calculated	6	—	—	Eggleton (1939)
	Germany	Calculated	—	2.6–3.0	—	Schlage and Wortberg (1972)
	Egypt	Calculated	8.0	5.5	—	Unpublished analysis

[a] Calculated on the basis of an average with consumption of 850 ml/day.
[b] Assume school lunches provide one-third day's zinc.

was partially caused by consumption of larger amounts of food by the school children, since the iron intakes calculated in relation to energy intakes were quite similar. The iron contents of the families' diets was not appreciably different from those reported in Interdepartmental Committee on Nutrition for National Development studies for calculated iron intakes in lesser developed countries (Table III), but it was higher than calculated household intake values for some Western European countries.

The calculated zinc intakes, 8 mg/day, were also lower in the families of children with malnutrition than were the chemically determined values for the diets of Egyptian teenage school boys, 11.5 mg/day (Carter et al., 1969). But again, there was no difference when the values were expressed per 1000 kcal. Zinc intakes of the households were lower than chemically determined values reported for adults from Iran (Reinhold et al., 1973) and India (Soman et al., 1969) and from most developed countries (Table IV), but were comparable to these values when expressed per 1000 kcal.

The calculated selenium values for households, 21 μg, and the assayed value for hospital diets, 29.4 μg, were not unlike the 31 μg found by Schroeder (1971) in one adult's hospital diet in the United States. The range was also quite similar to the range of 6–70 μg observed for thirteen New Zealand women (Griffiths, 1973). Selenium intakes of greater than 40 μg can be calculated for children receiving only cow's milk in seleniferous areas of Venezuela (Mondragon and Jaffee, 1971). However, these are the only values for selenium intake in the literature, and a great deal more dietary information on this trace element is needed before a comparison of selenium intake can be made.

The chromium intake by hospitalized Egyptian children, 129 μg, was approximately midway in a fifteen-fold range of mean values (60 to >1000 μg/day) for North American and Russian children (Table V). In fact, it is also midway in the nearly equally wide range of means for normal North American and Russian adults (52–820 μg). Thus, though the value calculated for poor Egyptian family members is one-third of that for the hospital diet of Egyptian children, it too is not sufficiently different from this wide range of reported values to be considered abnormal.

The intake of no other trace elements has been determined for Middle Eastern diets. However, comparison of values reported from developed and lesser developed countries indicates that such estimates might be important for copper and manganese. In data collected on the copper content of the diet of 377 babies from the United States, there was a twenty-fivefold range of 7–170 μg/kg body weight, or 18–92 mg/day.

39. HUMAN INTAKE OF TRACE ELEMENTS 357

TABLE V Chromium in Diets

Group	Country	Type of study	Diet chromium μg/day	Diet chromium μg/1000 kcal	Diet chromium μg/kg body wt	References
Infants (months)						
0–6	Germany	Cow's milk	11[a]	—	—	Underwood (1962)
0–6	USA	Breast milk	34–68[a]	—	—	Underwood (1971)
Children (years)						
1–3	Egypt	Hospital diet	129	72	14.8	Maxia et al. (1972)
1–11	USSR	Children's home			2.2	Schlettwein-Gsell and Mommsen-Straub (1971a)
9–12	USA	Children's home	632			Murphy et al. (1971)
10–12	USA	School lunch	60[b]	26		Murphy et al. (1971)
14–18 F	USA	Self-selected	<1000			White (1969)
Adults						
M	USA	Balance study	200–290			Tipton et al. (1969)
M	USA	Balance study	330–400			Tipton et al. (1966)
M	USA	Institution	52			Schlettwein-Gsell and Mommsen-Straub (1971a)
M–F	USA	Institution	78			Schroeder et al. (1962)
M–F	USA	Institution (summer)	<460			Gormican (1970)
M–F	USA	Institution (winter)	<890			Gormican (1970)
M–F	USA	Hospital	102	42		Deutsch et al. (1963)
M	USA	Hospital	123			Schroeder (1971)
F	USA	Self-selected	65			Schlettwein-Gsell and Mommsen-Straub (1971a)
M	USA	Self-selected	<860	<580		White (1969)
M–F	Japan	Self-selected	231			Murphy et al. (1971)
M–F	Japan	Self-selected	170			Soman et al. (1969)
M–F	India	Self-selected	130–140			Murakami et al. (1965)
M–F	USSR	Self-selected	150			Soman et al. (1969)
F	New Zealand	Self-selected	690–820			Schlettwein-Gsell and Mommsen-Straub (1971a)
			39–190			Gutherie (1973)
M–F	Italy	Representative	64			Sandstead (1967)
M–F	USA	Calculated	30–140			Schroeder et al. (1962)
M–F	USA	Calculated	30–80			Sandstead (1967)
Households	Egypt	Calculated	48	33		Maxia et al. (1972)

[a] Calculated on the basis of an average milk consumption of 850 ml/day.
[b] Assume school lunch provides one-third of day's chromium.

TABLE VI Copper in Diets

Group	Country	Type of study	Diet copper mg/day	mg/1000 kcal	mg/kg body wt	References
Infants						
Newborn	—	Balance study	—	—	0.015	Schlettwein-Gsell and Mommsen-Straub (1971c)
7–14 day	USSR	—	—	—	0.058	World Health Organization (1973)
7–14 day	UK	—	—	—	0.1	World Health Organization (1973)
Premature	—	—	—	—	0.059	World Health Organization (1973)
1 month	USA	Calculated	0.16	—	—	R. A. Stewart (personal communication, 1974)
3 months	USA	Calculated	0.25	—	—	R. A. Stewart (personal communication, 1974)
6 months	USA	Calculated	0.38	—	—	R. A. Stewart (personal communication, 1974)
4–6 months	Australia	Human milk	0.13–0.14[a]	—	—	World Health Organization (1973)
Children (years)						
1½–3	USSR	Institution	0.97–1.2	—	—	Vorob'eva (1965)
3–6	USSR	Balance study	—	—	0.053–0.085	Schlettwein-Gsell and Mommsen-Straub (1971c)
3–7	USSR	Institution (winter)	0.88	—	—	Kerimova (1968)
3–7	USSR	Institution (summer)	1.06	—	—	Kerimova (1968)
3–7	USSR	Institution	1.7–2.2	—	—	Vorob'eva (1965)
6–10	USA	—	—	—	0.04	World Health Organization (1973)
8	USA	Balance study	—	—	0.1	Schlettwein-Gsell and Mommsen-Straub (1971c)
11	USA	Balance study	—	—	0.08	Schlettwein-Gsell and Mommsen-Straub (1971c)
School children	USSR	Institution	2.3–4.6	—	—	Vorob'eva (1965)
Adults						
M–F	USA	Hospital (summer)	0.425	—	—	Gormican (1970)
M–F	USA	Hospital (winter)	<0.296	—	—	Gormican (1970)
M–F	USSR	Hospital	1.3–4.0	—	—	Soroka (1966)
M–F	USSR	Hospital	2.0–4.3	—	—	Soroka (1970)

M–F	USA	Institution	3.2	—	—	Schroeder et al. (1966)
M–F	USA	Institution	2.3	—	—	Schroeder et al. (1966)
F	New Zealand	Self-selected	2.4	—	—	Gutherie (1973)
M–F	UK	Self-selected	1.7	—	—	Soman et al. (1969)
M–F	India	Self-selected	5.8	—	—	Soman et al. (1969)

[a] Calculated on the basis of an average milk consumption of 850 ml/day.

TABLE VII Manganese in Diets

Group	Country	Type of study	Diet manganese mg/day	mg/1000 kcal	mg/kg body wt	References
Infants (months)						
Newborn	—	Human milk	—	—	0.003–0.004	Schlettwein-Gsell and Mommsen-Straub (1971b)
1	USA	Calculated	0.06	—	—	R. A. Stewart (personal communication, 1974)
3	USA	Calculated	0.18	—	—	R. A. Stewart (personal communication, 1974)
6	USA	Calculated	0.13	—	—	R. A. Stewart (personal communication, 1974)
0–6	USA	Human milk	0.006–0.34[a]	—	—	World Health Organization (1973)
0–6	USA	Cow's milk	—	—	0.003–0.025	World Health Organization (1973)
Children (years)						
1–3	USA	Self-selected	2.5	—	0.15–0.25	World Health Organization (1973)
2	USSR	Institution	3.2	—	0.273	Schlettwein-Gsell and Mommsen-Straub (1971b)
7–9	Holland	Calculated	1.7	—	—	Schlettwein-Gsell and Mommsen-Straub (1971b)
9	USSR	Institution	9.5	—	0.31	Schlettwein-Gsell and Mommsen-Straub (1971b)
9–12	USA	Institution	2.0	—	—	Murthy et al. (1971)
14–16	USA	Self-selected	<0.24–1.5	—	—	Schlettwein Gsell and Mommsen-Straub (1971b)
Schoolgirls	USSR	Institution	—	—	0.12	Schlettwein-Gsell and Mommsen-Straub (1971b)

							Reference
Schoolboys	USSR	Institution summer		—	—	0.10	Schlettwein-Gsell and Mommsen-Straub (1971b)
		winter		—	—	0.11	Schlettwein-Gsell and Mommsen-Straub (1971b)
Adults							
M–F	USA	Balance study	3.0	—	—		Schlettwein-Gsell and Mommsen-Straub (1971b)
M–F	India	Balance study	2.5–10.7	—	—		World Health Organization (1973)
M–F	USA	Hospital (summer)	0.9	—	—		Gormican (1970)
		Hospital (winter)	1.8	—	—		Gormican (1970)
F	New Zealand	Self-selected	2.9	—	—		Gutherie (1973)
M–F	UK	Self-selected	7.0	—	—		Soman et al. (1969)
M–F	India	Self-selected	9.7–10.5	—	—		Soman et al. (1969)
M–F	India	Self-selected	8.3	—	—		Soman et al. (1969)
M–F	Japan	Self-selected	2.3	—	—		Soman et al. (1969)
M–F	Japan	Self-selected	2.8	—	—		Murakami et al. (1965)
M–F	USA	Self-selected	0.9	—	—		Schlettwein-Gsell and Mommsen-Straub (1971b)
F	USA	Self-selected	<0.4–1.4	—	—		Schlettwein-Gsell and Mommsen-Straub (1971b)
M–F	Japan	Calculated	6–10	—	—		Nakagawa (1968)
M–F	USA	Calculated	2–5	—	—		Schlettwein-Gsell and Mommsen-Straub (1971b)
M–F	Holland	Calculated	2.3	—	—		Schlettwein-Gsell and Mommsen-Straub (1971b)

[a] Calculated on the basis of an average milk consumption of 850 ml/day.

TABLE VIII Miscellaneous Trace Elements in Diets

Group	Country	Type of study	Trace element in diet per day	per 1000 kcal	per kg body wt	References
			Arsenic			
0–6 months	—	Cow's milk	26–51 mg[a]	—	—	World Health Organization (1973)
			Barium			
Adults	USA	Hospital (summer)	<0.303 mg	—	—	Gormican (1970)
			<0.592 mg	—	—	Gormican (1970)
			Boron			
0–6 month	Australia	Cow's milk	0.4–0.85 mg[a]	—	—	World Health Organization (1973)
School children	USA	School lunch	1.5 mg[b]	—	—	World Health Organization (1973)
Adults	USA	Hospital (summer)	1.6 mg	—	—	Gormican (1970)
		Hospital (winter)	1.2 mg	—	—	Gormican (1970)
Adults	USA	Representative	3.0 mg	0.7 mg	—	World Health Organization (1973)
			Cobalt			
0–6 months	—	Human milk	0.4–23 μg[a]	—	—	World Health Organization (1973)
2–6 years	USSR	Institution	64–71 μg	—	—	Vorob'eva and Osmolovskaya (1970)
6–7 years	USSR	Balance study	40–42 μg	—	1.6 μg	Ripak (1961)
6–12 years	USA	Institution	880 μg	—	—	Murthy et al. (1971)
Adults	USA	Hospital	166 μg	—	—	Schlettwein-Gsell and Mommsen-Straub (1970)
Adults	USSR	Hospital	16–32 μg	—	—	Soroka (1966)
Adults	USSR	Hospital	22–39 μg	—	—	Soroka (1970)
Adults	USA	Institution	436 μg	—	—	Schlettwein-Gsell and Mommsen-Straub (1970)

Age	Country	Diet	Intake			Reference
Adults	Germany	Self-selected	360–920 µg	—	—	Schlettwein-Gsell and Mommsen-Straub (1970)
Adults	USA	Self-selected	150–600 µg	—	—	World Health Organization (1973)
Lead						
0–6 months	USA	Cow's milk	34 µg[a]	—	—	Lamm et al. (1973)
0–6 months	USA	Human milk	17 µg[a]	—	—	Lamm et al. (1973)
0–6 months	Australia	Cow's milk	17–68 µg[a]	—	—	World Health Organization (1973)
Adults	USA	Balance study	220 µg	—	—	Schroeder et al. (1962)
Adults	UK	Balance study	310 µg	—	—	Schroeder et al. (1962)
Adults	USA	Institution	258 µg	126 µg	—	Schroeder et al. (1962)
Adults	Germany	Self-selected	—	—	—	Lehnert et al. (1969)
Adults	USA	Representative	200–300 µg	—	—	World Health Organization (1973)
Adults	Europe	Representative	>400 µg	—	—	World Health Organization (1973)
Adults	USA	Calculated (low)	140 µg	61 µg	—	Schroeder et al. (1962)
Adults	USA	Calculated	275 µg	—	—	Bogen (1968)
Lithium						
Adults	UK	Self-selected	2.0 mg	—	—	Soman et al. (1969)
Adults	India	Self-selected	<0.1 mg	—	—	Soman et al. (1969)
Mercury						
Adults	England	Representative	14 µg	—	—	Vostal and Clarkson (1973)
Adults	Sweden	Representative	4 µg	—	—	Vostal and Clarkson (1973)
Adults	Germany	Representative	5 µg	—	—	Vostal and Clarkson (1973)
Adults	USSR	Representative	5–7 µg	—	—	Vostal and Clarkson (1973)
Adults	USA	Representative	20 µg	—	—	Vostal and Clarkson (1973)
Molybdenum						
0–6 months	—	Cow's milk	15–102 µg[a]	—	—	World Health Organization (1973)
2 years	USSR	Self-selected	—	—	1.3 µg	World Health Organization (1973)
2–6 years	USSR	Self-selected	159 µg	—	—	Vorob'eva and Osmolovskaya (1970)
Adult	USA	Institution	—	—	13.7 µg	World Health Organization (1973)

TABLE VIII (Continued)

Group	Country	Type of study	Trace element in diet per day	per 1000 kcal	per kg body wt	References
			Nickel			
0–6 months	—	Cow's milk	26 µg[a]	—	—	World Health Organization (1973)
Adults	USA	Institution	472 µg	231 µg	—	Schroeder et al. (1961)
Adults	USA	Self-selected	305–480 µg	—	—	Schroeder et al. (1961)
			Rubidium			
Adults	Japan	Self-selected	1.5 mg	—	—	Soman et al. (1969)
Adults	India	Self-selected	2.7 mg	—	—	Soman et al. (1969)
			Strontium			
Adults	USA	Hospital (summer)	1.24 mg	—	—	Gormican (1970)
Adults	UK	Hospital (winter)	1.89 mg	—	—	Gormican (1970)
Adults	India	Self-selected	1.4 mg	—	—	Soman et al. (1969)
Adults	India	Self-selected	3.5–4.2 mg	—	—	Soman et al. (1969)
Adults	India	Self-selected	4.0 mg	—	—	Soman et al. (1969)
			Tin			
0–6 months	—	Cow's milk	85–170 µg	—	—	World Health Organization (1973)
Adults	USA	Institutional	17,000 µg	—	—	World Health Organization (1973)
Adults	USA	Self-selected	3,500 µg	—	—	World Health Organization (1973)
			Vanadium			
Adults	USA	Calculated (low)	—	<34 ng	—	Nielsen (1974)

[a] Calculated on the basis of an average milk consumption of 850 ml/day.

Total intakes of copper ranged from an average of 0.160 mg for 1-month-old children to 0.380 mg for 6-month-old babies, 50–60% of the intake coming from milk. Intakes of children participating in balance studies or living in institutions in the United States or the Soviet Union have mean copper intakes ranging from 0.9 to 2.2 mg/day, and similar studies in adults showed mean intakes from 1.2 to 4.3 mg. Self-selected intakes of adults in the United Kingdom and New Zealand were 1.7 and 2.4 mg, respectively. However, the average copper intake of 5.8 mg in the Indian diet, determined on composites made from self-selected diets at a dozen locations throughout the country, was more than double the mean found for diets in developed countries (Table VI).

The manganese intake of the same infants as in the study of copper ranged from 0.01 to 1.97 mg, a 200-fold variation. The average went from intakes at 1 month of 0.06 mg to nearly 0.2 at 6 months. Intakes from children in the United States, the Soviet Union, and Holland ranged from a low of 0.8 for North American teenagers on a self-selected diet to a high of 9.5 for 9-year-old children from an institution in Russia. Self-selected intakes for adults from these same countries, New Zealand, and Japan ranged from 1 to 7. But Indian diets in two different studies of self-selected intakes had values ranging from 8 to 10 mg. (See Table VII.)

Information on the intake of other essential trace elements (Table VIII) is meager, and none is available on their intake in developing countries, where subsistence agriculture is more likely to result in localized deficiencies. The problem of consumption of excess amounts of the toxic trace element mercury has been alluded to by Smith and Brown in Chapter 38. Cadmium and lead toxicity may also be a problem, as there is no mechanism for monitoring or controlling their level in developing countries.

III. RESEARCH NEEDS

The first priority in assessing intake of trace elements is to develop reliable assay procedures that are suitably sensitive and do not introduce any contamination or losses of the nutrients under investigation. A great deal of confusion exists in the literature on the trace element content of foods and is caused in part by differences in technique but also by differences in sample preparation. Assessment of actual intake is further complicated by differences in food preparation used by the population under study. Thus, it is necessary to assay foods as eaten by a large representative sample of the population, such as has been done by the ICNND for dietary iron.

Simultaneous with determination of trace element content of foods, assessments should be made of accessory factors such as phytate and fiber that may influence absorption or utilization.

When suitable assay procedures become available, the diet of populations that might be susceptible to trace element deficiencies should be monitored, much as is currently done in the United States for cadmium, mercury, and lead. Although most people in developed countries probably are not at risk of trace element deficiency, there are individuals who may require abnormally large amounts of an essential trace element or who are sensitive to small amounts of a toxic element. In addition, changes in a nation's food supply can be caused by differences in food processing or food selection, which should be noted and corrected by appropriate fortification. In lesser-developed countries, where the food supply is less varied and where a majority of the population exists on subsistence agriculture, local soil and water conditions can cause a significant trace element problem.

Lastly, when suitable techniques have been developed, clinical studies should be done with typical diets to determine appropriate references for comparison of intakes.

REFERENCES

Allen, R. E., and Pierce, J. O. (1968). Determination of zinc in food, urine, air, and dust by atomic absorption. Amer. Ind. Hyg. Ass., J. 29, 469–473.

Bogen, D. C. (1968). Stable lead investigations at HASL. U.S. At. Energy Comm. UCRL 18140, 4–12.

Carter, J. P., Grivetti, L., Davis, J., Nasiff, S., Mansour, A., Mousa, W. A., Atta, A., Patwardhan, V. N., Abdel Moneim, A., Abdou, I. A., and Darby, W. J. (1969) Growth and sexual development of adolescent Egyptian village boys. Amer. J. Clin. Nutr. 22, 59–78.

Caughey, J. E., and Follis, R. H. (1965). Endemic goiter and iodine malnutrition in Iraq. Lancet 1, 1032–1034.

Caughey, J. E., Barakat, R., and Nourmand, I. (1970). Endemic goiter and iodine malnutrition in Southern Iran. Proc. Symp. Food Sci. Nutr. Dis. Mid. East, April 27–30, p. 30.

Coble, Y., Davis, J., Schulert, A., Heta, F., and Awad, A. Y. (1968). Goiter and iodine deficiency in Egyptian oases. Amer. J. Clin. Nutr. 21, 277–287.

Deutsch, M. J., Duffy, D., Pillsbury, H. C., and Lay, H. W. (1963). Total diet study. Section B. Nutrient content. J. Ass. Offic. Agr. Chem. 46, 759–762.

Eggleton, W. G. E. (1939). LI. The zinc content of epidermal structures in beri-beri. Biochem. J. 33, 403–410.

Engel, R. W., Miller, R. F., and Price, N. O. (1966). Metabolic patterns in adolescent children. XIII. Zinc balances. In "Zinc Metabolism" (A. S. Prasad, ed.), pp. 326–337. Thomas, Springfield, Illinois.

Flores, N., Flores, Z., and Lara, M. Y. (1966). Food intake of Guatemalan Indian children. *J. Amer. Diet. Ass.* **48**, 480–487.

Gormican, A. (1970). Inorganic elements in foods used in hospital menus. *J. Amer. Diet. Ass.* **56**, 397–403.

Griffiths, N. M. (1973). Daily dietary intake of selenium by some New Zealand women. *Proc. Univ. Otago Med. Sch.* **51**, 8–10.

Gutherie, B. (1973). Daily dietary intake of zinc, copper, manganese, chromium, and cadmium by some New Zealand women. *Proc. Univ. Otago Med, Sch.* **51**, 47–49.

Hampton, M. C., Heunemann, R. L., Shapiro, L. R., and Mitchell, B. W. (1967). Caloric and nutrient intakes of teen-agers. *J. Amer. Diet. Ass.* **50**, 385–396.

Hauck, H. M. (1961). Dietary study in a Nigerian secondary school. *J. Amer. Diet. Ass.* **39**, 467–473.

Hopkins, L. L., and Majaj, A. S. (1966). Selenium in human nutrition. *Proc. Symp. Selenium Biomed., 1967*, p. 200.

ICNND. (1959). "Nutrition Survey—Ethiopia." HEW-PHS, Washington, D.C.

ICNND. (1960a). "Nutrition Survey—Eucador." HEW-PHS, Washington, D.C.

ICNND. (1960b). "Nutrition Survey—Columbia." HEW-PHS, Washington, D.C.

ICNND. (1961). "Nutrition Survey—The Kingdom of Thailand." HEW-PHS, Washington, D.C.

ICNND. (1962a). "Nutrition Survey—Republic of Lebanon." Nutr. Sec. Off. Int. Res., NIH, HEW-PHS, Washington, D.C.

ICNND. (1962b). "Nutrition Survey—The West Indies." HEW-PHS, Washington, D.C.

ICNND. (1963). "Nutrition Survey—Venezuela." HEW-PHS, Washington, D.C.

ICNND. (1964a). "Nutrition Survey—Federation of Malaya." HEW-PHS, Washington, D.C.

ICNND. (1964b). "Nutrition Survey—Bolivia." HEW-PHS, Washington, D.C.

ICNND. (1966). "Nutrition Survey—East Pakistan." Off. Int. Res., NIH, HEW-PHS, Washington, D.C.

ICNND. (1967a). "Nutrition Survey—Federal Republic of Nigeria." Off. Int. Res., NIH, HEW-PHS, Washington, D.C.

ICNND. (1967b). "Nutrition Survey—Republic of Paraguay." HEW-PHS, Washington, D.C.

Jelliffe, D. B. (1966). "The Assessment of the Nutritional Status of the Community," p. 221. World Health Organ., Geneva.

Johnson, F. A., Frenchman, R., and Burroughs, E. D. (1951). The absorption of iron from spinach by six women and the effect of beef upon the absorption. *J. Nutr.* **44**, 383–389.

Kerimova, M. G. (1968). Seasonal variations in copper and zinc in the food of preschool age children. *Mater. Respub. Kohf. Probl., Mikroelem. Med. Zhivotnovod.* pp. 52–53.

Lamm, S., Cole, B., Glynn, B., and Ullmann, W. (1973). Lead content of milks fed to infants 1971–1972. *N. Engl. J. Med.* **289**, 574–575.

Lehnert, G., Stadelmann, G., Schaller, K. H., and Szadkowski, D. (1969). *Arch. Hyg. Bakteriol.* **153**, 403–412.

Mann, G. V. (1962). The health and nutritional status of Alaskan Eskimos—a survey of the ICNND—1958. *Amer. J. Clin. Nutr.* **11**, 31–76.

Maxia, V., Meloni, S., Rollier, M. A., Brandone, A., Patwardhan, V. N., Waslien, C. I., and El-Shami, S. (1972). Selenium and chromium assays of Egyptian foods and in blood of Egyptian Children by activation analysis. *Sym. Nuclear Activation Tech. in Life Sci.*, Bled, Yugoslavia, April 10–14, 1972.

Mondragon, M. C, and Jaffee, W. G. (1971). Selenium in foods and urine of school children in different regions of Venezuela. *Arch. Lationamer. Nutr.* 21, 185–195.

Monier-Williams, G. W. (1950). "Trace Elements in Foods." Chapman & Hall, London.

Murakami, Y., Suzuki, T., Yamagata, T., and Yamagata, N. (1965). Chromium and manganese in the Japanese diet. *J. Radiat. Res.* 6, 105–110.

Murphy, E. W., Page, L., and Watt, B. K. (1971). Trace elements in Type A school lunches. *J. Amer. Diet. Ass.* 58, 115–117.

Murthy, G. K., Rhea, U., and Peeler, J. T. (1971). Levels of antimony, cadmium, chromium, cobalt, manganese, and zinc in institutional total diets. *Environ. Sci. Technol.* 5, 436–442.

Murthy, G. K., Rhea, U., and Peeler, J. T. (1972). Copper, iron, magnesium, strontium, and zinc content of market milk. *J. Dairy Sci.* 55, 1666–1674.

Nakagawa, T. (1968). Daily manganese consumption in the food in Japan. *Osaka Shiritsu Daigaku Igaku Zasshi* 17, 401–424.

Nielsen, F. H. (1974). "Newer" trace elements in human nutrition. *Food Technol.* 28, 38–44.

Patwardhan, V. N., and Darby, W. J. (1972). "The State of Nutrition in the Arab Middle East." Vanderbilt Univ. Press, Nashville, Tennessee.

Prasad, A. S., Halsted, J. A., and Nadimi, M. (1961). Syndrome of iron deficiency anemia, hepatosplenomegaly, hypogonadism, dwarfism, and geophagia. *Amer. J. Med.* 31, 532–538.

Prasad, A. S., Miale, A., Farid, Z., Sandstead, H. H., Schulert, A. R., and Darby, W. J. (1963). Biochemical studies on dwarfism, hypogonadism, and anemia, *Arch. Intern. Med.* 111, 407–428.

Price, N. O., and Bunce, G. E. (1972). Effect of nitrogen and calcium on balance of copper, manganese, and zinc in pre-adolescent girls. *Nutr. Rep. Int.* 5, 275–279.

Price, N. O., Bunce, G. E., and Engel, R. W. (1970). Copper manganese, and zinc balance in pre-adolescent girls. *Amer. J. Clin. Nutr.* 23, 258–260.

Reinhold, J. G., Lahimgarzadeh, A., Nasr, K., and Hedayati, H. (1973). Effects of purified phytate and phytate-rich bread upon metabolism of zinc, calcium, phosphorus, and nitrogen in man. *Lancet* 1, 283–288.

Reshetkina, L. P. (1968). Iron in infant foods and the dietary iron supply of young children. *Pediatrija (Moscow)* 12, 64–65.

Reshetkina, L. P. (1969). Zinc requirement of children and its content in baby food. *Vop. Pitan.* 28, 62–64.

Ripak, E. N. (1961). Cobalt balance in pre-school children. *Vop. Pitan.* 20, 19–23.

Sandstead, H. H. (1967). Present knowledge of the minerals. In "Present Knowledge of Nutrition," pp. 117–125. Nutr. Found., New York.

Sandstead, H. H. (1973). Zinc nutrition in the United States. *Amer. J. Clin. Nutr.* 26, 1251–1260.

Schlage, C., and Wortberg, B. (1972). Zinc in the diet of healthy preschool and school children. *Acta Paediat. Scand.* 61, 421–425.

Schlaphoff, D. M., and Johnson, F. A. (1949). The iron requirement of six adolescent girls. *J. Nutr.* 39, 67–82.

Schlettwein-Gsell, D., and Mommsen-Straub, S. (1970). Spurenelemente in Lebensmitteln. III. Cobalt. *Int. Z. Vitaminforsch.* **40**, 674–683.

Schlettwein-Gsell, D., and Mommsen-Straub, S. (1971a). Ubersicht Spurenelemente in Lebensmitteln, III. Chrom. *Int. Z. Vitaminforsch.* **41**, 116–123.

Schlettwein-Gsell, D., and Mommsen-Straub, S. (1971b). Ubersicht Spurenelemente in Lebensmitteln. IV. Mangan. *Int. Z. Vitaminforsch.* **41**, 268–285.

Schlettwein-Gsell, D., and Mommsen-Straub (1971c). Ubersicht Spurenelemente in Lebensmitteln. VI. Kupfer. *Int. Z. Vitamin-forsch.* **41**, 554–581.

Schroeder, H. A. (1971). Losses of vitamins and trace minerals resulting from processing and preservation of foods. *Amer. J. Clin. Nutr.* **24**, 562–573.

Schroeder, H. A., Balassa, J. J., and Tipton, I. H. (1961). Abnormal trace elements in man-nickel. *J. Chronic Dis.* **15**, 51–65.

Schroeder, H. A., Balassa, J. J., and Tipton, I. H. (1962). Abnormal trace elements in man—chromium. *J. Chronic Dis.* **15**, 941–964.

Schroeder, H. A., Nason, A. P., Tipton, I. H., and Balassa, J. J. (1966). Essential trace metals in man: Copper. *J. Chronic Dis.* **19**, 1007–1037.

Schroeder, H. A., Nason, A. P., Tipton, I. H., and Balassa, J. J. (1967). Essential trace elements in man: Zinc, relationship to environmental cadmium. *J. Chronic Dis.* **20**, 179–200.

Soman, S. D., Panday, V. K., Joseph, K. T., and Raut, S. J. (1969). Daily intake of some major and minor trace elements. *Health Phys.* **17**, 36–40.

Soroka. N. V. (1966). Copper and cobalt contents in the hospital dietaries of the city Ivano-Frankovsk and foods of local origin. *Vop. Pitan.* **25**, 80–83.

Soroka, N. V. (1967). Content of iron and zinc in dietetic rations and foods of the precarpathian region. *Vop. Pitan.* **26**, 80–81.

Soroka, N. V. (1970). Chemical composition of dietetic rations in medical institutions of the Ivano-Frankov region. *Vop. Ratsion. Pitan.* **6**, 103–106.

Tipton, I. H., Stewart, P. L., and Martin, P. G. (1966). Trace elements in diet and excreta. *Health Phys.* **12**, 1683–1689.

Tipton, I. H., Stewart, P. L., and Dickson, J. (1969). Patterns of elemental excretion in long-term balance studies. *Health Phys.* **16**, 455–462.

Underwood, E. J. (1962). Miscellaneous elements. *In* "Trace Elements in Human and Animal Nutrition," 2nd ed., pp. 325–362. Academic Press, New York.

Underwood, E. J. (1971). "Trace Elements in Human and Animal Nutrition," 3rd ed. Academic Press, New York.

Valassi, K. V., and Reyonlds, J. W. (1966). Dietary studies of the civilian population of Uruguay. *Amer. J. Clin. Nutr.* **18**, 203–228.

Vorob'eva, A. I. (1965). Copper content of the food rations of the Tomsk Pediatric institutions. *Vop. Pitan.* **24**, 81–82.

Vorob'eva, A. I. (1967). Copper and zinc balances in children aged 2, 6, and 8–10 years. *Vop. Pitan.* **26**, 28–30.

Vorob'eva, A. I., and Bol'sanina, N. A. (1964). Zinc and iron in the rations of children in institutions in Tomsk. *Vop. Pitan.* **23**, 78–79.

Vorob'eva, A. I., and Osmolovskaya, E. V. (1970). Molybdenum and cobalt balance in pre-school children. *Gig. Sanit.* **35**, 108–109.

Vostal, J. J., and Clarkson, T. W. (1973). Mercury as an environmental hazard. *J. Occup. Med.* **15**, 649–656.

Waslien, C. I., Yacoub, N. Z., and Rizk, M. E. (1972). The diet of families with children having protein-calorie malnutrition. *Proc. 6th Symp. Nutr. Health Near East,* pp. 402–407.

Wharton, M. A. (1963). Nutritive intake of adolescents. *J. Amer. Diet. Ass.* **42,** 306–310.

White, H. S. (1969). Inorganic elements in weighed diets of girls and young women. *J. Amer. Diet. Ass.* **55,** 38–43.

World Health Organization Expert Committee. (1973). Trace elements in human nutrition. *World Health Organ., Tech. Rep. Ser.* **532.**

Wretlind, A. (1970). Food iron supply. *In* "Iron Deficiency: Pathogenesis, Clinical Aspects, Therapy" (L. Hallberg, H.-G. Harwerth, and A. Vannotti, eds.), pp. 39–69. Academic Press, New York.

Zook, E. G., and Lehmann, J. (1965). Total diet study: Content of ten minerals—aluminum, calcium, phosphorus, sodium, potassium, boron, copper, iron, manganese, magnesium. *J. Ass. Offic. Agr. Chem.* **48,** 850–855.

40

Basis of Recommended Dietary Allowances for Trace Elements

A. E. Harper

I. INTRODUCTION

Iron and iodine have long been recognized as nutritionally essential elements that may not be present in adequate amounts in the diet of man. Fluoride has long been recognized as an important agent for the control of dental caries. However, only during the past decade has there been serious concern about the significance for human health of the entire group of essential trace elements. Despite this concern, recommended dietary allowances (RDA) for only three trace elements are included in the table of allowances, with values for zinc being given for the first time in the latest edition of the RDA bulletin (Food and Nutrition Board, 1974). With evidence (1) that some fourteen trace elements are nutritionally essential, the nutritional importance of five of these being demonstrated since 1968; (2) that zinc, copper, and possibly selenium inadequacy may be encountered in malnourished children; and, (3) that marginal zinc and chromium nutriture may occur in the United States (Mertz, 1972); the time seems appropriate for discussion of the basis for establishing RDA for trace elements and to consider what additional information must be obtained before RDA can be established for more of the trace elements.

II. WHAT IS A RECOMMENDED DIETARY ALLOWANCE?

The definition given in the RDA bulletin is: "The Recommended Dietary Allowances are the levels of intake of essential nutrients considered, in the judgment of the Food and Nutrition Board on the basis of available scientific knowledge, to be adequate to meet the known nutritional needs of practically all healthy persons." In other words, *RDA are estimates of amounts of essential nutrients each person in a healthy population must consume in order to provide reasonable assurance that the physiological needs of all will be met.* This concept is not as well understood as it should be (Harper, 1974a,b). It is a public health concept based on the premise that if the requirement of each individual in a population is not known, the allowance must be high enough to meet the needs of those with the highest requirements. RDA for essential nutrients cannot, therefore, be equated with average requirements; they must exceed the requirements of most members of the population group for whom the recommendation is made.

The Food and Agriculture Organization (1973) and the World Health Organization of the United Nations refer to their very similar recommendations as "safe intakes" of nutrients. The Canadians refer to theirs as "dietary standards" (Department of National Health and Welfare, Ottawa, 1964). Unlike the term recommended dietary allowances, these terms carry no implication of being either nutritional requirements or recommendations for the ideal diet. I would prefer the term "acceptable nutrient intakes," which in my view implies safe intake and yet at the same time suggests that the recommendations are tentative, subject to revision, and not necessarily optimal or ideal intakes (Harper, 1974a).

III. CONSIDERATIONS IN SETTING RDA

A. Estimates of Human Requirements

The factors that are considered in setting RDA for trace elements are the same as for other essential nutrients. The starting point is the scientific evidence about requirements of man. For very few trace elements is there direct information about requirements from experiments on human subjects. For iron, there are estimates of iron losses of about 1 mg/day for adult man, mainly from estimates of the loss of iron in cells that are sloughed off. For women of child-bearing age, losses in menstrual fluid are estimated to represent an additional 0.5 mg/day. For children, estimates have been made of the amount of iron stored in tissues formed during growth. These values provide estimates of minimum metabolic needs. For zinc, there have been balance studies indicating that 8–10 mg of zinc is required to maintain zinc equilibrium in an adult man and estimates of turnover of body zinc using radioisotopes indicating that young children require about 6 mg/day. For iodine, the deficiency disease goiter is of worldwide importance, and the intake required to prevent goiter has been established at about 1 μg/kg of body weight per day. For copper, balance studies indicate that young girls require about 1.3 and adults about 2 mg/day to maintain copper balance (Food and Nutrition Board, 1974). But for most other trace elements there is little direct information about human requirements.

Another source of information that provides a rough estimate of human needs is knowledge of nutrient consumption by populations that show no evidence of nutritional deficiency. Nutritional needs would be unlikely to exceed the lowest intake values observed for a population that is healthy. Iron intake in the United States is estimated to be about 6 mg/1000 kcal of food, but this is associated with the occurrence of marginal iron deficiency in segments of the population, indicating that the iron needs of some groups in this country are not met by the quantities of iron they obtain from foods (Mertz, 1974). Estimates of zinc intake of 10–15 mg/day for adults exceed by relatively little the estimates of zinc needs from balance studies. Estimates of copper intake in the United States of about 2 mg/day correspond quite closely with estimates of copper requirements from balance studies. Chromium intakes have been estimated at about 60 μg/day, but chromium content of the body is known to decline with age. The amounts estimated to maintain chromium balance exceed average intakes, and there is evidence that impaired glucose tolerance in some older people is associated with chromium inadequacy. Although this type of information permits an estimate of the range within which trace element needs fall, the information is not precise enough to serve by itself as the basis for RDA. Also, information about the trace element content of foods is sparse, and for many trace elements, food analyses are not highly reliable, so this approach to establishing human needs is of limited value.

B. Age–Weight–Sex Groups

Information about the requirements of only one or two age groups is insufficient for developing RDA. Knowledge of how requirements change with age, sex, body size, physiological state, and activity is also needed to permit estimation of allowances for different population groups. For most age groups, it is usually necessary to interpolate from information about the nutritional needs of infants and adults, the two groups for whom information is most frequently available. This is usually done on the basis of average growth rates and knowledge of the composition of the tissue deposited, or on the basis of information about changes in food intake or energy needs with changing age and body size. A minimum estimate of the additional need during lactation can be obtained from measurements of the amount of nutrient secreted in the milk. A minimum estimate of the additional need during pregnancy can be made from knowledge of the amount of a nutrient that is deposited in the newly-formed tissues.

C. Estimates of Individual Variability

In extrapolating from an average requirement to derive an allowance, it is essential that individual variability be taken into account. If studies of the requirements of enough individuals have been done, the coefficient of variation can be calculated. Then, on the assumption that the distribution of individual requirements follows a normal distribution pattern, a value equal to the mean plus twice the coefficient of variation should include the requirements of 97.5% of the population. This is based on the accepted relationship that requirements of 95% of the population should fall within the range of plus or minus twice the coefficient of variation and that 2.5% of the population should have requirements below this range (Beaton, 1972). This is illustrated in Fig. 1. Although 2.5% of the population may have requirements above this range, the human body has great capacity to adapt, even to what are considered by many to be inadequate intakes of nutrients. Therefore, it seems reasonable to assume that those with the highest requirements should be able to adapt to intakes so close to their needs (Mitchell, 1944).

The RDA committee accepted the mean plus twice the coefficient of variation as a satisfactory approach to allowing for individual variability in estimating the RDA for protein, but there are insufficient data to permit such a calculation for many other nutrients. Beaton has done this for iron (1972). For many nutrients, however, the extra amount above the requirement that should be allowed for individual variation

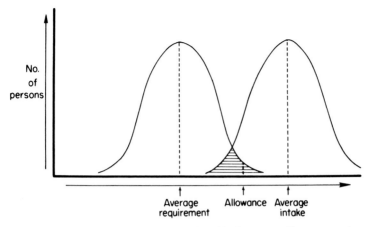

FIG. 1. Schematic representation of relationship between allowance and require-ment. Assuming that requirements of individuals follow a statistically normal distribu-tion, requirements of 97.5% of a healthy population should be met by an allowance equal to the average requirement plus twice the standard deviation. As intakes of nutri-ents among individuals are also highly variable (they tend to be skewed toward the right rather than following the normal distribution depicted), it is not valid to assume that the requirements of all individuals have been met when the average intake of a population exceeds the allowance. (From Harper, 1974a. Copyright The American Die-tetic Association. Reprinted by permission from the Journal of The American Dietetic Association **64**, 151, 1974.)

must be based on the assumption that the coefficients of variation for different nutrient requirements are similar.

D. Estimates of Biological Availability

Estimates of requirements for specific, highly available compounds; estimates of body losses; or estimates of turnover of a nutrient, even after addition of an increment to allow for individual variability, are insufficient for establishing RDA. Another increment must be added for efficiency of utilization of the nutrient as it occurs in foods. The problem of estimating efficiency of absorption or the availability of nutri-ents from foods is a major one in formulating dietary allowances. For iron, the amount required for body function and to allow for body losses is fairly well established as 1 mg/day for mature men and post-menopausal women and 1.5 mg/day for women of child-bearing age. However, with estimates of absorption of iron from foodstuffs ranging from negligible to about 30% and with an average figure of 10%, the allowances become 10 mg/day and 18 mg/day for these two groups. The availability of zinc from foodstuffs is also highly variable. The same is true for chromium and probably for other trace elements. However, if estimates of dietary allowances are based on measurements, such as balance studies, in which the nutrient is provided from foods or on intakes of the nutrient from foodstuffs by population groups exhibiting no signs of deficiency, availability of the nutrient from foods has already been taken into consideration.

The biological availability of trace elements may depend upon (1) the form in which the element occurs in foods; (2) the presence of phytates and other substances that bind the element; (3) the presence of substances that facilitate absorption, e.g., ascorbic acid, which improves the absorption of iron; (4) the occurrence of antagnostic compounds, such as goitrogens, which may reduce the effectiveness of iodine; and (5) the occurrence of heavy metal contaminants, which may act as antagonists to essential trace minerals. The health significance of imbalances of this last type or even imbalances among the trace elements themselves is not known (Mertz, 1972, 1974). Knowledge of the biological availability of nutrients, especially of the trace elements, is a major stumbling block to establishing accurate recommended allowances.

IV. RDA FOR TRACE ELEMENTS

In general, the establishment of RDA depends on:

1. being able to obtain a satisfactory quantitative estimate of the metabolic need for the nutrient;

2. being able to obtain an adequate estimate of variability among the requirements of individuals;

3. being able to estimate how requirements change with changes in physiological state;

4. being able to assess with a reasonable degree of accuracy the biological availability of the nutrient as it occurs in foodstuffs;

5. all of these measurements depend upon the development of analytical methods that permit accurate determination of the nutrient content of foods and body fluids.

At present, there are RDA for iron, iodine, zinc, and copper. The RDA for iron depend upon crude estimates of average availability of iron from foodstuffs and on the appropriateness of the criteria, such as estimates of iron stores, used as evidence of deficiency. The RDA for iodine depend mainly on evidence of minimal intakes of this element that are associated with the absence of goiter and knowledge of minimal amounts needed to cure the disease. The RDA for zinc are based on evidence from metabolic studies and intakes that do not result in appreciable evidence of deficiency. The RDA for copper are based on balance studies, but as the amount of information available is limited, they are not included in the table. The RDA for zinc are tentative; even for iron, the trace element that has been studied most extensively, the estimates are controversial. For most other trace elements, information is too scanty to permit estimation of an allowance—or even of a requirement.

V. NEED FOR MORE KNOWLEDGE ON WHICH TO BASE RDA

With (1) increasing use of fabricated foods, such as products prepared from purified soybean proteins, as substitutes for meat products which are known to be excellent sources of trace elements; (2) increasing use of highly refined foods from which a large proportion of many of the minor nutrients have been removed in processing; and, (3) the relatively low energy expenditure, and hence low food intake, of the United States population, the potential for creating health problems as a result of inadequate intakes of trace nutrients is increasing. It is therefore important that our knowledge of human needs for these substances be established accurately.

What stands out in reviewing this subject is how great the need is for more quantitative information about human requirements and the biological availability of trace elements. Unfortunately, much of the research required to provide this information does not promise the high degree of excitement associated with the discovery of unrecognized essential nutrients or new metabolic functions. Nevertheless, it is important from a very practical viewpoint if we are to circumvent potential public health problems and insure the future nutritional health of the population.

If I were a government administrator disbursing research funds and had to list priorities in trace element research, I would place at the top of the list support for the development of accurate and reproducible methods of analysis for the trace element content of foodstuffs. I would place second the development of methods for assessing the biological availability of trace elements and for determining the significance of factors that influence their availability. I would place third metabolic studies to assess the requirements for man of trace elements. But in setting these priorities, I would do my best to insure that investigations on these subjects involved a fundamental scientific approach that would improve our understanding of the role of trace elements in health and disease. Before it will be possible to establish RDA for additional trace elements, and even to assess the validity of those now established, considerable attention will have to be given to each of these subjects.

REFERENCES

Beaton, G. H. (1972). The use of nutritional requirements and allowances. *Proc. West. Hemisphere Nutr. Congr., 3rd, 1971* pp. 356–363.

Department of National Health and Welfare, Ottawa. (1964). Dietary standard for Canada. *Can. Bull. Nutr.* **6**, No. 1.

Food and Agriculture Organization. (1973). "Energy and Protein Requirements." FAO/WHO, Rome.

Food and Nutrition Board. (1974). "Recommended Dietary Allowances," 8th ed. Nat. Acad. Sci., Washington, D.C.

Harper, A. E. (1974a). Recommended dietary allowances—are they what we think they are? *J. Amer. Diet. Ass.* **64**, 151–156.

Harper, A. E. (1974b). Those pesky RDA's. *Nutr. Today* **9**, 15–28.

Mertz, W. (1972). Human requirements: Basic and optimal. *Ann. N.Y. Acad. Sci.* **199**, 191–201.

Mertz, W. (1974). Recommended dietary allowances up to date—trace minerals. *J. Amer. Diet. Ass.* **64**, 163–167.

Mitchell, H. H. (1944). Adaptation to undernutrition. *J. Amer. Diet. Ass.* **20**, 511–515.

41

Newer Trace Elements and Possible Application in Man

F. H. Nielsen

I. INTRODUCTION

Advancements in the past few years have clearly demonstrated the importance of certain trace elements in human health and disease. Yet, less than twenty years ago, trace elements such as zinc, copper, and chromium were thought to be esoteric considerations for human nutrition. The elements to be discussed in this chapter appear to be at the same level of consideration today. However, this opinion may change in the near future as people continue to consume more highly refined foods, food product analogs, and empty calories, which are often lacking in trace elements. The use of fad diets, defined diets, or total parenteral feeding may also reveal the importance of some "newer" trace elements. As dietary manipulations increase, a sense of urgency is created, because at present, knowledge of man's requirements for trace elements is incomplete. This is especially true for five elements—nickel, vanadium, silicon, fluorine, and tin—which recently have been found to be essential, or at least beneficial, in the diets of laboratory animals. It seems probable that some of these elements are also essential or beneficial for man. For the purpose of this report, silicon has been included with the trace elements, even though it is present in the body in relatively large amounts.

II. REVIEW AND DISCUSSION

A. Nickel

1. Essentiality

Nickel has been suspected of having some physiological role in animals or in man since the 1920s, when it was found to be present in animal tissue. Indirect evidence for such a role has been reviewed (Nielsen, 1971, 1974; Nielsen and Ollerich, 1974), so it will not be presented here. Direct evidence that nickel is essential for animals is a recent finding. Pathological signs consistent with nickel deficiency have been produced in chicks, rats, and swine.

The first direct evidence for the essentiality of nickel was reported in 1970 (Nielsen and Sauberlich, 1970). However, the findings of that study and of those that followed (Nielsen, 1971, 1974; Nielsen and Higgs, 1971; Nielsen and Ollerich, 1974; Nielsen et al., 1974; Sunderman et al., 1972b) were obtained under conditions that produced suboptimal growth in chicks. Also, some of the signs thought to be the result of nickel deficiency were inconsistent.

During the past year, with improved methodology for the study of nickel deficiency, day-old chicks grew to over 600 gm in 4 weeks—a highly satisfactory and apparently optimal growth rate. The diet used was based on dried skim milk, EDTA-extracted soy protein, acid-washed ground corn, and corn oil. It contained 2.2 ng nickel/gm on an air dried basis. The chicks were raised in a trace-element-controlled environment (Nielsen, 1974). Some of our observations to date with these chicks are reported here.

Grossly, at $3\frac{1}{2}$–4 weeks of age, the legs of deficient chicks were different from those of controls (supplemented with 3 μg nickel/gm diet). Deficiency resulted in less pigmentation of the shank skin. The legs also appeared to be shorter and thicker. Attempts were made to assess these observations objectively. The yellow lipochrome pigments were extracted from a defined area of the shank skin with acetone. Absorbance at 420 mμ was divided by the weight of the shank skin and multiplied by 100. The values given in Table I show that the shank skin of deficient chicks contained significantly lower amounts of the yellow pigments measured. Leg structural changes were assessed by the greatest length–smallest width ratios of the femurs and tibias. Significantly lower ratios were obtained with the deficient chicks (Table I).

Other obtainable signs of nickel deficiency in chicks are shown in Table II. These include significantly decreased hematocrits and decreased plasma cholesterol.

TABLE I Shank-Skin YELP[a] and Length–Width Ratios of Femurs and
Tibiae of Nickel-Deficient and Supplemented Chicks

Group	No. of chicks	Shank-skin YELP [(O.D. units/gm × 100) ± SEM]	Length–width ratio ± SEM	
			Femur	Tibia
Ni deficient	15	196[b] ± 6	9.46[c] ± 0.14	14.95[d] ± 0.28
+3 ppm Ni	15	230 ± 6	9.85 ± 0.12	15.59 ± 0.25

[a] Yellow lipochrome pigments. See text for method.
[b] Significantly different ($P < 0.001$) from +3 ppm Ni group.
[c] Significantly different ($P < 0.05$) from +3 ppm Ni group.
[d] Significantly different ($P < 0.10$) from +3 ppm Ni group.

Ultrastructural abnormalities in the hepatocytes were also a consistent finding (Figs. 1 and 2). They included pyknotic nuclei and the swelling of the mitochondria. The swelling of the mitochondria was in the compartment of the matrix and was associated with less clearly defined cristae. Other ultrastructural changes were ribosomal draping around the mitochondria and dilation of the cisterns of the rough endoplasmic reticulum.

Studies have been initiated with rats by using basically the same diet and a similar controlled environment. Successive generations are being raised so that the animals will be exposed to deficiency throughout fetal, neonatal, and adult life. Thus far, one generation has been completed. During the suckling stage, the nickel-deficient pups generally had a less thrifty appearance, characterized by a rougher hair coat and less active appearance. They also had a slower growth rate (Table III), and some actually seemed malnourished. Approximately 17% of the deficient pups died during the last few days of the suckling period. There

TABLE II Blood Analyses of Nickel-Deficient and
Supplemented Chicks

Group	No. of chicks	Hematocrit (% ± SEM)	Plasma cholesterol (mg% ± SEM)
Ni deficient	15	29.0[a] ± 0.5	150[a] ± 3
+3 ppm Ni	15	30.7 ± 0.5	160 ± 2

[a] Significantly different ($P < 0.05$) from +3 ppm Ni group.

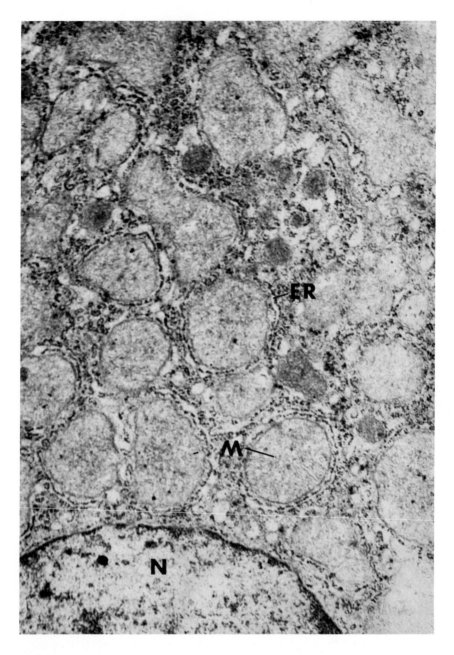

FIG. 1. Hepatic cell from nickel-deficient chick (2.2 ppb nickel). Swelling of mitochondria (M) was evident in numerous cells. The swelling was in the compartment of the matrix and was associated with less clearly defined cristae. Pyknotic nuclei (N) were also evident in numerous cells. Note the draping of ribosomes around the mitochondria and dilated cisterns of the rough endoplasmic reticulum (ER). Uranyl acetate and lead citrate, × 32,000.

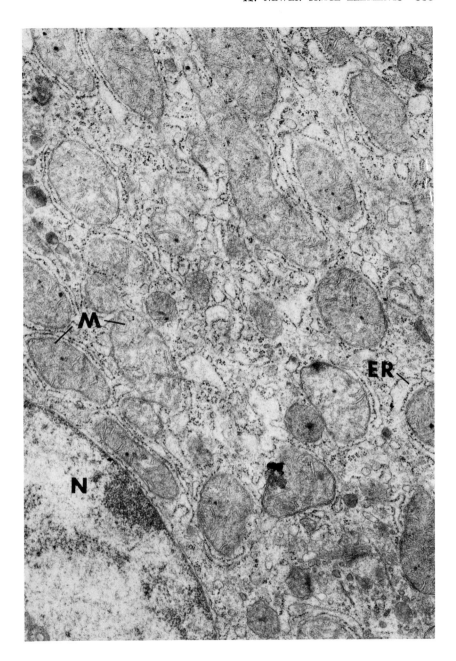

FIG. 2. Hepatic cell from nickel-supplemented chick (+3 ppm nickel). Compare mitochondria (M) and nucleus (N) with those in Fig. 1. Endoplasmic reticulum (ER). Uranyl acetate and lead citrate, × 32,000.

TABLE III   Growth and Mortality in First Generation Nickel-Deficient and Supplemented Rats

Group (no. of litters)	Mor- tal- ity[a] (%)	Weight (gm) ± SEM (no. of animals)			
		4 days	24 days[b]	40 days	
				Male	Female
Ni deficient (4)	17	10.3[c] ± 0.2 (41)	59[d] ± 1 (35)	159 ± 3 (17)	132 ± 3 (17)
+3 ppm Ni (4)	0	11.2 ± 0.2 (37)	66 ± 1 (37)	165 ± 3 (18)	136 ± 2 (18)

[a] Deaths between 4 and 24 days of age.
[b] Pups were weaned at this age.
[c] Significantly different ($P < 0.005$) from +3 ppm Ni group.
[d] Significantly different ($P < 0.001$) from +3 ppm Ni group.

was no mortality in the controls at this age. After being weaned, the appearance, activity, and growth of the deficient animals improved.

Nickel-deficient rats at 6–8 weeks of age showed some alterations in liver metabolism. Their livers weighed less (Table IV) than those of controls and were muddy brown color compared with a red-brown color for controls. Homogenates of the deficient livers exhibited an increased oxidative ability in the presence of α-glycerophosphate (Table IV). Nickel-deficient livers also contained significantly lower levels of liver glycogen.

Previous studies showed that with nickel deficiency, sucrose density

TABLE IV   Liver Analyses of Nickel-Deficient and Supplemented Female Rats

Group	No. of ani- mals	Liver weight (gm ± SEM)	Oxygen uptake[a] (μl/hr/mg protein ± SEM)	Glycogen[b] (mg/gm ± SEM)
Ni deficient	5	5.5[c] ± 0.18	6.07[c] ± 0.27	4.2[d] ± 0.7
+3 ppm Ni	5	6.1 ± 0.03	4.63 ± 0.15	7.0 ± 0.4

[a] Using liver homogenates and with α-glycerophosphate as the substrate.
[b] Fresh weight basis.
[c] Significantly different ($P < 0.05$) from comparable +3 ppm Ni group.
[d] Significantly different ($P < 0.025$) from comparable +3 ppm Ni group.

gradients of liver postmitochondrial supernates were consistent with a decrease in polysomes and an increase in monosomes (Nielsen, 1974; Nielsen and Ollerich, 1974; Nielsen et al., 1974).

Signs of nickel deficiency have been produced in swine as well as chicks and rats (Anke et al., 1974). Some of the findings include impaired reproduction and a sparse, rough hair coat. First generation piglets grew poorly.

Thus, a substantial amount of direct evidence exists that shows nickel is an essential element. However, no experimental evidence has been published that shows the level of nickel required by animals to maintain health, so this can only be approximated. An intake of 50–80 ng nickel/gm experimental diet is probably adequate for chicks and rats (F. H. Nielsen, unpublished observations). The experimental diet contained approximatly 20% protein, 12% fat, 52% carbohydrate, and 16% fiber, minerals, and vitamins.

2. Biological Function

The evidence that shows that nickel is essential has provided only meager insights as to its metabolic function. An attractive hypothesis is that nickel has a role in the metabolism or in the structure of membranes. The liver ultrastructural changes occur mainly in the membraneous organelles.

Another possibility is that nickel may have some role in hormonal control. Recent reports indicate that nickel may be important in the regulation of prolactin (LaBella et al., 1973). Since prolactin influences milk production, the finding that nickel deficiency appears to affect the suckling pup most severely lends support to the concept that nickel plays a role in lactation at the pituitary level. Moreover, many of the changes observed in nickel deficiency could be explained by changes in hormone actions. These include changes in liver glycogen, liver mitochondrial morphology and, shank skin yellow pigments, and plasma cholesterol.

Nickel may have a role in RNA, DNA, and/or protein structure or function. A nickel metalloprotein named "nickeloplasmin" has been isolated from human and rabbit serum (Nomoto et al., 1971; Sunderman et al., 1972a). The function of this protein is unclear at present. Significant concentrations of nickel are present in DNA and RNA (Wacker and Vallee, 1959; Eichhorn, 1962; Wacker et al., 1963; Sunderman, 1965). It was suggested that nickel and the other metals present may contribute to the stabilization of the structure of the nucleic acids. Nickel can preserve the compact structure of ribosomes against thermal denaturation

(Tal, 1968, 1969a,b) and will restore the sedimentation characteristics of *Escherichia coli* ribosomes that have been subjected to EDTA denaturation. The findings on rat liver polysomes described in this chapter, in addition to this *in vitro* evidence, suggest that nickel does have a structural role in nucleic acids.

The possibility that nickel may be an important cofactor in some enzyme system should not be precluded, as nickel can activate numerous enzymes *in vitro*, including desoxyribonuclease (Miyaji and Greenstein, 1951), acetylcoenzyme A synthetase (Webster, 1965), and phosphoglucomutase (Ray, 1969).

3. Possible Human Requirements

Because nickel is essential for animals, it is highly probable that it is also essential for man. However, at present it appears that nickel nutriture is not a practical problem for man. If animal data can be extrapolated to man, then the dietary requirement is probably in the range of 50–80 ng/gm diet. Most diets will provide this amount because grains and vegetables appear to be good sources of dietary nickel. This statement must be qualified, as knowledge concerning the chemical form of nickel in foods of plant origin is limited. It has been shown that nickel translocates in plants as a stable anionic amino acid complex (Tiffin, 1971). Whether organic nickel complexes are the usual compounds of nickel in plant tissues, and whether they in any way influence the bioavailability of nickel remains to be determined. Decsy and Sunderman (1974) have evidence that suggests that nickeloplasmin preferentially binds nickel in the form of an organic complex that is not synthesized, or is synthesized poorly, by the rabbit *in vivo*. Also, grains which are rich in nickel, are also usually high in phytin. Nickel can form a stable complex with phytic acid (Vohra *et al.*, 1965). Thus, it may be possible that the phytate in grains and other vegetables could decrease the availability of dietary nickel for intestinal absorption. Another possibility is that nickel may complex with fiber in these foods and could thereby decrease the availability of dietary nickel. In contrast to foods of plant origin, foods of animal origin contain relatively little nickel.

Diets based on foods of animal origin, or fats, or both may be low in nickel. A human diet containing 7–22 ng nickel/gm was prepared from meat, milk, eggs, refined white bread, butter, and corn oil (Schroeder *et al.*, 1962). Protein supplied 17.4% of the calories; carbohydrate, 43.5%; and fat, 39.1%.

Nickel nutriture may be of concern in individuals with diseases that interfere with intestinal absorption, or those who are under extreme physiological stress. It is known that the level of nickel in plasma is decreased in patients with cirrhosis of the liver, chronic uremia, or chronic renal insufficiency (McNeely *et al.*, 1971). Perhaps these findings are indicative of nickel depletion. Another consideration is the relatively high concentrations of nickel in sweat (Hohnadel *et al.*, 1973). Conditions that result in large losses of sweat may conceivably increase the need for nickel.

B. Vanadium

1. Essentiality

Data supporting the view that vanadium is an essential element for animals was first reported in 1971. Hopkins and Mohr (1971a,b) found significantly reduced growth of wing and tail feathers in chicks fed a diet containing less than 10 ng vanadium/gm. Strasia (1971) found that rats fed less than 100 ng vanadium per gram of diet exhibited reduced body growth and a significantly increased blood packed cell volume when compared with controls receiving at least 0.5 μg vanadium/gm. He also noted an increase in blood and bone iron in deficient rats. Schwarz and Milne (1971) found that rats fed highly purified amino acid diet (containing an unknown amount of vanadium) demonstrated a growth response to 50–100 ng of supplemental vanadium per gram of diet. In addition to these, several other deficiency symptoms attributable to low levels of dietary vanadium have been reported in rats and chicks.

As shown in Table V, vanadium deficiency has an effect on plasma

TABLE V   Effect of Vanadium Deficiency on Chick Plasma Lipids

Lipid	Vanadium-deficient diet[a]	Vanadium-supplemented diet[a]
Cholesterol (mg%)		
28 days[b]	178	206
49 days[b]	249	224
28 days[c]	158 (12)	145 (12)
28 days[c]	182 (10)	163 (10)
Triglycerides (mg%)[d]	48.7 (9)	25.4 (9)

[a] Number of chicks is given in parentheses.
[b] Hopkins and Mohr (1971a,b).
[c] Nielsen and Ollerich (1973; unpublished data).
[d] Hopkins and Mohr (1974).

lipids in chicks. Hopkins and Mohr (1971a,b) found that vanadium-deficient chicks had decreased plasma levels of cholesterol at 28 days of age, but at 49 days, their plasma cholesterol concentrations were greater than those of control chicks. Nielsen and Ollerich (1973; unpublished data) found increased plasma cholesterol levels in deficient chicks after only 28 days of deficiency. Recent data show that plasma triglyceride levels are also significantly increased in vanadium-deficient chicks (Hopkins and Mohr, 1974).

Vanadium deficiency also has adverse effects on bone development in the chick (Nielsen and Ollerich, 1973). In deficient chicks, the tibiae revealed increased epiphyseal plate and decreased primary spongiosa as judged by weight ratios and microsopic examination.

In rats, reproductive performance is impaired by vanadium deprivation (Hopkins and Mohr, 1974). When five fourth-generation female rats were mated, there were significantly fewer live births and significantly more deaths of neonatal pups than with vanadium-supplemented controls.

These data from four different laboratories and on two different species have established that vanadium is an essential nutrient for experimental animals. Due to limited data, the level of vanadium required by rats and chicks to maintain health can only be estimated. Schwarz (1974) has reported a requirement of 100 ng of supplemental vanadium per gram of diet containing an unknown amount of vanadium for an optimal growth response in rats. However, an additional increment of growth was observed when 500 ng of vanadium was supplemented per gram of diet. Hopkins and Mohr (1974) have suggested that the requirement is between 50 and 500 ng/gm when a purified diet is fed. Moreover, they stated the requirement may be even higher if natural feeds are used. With an experimental diet composed of 26% protein, 6% fat, and 57% carbohydrate (balance minerals, vitamins, and non-nutritive fiber), an intake of approximately 100 ng/gm for chicks is probably adequate (F. H. Nielsen, unpublished observations).

2. Biological Function

As with nickel, very little is known about the specific biological function or functions of vanadium. Most likely, vanadium is an important cofactor in controlling one or more enzymatic or calatytic reactions. Schwarz (1974) speculated that vanadium functions as an oxidation–reduction catalyst. It was reported that added vanadium markedly increased the oxidation of phospholipids by washed liver suspensions in vitro (Bernheim and Bernheim, 1939). Further evidence that vanadium can act as an oxidation–reduction catalyst in biological systems was obtained from a lower group of organisms known as the ascidians. Schroeder *et al.* (1963) and Underwood (1971) have briefly reviewed these data. Ascidians contain green blood cells called vandocytes. Vandocytes contain hemovanadin, a pigment composed of pyrrole rings and a protein. Hemovanadin is a strong reducing agent.

Studies involving vanadium and its effect on cholesterol metabolism have revealed that pharmacological levels of vanadium can affect tissue cholesterol levels. Curran and Burch (1967) have been able to relate these altered cholesterol levels to vanadium inhibition of the microsomal enzyme system known as squalene synthetase, and to the vanadium stimulation of acetoacetyl-CoA deacylase in liver mitochondria. The findings of altered lipid metabolism in vanadium deficiency are consistent with an enzymatic role for vanadium in lipid metabolism.

Vanadium may also have a catalytic or enzymatic function in hard tissue metabolism or formation. The finding of abnormal bone growth in vanadium deficiency suggests such a possibility. Further evidence for such a function is that when radiovanadium was injected subcutaneously into young rats, the highest uptake was in areas of rapid mineralization in the dentine and bone (Soremark *et al.*, 1962). Moreover, radiovanadium injected intravenously into adult mice was also taken up by the teeth and bones. After 24–48 hr, the bones and teeth were the tissues having the highest concentration, with the zones of mineralization showing an especially high uptake (Soremark and Ullberg, 1962).

3. Possible Human Requirements

Information as to the amount of vanadium in dietary items is limited. This is partly due to the difficulty in accurately analyzing for low levels of vanadium. Soremark (1967) reported values obtained by activation analysis. These ranged from less than 0.1 ng vanadium/gm in peas, beets, carrots, and pears to 52 ng/gm in radishes. Milk generally contained less than 0.1 ng/gm (fresh basis) and liver, fish, and meat contained up to 10 ng/gm. Some foods that are apparently good sources of vanadium are bread, some grains and nuts, vegetable oils, and a few root vegetables (Schroeder *et al.*, 1963). However, these limited data indicate that many dietary items contain amounts of vanadium below 50 ng/gm. Also, information as to the availability of vanadium from foods is limited. The toxicity of vanadium compounds has been found to be greater when the compounds are fed in a purified diet than when these compounds are given in a natural diet (Berg, 1966).

Obviously, many additional data are needed before firm conclusions can be drawn; however, if man has a vanadium requirement that is similar to that of rats and chicks, adequate vanadium nutrition should not be taken for granted. A diet exclusively of milk, meat, and certain vegetables could contain less than 50 ng vanadium/gm.

C. Silicon

1. Essentiality

Silicon is one of the newest elements to be shown essential for animals. Although it was reported earlier (Carlisle, 1970, 1971) that silicon may be necessary for an early stage of bone calcification, the first clear evidence for the essentiality of silicon was given in 1972 (Carlisle, 1972a,b; Schwarz and Milne, 1972a). Studies with chicks (Carlisle, 1972a,b) showed that feeding a silicon-deficient diet resulted in depressed growth. Pallor of the legs, comb, skin, and mucous membranes occurred. The subcutaneous tissue was a muddy yellowish color in contrast to the white-pinkish subcutaneous tissue of the silicon-adequate controls. The deficient chicks had no wattles, and their combs were severely attenuated. Feathering was retarded. Leg bones had thinner cortexes and were shorter and of smaller circumference than were those of controls. Femurs and tibiae fractured more easily. Cranial bones were flatter and beaks were more flexible.

In rats, 500 μg of silicon per gram of amino acid diet gave a growth response (Schwarz and Milne, 1972a). Initially, because of the high level of silicon supplementation as sodium metasilicate, some reservation existed to the idea that this growth response demonstrated silicon essentiality. However, the unsupplemented animals had skull deformations and poor incisor pigmentation. Also, later studies (Schwarz, 1974) showed that some silicon substances other than sodium metasilicate were five to ten times as active per atom of silicon in producing responses in rats. Thus, it is apparent that silicon is acting as an essential element in the rat.

More recently, it was shown (Carlisle, 1973) that the skeletal alterations involve the cartilage matrix. In the silicon-deficient chick metatarsus and tibial epiphyses, epiphyseal plates, and spongiosae there is a significant decrease in hexosamines.

The level of silicon required by animals is still uncertain. Schwarz (1974) found that for optimal response the rat requires 500 μg silicon per gram of diet as sodium metasilicate, but, as indicated, other forms can be more potent. E. M. Carlisle (personal communication) estimated that the chick requirement for silicon as sodium metasilicate is in the range of 100–200 μg per gram of experimental diet containing 26% amino acids, 5% fat, 62% carbohydrate, and 7% minerals and vitamins. It is probable that other forms of silicon are more available than the silicate for the chick as they are for the rat. Thus, the absolute requirement for the chick probably is lower than 100–200 μg/gm.

2. Biological Function

Latest studies have given evidence that silicon is an essential cross-linking agent in connective tissue. Both the distribution of silicon in the organism and the effect of silicon deficiency on connective tissue form and composition strongly suggest such a role. Table VI shows the silicon content of various connective tissue components. The data of Schwarz (1973) show 331–554 μg of bound silicon per gram of purified hyaluronic acid from human umbilical cord, chondroitin 4-sulfate, dermatan sulfate, and heparan sulfate. These levels correspond to one atom of silicon per 50,000 to 85,000 molecular weight, or 130 to 280 repeating units. Lesser amounts (57–191 μg/gm) were found in chondroitin 6-sulfate, heparin, and keratan sulfate-2 from cartilage. Hyaluronic acid from vitreous humor and keratan sulfate-1 from cornea were silicon-free. As seen in Table VI, collagen in connective tissue contains silicon. Schwarz and Chen (1974) gave evidence that indicates the presence of at least three to six atoms of silicon per each α-protein chain in the collagen molecule. Carlisle (1974a) found lesser amounts of silicon in collagen, but it is still apparent that silicon may have a fundamental role in collagen cross-linking mechanisms.

Numerous experiments carried out (Schwarz, 1973, 1974) to characterize the form in which silicon may be present indicate that the silicon atom is bound over oxygen to the carbon skeleton of mucopolysaccharides: —Si—O—C—. It was concluded that silicon is present as a silanolate, an etherlike or esterlike derivative of silicic acid. Silicon may link portions of the same polysaccharide to each other, or acid mucopolysaccharides to proteins. The possible biochemistry of silicon that may contribute to the structure and resilience of connective tissue has been reviewed by Schwarz (1973, 1974).

In addition to a structural function, silicon may have a matrix, or catalytic, function in bone calcification. Using electron microprobe techniques, Carlisle (1970, 1971, 1974b) observed that as mineralization progresses the silicon and calcium contents rise congruently in osteoid tissue. In the more advanced stages of mineralization, the silicon concentration falls markedly, whereas calcium concentrations approach proportions found in bone apatite. In the metaphysis of young bone, minute

TABLE VI Silicon Content of Selected Connective Tissue Components

Substance and source	Silicon content (μg/gm)		
	Free	Total	Bound (total minus free)
Hyaluronic acid			
Human umbilical cord[a]	1533	1892	359
Bovine vitreous humor[a]	980	949	(0)
Chondroitin 4-sulfate			
Notocord of rock sturgeon[a]	44	598	554
Rat costal cartilage[a]	30	361	331
Chondroitin 6-sulfate			
Human umbilical cord[a]	45	123	78
Human cartilage[a]	36	227	191
Sturgeon cartilage[a]	64	121	57
Dermatan sulfate			
Hog mucosal tissue[a]	46	548	502
Heparan sulfate			
Beef lung[a]	39	466	427
Heparin			
Hog mucosal tissue[a]	33	175	142
Keratan sulfate-1			
Bovine cornea[a]	31	37	(0)
Keratan sulfate-2			
Human costal cartilage[a]	37	105	68
Collagen, salt soluble			
Rat skin[b]	—	547–897	—
Chick skin[c]	—	127	—
Collagen, acid soluble			
Rat skin[b]	—	479–1997	—
Calf skin[b]	—	3296	—
Bovine achilles' tendon[b]	—	90–496	—
Bovine articular cartilage[b]	—	307–979	—
Collagen, insoluble			
Chick skin[c]	—	43	—

[a] Schwarz (1973, 1974).
[b] Schwarz and Chen (1974).
[c] Carlisle (1974a).

silicon-rich sites were found that corresponded with the margin of trabeculae and bony spicules during bone formation. Silicon was also found in blood vessels between metaphyseal trabeculae. Carlisle stated that "the fact that silicon occurs both in metaphyseal blood vessels and in the silicon-rich sites, along with the observations by earlier workers that invasion of the metaphysis by blood vessels triggers the sequence of matrix alterations leading to calcification, suggests that silicon takes part in the sequence of events leading to calcification."

3. Possible Human Requirements

Silicon deficiency has not been described in man. However, from the previous discussion, it is apparent that silicon has important functions in man. Mucopolysaccharides, collagen, and silicon are probably inter-related in human growth and maintenance of connective tissues. Silicon content has been found to decrease in the arterial wall with the development of atherosclerosis (Loeper and Loeper, 1961). Aging results in diminished silicon concentrations in human skin (dermis) (Brown, 1927; MacCardle et al., 1943) and in normal human aorta (Loeper and Loeper, 1961).

The form and absolute requirement of silicon for animals has not been ascertained, so nothing can be said about probable human requirements. Silicon is probably not a major dietary problem, as many foods contain high levels of silicon. Such foods include those high in fiber (e.g., some cereal grains) and pectin (e.g., citrus fruits). Dietary items of animal origin, except skin (e.g., chicken) are relatively low in silicon, so diets relatively low in silicon would be possible. Thus, adequate silicon nutrition should not be taken for granted.

D. Fluorine

1. Essentiality

A beneficial function of fluorine has been known since the late 1930s, when it was discovered that the fluoride ion can play a significant role in the prevention of human dental caries. In 1960, evidence was presented that indicates fluoride is also beneficial for the maintenance of a normal skeleton in the adult. These effects of fluoride have been reviewed by Underwood (1971) and probably will be updated elsewhere in this treatise by Navia et al. (Chapter 34).

Recently, interest in fluorine has been stimulated by unconfirmed reports that fluoride may be necessary for normal hematocrit levels, fertility, and growth. It was found that during the stress of pregnancy, feeding diets low in fluoride resulted in decreased hematocrits in mice (Messer et al., 1972b). Also, the number of litters produced by first and second generation females was reduced, but litter size was not affected (Messer et al., 1972a, 1973). These abnormalities were prevented by the addition of 50 μg fluoride per milliliter of drinking water. Although this amount is toxic for man, it is not an unusual amount to be fed to rodents. However, such high levels of supplemental fluoride give rise to the question as to whether fluoride was acting physiologically or pharmacologically. Thus, although these results strongly indicate an essential role for fluoride, it may be that fluoride was acting as a pharmacological agent in correcting some dietary imbalance or deficiency. Both infertility and anemia are not unusual findings in trace element and vitamin deficiencies.

Schwarz and Milne (1972b) reported that fluoride stimulates the growth of rats fed a highly purified amino acid diet and maintained in trace element-controlled isolators. This observation must also, until confirmed, be viewed with reservation for the following reasons: (1) Other investigators were not able to obtain this finding even though they fed diets containing less fluoride (Maurer and Day, 1957; Doberenz et al., 1964). (2) The control rats grew suboptimally, even with fluoride supplementation. Here too, as was suggested in the previous paragraph, fluoride may have been acting just to correct, or partially correct, some dietary imbalance or deficiency. The growth rate of the controls is strongly indicative of some dietary inadequacies, and if these were eliminated, it might be possible that fluoride would give no growth response, as other investigators have found.

At present, because of these uncertainties, a requirement for fluoride cannot be estimated. However, 1–2 μg per gram of diet appears beneficial for rats (Schwarz and Milne, 1972b).

2. Biological Function

Determining a possible function for fluoride by using the previously discussed studies is difficult. It is suggestive that fluoride may have a role interrelated with absorption or utilization of some other dietary nutrient. Additional evidence for this is that fluoride can enhance the intestinal absorption of iron (Ruliffson et al., 1963). Fluoride can activate some enzyme systems, most notably adenyl cyclase (Drummond et al., 1971). Thus, a role in the mediation of hormone effects is possible for fluoride.

3. Possible Human Requirements

On the basis of the above experimental studies in animals, it seems possible that fluoride is beneficial in ways other than in the prevention of dental caries.

Foods high in fluorine (Underwood, 1971) include sea foods (5–10

μg/gm) and tea (100 μg/gm). Cereal and other grains contain 1–3
μg/gm. Cow's milk usually contains 1–2 μg/gm (dry basis). An important
source of fluoride is fluoridated drinking water.

E. Tin

1. Essentiality

Trace amounts of tin occur in many tissues and dietary items, but
until recently the element had been considered an environmental contaminant instead of a possibly essential dietary factor. In 1970, it was
reported that tin is essential for the growth of rats maintained on purified
amino acid diets in a trace-element-controlled environment (Schwarz
et al., 1970). Tin also gave significant improvement in incisor pigmentation (Milne and Schwarz, 1972). These observations have not been
confirmed.

2. Biological Function

Tin has a number of chemical properties that offer possibilities for
biological function. Tetravalent tin has a strong tendency to form coordination complexes with four, five, six, and possibly eight ligands. Thus,
Schwarz et al. (1970) suggested that tin may contribute to the tertiary
structure of proteins or other components of biological importance. They
also speculated that tin may participate in oxidation–reduction reactions
in biological systems because the $Sn^{2+} \leftrightarrows Sn^{4+}$ potential of 0.13 V is within
the physiological range. In fact, it is near the oxidation–reduction poten-
tial of flavine enzymes.

3. Possible Human Requirements

Since so little is known about the metabolism of tin, it is impossible
to state any possible needs for it in man. The levels of tin found to
promote growth in rats are similar to the amounts found in many foods
of plant and animal origin (Schwarz et al., 1970). Therefore, tin nutriture
is not of much concern at present. Increased use of highly refined foods
or food product analogs containing little or no tin may alter this judge-
ment in the future.

III. RESEARCH NEEDS

In summary, three new elements (vanadium, nickel, and silicon) have
been found essential and two (fluorine and tin) possibly essential for

animals. To date, these elements have not been shown essential for man. However, by extrapolation from animal data, it is possible to postulate their importance in human nutrition. Moreover, the recognition of human deficiencies of other trace elements, such as zinc and copper, in certain populations and in patients with specific diseases supports the concept that these less understood trace elements are probably also important for man. Thus, the following research is needed:

1. To confirm the essentiality of fluorine and tin and determine whether there are yet other undiscovered essential trace elements.

2. To ascertain the specific biological functions of nickel, vanadium, fluorine, and tin.

3. To determine whether nickel, vanadium, silicon, fluorine, and tin are essential to humans, and whether deficiencies or subclinical or marginal deficiencies occur.

4. To establish requirement levels for nickel, vanadium, silicon, fluorine, and tin in animals and humans.

5. To determine the chemical nature of nickel, vanadium, silicon, fluorine, and tin in feeds and foods, the forms of these that are available to meet dietary requirements, and the factors that can increase or decrease the requirement for these trace elements.

Above all, this review should indicate to those who are concerned with human and animal nutrition that they should be open minded concerning the possible practical importance of the more recently established essential (and undiscovered essential) trace elements.

REFERENCES

Anke, M., Grun, M., Dittrich, G., Groppel, B., and Hennig, A. (1974). Low nickel rations for growth and reproduction in pigs. In "Trace Element Metabolism in Animals-2" (W. G. Hoekstra et al., eds.), pp. 715–718. Univ. Park Press, Baltimore, Maryland.

Berg, L. R. (1966). Effect of diet composition on vanadium toxicity for the chick. Poultry Sci. 45, 1346–1352.

Bernheim, F., and Bernheim, M. L. C. (1939). The action of vanadium on the oxidation of phospholipids by certain tissues. J. Biol. Chem. 127, 353–360.

Brown, H. (1927). The mineral content of human skin. J. Biol. Chem. 75, 789–794.

Carlisle, E. M. (1970). Silicon: A possible factor in bone calcification. Science 167, 279–280.

Carlisle, E. M. (1971). A relationship between silicon, magnesium, and fluorine in bone formation in the chick. Fed. Proc., Fed. Amer. Soc. Exp. Biol. 30, 462 (abstr.).

Carlisle, E. M. (1972a). Silicon: An essential element for the chick. Fed. Proc., Fed. Amer. Soc. Exp. Biol. 31, 700 (abstr.).

Carlisle, E. M. (1972b). Silicon: An essential element for the chick. *Science* **178**, 619–621.

Carlisle, E. M. (1973). A skeletal alteration associated with silicon deficiency. *Fed. Proc., Fed. Amer. Soc. Exp. Biol.* **32**, 930 (abstr.).

Carlisle, E. M. (1974a). A relationship between silicon, glycosaminoglycan and collagen formation. *Fed. Proc., Fed. Amer. Soc. Exp. Biol.* **33**, 704 (abstr.).

Carlisle, E. M. (1974b). Silicon as an essential element. *Fed. Proc., Fed. Amer. Soc. Exp. Biol.* **33**, 1758–1766.

Curran, G. L., and Burch, R. E. (1967). Biological and health effects of vanadium. *In* "Trace Substances in Environmental Health" (D. D. Hemphill, ed.), Vol. I, pp. 96–102. University of Missouri, Columbia.

Decsy, M. I., and Sunderman, F. W., Jr. (1974). Binding of ^{63}Ni to rabbit serum α_1-macroglobulin in vivo and in vitro. *Bioinorg. Chem.* **3**, 95–105.

Doberenz, A. R., Kurnick, A. A., Kurtz, E. B., Kemmerer, A. R., and Reid, B. L. (1964). Effect of a minimal fluoride diet on rats. *Proc. Soc. Exp. Biol. Med.* **117**, 689–693.

Drummond, G. I., Severson, D. L., and Duncan, L. (1971). Adenyl cyclase. Kinetic properties and nature of fluoride and hormone stimulation. *J. Biol. Chem.* **246**, 4166–4173.

Eichhorn, G. L. (1962). Metal ions as stabilizers or destabilizers of the deoxyribonucleic acid structure. *Nature (London)* **194**, 474–475.

Hohnadel, D. C., Sunderman, F. W., Jr., Nechay, M. W., and McNeely, M. D. (1973). Atomic absorption spectrometry of nickel, copper, zinc, and lead in sweat collected from healthy subjects during sauna bathing. *Clin. Chem.* **19**, 1288–1292.

Hopkins, L. L., Jr., and Mohr, H. E. (1971a). The biological essentiality of vanadium. *In* "Newer Trace Elements in Nutrition" (W. Mertz and W. E. Cornatzer, eds.), pp. 195–213. Dekker, New York.

Hopkins, L. L., Jr., and Mohr, H. E. (1971b). Effect of vanadium deficiency on plasma cholesterol of chicks. *Fed. Proc., Fed. Amer. Soc. Exp. Biol.* **30**, 462 (abstr.).

Hopkins, L. L., Jr., and Mohr, H. E. (1974). Vanadium as an essential nutrient. *Fed. Proc., Fed. Amer. Soc. Exp. Biol.* **33**, 1773–1775.

LaBella, F. S., Dular, R., Lemon, P., Vivian, S., and Queen, G. (1973). Prolactin secretion is specifically inhibited by nickel. *Nature (London)* **245**, 330–332.

Loeper, J., and Loeper, J. (1961). Role of silicon in the arterial wall. *C. R. Soc. Biol.* **155**, 468–470.

MacCardle, R. C., Engman, M. F., Jr., and Engman, M. F., Sr. (1943). Mineral changes in neurodermatitis revealed by microincineration. *Arch. Dermatol. Syphilol.* **47**, 335–372.

McNeely, M. D., Sunderman, F. W., Jr., Nechay, M. W., and Levine, H. (1971). Abnormal concentrations of nickel in serum in cases of myocardial infarction, stroke, burns, hepatic cirrhosis, and uremia. *Clin. Chem.* **17**, 1123–1128.

Maurer, R. L., and Day, H. G. (1957). The non-essentiality of fluorine in nutrition. *J. Nutr.* **62**, 561–573.

Messer, H. H., Armstrong, W. D., and Singer, L. (1972a). Fertility impairment in mice on a low fluoride diet. *Science* **177**, 893–894.

Messer, H. H., Wong, K., Wagner, M., Singer, L., and Armstrong, W. D. (1972b). Effect of reduced fluoride intake by mice on haematocrit values. *Nature (London), New Biol.* **240**, 218–219.

Messer, H. H. Armstrong, W. D., and Singer, L. (1973). Influence of fluoride intake on reproduction in mice. *J. Nutr.* 103, 1319–1326.

Milne, D. B., and Schwarz, K. (1972). Effect of newer essential trace elements on rat incisor pigmentation. *Fed. Proc., Fed. Amer. Soc. Exp. Biol.* 31, 700 (abstr.).

Miyaji, T., and Greenstein, J. P. (1951). Cation activation of desoxyribonuclease. *Arch. Biochem. Biophys.* 32, 414–423.

Nielsen, F. H. (1971). Studies on the essentiality of nickel. In "Newer Trace Elements in Nutrition" (W. Mertz and W. E. Cornatzer, eds.), pp. 215–253. Dekker, New York.

Nielsen, F. H. (1974). Essentially and function of nickel. In "Trace Element Metabolism in Animals-2" (W. G. Hoekstra et al., eds.), pp. 381–395. Univ. Park Press, Baltimore, Maryland.

Nielsen, F. H., and Higgs, D. J. (1971). Further studies involving a nickel deficiency in chicks. In "Trace Substances in Environmental Health" (D. D. Hemphill, ed.), Vol. IV, pp. 241–246. University of Missouri, Columbia.

Nielsen, F. H., and Ollerich, D. A. (1973). Studies on a vanadium deficiency in chicks. *Fed. Proc., Fed. Amer. Soc. Exp. Biol.* 32, 929 (abstr.).

Nielsen, F. H., and Ollerich, D. A. (1974). Nickel: A new essential trace element. *Fed. Proc., Fed. Amer. Soc. Exp. Biol.* 33, 1767–1772.

Nielsen, F. H., and Sauberlich, H. E. (1970). Evidence of a possible requirement for nickel by the chick. *Proc. Soc. Exp. Biol. Med.* 134, 845–849.

Nielsen, F. H., Ollerich, D. A., Fosmire, G. J., and Sandstead, H. H. (1974). Nickel deficiency in chicks and rats: Effects on liver morphology, function and polysomal integrity. In "Protein–Metal Interactions," *Advan. Exp. Med. Biol.* (M. Friedman, ed.), vol. 48, pp. 389–403. Plenum Press, New York.

Nomoto, S., McNeely, M. D., and Sunderman, F. W., Jr. (1971). Isolation of a nickel α_2-macroglobulin from rabbit serum. *Biochemistry* 10, 1647–1651.

Ray, W. J., Jr. (1969). Role of bivalent cations in the phosphoglucomutase system. I. Characterization of enzyme-metal complexes. *J. Biol. Chem.* 244, 3740–3747.

Ruliffson, W. S., Burns, L. V., and Hughes, J. S. (1963). The effect of fluorine ion on Fe[59] iron levels in blood of rats. *Trans. Kans. Acad. Sci.* 66, 52–58.

Schroeder, H. A., Balassa, J. J., and Tipton, I. H. (1962). Abnormal trace metals in man—nickel. *J. Chronic Dis.* 15, 51–65.

Schroeder, H. A., Balassa, J. J., and Tipton, I. H. (1963). Abnormal trace metals in man—vanadium. *J. Chronic Dis.* 16, 1047–1071.

Schwarz, K. (1973). A bound form of silicon in glycosaminoglycans and polyuronides. *Proc. Nat. Acad. Sci. U.S.* 70, 1608–1612.

Schwarz, K. (1974). Recent dietary trace element research, exemplified by tin, fluorine, and silicon. *Fed. Proc., Fed. Amer. Soc. Exp. Biol.* 33, 1748–1757.

Schwarz, K., and Chen, S. C. (1974). A bound form of silicon as a constituent of collagens. *Fed. Proc., Fed. Amer. Soc. Exp. Biol.* 33, 704 (abstr.).

Schwarz, K., and Milne, D. B. (1971). Growth effects of vanadium in the rat. *Science* 174, 426–428.

Schwarz, K., and Milne, D. B. (1972a). Growth promoting effects of silicon in rats. *Nature (London)* 239, 333–334.

Schwarz, K., and Milne, D. B. (1972b). Fluorine requirement for growth in the rat. *Bioinorg. Chem.* 1, 331–338.

Schwarz, K., Milne, D. B., and Vinyard, E. (1970). Growth effects of tin compounds in rats maintained in a trace element controlled environment. *Biochem. Biophys. Res. Commun.* 40, 22–29.

Soremark, R. (1967). Vanadium in some biological specimens. *J. Nutr.* **92,** 183–190.

Soremark, R., and Ullberg, S. (1962). Distribution and kinetics of $^{48}V_2O_5$ in mice. *In* "Use of Radioisotopes in Animal Biology and the Medical Sciences" (M. Fried, ed.), pp. 103–114. Academic Press, New York.

Soremark, R., Ullberg, S., and Appelgren, L.-E. (1962). Autoradiographic localization of vanadium pentoxide ($V_2^{48}O_5$) in developing teeth and bones of rats. *Acta Odontol. Scand.* **20,** 225–232.

Strasia, C. A. (1971). Vanadium: Essentiality and toxicity in the laboratory rat. Ph.D. Thesis, University Microfilms, Ann Arbor, Michigan.

Sunderman, F. W., Jr. (1965). Measurements of nickel in biological materials by atomic absorption spectrometry. *Amer. J. Clin. Pathol.* **44,** 182–188.

Sunderman, F. W., Jr., Decsy, M. I., and McNeely, M. D. (1972a). Nickel metabolism in health and disease. *Ann. N.Y. Acad. Sci.* **199,** 300–312.

Sunderman, F. W., Jr., Nomoto, S., Morang, R., Nechay, M. W., Burke, C. N., and Nielsen, S. W. (1972b). Nickel deprivation in chicks. *J. Nutr.* **102,** 259–267.

Tal, M. (1968). On the role of Zn^{2+} and Ni^{2+} in ribosome structure. *Biochim. Biophys. Acta* **169,** 564–565.

Tal, M. (1969a). Thermal denaturation of ribosomes. *Biochemistry* **8,** 424–435.

Tal, M. (1969b). Metal ions and ribosomal conformation. *Biochim. Biophys. Acta* **195,** 76–86.

Tiffin, L. O. (1971). Translocation of nickel in xylem exudate of plants. *Plant Physiol.* **48,** 273–277.

Underwood, E. J. (1971). "Trace Elements in Human and Animal Nutrition," 3rd ed., pp. 369 and 416. Academic Press, New York.

Vohra, P., Gray, G. A., and Kratzer, F. H. (1965). Phytic-acid-metal complex. *Proc. Soc. Exp. Biol. Med.* **120,** 447–449.

Wacker, W. E. C., and Vallee, B. L. (1959). Nucleic acids and metals. I. Chromium, manganese, nickel, iron, and other metals in ribonucleic acid from diverse biological sources. *J. Biol. Chem.* **234,** 3257–3262.

Wacker, W. E. C., Gordon, M. P., and Huff, J. W. (1963). Metal content of tobacco mosaic virus and tobacco mosaic virus RNA. *Biochemistry* **2,** 716–718.

Webster, L. T., Jr. (1965). Studies of the acetyl coenzyme A synthetase reaction III. Evidence of a double requirement for divalent cations. *J. Biol. Chem.* **240,** 4164–4169.

42

Cadmium Metabolism—A Review of Aspects Pertinent to Evaluating Dietary Cadmium Intake by Man

M. R. Spivey Fox

I. INTRODUCTION

There are several recent reviews that deal entirely or in part with the metabolism of cadmium (Nilsson, 1970; Flick *et al.*, 1971; Friberg *et al.*, 1971, 1973; Cheftel *et al.*, 1972; Fassett, 1972; Vallee and Ulmer, 1972; Albert *et al.*, 1973; Fleischer *et al.*, 1974; Fox, 1974). Since the purpose of this treatise is to consider trace elements and human disease, this review will focus on those aspects of cadmium metabolism that are particularly important in evaluating the tolerance of human beings to cadmium in the diet. The design of appropriate experimental animal models will also be discussed. Due to the scope of even these limited aspects, many topics can be treated only superficially.

401

We have been fortunate, perhaps lucky, in this country in that no overt disease problems due to cadmium exposure have occurred. In Japan, a severe and painful disease, *itai itai byo*, has been related causally to prolonged ingestion of food and water containing high concentrations of cadmium. The total daily intake of cadmium was approximately ten times greater than that typical in most parts of the world. The sensitive population group consisted of postmenopausal women who had borne several children. From the disease syndrome in these patients and the changes observed in industrially exposed workers, it is clear that cadmium intake from foods and water is an appropriate matter for serious consideration.

II. PRESENT KNOWLEDGE OF CADMIUM METABOLISM

A. General Outline of Cadmium Metabolism

1. Important Anatomical Sites and Physiological Processes

Cadmium has no known essential function, so at this time its presence in any cell must be regarded as something to be minimized. The movement of cadmium into and within the body appears to be very precisely regulated within certain constraints that will be discussed later. Some tissues and organs are of special significance with respect to metabolism of cadmium and its adverse effects. A summary of these sites and processes appears in Table I.

The gastrointestinal tract provides a passageway for food and its residues through the body. During transit, digestion releases many types of metal-binding ligands, some of which may bind cadmium, typically in competition with other divalent elements. For example, cadmium and zinc are usually found together in geological and biological systems. Of the two, zinc binds more firmly to nitrogen and oxygen ligands, whereas cadmium binds more firmly to mercapto groups.

Cadmium concentrates to a marked extent in the small intestinal wall, presumably in the absorptive mucosal cells. At dietary levels below 10 mg cadmium per kilogram of diet, the duodenums of our young Japanese quail accumulated cadmium to concentrations (fresh weight basis) ten to twenty times greater than the concentration in the dry purified diet (Harland *et al.*, 1973). Many investigators have found that concentrations of cadmium in the liver and kidney are related to the oral dose of cadmium under given conditions (Decker *et al.*, 1958; Anwar *et al.*,

TABLE I Important Sites and Processes in the Metabolism of Cadmium

Anatomical site	Physiologically significant process
Gastrointestinal tract:	(1) Passage of food and its residue through the body; (2) digestion of foods with the release of metal-binding ligands; (3) binding of cadmium with other components of the diet
Small intestinal wall:	(1) Concentration of cadmium in the mucosal cells; (2) barrier to transport into the body; (3) competition by cadmium with essential elements for ligands required for storage and transport; (4) enteropathy from high cadmium, affecting absorption of cadmium and nutrients
Blood	Cadmium transport between tissues
Liver	Long-term storage of cadmium
Kidney	(1) Long-term storage of cadmium; (2) renal tubule damage from high cadmium preceding adverse physiological changes
Placenta	Barrier to cadmium transport to the fetus
Mammary gland	Barrier to cadmium transport into milk

1961; Harland *et al.*, 1973; Cousins *et al.*, 1973; Doyle *et al.*, 1974). These and other data suggest control at the gut level prior to transport into the body; however, the exact nature of the regulation is not known.

Due to the rapid turnover of intestinal mucosal cells, most of this cadmium is lost from the body when the cells are sloughed from the tip of the villus. The extent to which cadmium from these shed cells is taken up by mucosal cells lower in the gastrointestinal tract is unknown. An enteropathy was observed in patients with *itai itai* disease (Murata *et al.*, 1969) and in experimental animals fed cadmium (Wilson *et al.*, 1941; Yoshikawa *et al.*, 1960; Stowe *et al.*, 1972; Richardson *et al.*, 1974). It appears that under given conditions a critical cadmium concentration in the mucosal cell produces structural damage that probably is accompanied by marked changes in absorption of cadmium and other dietary components.

Blood is the obvious means of cadmium transport within the body. The concentrations of cadmium are normally very small, less than 1 μg/100 ml of whole blood in persons not exposed to high amounts of cadmium. This small amount is difficult to assay accurately.

The liver and kidney are the principal sites of long-term storage in the body. It has not been possible to determine the biological half-life of dietary cadmium accurately for either organs or the whole body; however, it is certain that it is a matter of years for man. From estimates of intake and cross-sectional age data on organ concentrations, estimates of half-life for the kidney of man range from 16 to 33 years (Kjellström, 1971; Tsuchiya and Sugita, 1971).

The critical organ in man appears to be the kidney (Friberg *et al.*, 1971). They postulated that when the concentration of cadmium reaches a critical level in the renal cortex, 200 μg/gm fresh weight, renal tubular damage occurs, cadmium is lost from the kidney, and a series of adverse physiological events can ensue. These and other toxicological effects are to be considered in other chapters of this treatise. A variety of compounds have been used in an attempt to flush cadmium from the tissues; however, no means of accomplishing this has been devised that does not enhance the probability of kidney damage.

The placenta and the mammary gland have been shown to act as barriers to cadmium transport into the fetus and newborn, respectively (Lucis *et al.*, 1972). Concentrations of cadmium in the human newborn are extremely small (Henke *et al.*, 1970; Chaube *et al.*, 1973).

2. Metallothionein and Other Cadmium-Binding Proteins

A protein containing large amounts of cadmium was first isolated from equine renal cortex (Kägi and Vallee, 1960) and later from human renal cortex (Pulido *et al.*, 1966). This protein was named metallothionein, and the metal-free protein was designated thionein. Metallothionein has now been characterized by several investigators. The metal content may vary somewhat with different preparations. Typical values are: cadmium 6%; zinc 2.2%; small amounts of copper, iron and mercury; sulfur 8%, from cysteinyl residues; 20 mercapto groups with 3 mercapto groups per atom of zinc or cadmium; and no aromatic amino acids. The molecular weight is 7000. The cadmium mercaptide is a chromophore with an absorption maximum at 250 nm.

Nordberg *et al.* (1972) injected large amounts of cadmium into rabbits. By isoelectric focusing, they were able to resolve metallothionein into two main protein peaks, which differed in amino acid content. Both proteins contained cadmium, but only one contained significant amounts of zinc. Other evidence for two forms of cadmium-binding protein in liver and kidney have been reported (Shaikh and Lucis, 1971, 1972).

Nordberg *et al.* (1971) reported that very soon after injection, cadmium was bound in the liver to high molecular weight proteins. By 24 hr after injection, the cadmium was found bound entirely to low molecular weight proteins. It has also been shown that with repeated injection of cadmium, there is a marked increase in the amount of low molecular weight cadmium-binding proteins present in the liver (Wiśniewska-Knypl and Jablońska, 1970; Winge and Rajagopolan, 1972).

A low molecular weight protein similar to metallothionein, which binds copper, has been isolated from the duodenum of the chick (Starcher, 1969) and from bovine duodenum and liver (Evans *et al.*, 1970). In both papers, evidence was presented that cadmium and zinc could displace copper from the protein, providing evidence to explain the antagonism of copper by these two elements.

3. Biochemical Changes Produced by Cadmium

Vallee and Ulmer (1972) have reviewed the biochemical effects of cadmium. It is difficult at this point to explain the toxicity of cadmium in entirely precise biochemical terms. A large number of *in vitro* studies have shown that cadmium can replace zinc in many of its metalloenzymes, with resultant changes in activity. As noted above, cadmium binds readily to mercapto groups, and these are frequently important in enzyme systems. Cadmium also binds to phospholipids and nucleic acids and has been shown to uncouple oxidative phosphorylation.

In general, cadmium can compete with some of the essential divalent elements for ligands. The displacement of the essential element may affect its transport, storage, or function at the active site of an enzyme, or effect a change in the conformation of proteins or nucleic acids required for normal function.

4. Relevance of Existing Animal Data to Man

The greater part of our knowledge of cadmium metabolism is derived from animal experiments in which massive amounts of inorganic cadmium salts were injected or in a few experiments wherein cadmium salts were administered orally, usually in the drinking water. These studies have provided some interesting and important insights into the behavior of cadmium under these conditions; however, they are of very limited usefulness in evaluating the quantitative effects of low-level long-term exposure to cadmium, such as occurs from the diet of human beings.

B. Human Exposure to Cadmium

1. Food and Water

The Food and Drug Administration monitors the quantities of pesticides and certain inorganic elements present in the United States diet. Samples of food to represent maximal food intake, the diet of a 16–19 year old male, are collected six times per year in five geographic regions of the

United States and are cooked by a dietitian according to local customs. The foods are composited by twelve food groups; thus, 360 composites are analyzed annually.

In the most recent report (Mansko and Corneliussen, 1974), which covered food collected from June 1970 through April 1971, cadmium was detectable in 213 of 360 composites. The limit of detection was approximately 0.01 μg/gm. The annual mean for food composites in given geographic areas ranged between 0.01 and 0.03 μg/gm. Higher values in some areas were obtained for dairy products, potatoes, and leafy vegetables. The single highest value was 0.2 μg/gm for leafy vegetables.

The concentrations of cadmium found during this interval were similar to those reported previously (Corneliussen, 1972). From these earlier data, the contribution of each food class to the total daily cadmium intake in the United States was estimated (Duggan and Corneliussen, 1972). From these calculations, grain and cereals supplied the largest amount, 14 μg cadmium per day. Potatoes supplied 7 μg and amounts between 4 and 5 μg were supplied by each of the following food groups: beverages, leafy vegetables, dairy products, fruits and meats, fish and poultry. The remaining food groups each supplied 1–2 μg per day. From these data it is estimated that the average daily cadmium intake in the United States is approximately 50 μg. The total daily intake of cadmium in Canada has recently been estimated to be 67 μg, based on analysis of foods sampled during 1970–1971 (Kirkpatrick and Coffin, 1974).

Oysters, liver, and kidney are known to contain amounts of cadmium that may be appreciably higher than most foods, depending on the amount of cadmium available to the growing organism. It is estimated that single servings of these foods could supply the following amounts of cadmium: beef liver, 20 μg; beef kidney, 40 μg; and oysters, 50 μg. The food composites assayed by the Food and Drug Administration contained liver but no kidneys and oysters.

The Joint FAO/WHO Expert Committee on Food Additives (Cheftel et al. 1972) reported a "provisional tolerable weekly intake" of dietary cadmium, lead, and mercury for a 60 kg man. The values were expressed on a weekly basis because of the wide variation possible on a daily basis. The weekly and daily values for cadmium are 400–500 μg and 57–71 μg, respectively. Thus, there is probably a narrow margin between the present typical United States intake and the "provisional tolerable intakes."

The intake of cadmium from water must also be considered in conjunction with that in food. The tentative upper limit set in the WHO International Standards for drinking water (World Health Organization, 1971) is 10 μg/liter. The amounts in drinking water for most industrialized countries are less; however, additional amounts may be dissolved from home plumbing, particularly from galvanized pipes. Daily intakes up to 10 μg from water do not seem unreasonable.

2. Other Sources

There are very small amounts of cadmium in the air. It is estimated that approximately 0.02 μg may be inhaled daily by an adult man. Cigarette smoke can contribute significant amounts of cadmium to the total body burden. Menden et al. (1972) estimated that approximately 0.1 μg cadmium was inhaled from the mainstream smoke of each cigarette. The sidestream smoke contained a higher concentration of cadmium; however, the amount inhaled would be quite variable. It has been shown that the livers and kidneys of long-term smokers contain much higher than average amounts of cadmium (Lewis et al., 1972).

There is a vast amount of literature showing that very little cadmium from food is absorbed past the gut wall. If the particle size is sufficiently small, inhaled cadmium is retained very efficiently. Moore et al. (1973) compared whole body retention of cadmium-115m in rats after various routes of administration. Following the early rapid clearance phase, the initial retention values were 93%, 91%, 41%, and 2.3% of the dose for administration by intraperitoneal, intravenous, inhalation, and oral routes, respectively. The rate of elimination of the slower component of the curve was unaffected by route of administration. The amount absorbed from food can be modified by other dietary components as discussed below.

C. Responses to Dietary Cadmium in Experimental Animals

1. Toxic Responses

In order to evaluate the hazards of cadmium in foods to man, good experimental models are required. Two types of parameters have proved useful in cadmium studies, namely, adverse physiological effects and tissue accumulation of cadmium. The minimal dietary concentrations to produce meaningful data are shown in Table II. These levels apply to relatively short-term experiments, 2–8 weeks in duration.

In order to produce adverse physiological effects with an adequate

TABLE II Minimal Dietary Cadmium Concentrations for
Measurable Responses in Short-Term
Experiments[a]

Response	Dietary cadmium (mg/kg)
Physiological abnormalities	5
Tissue accumulation	
Cadmium-109	0.02[b]
Duodenal cadmium by atomic absorption spectrophotometry	0.05
Liver and kidney cadmium by atomic absorption spectrophotometry	5

[a] For comparison, the concentration of cadmium in the normal human diet is 0.08 mg/kg of dry fiber-free diet, assuming 50 μg cadmium/600 gm dry fiber-free diet per day.
[b] The lower limit is restricted to the minimal background level obtainable with each diet.

diet, 5 mg cadmium per kilogram of diet are usually required. Some types of adverse effects, the severity of which are either known or thought to be dose related, include reduced growth rate, anemia, poor bone mineralization, and pathological changes in several tissues.

No human food contains sufficient cadmium to permit a bioassay based on evaluation of toxic responses. Oysters are a food that is apt to contain a high amount of cadmium, on the average about 50 μg/100 gm serving, or 3.3 μg/gm dry weight. Even this is too low for a bioassay based on parameters of toxicity.

It is possible to expose oysters to water containing high levels of cadmium and rapidly increase the concentration of cadmium in the oysters. With this type of freeze-dried oyster meat, the toxic effects of cadmium incorporated into oysters were compared with those produced by inorganic cadmium at dietary levels of 5 and 10 mg/kg of diet (Fox et al., 1973a). The effects of the two sources of cadmium were similar. The results must be regarded as somewhat equivocal, however, because it was not known whether the cadmium in the oyster containing an unusually high concentration was present in the same molecular form(s) as in oysters containing more typical, lower amounts of cadmium. Furthermore, with the high-cadmium oysters, the ratios of cadmium to various essential minerals were lower than with average oysters. This is another consideration that could lead to an erroneous interpretation.

The young growing animal is typically more responsive to the toxic effects of cadmium than the adult animal. The characteristic toxicity syndrome in young Japanese quail has been observed by 7 days of age (M. R. S. Fox, unpublished data), whereas between 4 and 6 weeks of age some of the toxic manifestations decrease (Richardson et al., 1974).

2. Tissue Accumulation

The whole-body accumulation of cadmium or that in the liver and kidney or duodenum of experimental animals can be determined in a very precise manner in a fairly short-term experiments by the use of radioisotopes (Table II). Cadmium-115m is suitable for whole-body counting, whereas either cadmium-109 or cadmium-115m is satisfactory for counting individual tissues following solubilization. Cadmium-109 is available in carrier-free form, so very small amounts of stable cadmium accompany the tracer. Thus, when foods are labeled with cadmium-109, it is possible to develop bioassays based on metabolism and tissue accumulation of cadmium at dietary levels similar to those of man.

If one assumes a daily intake for an adult man of 50 μg cadmium and approximately 600 gm of dry fiber-free diet, this is a dietary concentration of 0.08 mg cadmium/kg dry fiber-free diet. Apart from differences in food intake related to differences in body size, the dry fiber-free basis seems to be reasonable for comparisons between man and experimental animals fed purified diets.

The duodenum of the Japanese quail rapidly and markedly concentrates cadmium from the diet (Jacobs et al., 1974a). With dietary levels beginning at 0.05 μg/gm, it is possible to assay the amount of cadmium in the 0.5 gm of duodenal tissue from the 2-week old Japanese quail by conventional flame atomic absorption spectrophotometry. With cadmium chloride, the log of the duodenal concentration is linearly related to the log concentration of dietary cadmium. This provides a useful means of investigating differences in metabolism of cadmium supplied in the diet by different foods. The problem cannot be approached so simply with this degree of sensitivity by any other means. Taken alone, duodenal cadmium level is not a definitive basis for comparison; however, it provides a useful screening procedure for identifying foods that are unusual and that should be labeled with cadmium-109 for detailed study.

The concentration of cadmium in livers and kidneys of experimental animals fed 5 mg cadmium/kg of diet can also be determined by atomic absorption spectrophotometry. This dietary level is far in excess of concentrations found in foods.

D. Effects of Essential Nutrients on Cadmium Metabolism

1. Nutrients That Alter the Effects of Cadmium

The multiplicity of relationships between cadmium and essential minerals has recently been reviewed (Fox, 1974). It has been recognized for several years that cadmium can markedly alter the metabolism and function of some essential elements. These include zinc, iron, manganese, copper, selenium, and calcium. With individual deficiencies of zinc, iron, copper, calcium, vitamin D, or protein, the toxicity of cadmium and sometimes tissue accumulation are markedly increased.

An excess above the requirement of zinc, iron(II), copper, selenium, ascorbic acid, or protein has been shown to protect against various effects of cadmium. Fox et al. (1973b) reported that the toxicity of cadmium was decreased when the dietary protein was supplied by dried egg white as compared with either isolated soybean protein or the combination of casein plus gelatin. The adverse effects produced by cadmium that were less severe with the dried egg white diet included growth depression, anemia, and low tissue concentrations of zinc and iron. On the other hand, Stowe et al. (1974) reported that high dietary pyridoxine levels increased the severity of the anemia produced by dietary cadmium.

Most of the above results were obtained with relatively high levels of cadmium fed in short-term studies. Many of these findings are consistent with the toxic manifestations and nutritional component associated with the etiology of *itai itai* disease. This human disease occurred following consumption of much smaller amounts of cadmium in food and water for many years.

2. Effects of Zinc, Copper, and Manganese on Tissue Accumulation of Cadmium from Low Levels of Cadmium in the Diet

As noted above, most studies of nutrient–cadmium interrelationships have been carried out with amounts of cadmium far in excess of the daily intake of man. It has been found that simultaneously supplementing a diet with amounts of zinc, copper, and manganese appreciably above the requirement level of each resulted in decreased concentrations of cadmium in the kidneys of young Japanese quail (M. R. S. Fox, unpublished data). This effect was observed with dietary concentrations of 10, 20 and 40 mg cadmium/kg of diet.

More recently, Jacobs et al. (1974a) studied the effect of more modest excesses of these three elements above requirement levels in the diet. The excess of each (milligrams per kilogram of diet) was zinc 30, manganese 12, and copper 4. Jacobs *et al.* (1974b) determined the effects of the combined elemental supplement on the tissue accumulation of very small amounts of dietary cadmium. These were the background level of 0.02 mg/kg of diet and five additional levels to 1.02 mg/kg of diet. With carrier-free cadmium-109, it was found that the liver and kidney concentrations of cadmium in young Japanese quail were significantly decreased by the supplement of zinc, manganese, and copper. This was true for the background level of cadmium and higher concentrations to 1.02 mg cadmium/kg of diet. The data are impressive for (1) the precise regulation of cadmium metabolism that exists down to the very low level of 0.02 mg/kg of diet and (2) for the effect of supplemental essential minerals that was observed with each of the very low levels of dietary cadmium.

The need for protecting against unavoidable exposure to toxic elements may make it desirable for man to consume slightly more than the requirement levels of some nutrients. As more information is obtained, it is reasonable to expect that the quantities of essential nutrients that provide protection against toxic elements will be a consideration in establishing requirements for man.

E. Design of Control Diets for Cadmium Studies

From the above discussion of cadmium–nutrient interrelationships and cadmium dose levels, it is apparent that quite a range of results could be obtained through intentional or accidental variations with the "normal" compositional range of nutrients in the control diet of a given study. In order to minimize variation between experiments, laboratories, and species, and to provide the most meaningful data pertinent to man, the composition of controls diets merits very careful consideration. Stemming from studies of cadmium and essential trace elements, some criteria have evolved that have proven useful in designing control diets for trace mineral studies; these diets should be composed of the nutritional minimum that supports normal physiological function.

Insofar as possible, diets composed of purified components are desirable. This permits better control of dietary composition over a long period. Many experimental options are possible in varying the composition of the diet with respect to one or more nutrients from deficient to excess levels.

In order to define meaningful response thresholds for elemental antagonisms and toxicity, it is very important that the diet supply essential nutrients as near to the requirement level as possible. The requirement, at least for some trace elements, needs to be defined with respect to each protein source. It is well recognized that the level of some individual amino acids and the presence of nonprotein components, such as phytic acid, accompanying a purified protein can alter the availability of some trace minerals. Most purified proteins contain significant amounts of trace and macroelements. The amounts and biological availability of these background elements must be taken into consideration.

For trace element studies, the levels of most vitamins are perhaps less critical. A moderate margin of excess should be permissable to allow for possible destruction in the diet during the course of the experiment. Components that are not required should be deleted or minimized whenever possible.

It is desirable that elements be present in stable form so that they are not lost or converted to unavailable forms and that they do not adversely affect other components of the diet. Individual compounds of average biological availability are desirable. When the concentrations of individual micronutrients are limited to the required amount, the uniformity of distribution within the diet becomes critical.

III. RESEARCH AND INFORMATION NEEDS

A. Tissue Accumulation with Low Levels of Dietary Cadmium—Medium- to Short-Term Radioisotope Studies

With the use of cadmium-109, it is possible to study very precisely the absorption and tissue retention of cadmium at very low dietary levels similar to those in the diet of man. Information is needed with "requirement" diets per se in order to establish normative, quantitative reference points with respect to absorption and biochemical details of cadmium metabolism and retention. These studies should involve evaluation of varying dose levels over varying periods of time.

In changing the basic experimental model to evaluate further factors important to man, several variables are of particular significance. Some foods are so high in cadmium, as noted above, that it is possible to double the day's intake by a single serving of a high-cadmium food, but the effect of such a marked variation of intake on the absorption and retention of cadmium has not been established. Also, little is known about bioavailability of cadmium in foods at any level of intake. These types of information are required for setting limits of cadmium allowed in given foods.

Nutrient deficiencies and excesses are known to alter the toxicity of cadmium, but very little is known about the effects of these nutrients on retention of very low levels of dietary cadmium. Similarly, there are many nonrequired nutrients and other components in the human diet whose effects on cadmium have not been ascertained. The physiological variables of age, pregnancy, and lactation merit special consideration.

B. Adverse Physiological Effects with Low-Level Dietary Dosage of Cadmium—Long-Term Studies

There are relatively few experimental studies of long-term dietary exposure of experimental animals to cadmium. Such studies need to be carried out, taking into account the best designs of experimental diets and models of human problems as discussed above. Tissue accumulation of cadmium should be closely correlated with microscopic integrity of critical tissues, appropriate biochemical measurements, and tests of physiological function.

C. Surveillance of Cadmium Exposure in the General Population

The movement and dissemination of cadmium from the earth need to be followed rather closely to avoid a hazard to the health of either small groups or the general population. Monitoring the concentrations of cadmium in foods and water will be required into the foreseeable future.

A check against relatively recent cadmium exposure is provided by determination of cadmium in tissues of accidental death victims. Collection of data for different age groups at regular intervals provides at least some basis for development of historical cause and effect relationships that is not possible from a single cross-sectional age study.

REFERENCES

Albert, R., Berlin, M., Finklea, J., Friberg, L., Goyer, R. A., Henderson, R., Hernberg, S., Kazantzis, G., Kehoe, R. A., Kolbye, A. C., Magos, L., Miettinen, J. K., Nordberg, G., Norseth, T., Pfitzer, E. A., Piscator, M., Shibko, S. I., Singerman, A., Tsuchiya, K., and Vostal, J. (1973). Accumulation of toxic metals with special reference to their absorption, excretion, and biological half-times. *Environ. Physiol. Biochem.* 3, 65–107.

Anwar, R. A., Langham, R. F., Hoppert, C. A., Alfredson, B. V., and Byerrum, R. U. (1961). Chronic toxicity studies. III. Chronic toxicity of cadmium and chromium in dogs. *Arch. Environ. Health* 3, 456–460.

Chaube, S., Nishimura, H., and Swinyard, C. A. (1973). Zinc and cadmium in normal human embryos and fetuses. *Arch. Environ. Health* **26**, 237–240.

Cheftel, H., Cotta-Ramusino, F., Egan, H., Kojima, K., Miettinen, J. K., Smith, D. M., Berglund, F., Blumenthal, H., Goldberg, L., Kazantzis, G., Piscator, M., Truhaut, R., Tsubaki, T., and Najcev, A. N. (1972). Evaluation of certain food additives and the contaminants mercury, lead, and cadmium. *World Health Organ., Tech. Rep. Ser.* **505**, 20–24 and 32.

Corneliussen, P. E. (1972). Pesticide residues in total diet samples (VI). *Pestic. Monit. J.* **5**, 313–330.

Cousins, R. J., Barber, A. K., and Trout, J. R. (1973). Cadmium toxicity in growing swine. *J. Nutr.* **103**, 964–972.

Decker, L. E., Byerrum, R. U., Decker, C. F., Hoppert, C. A., and Langham, R. F., (1958). Chronic toxicity studies, I. Cadmium administered in drinking water to rats. *AMA Arch. Ind. Health* **18**, 228–231.

Doyle, J. J., Pfander, W. H., Grebing, S. E., and Pierce, J. O., II. (1974). Effect of dietary cadmium on absorption and cadium tissue levels in growing lambs. *J. Nutr.* **104**, 160–166.

Duggan, R. E., and Corneliussen, P. E. (1972). Dietary intake of pesticide chemicals in the United States (III), June, 1968–April, 1970. *Pestic. Monit. J.* **5**, 331–341.

Evans, G. W., Majors, P. F., and Cornatzer, W. E. (1970). Mechanism for cadmium and zinc antagonism of copper metabolism. *Biochem. Biophys. Res. Commun.* **40**, 1142–1148.

Fassett, D. W. (1972). Cadmium. *In* "Metallic Contaminants and Human Health" (D. H. K. Lee, ed.), pp. 98–117. Academic Press, New York.

Fleischer, M., Sarofim, A. F., Fassett, D. W., Hammond, P., Shacklette, H. T., Nisbet, I. C. T., and Epstein, S. (1974). Environmental impact of cadmium: a review by the panel on hazardous trace substances. *Environ. Health Perspect., Exp. Issue* No. 7, pp. 253–323.

Flick, D. F., Kraybill, H. F., and Dimitroff, J. M. (1971). Toxic effects of cadmium: A review. *Environ. Res.* **4**, 71–85.

Fox, M. R. S. (1974). Effects of essential minerals on cadmium toxicity. A review. *J. Food Sci.* **37**, 321–324.

Fox, M. R. S., Jacobs, R. M., Fry, B. E., Jr., Harland, B. F., and Story, A. H. (1973a). Comparative effects in quail of cadmium supplied by oysters and cadmium chloride. *Abstr., Int. Congr. Nutr., 9th, 1972* p. 137.

Fox, M. R. S., Jacobs, R. M., Fry, B. E., Jr., and Harland, B. F. (1973b). Effect of protein source on response to cadmium. *Fed. Proc., Fed. Amer. Soc. Exp. Biol.* **32**, 924.

Friberg, L., Piscator, M., and Nordberg, G. (1971). "Cadmium in the Environment." Chem. Rubber Publ. Co., Cleveland, Ohio.

Friberg, L., Piscator, M., Nordberg, G., and Kjellström, T. (1974). "Cadmium in the Environment," (2nd ed.) Chem. Rubber Publ. Co., Cleveland, Ohio.

Harland, B. F., Fry, B. E., Jr., Jacobs, R. M., and Fox, M. R. S. (1973). Response of young Japanese quail to graded levels of dietary cadmium. *Abstr., Int. Congr. Nutr., 9th, 1972* p. 53.

Henke, G., Sachs, H. W., and Bohn, G. (1970). Cadmium-bestimmungen in leber und nieren von kindern und jugendlichen durch neutronenaktivierungsanalyse. *Arch. Toxikol.* **26**, 8–16.

Jacobs, R. M., Fox, M. R. S., Lee, A. O., Harland, B. F., and Fry, B. E., Jr. (1974a). Increased duodenal and decreased hepatic and renal Cd in Japanese quail fed supplements of Zn, Mn, and Cu. *Fed. Proc., Fed. Amer. Soc. Exp. Biol.* 33, 668.

Jacobs, R. M., Fox, M. R. S., Fry, B. E., Jr., and Harland, B. F. (1974b). The effect of two day exposure to dietary cadmium on the concentration of elements in tissues of Japanese quail. *In* "Trace Element Metabolism in Animals" (W. G. Hoekstra *et al.*, eds.), 2nd Int. Symp., pp. 684–686. Univ. Park Press, Baltimore, Maryland.

Kägi, J. H. R., and Vallee, B. L. (1960). Metallothionein: A cadmium- and zinc-containing protein from equine renal cortex. *J. Biol. Chem.* 235, 3460–3465.

Kirkpatrick, D. C., and Coffin, D. E. (1974). The trace metal content of representative Canadian diets in 1970 to 1971. *Can. Inst. Food Sci. Technol. J.* 7, 56–58.

Kjellström, T. (1971). A mathematical model for the accumulation of cadmium in human kidney cortex. *Nord. Hyg. Tidskr.* 53, 111–119.

Lewis, G. P., Jusko, W. J., Coughlin, L. L., and Hartz, S. (1972). Contribution of cigarette smoking to cadmium accumulation in man. *Lancet* 1, 291–292.

Lucis, O. J., Lucis, R., and Shaikh, Z. A. (1972). Cadmium and zinc in pregnancy and lactation. *Arch. Environ. Health* 25, 14–22.

Mansko, D. D., and Corneliussen, P. E. (1974). Pesticide residues in total diet samples (VII). *Pestic. Monit. J.* 8, 110–124.

Menden, E. E., Elia, V. J., Michael, L. W., and Petering, H. G. (1972). Distribution of cadmium and nickel of tobacco during cigarette smoking. *Environ. Sci. Technol.* 6, 830–832.

Moore, W., Jr., Stara, J. F., Crocker, W. C., Marachuk, M., and Iltis, R. (1973). Comparison of [115m]cadmium retention in rats following different routes of administration. *Environ. Res.* 6, 473–478.

Murata, I., Hirono, T., Saeki, Y., and Nakagawa, S. (1969). Cadmium enteropathy, renal osteomalacia ("Itai Itai" disease). *Bull. Soc. Int. Chir.* 29, 34–42.

Nilsson, R. (1970). "Aspects on the Toxicity of Cadmium and Its Compounds," Ecol. Res. Comm. Bull. No. 7. Swed. Nat. Sci. Res. Counc., Stockholm.

Nordberg, G. F., Piscator, M., and Lind, B. (1971). Distribution of cadmium among protein fractions of mouse liver. *Acta Pharmacol. Toxicol.* 29, 456–470.

Nordberg, G. F., Nordberg, M., Piscator, M., and Vesterberg, O. (1972). Separation of two forms of rabbit metallothionein by isoelectric focusing. *Biochem. J.* 126, 491–498.

Pulido, P., Kägi, J. H. R., and Vallee, B. L. (1966). Isolation and some properties of human metallothionein. *Biochemistry* 5, 1768–1777.

Richardson, M. E., Fox, M. R. S., and Fry, B. E., Jr. (1974). Pathological changes produced in Japanese quail by ingestion of cadmium. *J. Nutr.* 104, 323–338.

Shaikh, Z. A., and Lucis, O. J. (1971). Isolation of cadmium-binding proteins. *Experientia* 27, 1024–1025.

Shaikh, Z. A., and Lucis, O. J. (1972). Cadmium and zinc binding in mammalian liver and kidneys. *Arch. Environ. Health* 24, 419–425.

Starcher, B. C. (1969). Studies on the mechanism of copper absorption in the chick. *J. Nutr.* 97, 321–326.

Stowe, H. D., Wilson, M., and Goyer, R. A. (1972). Clinical and morphologic effects of oral cadmium toxicity in rabbits. *Arch. Pathol.* 94, 389–405.

Stowe, H. D., Goyer, R. A., Medley, P., and Cates, M. (1974). Influence of dietary pyridoxine on cadmium toxicity in rats. *Arch. Environ. Health* 28, 209–216.

Tsuchiya, K., and Sugita, M. (1971). A mathematical model for deriving the biological half-life of a chemical. *Nord. Hyg. Tidskr.* 53, 105–110.

Vallee, B. L., and Ulmer, D. D. (1972). Biochemical effects of mercury, cadmium and lead. *Annu. Rev. Biochem.* **41**, 91–128.

Wilson, R. H., DeEds, F., and Cox, A. J., Jr. (1941). Effects of continued cadmium feeding. *J. Pharmacol. Exp. Ther.* **71**, 222–235.

Winge, D. R., and Rajagopalan, K. V. (1972). Purification and some properties of Cd-binding protein from rat liver. *Arch. Biochem. Biophys.* **153**, 755–762.

Wiśniewska-Knypl, J. M., and Jablońska, J. (1970). Selective binding of cadmium *in vivo* in metallothionein in rat's liver. *Bull. Acad. Pol. Sci. Biol.* **18**, 321–327.

World Health Organization (1971). "International Standards for Drinking Water," 3rd ed. World Health Organ., Geneva.

Yoshikawa, H., Hara, N., and Kawai, K. (1960). Experimental studies on cadmium stearate poisoning. I. Dissociation curve and toxicity. *Bull. Nat. Inst. Ind. Health, Kawasaki* **3**, 61–69.

43

Review of Hypertension Induced in Animals by Chronic Ingestion of Cadmium

H. Mitchell Perry, Jr.

I. INTRODUCTION

Some twenty years ago, when the drug treatment of hypertension was in its infancy, Harry Schroeder and I became interested in a group of antihypertensive compounds which apparently acted by reducing peripheral resistance. These compounds were a diverse group, and their only obvious common characteristic was their ability to bind transition trace metals. At about this same time, Isabel Tipton first emphasized the surprisingly high levels of cadmium which were found in virtually all adult human kidneys. Combining the concept of metal-binding antihypertensive agent with the observed accumulation of renal cadmium led to speculation regarding a possible role for cadmium in the pathogenesis of human essential hypertension. Since then, both Schroeder's laboratories in Brattleboro, Vermont, and the laboratories of the Hypertension Division at Washington University in St. Louis have devoted considerable effort to studying the effects of cadmium on the cardiovascular system and blood pressure.

As a result of these investigations, Schroeder has reported that hypertensive subjects have abnormally high concentrations of renal cadmium, and both his laboratory and ours have reported elevated blood pressures in animals following chronic cadmium feeding. This pair of observations provides support for early speculations relating cadmium to hypertension, but does not prove a relationship. Unfortunately methodologic problems obscure the first observation, and I shall not comment further except to note that Schroeder's original report of elevated renal cadmium concentrations in two quite different populations of hypertensive subjects (Schroeder, 1965) has been both confirmed (Lener and Bibr, 1971) and denied (Morgan, 1969).

On the other hand, the evidence that cadmium can increase blood pressure in animals seems incontrovertible. Certainly, parenteral cadmium can induce acute transient hypertension in animals (Perry and Erlanger, 1971b; Schroeder et al., 1966), however that topic will not be further considered, since injected cadmium plays no part in human hypertension. Rather, I propose to review what is known regarding the hypertensive effects of chronic low-level exposure to oral cadmium. The existence of hypertension induced by ingested cadmium is a critical point and the pertinent data deserve thorough evaluation. A considerable amount has been written on this subject, but it is difficult to comprehend fully some of the complex reports without exhaustive study. Fortunately the problems of review are greatly simplified because all of the early positive observations originated in Schroeder's laboratory; recently our laboratory has also made contributions.

The induction of hypertension in animals by feeding cadmium was first reported by Schroeder and Vinton (1962). During the next twelve years, Schroeder extended his initial observations in numerous reports (Schroeder, 1964; Schroeder and Buckman, 1967; Schroeder et al., 1968a,b, 1970; Kanisawa and Schroeder, 1969). In 1971, our laboratory confirmed, in an abstract, that chronically fed cadmium could raise systolic pressure (Perry and Erlanger, 1971a), and a more detailed report has just been published (Perry and Erlanger, 1974). Superficially, our results have apparently differed from Schroeder's in that we have only induced a mild elevation in blood pressure, whereas he has reported very marked hypertension. There does seem to be some real difference in the magnitude of the induced hypertension, but much of the apparent difference seems to involve the manner of reporting results. Differences and similarities in the hypertension induced in the two laboratories are important, and an effort has been made to define them and generally clarify the situation. Recently, a preliminary communication from a third laboratory has reported mild hypertension following cadmium feeding (Petering and Sorenson, 1974). On the other hand, two groups of investigators have indicated their inability to induce hypertension with fed cadmium (Friberg et al., 1971, p. 118).

II. REVIEW OF HYPERTENSION INDUCED BY CADMIUM FEEDING

Schroeder's original definitive work on the induction of hypertension by cadmium feeding was largely done using one particular set of conditions which became standard for his laboratory. The most important of these conditions are: (1) one dose level of cadmium, 5 ppm, dissolved in the only water available for drinking; (2) special "low contamination" animal quarters on a hilltop in Vermont, where air pollution is minimal; (3) a low-cadmium diet manufactured in his laboratory; (4) *ad libitum* "basic" (i.e., fortified) drinking water containing both cadmium, if it was exhibited, and invariant quantities of five essential metals, including 50 ppm of zinc and small amounts of copper, cobalt, molybdenum, and manganese; (5) acrylic plastic cages with stainless steel tops and bedding of kiln-dried soft wood chips; (6) female weanling Long-Evans rats obtained from a single source, and eventually raised in his own laboratory; and finally (7) indirectly measured systolic pressures obtained during cuff occlusion of the tail artery of rats lightly anesthetized with pentobarbital. Unless otherwise indicated, these conditions were maintained in the experiments described here. The critical data for Schroeder's three initial experiments are summarized in Fig. 1, which indicates average systolic pressures of animals exposed to 5 ppm cadmium and of control animals without cadmium exposure.

Schroeder's first experiment began in 1960; after six months, the pressures of the control and cadmium-fed groups were 106 and 218 Torr, respectively (Schroeder and Vinton, 1962). Three comments can be made regarding significant limitations of this experiment. First, the cited averages involved groups of only eight rats each, and for the cadmium-fed group the corresponding standard deviation was very large (>40 Torr). Second, there were more rats than this in each group, and no mention is made of precisely how the eight animals were chosen. Third, the marked lability of the cadmium-induced hypertension was emphasized, and multiple pressures were obviously obtained on each animal; however, nothing is mentioned about the schedule and rules according to which these multiple pressures were taken, although such things could drastically alter the final average pressures.

Schroeder's second report (1964) considers the pressures obtained after 18, 24, and 30 months of cadmium exposure to these same animals. Again, the marked hypertension in the cadmium-exposed rats in comparison to the control rats is evident at all three times (Fig. 1). Three comments can again be made. First, because of unexplained deaths during the course of the experiment, many rats were added from available

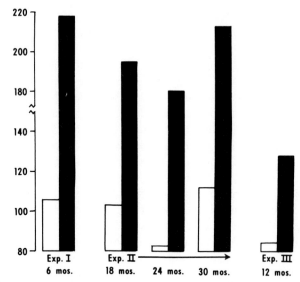

FIG. 1. Average systolic pressure (in Torr) for three of Schroeder's experiments (1962, 1964, and 1967). Note that the scale is broken between 140 and 180 Torr. On this and the next two figures, large differences between cadmium and control values are statistically significant at least at a level of $p < 0.005$. White bars = controls, black bars = 5 ppm cadmium.

"pools" of similarly handled animals in order to maintain adequately large experimental groups. In fact, between the seventeenth and twenty-fourth month, the number of added rats approximated the number of rats in the study initially. Second, the change in the average control pressure from 103 to 85 Torr between the seventeenth and twenty-fourth month and its rise again by the thirtieth month is obvious, but the reason for it is not. Third, variability of pressure in the cadmium-fed rats was again stressed, suggesting that numerous readings were made, again without any indication of the schedule.

Schroeder's third experiment (Schroeder and Buckman, 1967) involved animals that began their cadmium exposure some five years later, in 1965. For the first time, data are presented for two groups of cadmium-exposed rats—so-called hypertensive and normotensive groups, for which the average systolic pressures were 169 and 98 Torr, respectively. Since there were nine rats in the former group and thirteen in the latter, the average systolic pressure for all twenty-two rats exposed to 5 ppm cadmium was 127 Torr (Fig. 1). This value is strikingly similar to the average pressures we have subsequently obtained for similarly exposed animals (Perry and Erlanger, 1974). The average systolic pressure of Schroeder's control group was 84 Torr, which was about 20 Torr below the control averages in his first two experiments; since this report, the lower pressures have been characteristic of his control groups.

Schroeder's next report (Schroeder *et al.*, 1968b) does not provide an average systolic pressure for cadmium-fed animals comparable to those cited above. Nonetheless, the description of the hypertension was significant, since the fraction of the rats with systolic pressures greater than 140 Torr was stated, and it proved to be very similar to what we subsequently observed. After 12 months of cadmium ingestion, 38% of Schroeder's animals had systolic pressures greater than 140 Torr, whereas after a similar exposure, 28% of our animals had pressures greater than 138 Torr (Perry and Erlanger, 1974).

Schroeder's last report (Schroeder *et al.*, 1970), which is considered here, compares the effect of the low-cadmium diet manufactured in his laboratory (containing 0.02 µg of cadmium per gram) with a commercial diet (containing thirty-one times as much cadmium) on the systolic pressure of rats born and raised in his laboratory. The average systolic pressure with his laboratory diet varied between 81 and 87 Torr and with the commercial diet between 109 and 115 Torr, suggesting that the pressures of his original control animals may not have been truly basal because of minimal and unrecognized cadmium exposure. During the first 18 months of exposure, our control rats housed in stainless steel cages have characteristically had average systolic pressures of 110–115 Torr. For our control rats housed in plastic cages, and therefore presumably somewhat less exposed to environmental contamination, the average pressures were about 10 Torr lower (Perry and Erlanger, 1974).

Work in our laboratory began soon after Schroeder's initial report on hypertension induced by fed cadmium. From the first, we considered his observations to be very significant and their confirmation very important. During the late 1960s, we tried to repeat his work without having access to comparable animal facilities. We had some partial successes but were unable to obtain consistent results. Groups of cadmium-exposed animals that remained entirely healthy throughout the experiment had higher pressures than controls, but our animals often became sick, and sick rats did not seem to have elevated pressures. In 1970, we obtained much improved animal facilities where we could maintain the animals in excellent health and closely control their environment. We tried again to repeat Schroeder's work, adhering as closely as possible to his conditions, and this time we consistently found a higher pressure in rats fed cadmium; however, we could not control ambient air as well as he had done, and we put somewhat less energy into obtaining food with low-cadmium content.

We have now followed four separate groups of rats for a year or more in our improved animal facilities. The systolic pressure data are summarized in Table I. The first group began its cadmium exposure in October of 1970, and the last one began in May of 1973. The first two groups were followed for 24 months. The last two are still being followed, with data available for 18 months in one and 12 months in the other. These four experiments have involved a total of 129 control and 331 cadmium-fed animals. Individual systolic pressures were measured essentially as described by Schroeder; they were measured three times for each animal during each period of anesthesia, and the results averaged, but an animal was anesthetized only once every 3 or 6 months (Perry and Erlanger, 1974). Further data on the first two of these experiments follow.

Our first experiment, involving 32 control and 32 cadmium-fed rats,

TABLE I   Summary of Hypertension Induced by Cadmium Feeding

Experi- ment no.[a]	Date	No. of rats	Cd (ppm)	Average systolic pressure (Torr)			
				6 months	12 months	18 months	24 months
1	October 1970	32	0	106	101	108	118
		32	5	122	118	120	147
2	October 1970	64	0	112	110	114	132
		16	1	111	129	128	157
		16	2.5	125	124	130	156
		32	5	125	127	131	149
		16	10	125	115	110	121
		16	25	125	119	97	112
		16	50	122	98	102	108
3	October 1972	5	0	116	103	112	
		5	1	134	125	131	
		5	2.5	131	118	125	
		5	5	116[b]	122	125	
		5	10	126	117	123	
		5	25	126	118	107	
		5	50	126	93	98	
4	May 1973	28	0	117	113		
		14	2.5	126	128		
		14	10	131	128		

[a] Plastic cages were used in Experiment 1 and stainless steel cages in the other three experiments; otherwise the rats were treated similarly in all experiments.
[b] One of five animals had a pressure of 87 Torr.

is summarized in Fig. 2. Schroeder's experimental conditions, including acrylic plastic cages, were used. During the first 18 months of the experiment, the average systolic pressures of the cadmium-exposed rats remained relatively constant. Although the differences in pressure were small, cadmium-feeding was associated with a significant increase ($p < 0.001$). The average systolic pressures of control rats cited in the first three panels of Fig. 2 are slightly higher than, but thoroughly comparable to, what Schroeder found for control rats in his first two experiments (Schroeder and Vinton, 1962; Schroeder, 1964); the average systolic pressures for cadmium-fed rats are comparable to what he found for cadmium-fed rats in his next two experiments (Schroeder and Buckman, 1967; Schroeder et al., 1968b). By 24 months, the average pressures of both our cadmium-fed and control groups seemed to have increased, and the difference between them increased to 29 Torr (Perry and Erlanger, 1974).

Our second experiment was conducted simultaneously. It involved considerably more animals and a wide range of cadmium exposures. The rats were housed in stainless steel rather than plastic cages, so that the same personnel were able to handle several times as many animals; otherwise Schroeder's standardized conditions continued to be used. The average pressures of the control group of rats and the groups exposed to 1 and 5 ppm cadmium are shown in Fig. 3. During the

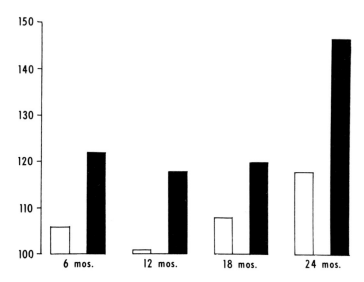

FIG. 2. Average systolic pressure (in Torr) for our first experiment (Perry and Erlanger, 1974) in which animals were housed in plastic cages and otherwise handled as described by Schroeder. White bars = controls, black bars = 5 ppm cadmium.

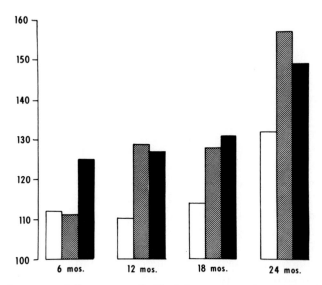

FIG. 3. Average systolic pressure (in Torr) for our second experiment (Perry and Erlanger, 1974) in which animals were housed in stainless steel cages but otherwise handled as described by Schroeder. White bars = control, hatched bars = 1 ppm cadmium, black bars = 5 ppm cadmium.

first 18 months, the average pressures for both the control and the 5 ppm cadmium groups were somewhat above the comparable averages for rats in plastic cages. More important, however, the difference between the control and cadmium-fed groups was significant, with $p < 0.001$, for rats in steel cages as it had been for rats in plastic cages. The 1 ppm cadmium group resembled the control group during the first 6 months; thereafter it resembled the 5 ppm cadmium group. By 24 months, the pressures of all three groups had increased for unexplained reasons, but the cadmium fed animals continued to have significantly higher pressures.

The second experiment involved exposures to 1, 2.5, 5, 10, 25, and 50 ppm cadmium; dose-related differences in response are indicated in Table I. In brief, high doses rapidly produced a transient hypertension, while lower doses had a slower but more prolonged effect. Thus 10 and 25 ppm cadmium induced significant elevations in pressure at 6 months but were no longer hypertensive after a year of exposure, whereas 1 ppm had no effect at 6 months but was hypertensive at 1 year.

One additional confirmatory, but preliminary, report and two brief negative reports should also be mentioned. The confirmatory report involves weanling Sprague-Dawley rats housed in stainless steel cages and provided *ad libitum* with Purina Rat Chow and deionized distilled water containing 0, 4.3, 8.6, or 17.2 ppm cadmium; systolic pressure was measured indirectly in anesthetized animals four times between the twenty-ninth and thirty-ninth weeks of exposure. For male rats, systolic pressure was directly related to the intensity of cadmium exposure, with only the highest exposure producing a significant increase in pressure. After 36 weeks, when the maximum effect and stability had been achieved, the mean systolic pressure for twelve control males was 117 Torr while for eight males receiving 17.2 ppm cadmium, it was 132. The difference was significant ($p < 0.005$). There was no comparable cadmium-induced hypertension among female rats, which weighed only half as much as males; the mean systolic pressures of both control and cadmium-fed females approximated 100 Torr (H. G. Petering and J. R. J. Sorenson, personal communication, 1974).

In the first of the two brief negative reports, Castenfors and Piscator (unpublished data referred to in Friberg et al., 1971a) gave Schroeder's usual dose, 5 ppm cadmium in drinking water, to Sprague-Dawley rats for 1 year and determined blood pressures by a direct method at monthly intervals; they found average systolic pressures of 153 Torr for thirteen cadmium-exposed and 151 Torr for nine control rats. The average pressures of these control animals were much higher than those found by Schroeder or by our group and may have been associated with less rigid control of contamination. In addition, it is difficult to assess the effect of stressful procedures such as monthly direct blood pressure determinations with their associated anesthesia and surgery.

In the second negative report, Lener and Bibr (1970) failed to induce hypertension in Wistar rats given 5 ppm cadmium in deionized drinking water for 16 months, while control animals apparently received water with 1% sodium chloride and small amounts of cobalt, copper, manganese, molybdenum, and zinc. Obviously, the control and cadmium-fed groups differed in more than just cadmium exposure, and this difference makes the experiment difficult to interpret.

Some related observations by both Schroeder and our own group, involving hypertension induced by fed cadmium, deserve to be noted briefly and without in-depth evaluation. Schroeder reported that 1% sodium chloride in the drinking water had no significant effect on the hypertension induced by 5 ppm cadmium; likewise, the cadmium exposure did not increase the intake of sodium chloride (Schroeder et al., 1966). He suggested that cadmium enhanced the production of hypertension in rats with renal ischemia and concluded that cadmium and renal ischemia produced hypertension by different mechanisms; however, the data are difficult to evaluate, since the cadmium (5 ppm) was given in deionized water, rather than in his standard "basic" water fortified with trace metals (Schroeder *et al.*, 1968a). He also reported that one injection of cyclohexane-1,2-diamine-NNN'N'-tetra-acetic acid (CDTA) containing 9 mg of zinc temporarily lowered the pressure to normal in all of nine yearling rats with cadmium-induced (5 ppm) hypertension (thirteen of the original twenty-two rats did not become hypertensive and did not receive CDTA); the nine continued their cadmium intake, and within 6 months, half of them were hypertensive again (Schroeder and Buckman, 1967). Finally, he reported that after 3 months of 10 ppm cadmium, rats with the expected elevations in systolic pressure had depressed responses to norepinephrine and angiotensin (Schroeder *et al.*, 1970).

Our recent experiments have investigated potential inhibitors of cadmium-induced hypertension. In brief, our results, which are preliminary and have yet to be repeated, indicate first that cadmium does not induce hypertension when the cadmium is administered with half as much selenium, and second, that dissolving the cadmium in a local hard water also prevented the appearance of hypertension (Perry *et al.*, 1974). The latter result seems explicable, since the cadmium was found to precipitate rapidly out of the hard water. Additional preliminary experiments suggest, as might be expected, that zinc can strongly influence the effects of cadmium; diminishing zinc exposure can lessen the cadmium-induced

TABLE II   Renal Cadmium Concentration of Cadmium-Fed Rats μg/gm Ash

Investigator	Cd (ppm)	1 year	$2\frac{1}{2}$ years
Perry	0	16.8	30.1
	1	801	1070
	5	2860	4850
Schroeder	0	—	0
	5	—	4290[a]

Column header note: Cadmium concentration (μg/gm ash)

[a] These "ash weight" figures are approximations, having been obtained from the original wet weight data by multiplying the latter by 100. Schroeder's data are not on animals that were sacrificed; rather, they are from animals that died in their cages. Hence, the exposure time of $2\frac{1}{2}$ years is only approximate.

hypertension and sufficient zinc is apparently able to induce hypertension without added cadmium (H. M. Perry, Jr., unpublished observation).

Renal cadmium concentrations in rats following exposure to 5 ppm cadmium are comparable to the renal cadmium concentrations of the average American adult without known exposure. Typical data for our exposed animals are summarized in Table II. The data for "$2\frac{1}{2}$ years" of exposure in our laboratory were obtained from the previously described groups of animals in which we first successfully induced cadmium hypertension. The results were as might be expected—there was very little in the control animals, and there were large amounts in old and heavily exposed rats. Not surprisingly, Schroeder's controls have less cadmium than ours. For purposes of comparison, the average American adult has approximately 3000 μg of cadmium per gram of renal ash.

III. DISCUSSION

On the basis of the available data, it seems that fed cadmium can indeed induce increases in the systolic pressure of rats. In our hands, the average systolic pressure of cadmium-fed rats has approximated 125 to 130 Torr and has been normally distributed, with a quarter of the exposed animals having pressures in the 140 Torr range and higher. Our average value for control rats has ranged from 110 to 115 Torr, and the difference between the cadmium-fed and control averages has consistently been significant (Perry and Erlanger, 1974). In at least one of Schroeder's experiments, the average systolic pressure of his whole group of cadmium-fed rats was in the 125–130 range, with a quarter of the animals having systolic pressures greater than 140 Torr. His control rats usually had average systolic pressures in the 80 Torr range (Schroeder and Buckman, 1967), making the cadmium-induced increase apparently greater for his animals.

Important questions remain to be answered before the induction of hypertension by feeding cadmium can be considered to be defined, even in a preliminary manner. Now that we feel able to induce elevated pressure reproducibly by feeding cadmium to rats, we are investigating several variables individually. Specifically, we are comparing the responses of male and female animals, and we are comparing the responses of other strains of rats with the Long-Evans strain. This last approach should be extended to an examination of the effect of cadmium in other species, but we are not now able to attempt that. In addition, we are currently feeding smaller amounts of cadmium than have been tested previously. The lowest concentration tested to date, 1 ppm cadmium, is maximally hypertensive; therefore, it seems reasonable to test still lower doses, especially since 1 ppm cadmium is many times the human intake, which is estimated at 50 μg daily (Friberg *et al.*, 1971). We are therefore evaluating the effect of $\frac{1}{2}$, $\frac{1}{4}$, and $\frac{1}{10}$ ppm cadmium. We are also attempting to define the effects of zinc and other elements that seem likely to have an effect on cadmium-induced hypertension.

The mechanism of cadmium-induced hypertension in animals remains obscure, although several suggestions have been made, of which the most likely involves an effect on salt and water metabolism. Several experiments indicate that cadmium may produce sodium retention. Vander has observed that cadmium injected into one renal artery decreased sodium excretion on that side acutely (Vander, 1962). In a chronic experiment, repeated subcutaneous injections of cadmium have produced an early sodium loss followed by sodium retention (Perry *et al.*, 1971). Hyperreninemia has been reported in cadmium-fed rats (Perry and Erlanger, 1973). Observations recently presented by Doyle and co-workers suggest that ingested cadmium induces significant retention of a single intravenous injection of radiosodium (Doyle *et al.*, 1974).

It is not clear why Schroeder's 12-year-old observation that cadmium can induce hypertension in rats has not been confirmed until recently. It may involve the large investment in time and energy needed for such long-term experiments plus the requirements for a very low-cadmium environment and for unusually good animal facilities. Preliminary experiments by others may have been laid aside when they failed to evoke hypertension. On the other hand, quite possibly, there may be unrecognized conditions that are needed for the induction of chronic hypertension by fed cadmium, such as the appropriate zinc or selenium requirements, which were fortuitously met in Schroeder's laboratory and in ours when we followed Schroeder's procedure but not in some other places.

IV. CONCLUSIONS

Cadmium-induced hypertension in rats, although real, may be relatively small in magnitude; however, that by no means demonstrates its insignificance or lack of importance. Most human hypertension is also mild. Of the 25 million Americans who are estimated to have hypertension, at least two-thirds have diastolic pressures below 105 Torr. Moreover, in man, at least, even such mild elevations in blood pressure can double the risk of heart attack or stroke, the major cardiovascular causes of disability and death. Moreover, like cadmium-induced hypertension in rats, mild human hypertension has no obvious associated findings. In rats, the small amounts of cadmium that induce hypertension produce none of the usual toxic manifestations of heavier exposure to cadmium, while in man, the complete absence of symptoms is a major part of the difficulty in identifying mild hypertension and convincing the involved individuals of its ominous prognostic significance.

Finally, there is no proof, pro or con, that cadmium is in any way involved in human hypertension. Since a role for cadmium in human hypertension cannot be excluded, and since cadmium, like many other things, is an increasingly prevalent and serious environmental pollutant, it becomes very pertinent to determine the maximum cadmium exposure that man can tolerate without affecting blood pressure. This level may be difficult to define. Obviously, cadmium does not produce an effect in a vacuum, and any hypertensive effect it has seems very likely to be conditioned not only by genetic and other constitutional factors, but also by complex interactions with other substances, particularly zinc and selenium, probably copper, and possibly many other things including hard water. Therefore, any such definition of permissible limits of cadmium exposure must take into account the rest of the environment and perhaps other factors as well.

REFERENCES

Doyle, J. J., Bernhoft, R. A., Vo-Khactu, K. P., and Sandstead, H. H. (1974). The effects of a low level of dietary cadmium on some biochemical and physiological parameters in rats. In "Trace Substances in Environmental Health" (D. D. Hemphill, ed.), 8th Annu. Conf. p. 403. University of Missouri, Columbia.

Friberg, L., Piscator, M., and Nordberg, G. (1971a). "Cadmium in the Environment," p. 118. CRC Press, Cleveland, Ohio.

Friberg, L., Piscator, M., and Nordberg, G. (1971). "Cadmium in the Environment," p. 25. CRC Press, Cleveland, Ohio.

Kanisawa, M., and Schroeder, H. A. (1969). Renal arteriolar changes in hypertensive rats given cadmium in drinking water. Exp. Mol. Pathol. 10, 81–98.

Lener, J., and Bibr, B. (1970). Cadmium content in some foodstuffs in respect to its biological effects. Vitalst. Zivilisationskr. 15, 139.

Lener, J., and Bibr, B. (1971). Cadmium and hypertension. Lancet 1, 970.

Morgan, J. M. (1969). Tissue cadmium concentration in man. Arch. Intern. Med. 123, 405–408.

Perry, H. M., Jr., and Erlanger, M. W. (1971a). Hypertension in rats induced by long-term low-level cadmium ingestion. Circulation 44, Suppl. II, 130.

Perry, H. M., Jr., and Erlanger, M. (1971b). Hypertension and tissue metal levels after intraperitoneal cadmium, mercury, and zinc. Amer. J. Physiol. 220, 808–811.

Perry, H. M., Jr., and Erlanger, M. (1973). Elevated circulating renin activity in rats following doses of cadmium known to induce hypertension. *J. Lab. Clin. Med.* **82**, 399–405.

Perry, H. M., Jr., and Erlanger, M. (1974). Metal-induced hypertension following chronic feeding of low doses of cadmium and mercury. *J. Lab. Clin. Med.* **83**, 541–547.

Perry, H. M., Jr., Perry, E. F., and Purifoy, J. E. (1971). Antinatriuretic effect of intramuscular cadmium in rats. *Proc. Soc. Exp. Biol. Med.* **136**, 1240–1244.

Perry, H. M., Jr., Perry, E. F., and Erlanger, M. (1974). Reversal of cadmium-induced hypertension by selenium, or hard water. *In* "Trace Substances in Environmental Health" (D. D. Hemphill, ed.), 8th Annu. Conf., p. 51. University of Missouri, Columbia.

Petering, H. G., and Sorenson, J. R. J. (1974). Personal communication.

Schroeder, H. A. (1964). Cadmium hypertension in rats. *Amer. J. Physiol.* **207**, 62–66.

Schroeder, H. A. (1965). Cadmium as a factor in hypertension. *J. Chronic Dis.* **18**, 647–656.

Schroeder, H. A., and Buckman, J. B. (1967). Cadmium hypertension. Its reversal in rats by a zinc chelate. *Arch. Environ. Health* **14**, 693–697.

Schroeder, H. A., and Vinton, E. H., Jr. (1962). Hypertension induced in rats by small doses of cadmium. *Amer. J. Physiol.* **202**, 515–518.

Schroeder, H. A., Kroll, S. S., Little, J. W., Livingston, P. O., and Meyers, M. A. G. (1966). Hypertension in rats from injection of cadmium. *Arch. Environ. Health* **13**, 788–789.

Schroeder, H. A., Nason, A. P., Prior, R. E., Reed, J. B., and Haessler, W. T. (1968a). Influence of cadmium on renal ischemic hypertension in rats. *Amer. J. Physiol.* **214**, 469–474.

Schroeder, H. A., Nason, A. P., and Mitchener, M. (1968b). Action of a chelate of zinc on trace metals in hypertensive rats. *Amer. J. Physiol.* **214**, 796–800.

Schroeder, H. A., Baker, J. T., Hansen, N. M., Size, J. G., and Wise, R. A. (1970). Vascular reactivity of rats altered by cadmium and a zinc chelate. *Arch. Environ. Health* **21**, 609–614.

Vander, A. J. (1962). Cadmium enhancement of proximal tubular sodium reabsorption. *Amer. J. Physiol.* **203**, 1005–1007.

44

The Chronic Toxicity of Cadmium

Magnus Piscator

I. INTRODUCTION

It has been known for more than a century that cadmium can cause acute poisoning in man. That cadmium could cause chronic poisoning was not established until about 25 years ago, when the chronic syndrome after long-term exposure to cadmium oxide dust was described (Friberg, 1949, 1950). Friberg made detailed examinations of cadmium-exposed workers and found that lung damage, mainly emphysema, and renal dysfunction were the major features. Since then, many similar investigations have been performed in several countries, and exposure to cadmium compounds is now recognized as a serious occupational hazard.

From being a problem only inside the industries, cadmium is now also recognized as a potential hazard to the general population. In Japan, large population groups are exposed to cadmium via food, especially rice. In several areas polluted by cadmium, a high prevalence of proteinuria has been found, and in at least one area, the exposure has been high enough to cause more severe damage—the itai-itai disease.

For evaluation of the health hazards of cadmium, the main emphasis must be on experience gained in studies on human beings. The metabolic peculiarities of cadmium, i.e., the slow selective accumulation in the kidney and the extremely long biological half-time, make it difficult

431

to extrapolate from results obtained in short-term animal studies. In the following, the toxic effects of cadmium will mainly be discussed as seen in man, and of the numerous papers on cadmium toxicity in animals, only a few with relevant application will be mentioned. Since the metabolism of cadmium is reviewed in another section of this book, metabolic aspects will be given only when needed in context. A special effect of cadmium documented in animals is hypertension. This effect, however, is also treated separately and will not be discussed in this chapter.

There have been many reports on acute cadmium posioning after ingestion of cadmium-contaminated food or drinks. Recent incidents in the United States and Sweden, where children got acute poisoning from sweets ("Love beads") and soft drinks from a vending machine, respectively, show that this hazard still is a reality. There are, however, no reports that indicate that there are any chronic effects from such acute episodes, and in the following only the chronic toxicity of cadmium as seen after long-term exposure will be reviewed, based mainly on two recent monographs on cadmium (Friberg et al.,.1974, 1975). Since the kidney is the critical organ, the emphasis will be on renal effects.

II. EFFECTS OF CADMIUM

A. General Picture of Chronic Cadmium Poisoning

1. Occupational Poisoning

In a Swedish factory producing alkaline batteries with nickel and cadmium electrodes, a number of deaths had occurred in the 1930s and early 1940s, and the causative agent was not known. There were also complaints about shortness of breath, fatigue, etc. Careful studies, both clinical and experimental, by Friberg revealed that cadmium oxide dust was responsible (Friberg, 1949, 1950). It caused emphysema of the lungs and renal damage, these two being the most prominent findings. Anemia, slight liver damage, anosmia, and a yellow coloring of the teeth were other significant findings. The exposure had been high, probably several milligrams per cubic meter of air for many years. (The present threshold limit values in most countries are 0.2 and 0.1 mg/m^3 for cadmium oxide dust and fumes, respectively, and these are regarded as too high.)

Friberg's findings were confirmed by studies in West Germany and the United Kingdom (Baader, 1951; Hunter, 1954). Further reports from these countries and during later years also from Japan, France, and Belgium have shown that renal damage is the most common finding, whereas lung damage and anemia are seldom reported. Improved working conditions and lower cadmium concentrations in air have caused less intense exposure. Most data are from studies on male workers. Already in 1942, however, osteomalacia was reported to have occurred in a French factory where there was exposure to cadmium (Nicaud et al., 1942). Of six cases, four were women. In a study in the Soviet Union, it was found that newborns from cadmium-exposed women had lower weights than children of nonexposed women. Since cadmium does not traverse the placenta to any significant extent, this effect might well be due to a zinc deficiency in the fetus caused by zinc retention in the mother.

2. Chronic Poisoning via Food

The most severe form of chronic cadmium poisoning is the itai-itai disease. It was first seen in women above 45 years of age in Fuchu, Toyama Prefecture, Japan. Exposure to cadmium had occurred through the ingestion of rice grown on fields irrigated by water from a river that had been contaminated by a mine many miles upstream. The concentration of cadmium in the rice may for many years have been around 1 μg/gm, and the daily intake of cadmium must have been 300 μg or more, which can be compared to present intakes in some European countries and the United States, where it is around 50 μg. Itai-itai disease is an osteomalacia and received its name from the severe pain caused by fractures of the softened bones. The renal dysfunction is severe, and an increase in the excretion of protein, glucose, amino acids, and phosphorus is seen, i.e., a complete so-called Fanconi syndrome. Cadmium concentrations in the liver are high, of the same magnitude as found in exposed workers, but renal concentrations of cadmium are often very low due to losses of cadmium caused by the renal dysfunction (Friberg et al., 1974). Predisposing factors are the low intakes of calcium and Vitamin D, and many pregnancies and lactation periods, which themselves cause depletion of calcium. Among the males in the area, proteinuria and glucosuria are common findings, but osteomalacia is uncommon, which may be explained by a better calcium balance. Itai-itai disease is an extreme manifestation of chronic cadmium poisoning, but in several other cadmium-polluted areas of Japan, tubular proteinuria has been found.

B. Effects on the Kidney

1. In Human Beings

Before Friberg began his studies, it had not been shown that cadmium could cause chronic renal dysfunction. The tests used for detection of proteinuria at that time were the boiling test, Esbach's test, or the nitric acid test, which generally were negative in examinations of urine from cadmium workers. Friberg found, however, by using trichloroacetic acid, that cadmium exposed workers had a high prevalence of proteinuria compared to controls. Further studies showed that this proteinuria was not of the classical type seen in chronic nephritis or nephrosis. The proteins had a different electrophoretic pattern and had lower molecular weight than albumin. A decreased ability to concentrate the urine and a reduction in inulin clearance were other signs of renal dysfunction (Friberg, 1949, 1950). At that time, it was not possible to further characterize and identify this type of proteinuria, but after Butler and Flynn (1958) had shown that some diseases with congenital or acquired renal tubular dysfunction had a typical urine protein pattern on electrophoresis, it could be demonstrated that the proteinuria in chronic cadmium poisoning was of the same type (Piscator, 1962, 1966).

This tubular proteinuria is characterized by the excretion of low molecular weight serum proteins in the urine, caused by a decrease in reabsorption of proteins from the glomerular filtrate (Piscator, 1966). Improved methods for the determination of total urine protein made it possible to show that the excretion of protein was related to exposure time, as shown in Table I. This low molecular weight proteinuria is regarded as the first sign of an effect of cadmium on renal function, and by using immunological methods for determination of specific proteins in combination with electrophoresis, it is now possible to detect small increases in excretion of such proteins, e.g., β_2-microglobulin. The other signs mentioned earlier in this section, e.g., glucosuria and aminoaciduria, generally appear later than the proteinuria. The renal dysfunction will also cause an increase in the urinary excretion of cadmium (Friberg et al., 1974). In investigations on population groups exposed to cadmium via rice in Japan, it has been shown that the proteinuria is of the same type as seen in cadmium-exposed workers and that cadmium excretion is considerably higher than in people from nonpolluted areas (Friberg et al., 1974).

The critical concentration of cadmium in the renal cortex, i.e., the concentration at which sensitive individuals may get tubular dysfunction, has been estimated to be 200 μg/gm wet weight (Friberg et al., 1974).

TABLE I Urinary Protein Excretion in
Cadmium-Exposed Workers in
Relation to Exposure Time[a]

| Exposure time (years) | N | Urinary protein excretion (mg/24 hr) | |
		Mean	Range
0	15	60	25–110
1–5	4	100	50–170
6–10	4	210	70–570
11–15	5	300	70–770
16–20	9	575	165–1300
21–25	6	460	160–1050
26–30	6	790	210–2600
31–	6	955	370–1800

[a] Exposure ceased 10 years before the examination. From Piscator (1962), *Arch. Environ. Health* (1962), **4**, 607–621, Copyright 1962, American Medical Association.

This estimate was based on data obtained from autopsies on former cadmium workers and agrees well with findings in animal studies, as will be shown below. In Table II, present mean levels at age 50 in "normal" populations are shown for comparison. In the United States and Europe, there is still a margin of safety, but in some Japanese areas not regarded as cadmium polluted, this margin is not large.

TABLE II Mean Cadmium Concentration in Renal Cortex at Age 50

Country	Sex	Cadmium (μg/gm wet weight)	Reference
East Germany	M	30	Anke and Schneider, 1971
East Germany	F	15	Anke and Schneider, 1971
Sweden (Stockholm)	M–F	30	Piscator and Lind, 1972
United States (large cities)	M–F	50	Schroeder and Balassa, 1961
United States (North Carolina)	M	25	Hammer et al., 1973
United States (North Carolina)	F	25	Hammer et al., 1973
Japan (Kobe)	M–F	60	Kitamura et al., 1970
Japan (Kanazawa)	M–F	85	Ishizaki et al., 1970
Japan (Tokyo)	M–F	125	Tsuchiya et al., 1972

2. In Animals

Experiments on animals have verified that exposure to cadmium causes renal tubular dysfunction (Axelsson and Piscator, 1966; Nordberg, 1972). Autoradiographic studies by Berlin et al. (1964) showed that cadmium accumulated mainly in the proximal part of the proximal tubule. This is the part of the tubule where protein reabsorption occurs. It has also been indicated that cadmium bound to the cadmium-binding protein metallothionein may be filtered through the glomeruli and reabsorbed (Nordberg, 1972). It is conceivable that cadmium originally bound to this protein in the liver will in that way be transported to the renal tubules and that cadmium will accumulate mainly at a site where there is reabsorption of protein. This also means that the first function to be disturbed when there is excessive accumulation of cadmium should be protein reabsorption, which fits well with the experience from investigations on human beings.

It has also been shown (Nordberg, 1972) that in mice exposed to cadmium, the urinary excretion was very low as long as the renal function was normal, whereas there was a sharp rise in cadmium excretion when the tubular proteinuria appeared. It was then also possible to demonstrate the presence of cadmium in a low molecular weight urine protein fraction, conceivably metallothionein. That means that the decreased reabsorption of proteins also causes a decrease in the reabsorption of metallothionein. This increase in cadmium excretion may eventually lead to a depletion of renal cadmium as seen in itai-itai patients.

Data from animal experiments also indicate that the critical level in renal cortex is around 200 $\mu g/gm$ wet weight (Axelsson and Piscator, 1966; Nordberg, 1972; Stowe et al., 1972). In calcium-deficient rats, however, the excretion of the low molecular weight enzyme ribonuclease was increased at a cadmium concentration in renal cortex of about 90 $\mu g/gm$ wet weight, indicating that under certain circumstances the critical level might be below 200 $\mu g/gm$ (Piscator and Larsson, 1972).

3. Cadmium and Zinc

The kidney is rich in zinc-dependent enzymes, and the renal dysfunction caused by cadmium is thought to be due to cadmium interfering with enzymes necessary for reabsorption and catabolism of proteins. Simultaneous administration of zinc to cadmium-exposed animals alleviates some of the renal symptoms caused by cadmium (Vigliani, 1969). Cousins et al. (1973) found that the activity in renal cortex of the zinc enzyme leucinaminopeptidase was decreased in swine exposed to high concentrations of cadmium in the diet. This decrease occurred at a cadmium concentration in the cortex of about 100 μg/gm wet weight.

In "normal" human beings, the increase in cadmium concentrations in renal cortex with age is accompanied by an equimolar increase in zinc concentrations (Piscator and Lind, 1972; Hammer et al., 1973), which has been shown to be valid for cadmium concentrations up to 75 μg/gm wet weight. However, human data for the range 75/200 μg/gm are lacking. The relationship between cadmium and zinc in this range has been studied in normal horses, and it has been found that whereas at cadmium concentrations below 75 μg/gm there was equimolar increase in zinc with increased cadmium, such a relationship could not be found in the higher range; i.e., zinc did not increase to the same extent as cadmium (Piscator, 1974). These findings indicate that there could be a progressive relative zinc deficiency in the renal cortex at cadmium concentrations between 100 and 200 μg/gm, and that with increasing zinc deficiency, tubular dysfunction might appear. The retention of zinc in liver and kidney caused by cadmium may also cause depletion in other organs. Thus, Petering et al. (1971) showed that when the intake of zinc in rats was marginal, exposure to cadmium caused a decrease in the zinc concentrations in the testes. Such an effect was not seen when the intake of zinc was increased. There is thus evidence for cadmium interference with metabolism and utilization of zinc, and it is obvious that in studies on effects of cadmium, the intake and organ levels of zinc also must be studied.

C. Effects on Bone

Since osteomalacia has been found both in exposed workers and in Japanese women exposed to cadmium via rice, special attention has during the last years been paid to different aspects of cadmium and mineral metabolism. The concentrations of cadmium in bone tissue are low even at high body burdens, and there is little evidence for a direct action of cadmium on bone. In short-term experiments on calcium-deficient rats given cadmium in drinking water (25 μg/gm for 2 months) and long-term experiments (7.5 μg/gm for 13 months), calcium accretion in bone was not decreased in cadmium-exposed animals (Larsson and Piscator, 1971; Piscator and Larsson, 1972). It was found, however, that cadmium accelerated the osteoporotic process caused by calcium deficiency alone, and both interference with intestinal absorption of calcium and endocrine disturbances might have caused this. In the short-term experiment, it was found that the increase in parathyroid volume, which is caused by calcium deficiency, was inhibited by cadmium. In the long-term experiment, there were signs of slight renal tubular damage already at a cadmium concentration in renal cortex of about 90 μg/gm wet weight, indicating that kidneys of calcium-deficient animals may be more sensitive to cadmium than normal animals.

The bone changes in itai-itai disease have occurred mainly in women with low intakes of calcium and losses due to multiple pregnancies. The exposure to cadmium has caused renal tubular dysfunction, which has caused further losses of minerals. In Swedish factory workers with renal tubular damage but high intakes of calcium, bone changes were not seen (Friberg, 1950).

Since the most active form of Vitamin D is produced in the kidney, it is also conceivable that the accumulation of cadmium may interfere with the synthesis of this form, which may further contribute to the disturbances in mineral metabolism.

D. Other Effects

Anemia has been seen in exposed workers, and animal experiments indicate that this may be due both to interference with the absorption of iron and slight hemolysis (Friberg *et al.*, 1974).

The liver may contain large amounts of cadmium, but clinical tests for signs of liver damage are often negative. Recent animal experiments by Stowe *et al.* (1972) indicate, however, that clinical tests generally used for studies of liver function, e.g., glutamic oxaloacetic transaminase (GOT) and glutamic pyruvic transaminase (GPT), may be negative even when morphological changes are manifest. Experiments by Sporn *et al.* (1970) on rats given small amounts of cadmium in drinking water for 1 year indicate that at liver levels of cadmium of the same magnitude as found in normal human beings some metabolic pathways in the liver may be affected.

III. NEEDS FOR FURTHER RESEARCH

Data on metabolism and effects of cadmium are rapidly accumulating, but there are still some gaps that have to be filled. The critical concentration in renal cortex has been established by relatively crude methods. There is a need for data on changes at the cellular level before renal dysfunction occurs, i.e., increased excretion of low molecular weight proteins. Such data may be obtained by renal biopsies on exposed human beings, a method that for practical reasons will be difficult to use. Animal experiments to obtain such data should be performed for long periods of time. Very few studies have been performed on monkeys, and it is conceivable that well controlled, long-term studies could give valuable information. Due to their short life spans, mice and rats are not ideal for experiments where one wants to reproduce the human long-term, low-level exposure via food. Special attention should be paid to enzymes that might be reduced in activity by cadmium replacing essential metals, especially zinc. Since cadmium exposure also may cause zinc depletion in some organs when the intake of zinc is marginal, enzyme activities may be decreased by decreased concentrations of zinc in some organs. The fetus may also become zinc deficient if the mother has a marginal zinc intake and is exposed to cadmium. This is an area that merits further studies.

In recent years, a large number of papers dealing with zinc-dependent enzymes and zinc deficiency have been published. By applying that knowledge, it should be possible to find suitable systems for testing the influence of cadmium on enzymatic activities in the renal cortex. It has been shown that the activity of leucinaminopeptidase can be decreased at relatively low renal concentrations of cadmium. It is necessary, however, also to study such enzymes under long-term exposure conditions to avoid the general effects of the high exposure used.

Changes in enzymatic activity may not only influence enzymes necessary for reabsorption and catabolism of proteins in the kidney. Studies are now in progress in several laboratories to study the *in vivo* effect of cadmium exposure on the formation of 1,25-dihydroxycholecalciferol in the kidney. This is the most active form of vitamin D and should in fact be regarded as a hormone.

Since deficiency of zinc and calcium are common among large populations, it is thus of great importance to study how cadmium may influence the metabolism of these two metals. Data on intake of cadmium, other metals, vitamins, and protein can be used for predicting risks for cadmium accumulation in different areas of the world.

There is also scarce knowledge of how cadmium affects endocrine functions. The acute effects of cadmium on the testes have been reported in more than one hundred publications, but these reports do not have bearing on the effects of long-term, low-level exposure in humans. Detailed studies on excretion of hormones, e.g., androgens and other steroids, in exposed workers would be of value, since cadmium in animal long-term experiments has been indicated to reduce testosterone synthesis (Nordberg, 1972).

Also, effects on the liver should be studied in more detail, since recent data indicate that some liver functions may be disturbed at relatively low concentrations.

It should thus be possible within this decade to obtain more accurate data on the critical concentration in the renal cortex also with regard to nutritional factors. It will probably also be possible to establish dose–response relationships for populations according to geographical location, since similar intakes of cadmium may in different areas have different responses depending on nutritional factors.

REFERENCES

Anke, M., and Schneider, H. J. (1971). Der Zink-, Kadmium- und Kupferstoffwechsel des Menschen. *Arch. Veterinaermed.* 25, 805–809.

Axelsson, B., and Piscator, M. (1966). Renal damage after prolonged exposure to cadmium. *Arch. Environ. Health* 12, 360–373.

Baader, E. W. (1951). Die Chronische Kadmiumvergiftung. *Deut. Med. Wochenschr.* 76, 484–487.

Berlin, M., Hammarström, I., and Maunsbach, A. B. (1964). Microautoradiographic localization of water-soluble cadmium in mouse kidney. *Acta Radiol.* 2, 345–352.

Butler, E. A., and Flynn, F. V. (1958). The proteinuria of renal tubular disorders. *Lancet* 2, 978–980.

Cousins, R. J., Barber, A. K., and Trout, J. R. (1973). Cadmium toxicity in growing swine. *J. Nutr.* 103, 964–972.

Friberg, L. (1949). Proteinuria and emphysema among workers exposed to cadmium and nickel dust in a storage battery plant. *Proc. Int. Congr. Ind. Med., 9th, 1948* pp. 641–644.

Friberg, L. (1950). Health hazards in the manufacture of alkaline accumulators with special reference to chronic cadmium poisoning. *Acta Med. Scand.* 138, Suppl. 240, p. 124.

Friberg, L., Piscator, M., Nordberg, G., and Kjellström, T. (1974). "Cadmium in the Environment," 2nd. edition, p. 248. CRC Press, Cleveland, Ohio.

Friberg, L., Kjellström, T., Nordberg, G., and Piscator, M. (1975). "Cadmium in the Environment, III," EPA-650/2-75-049 Off. Res. Devel., U.S. Environ. Protect. Ag., Washington, D.C.

Hammer, D. I., Colucci, A. V., Hasselblad, V., Williams, M. E., and Pinkerton, C. (1973). Cadmium and lead in autopsy tissues. *J. Occ. Med.* 15, 956–963.

Hunter, D. (1954). Cadmium poisoning, *Arh. Hig. Rada.* 5, 221–224.

Ishizaki, A., Fukushima, M., and Sakamoto, M. (1970). On the accumulation of cadmium in the bodies of itai-itai patients. *Jap. J. Hyg.* 25, 86.

Kitamura, M., Sumino, K., and Kamatani, N. (1970). Cadmium concentrations in livers, kidneys, and bones of human bodies. *Jap. J. Pub. Health* 17, 507.

Larsson, S.-E., and Piscator, M. (1971). Effect of cadmium on skeletal tissue in normal and calcium-deficient rats. *Isr. J. Med. Sci.* 7, 495–497.

Nicaud, P., Lafitte, A., and Gros, A. (1942). Les troubles de l'intoxication chronique par le cadmium. *Arch. Mal. Prof., Hyg. Toxicol. Ind.* 4, 192–202.

Nordberg, G. (1972). Cadmium metabolism and toxicity. *Environ. Physiol. Biochem.* 2, 7–36.

Petering, H. G., Johnson, M. A., and Stemmer, K. L. (1971). Studies of zinc metabolism in the rat. I. Dose-response effects of cadmium. *Arch. Environ. Health* 23, 93–101.

Piscator, M. (1962). Proteinuria in chronic cadmium poisoning. I. An electrophoretic and chemical study of urinary and serum proteins from workers with chronic cadmium poisoning. *Arch. Environ. Health* 4, 607–622.

Piscator, M. (1966). "Proteinuria in Chronic Cadmium Poisoning," p. 29. KL Beckmans Tryckerier AB Stockholm.

Piscator, M. (1974). Cadmium-zinc interactions. *Proc. CEC-EPA-WHO Int. Symp., Environ. Health, 1974* (in press).

Piscator, M., and Larsson, S.-E. (1972). Retention and toxicity of cadmium in calcium-deficient rats. *Proc. Int. Congr. Occup. Health, 17th, 1972* (in press).

Piscator, M., and Lind, B. (1972). Cadmium, zinc, copper and lead in human renal cortex. *Arch. Environ. Health* 24, 426–431.

Schroeder, H. A., and Balassa, J. J. (1961). Abnormal trace metals in man: Cadmium. *J. Chronic Dis.* 14, 236–258.

Sporn, A., Dinu, I., and Stoenescu, L. (1970). Influence of cadmium administration on carbohydrate and cellular energetic metabolism in the rat liver. *Rev. Roum. Biochim.* 7, 299–305.

Stowe, H. D., Wilson, M., and Goyer, R. A. (1972). Clinical and morphological effects of oral cadmium toxicity in rabbits. *Arch. Pathol.* 94, 389–405.

Tsuchiya, K., Seki, Y., and Sugita, M. (1972). Organ and tissue cadmium concentrations of cadavers from accidental deaths. *Proc. Int. Congr. Occup. Health, 17th, 1972* (in press).

Vigliani, E. C. (1969). The biopathology of cadmium. *Amer. Ind. Hyg. Ass. J.* 30, 329–340.

45

Metabolism and Toxicity of Lead

Jack L. Smith

I. INTRODUCTION

A study in the town of Hammond, Louisiana, which has a population of approximately 10,000, was conducted to determine the effects of iron-fortified foods on the iron nutriture of anemic 2–6-year-old children. The children were selected for the study by canvassing the neighborhoods to detect children between the ages of 2 and 6 years who had hemoglobin levels of 11 gm/dl or less. The families of these children were then brought into a clinic and given a more complete examination. The results for hemoglobin and hematocrit levels are shown in Tables I and II. The families of those children who met these criteria were

TABLE I Hemoglobin Levels of 2–6 Year-Old Children Participating in an Iron Intervention Study

	Number	Hemoglobin level (gm/dl) (mean ± SD)	Percent <11 gm/dl
Preintervention	115	10.51 ± 0.53	100
First intervention	127	11.35 ± 0.96	
Second intervention	115	11.37 ± 0.83	

TABLE II   Mean Hematocrit Values of 2–6-Year-Old Children
Participating in an Iron Intervention Study

	Number	Hematocrit value (%) (mean ± SD)
Preintervention	154	32.67 ± 1.70
First intervention	127	34.02 ± 2.60
Second intervention	115	33.67 ± 2.54

then provided certain food products that either had been fortified with additional iron or were equivalent products without additional fortification.

The criteria used to evaluate the iron nutriture of these children were hemoglobin, hematocrit, red cell count, serum B_{12}, serum folacin, serum iron, serum iron-binding capacity, transferrin saturation, and free erythrocyte protoporphyrin. Both iron deficiency anemia and lead toxicity could effect protoporphyrin levels; therefore, it was considered essential to analyze blood for lead levels as well. All blood samples were sent to the Nutritional Biochemistry Laboratory at the Center for Disease Control in Atlanta, Georgia, where Dr. Gordon McLaren and Mr. William Barthel ran protoporphyrin and lead assays, respectively (McLaren, *et al.*, 1973). The results of the iron fortification program will be reported elsewhere, as will be a more complete discussion of the lead, protoporphyrin, and iron assays. Table III shows the whole blood lead levels obtained from the 2–6-year-old children in the study. It was found that 40.3% of the children had levels greater than 40 μg/dl of whole blood. The intervention experiment was conducted in such a way that there were two separate periods in which food was provided. The results of a second lead assay, which followed the second intervention period, are also shown in Table III and indicate no substantial change in blood lead levels in that

TABLE III   Blood Lead Levels of 2–6-Year-Old Children Participating in
an Iron Intervention Study

	Number	Lead level (μg/dl) (mean ± SD)	Percent >40 μg/dl
First intervention period	115	40.6 ± 9.35	50.4
Second intervention period	111	37.8 ± 9.28	40.6

TABLE IV Free Erythrocyte Protoporphyrin Levels of
2–6-Year-Old Children Participating in an Iron
Intervention Study

	Number	Protoporphyrin level (μg/dl RBC) (mean $\pm$ SD)
First intervention period	113	104.4 $\pm$ 81.9
Second intervention period	109	74.3 $\pm$ 48.9

period. There were approximately the same number of individuals with blood levels greater than 40 μg/dl. The protoporphyrin levels were 104 μg/dl at the end of the first intervention period, as shown in Table IV. The mean protoporphyrin levels decreased to 73.3 μg/100 ml red blood cells in the same children after the second intervention period. These data include children who received iron-fortified food as well as those who did not, and the drop in protoporphyrin levels after the second intervention period is probably due to the change in the iron status of two-thirds of them rather than a change in their lead status, since the children in the groups that received iron-fortified food had significantly lower protoporphyrin levels than the children who did not. These data will be presented elsewhere. There was no difference in the mean lead levels. The data obtained for whole blood lead levels in each age group showed a decrease in levels with age, dropping from 41.2 μg/dl in the youngest age group to 23.3 μg/dl in the oldest age group. There was a general slight drop after the second intervention period, but the relatively high level was maintained. These data were surprising in that it was not consistent with the general belief that lead levels of this magnitude were generally found in children living in large urban areas and would be unexpected in a rural or semirural setting such as we were using.

II. SOURCES OF LEAD

Let us consider some of the sources of lead that these children may have encountered in order to obtain blood lead values observed. Our initial reaction was that exposure of the children to lead must have come from pica of lead-containing paint or plaster. However, peeling paint and cracked plaster were not found in examining many of the homes. In fact, some of the children were living in housing that was of recent construction, built under federal guidelines, so that it should not contain lead-based paint or lead-containing plaster. Other children did live in older, run-down housing that may at one time have been painted with lead-based paint. However, there was no consistency or correlation between their lead levels and their living conditions. The most common finding in an inspection of the housing was the amount of junk and debris in the yard. This consisted sometimes of old cars, refrigerators, and rusted parts. We were unable to perform any analysis of dirt or dust to clearly establish the source of the lead.

At one time, it was felt that the only significant exposure that increased lead ingestion was due to plaster, paint, or industrial exposure. This is probably true for acute poisoning with blood levels over 80 μg/dl, in which symptoms of toxicity are seen. It need not be true for the individual with signs of increased ingestion of lead. These are individuals who have lead levels between 40 and 80 μg/dl (Lin-Fu, 1973).

Other potential sources for exposure include house dust, in which the lead content can vary between 65 and 1000 μg per gram of dust (Fairey and Gray, 1970; Haar and Aronow, 1974; Sayre *et al.*, 1974). Another source is dirt. The lead content of dirt is usually higher in the inner city and around highways than in rural areas. The lead content of dirt is also higher the closer it is to a house that is painted with lead paint or a yard that contains old batteries and other types of junk (Haar and Aronow, 1974). An important source that causes much difficulty in some areas is airborne contamination, which has been a subject of a National Academy of Science Workshop (National Research Council, 1972). This is of particular importance in the vicinity of lead smelting, battery plants, or other industrial operations that involve lead. The importance of lead being obtained from gasoline additives is under dispute, although lead in dirt and dust near a highway is higher than further away. A decision has been made that all new cars require gasoline without lead-containing additives, which should alleviate this problem within a few years. There is no question about an increase in lead content of dirt and water around highways, which lead is most likely derived from tetraethyllead from exhaust.

Another source of lead is paper and newsprint (Lin-Fu, 1973). This can be a problem in children who chew paper or make spitballs, or in other conditions that would allow them to either ingest or have in their mouths newsprint or ink. Another source of lead available for ingestion is the soldering that is done on cans (Mitchell and Aldous, 1974). This is particularly true with acidic types of food and even more true if the acidic food is stored in the can after opening for a period of time at room temperature. The importance of this is difficult to evaluate, but the can contributes to an overall burden of lead. Another source that is available to children are tubes of toothpaste, which often contain lead, either by the direct chewing of the tube or from the lead being dissolved into the toothpaste (Berman and McKiel, 1972; Shapiro *et al.*, 1973). None of these sources in themselves, with the exception of the air around smelting and battery plants, is enough to cause acute toxic levels of lead, but they are likely to be involved in the cases in which evidence of increased lead burdens were found.

III. METABOLIC EFFECTS

The best known effect of lead is the inhibition of nearly all the enzymatic steps that lead to heme synthesis. All of these steps seem to be inhibited to some degree. This will be considered in more detail later.

One of the primary reactions to lead is with immature erythrocytes (Albahary, 1972). Lead appears to increase their production and reacts both on the reticulocyte membrane and intracellularly. Nearly all of the blood lead is found in red cells. One clinical characteristic of plumbism is the appearance of basophilic stippled red cells in both bone marrow and peripheral circulation. These stippled cells contain mitochondria and therefore resemble reticulocytes. The stippling is due to the agglutination of ribosomes (Jensen *et al.*, 1965). Mitochondria are not normally present in a mature red cell; however, their presence is required to provide the necessary enzymatic machinery for the synthesis of heme.

Another way in which lead effects the metabolism of the reticulocyte is by inhibiting the uptake of iron from transferrin. This inhibition is in addition to the more direct reaction of the ferrochelatase in effecting iron utilization (Morgan and Baker, 1969). There is also evidence that globin synthesis is inhibited in the presence of lead, although it is unclear what is the minimal amount of lead required for this inhibition to begin and whether it is related to stippling, which involves ribosomes. An additional effect on the erythrocyte is the red cell survival time. The exact cause for a decrease in the survival time is unknown; however, the decrease is shown by several different methods, including those involving the addition of tagged erythrocytes and use of internal tags.

Figure 1 shows an abbreviated scheme for heme synthesis, giving the essential enzymes and illustrating which steps occur within the mitochondria and which occur outside the mitochondria (Chisholm, 1964). The initial reaction in heme synthesis is the combination of succinyl-CoA with glycine to form δ-aminolevulinic acid (Kassenaar, 1957). This reaction is catalyzed by the enzyme δ-aminolevulinic acid synthetase (ALA-syn-

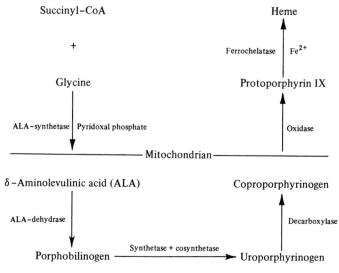

FIG. 1. Steps in the synthesis of heme.

thetase), which is a mitochondrial enzyme. One major source of toxicity of lead is the inhibition of this enzyme. However, the next step is a combination of the two δ-aminolevulinic acid molecules into porphobilinogen. This reaction is catalyzed by the enzyme δ-aminolevulinic dehydrase and is inhibited to an even greater extent by lead. This reaction occurs in the cytoplasm of the cell. The inhibition of this enzymatic step causes a urinary excretion and an increased blood level of δ-aminolevulinic acid. This occurs in spite of the fact that ALA-synthetase is also inhibited. The next step in the reaction is a combination of four porphobilinogens to form coproporphyrinogen. These reactions occur extramitochondrially and are synthesized by the enzymes synthetase and cosynthetase. There is an inhibition in these steps even though the level of porphobilinogen is decreased and coproporphyrinogen is excreted in the urine. The next step is the conversion of coproporphyrinogen to protoporphyrin IX, which occurs intramitochondrially, catalyzed by an oxidase. The final step is the addition of ferrous iron to protoporphyrin to form heme. The enzyme, in addition to ALA-dehydrase, that is nearly totally inhibited by lead is the ferrochelatase enzyme. This causes an increased level of free erythrocyte protoporphyrin. It is obvious that heme may not be synthesized either because of an insufficient protoporphyrin due to lead toxicity due to an inhibition in ferrochelatase or because of an absence of iron. The results are essentially the same even though determined by a different mechanism.

IV. CLINICAL SYMPTOMS

Now that we have discussed the sites of lead toxicity, let us discuss the methods of detection for lead toxicity, since they are certainly related to the metabolic site of lead interaction. We have primarily been discussing a chronic form of lead poisoning which is asymptomatic; however, for completeness, I will include items that indicate clinical manifestations of lead poisoning (Flink, 1971).

The clinical symptoms of lead poisoning, when they develop, are similar whether or not it is so-called acute or chronic poisoning; chronic poisoning refers to prolonged exposure to lead. The symptomatology has been divided into alimentary forms, neuromuscular forms, and encephalopathic forms. The symptoms that are common to all three are anemia, insomnia, headache, dizziness, irritability, and lead-line stippling of the retina. The alimentary form also has colicky pain. The neuromuscular form involves weakness of the muscle groups, with a characteristic wrist drop. In the encephalopathic form, which occurs primarily in children, the presenting manifestations include coma, convulsions, mania, or delirium. There often is a history of antecedent behavioral change, such as irritability, insomnia, restlessness, loss of memory, hallucinations, or confusion.

V. SCREENING METHODS

The laboratory methods of detection that are more commonly used for screening of populations for relatively high lead burdens involve the measurement of either blood or urine, certain precursor products of heme synthesis, or lead itself.

A sensitive method is a measure of δ-aminolevulinic acid in either urine or serum (Haeger-Aronson, 1960; Chisholm, 1964; Robinson, 1974). Reports using this technique have demonstrated that there is a correlation between lead levels and the δ-aminolevulinic acid levels of lead workers (Haeger-Aronson, 1960; Robinson, 1974).

Another method that can be used, is the measure of free erythrocyte protoporphyrin. Micro methods have been developed by Granick et al. (1972) and Piomelli et al. (1973) that permit the analysis of only 1–2 μl of whole blood using a simple fluorometric procedure. What has been found is that blood levels less than 80 μg/dl erythrocytes usually indicate very low exposure to lead, whereas levels between 80 and 100 would have moderate exposure to lead, and levels greater than 100 have more chronic exposure to lead. The values can reach as high as 1–2000 μg and correlate exponentially with lead levels.

A direct method for detecting lead toxicity and a useful method for detection of moderate exposure is the measure of whole blood lead levels. There are several techniques available for this, but primarily the use of atomic absorption spectrometry has made this a very simple assay using small quantities of blood. It is normally considered that blood levels of less than 40 μg/dl indicate a low lead burden, levels between 40 and 60 μg indicate a moderate lead burden, and acute lead toxicity does not appear until 80–100 μg/dl of whole blood. There have been some discrepancies in methodology that are beyond the scope of this paper, but in general these have been worked out.

VI. INTERACTION WITH OTHER NUTRIENTS

Let us now consider the interaction of other nutrients with the development of chronic or acute lead toxicity. One of the first considerations should be lead absorption. As with all trace metals, the mechanisms of absorption are very important; however, most studies, particularly radioactive studies, have been performed with adult animals or humans and indicate that in normal conditions between 1 and 10% of the lead ingested is absorbed. The exact percentage depends on the chemical form of the lead, such as whether it is organically bound, tied up in insoluble oxides, or physically bound in a way that it is difficult to obtain access, such as in large paint flakes. Obviously, more soluble forms are more readily absorbed than less soluble forms. However, recent studies indicate that a much higher rate of absorption might be present in children. Normal children may absorb as much as 50% of an ingested dose (Alexander, 1974). Another condition that can greatly effect iron deficiency, and one that has been discussed here previously, is that iron deficiency will increase the absorption of several trace minerals, lead included. This mechanism may be one of the causes for the apparent increase in lead burden in those children that have some indication of being iron deficient (Lin-Fu, 1973; Mahaffey, 1974). This interaction of lead and iron, relating to absorption, is in addition to the reduction in the iron uptake from transferrin into red cell precursors from lead-intoxicated animals and in addition to the inhibition of the enzyme ferrochelatase, which catalyzes the addition of iron into porphyrin. Another factor that can effect the absorption of lead is the metabolism and absorption of calcium. Recent studies indicate that more lead is absorbed in the presence of low calcium than in the presence of high calcium. Vitamin D plays a role in this as well. In animals low in vitamin D, less lead is absorbed. This implies a competitive interaction between the two divalent cations, lead and calcium. Lastly, more lead has been shown to be absorbed in the presence of low protein intake (Mahaffey, 1974; Lin-Fu, 1973).

VII. SUMMARY

The factors that may help explain the evidence of an increased lead burden in the children we studied in the small Louisiana community include:

1. Low iron—subjects were selected on the basis of low hemoglobin levels.

2. Low calcium—milk and other calcium-containing foods are not consumed by this population.

3. High levels of vitamin D—the high sunlight exposure would predict adequate vitamin D levels.

4. Exposure to lead—possibly due to dust and dirt as well as pica of paint and plaster.

REFERENCES

Albahary, C. (1972). Lead and hemopoiesis: The mechanism and consequences of the erythropathy of occupational lead poisoning. *Amer. J. Med.* **52**, 367–378.

Alexander, F. W. (1974). The uptake of lead by children· in differing environments. *Environ. Health Perspect.* **7**, 155–159.

Berman, E., and McKiel, K. (1972). Is that toothpaste safe? *Arch. Environ. Health* **25**, 64–65.

Chisholm, J. J., Jr. (1964). Disturbances in the bio-synthesis of heme in lead intoxication. *J. Pediat.* **64**, 174–187.

Fairey, F. S., and Gray, J. W., III. (1970). Soil lead and pediatric lead poisoning in Charleston, S.C. *J. S. C. Med. Ass.* **66**, 79–82.

Flink, E. B. (1971). Heavy metal poisoning. In "Cecil-Loeb: Textbook of Medicine" (C. B. Beeson and W. McDermott, eds.), 13th ed., p. 63. Saunders, Philadelphia, Pennsylvania.

Granick, S., Sassa, S., Granick, J. L., Levere, R. D., and Kappas, A. (1972). Assays for porphyrins, δ-aminolevulinic acid dehydratase, and porphyrinogen synthetase in microliter samples of whole blood: Applications to metabolic defects involving the heme pathway. *Proc. Nat. Acad. Sci. U.S.* **69**, 2381.

Haar, G. T., and Aronow, R. (1974). New information on lead in dirt and dust as related to the childhood lead problem. *Environ. Health Perspect.* **7**, 83–89.

Haeger-Aronson, B. (1960). Studies on urinary excretion of δ-aminolevulinic acid and other heme precursors in lead workers and lead-intoxicated rabbits. *Scand. J. Clin. Lab. Invest.* **12**, Suppl. 47, 1–128.

Jensen, W. N., Moreno, G. D., and Bessis, M. C. (1965). An electron microscopic description of basophilic stippling in red cells. *Blood* **25**, 933–943.

Kassenaar, A., Morell, H., and London, I. M. (1957). The incorporation of glycine into globin and the synthesis of heme *in vitro* in duck erythrocytes. *J. Biol. Chem.* **229**, 423–435.

Lin-Fu, J. S. (1973). Vulnerability of children to lead exposure and toxicity. *N. Engl. J. Med.* **289**, 1229–1233 and 1289–1293.

McLaren, G. D., Barthel, W. F., and Landrigan, P. (1973). Screening for lead poisoning: Measurements and methodology. *Pediatrics* **52**, 303–306.

Mahaffey, K. (1974). Nutritional factors and susceptibility to lead toxicity. *Environ. Health Perspect.* **7**, 107.

Mitchell, D. G., and Aldous, K. M. (1974). Lead content of foodstuffs. *Environ. Health Perspect.* **7**, 59–64.

Morgan, E. H., and Baker, E. (1969). The effect of metabolic inhibitors on transferrin and iron uptake and transferrin release from reticulocytes. *Biochim. Biophys. Acta* **184**, 442–454.

National Research Council. (1972). Biological effects of atmospheric pollutants. "Lead." Nat. Res. Counc., Washington, D.C.

Piomelli, S., Davidow, B., Guinee, V. P., Young, P., and Gay, G. (1973). The FEP (Free Erythrocyte Porphyrins) test: A screening micro-method for lead poisoning. *Pediatrics* **51**, 254.

Robinson, T. R. (1974). δ-aminolevulnic acid and lead in urine of lead anti-knock workers. *Arch. Environ. Health* **28**, 133–138.

Sayre, J. W., Charney, E., Bostal, J., and Pless, I. B. (1974). House and hand dust as a potential source of childhood lead exposure. *Amer. J. Dis. Child.* **127**, 167–170.

Shapiro, I. M., Cohen, G. H., and Needleman, H. L. (1973). The presence of lead in toothpaste. *J. Amer. Dent. Ass.* **86**, 394–395.

46

Quantitative Measures of the Toxicity of Mercury in Man

Thomas W. Clarkson

I. INTRODUCTION

In discussing the toxicity of mercury, it is necessary to distinguish between its different physical and chemical forms. According to an international committee (MAC committee, 1969), the various forms of mercury can be classified as "inorganic" and "organic." Examples of this classification are given in Table I, selected from those forms of mercury occurring most commonly in nature or from those that have an anthropogenic origin. Inorganic mercury consists of elemental mercury and of

TABLE I Organic and Inorganic Forms of Mercury

Inorganic	
Metallic	Hg^0
Mercurous salts	Hg_2Cl_2
Mercuric salts	$HgCl_2$
Organic	
Alkylmercury compounds	CH_3HgCl
Arylmercury compounds	C_6H_5HgCl
Alkoxarylmercury compounds	CH_3OCH_2HgCl

the dissociable salts of mercurous and mercuric mercury. Mercury present in molecules, where it is linked directly to a carbon atom, is referred to as organic mercury. The short-chain alkyl mercurials and the aryl and alkoxyalkyl mercurials belong in this category. The anion in Table I is depicted as chloride. In fact, a wide variety of anions may be found in combination with the mercury cation and have little effect on its toxic properties.

This physicochemical classification .does not correlate well with the toxic properties. For example, the toxicity of elemental mercury vapor is distinctly different from that of the mercurous and mercuric salts. The signs and symptoms of poisoning due to phenyl mercury compounds are different from those due to exposure to the short-chain alkyl mercurials. From the point of view of a toxicological classification, the short-chain alkyl mercurials occupy a unique position. They cause irreversible damage to the central nervous system and are fetotoxic. Exposure to metallic mercury vapor can also cause damage to the nervous system, but in general, these changes are reversible, especially at lower exposures. There is no evidence that elemental vapor is toxic to the fetus. Exposure to inorganic mercury as well as to the aryl and alkoxyalkyl compounds leads to accumulation of mercury in the kidneys, the primary target organs. Involvement of the central nervous system with these classes of compounds is minimal. The similarity of the toxic effects of the aryl and alkoxyalkyl compounds with those of inorganic mercury is due to the fact that these organic mercurials are rapidly converted to inorganic mercury in mammalian tissues (for review, see Clarkson, 1972). Space does not permit a full discussion of the toxicities of all these forms of mercury. This discussion will be restricted to the toxic effects of the alkyl mercury compounds and of elemental mercury vapor, the two forms of mercury that primarily affect the central nervous system.

II. DOSE–RESPONSE RELATIONSHIPS IN HUMAN POPULATIONS EXPOSED TO ELEMENTAL MERCURY VAPOR OR METHYLMERCURY COMPOUNDS

The toxicity of metallic mercury vapor and of methylmercury compounds exhibits remarkable species differences. For example, the pigeon can withstand an atmosphere of mercury vapor about 100 times greater than that which produces adverse effects in humans (Armstrong et al., 1963). Species differences in sensitivity to methylmercury are of the order of 10- to 100-fold (for review, see Berglund et al., 1971). Consequently, if we are to study the quantitative aspects of toxicity in man, we have no alternative other than to study human populations exposed to these forms of mercury. Data on human exposures to both methyl and elemental mercury are now available, since sizable numbers of people have been exposed to these forms of mercury in the past resulting in many cases of poisoning. Such studies are of considerable importance from the public health point of view, since it is likely that occupational exposure to elemental mercury vapor and exposure to methylmercury compounds in food (particularly food containing fish and fish products) will continue. The question of what is safe versus what is a hazardous exposure will therefore continue to be of considerable importance. Quantitative studies of the toxicity of these forms of mercury in man provide vital information in determining the degree of risk or hazard that is faced by exposure to these forms of compounds either in the working environment or in the food supply.

Quantitative studies on toxicity whether in animals or man usually take the form of establishing a dose–response relationship. The studies of Smith and his colleagues (1970) are an example as to how these measurements are made in man. The data in Fig. 1, taken from Smith *et al.* (1970), indicate a relationship between the frequency (incidence) of certain signs and symptoms in a population and the exposure to elemental mercury vapor as measured by concentrations of the vapor

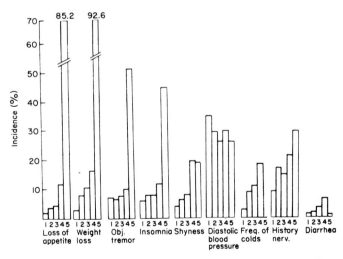

FIG. 1. Percentage incidence of certain signs and symptoms related to exposure of workers to elemental mercury vapor. Time-weighted average concentrations (mg/m³): (1) control, (2) 0.1–0.05, (3) 0.06–0.10, (4) 0.11–0.14, (5) 0.24–0.27. Reproduced from Smith *et al.* (1970) by permission.

in the working atmosphere. In this type of study, the population is divided into subgroups according to the average exposure to mercury vapor in air (Fig. 1). Group 1, the controls, work in an atmosphere virtually free of mercury vapor. The concentration is substantially less than 10 $\mu g/m^3$. People in Group 2 are working in an atmosphere having a time-weighted average concentration of from 10 to 50 $\mu g/m^3$. People in the Group 3 work in an atmosphere with concentration between 60 and 100 $\mu g/m^3$, and so on as specified in the figure. The various groups are matched as closely as possible so that the only significant variable from one group to the other is the concentration of mercury vapor in air. These data indicate certain important general features that apply to all studies attempting to quantify the toxic effects of mercury in man. In the first place, qualitative features, i.e., the presence or absence of certain signs and symptoms, depend on the level of exposure. For example, at the very lowest exposures (Group 2), there is a significant increase in complaints of loss of appetite. However, it is not until exposure rises to a level equivalent to Group 5 that the frequency of objective tremors shows a sharp increase. Indeed, the classic triad of symptoms of mercurialism, which are tremor, erethism, and gingivitis, appear only at exposures higher than those experienced by this population. A second important feature is that the effects of elemental mercury vapor become evident first in changes in the frequency of subjective complaints by the workers. The exposed person complains of certain maladies, but the physician cannot detect any organic signs of such an effect. In the study by Smith et al. (1970), the symptoms of loss of appetite and the complaint of loss of weight are the first to be affected. A third important general aspect is that, at very low exposures to metallic mercury vapor, the effects are generally nonspecific; that is to say that these effects, such as loss of appetite, could be caused by a variety of agents and disease states as well as by exposure to elemental mercury vapor. Thus, one is faced with the crucial problem of distinguishing between the background frequency of the symptoms, which may occur in any population and be unrelated to exposure to mercury, and the change in that frequency due to exposure to metallic mercury vapor. This raises important statistical and epidemiological questions; for example, were the studies made blind or double blind, was the control population appropriately matched to the exposed population, and so on.

   In view of these difficulties, there is not yet any general agreement as to the lowest air level of mercury that produces detectable adverse effects. Russian workers (for review, see Friberg and Nordberg, 1973) have claimed to see effects at very low concentration of mercury vapor in air (of the order of 10 $\mu g/m^3$). This claim is based mainly on subjective symptoms in workers, with all the attendant difficulties of quantifying these effects. On the other hand, the objective signs associated with mercurialism do not occur until air levels are substantially above 100 $\mu g/m^3$. It is the concentration range from 10 to 100 $\mu g/m^3$ about which there is so much controversy at the present moment over possible adverse health effects.

Quantitative studies on the toxicity of methylmercury have been reported recently from an outbreak of methylmercury poisoning in Iraq (Bakir *et al.*, 1973). This outbreak, involving over 6000 cases admitted to hospital, was due to the ingestion of homemade bread prepared from wheat treated with a methylmercury fungicide. People ingested contaminated bread for a period of approximately 2 months, after which signs and symptoms of methylmercury poisoning developed. The signs and symptoms were essentially similar to those described in previous cases of methylmercury poisoning (Methyl Mercury in Fish, 1971) and included paresthesia, ataxia, constriction of the visual fields, slurred speech, and hearing difficulties.

The approach to measuring the quantitative toxicity in this population was essentially similar to that adopted by Smith and his colleagues in their studies reviewed above. Groups of people were categorized according to the amount of methylmercury that they had ingested, ranging from a control group that had no ingestion of the contaminated bread to groups of people having graded exposures ranging from subtoxic to lethal. In these studies, the exposure to methylmercury was expressed in terms of the maximum amount of methylmercury that had accumulated in the body. The details as to how these estimates and calculations were made are given in the article by Bakir *et al.* (1973). Figure 2 shows the frequency of signs and symptoms in each of the exposure groups. The frequency is plotted vertically as the percentage in each group having a specified sign or symptom. The body burden is plotted horizontally in terms of milligrams of mercury present in the body. Two scales are used for the abscissa because of uncertainties in the calculation of the body burden. Each line in the figure refers to a specified sign or symptom. The same general features that we noted in the case of the Smith study are exhibited in the Iraq data. The qualitative picture depends on the body burden of mercury. At high body burdens, all the signs and symptoms of poisoning are evident, but at lower body burdens, only certain of these signs and symptoms are exhibited. Second, the effects of methylmercury are first evident with the symptoms rather than objective signs. For example, paresthesia, which is a complaint of loss of sensation or tingling in the extremities of the hands and feet or around the mouth, is the first of the effects due to methylmer-

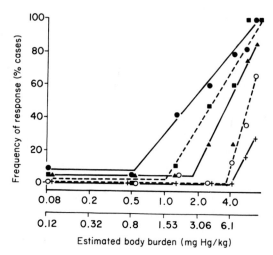

FIG. 2. The relationship between the frequency of signs and symptoms and the estimated maximum body burden of methylmercury. Key: ● = paresthesia, ■ = ataxia, ▲ = disarthria, ○ = deafness, + = death. The two scales on the abscissa are used because of alternative ways of estimating the maximum body burden (see Bakir *et al.,* 1973).

cury. Third, paresthesia is a nonspecific symptom with respect to methylmercury and could be caused by a variety of other agents or disease states. Thus, a common problem in this study and in the mercury vapor study is distinguishing between the background frequency of a symptom and the increase in that frequency due to methylmercury. On this graph, an attempt was made to determine the body burden at which the frequency of paresthesia exceeded that of the background frequency. This was achieved by joining the points in the way indicated in the figure so that the two straight-line portions of the graph intercepted at about 0.5 mg Hg/kg body weight according to the upper scale or 0.8 according to the lower scale. Thus, it was argued that the true threshold point at which the effects of methylmercury become detectable could lie anywhere between the 0.5 mg and 0.8 mg Hg/kg body weight.

It is clear that the accuracy of this dose–response relationship could be increased by increasing the number of individuals studied. In the study reported from Iraq, the number of people involved was over one hundred. Increasing the number to a thousand or more is a practical possibility, and the result may be a decrease in statistical errors. Nevertheless, the problem arising from the background frequency of the symptom, in this case paresthesia, will still be found and will always set the lower limit to the sensitivity at which one can detect the effects of methylmercury. The preliminary report from Iraq (Bakir *et al.*, 1973) suggests that effects become detectable above a body burden in the range of 0.5–0.8 mg Hg/kg. This conclusion agrees with a previous report by a Swedish expert committee examining data from the outbreaks of methylmercury poisoning in Japan (Methyl Mercury in Fish, 1971).

Studies of the distribution of tracer doses of radioactive methylmercury in man allow a rough calculation of the chronic daily intake of methylmercury from food necessary to produce a body burden of the order of 0.5 mg/kg. Without going into details of the calculation (see Clarkson, 1972), a steady daily intake of between 280 and 420 μg per day might be expected to yield a body burden in the range of about 25 mg in a 70 kg adult. These figures would compare to an average daily intake in the general population of less than 20 μg per day and the probable average of around 5 μg per day (Methyl Mercury in Fish, 1971).

III. FACTORS AFFECTING THE TOXICITY OF MERCURY IN MAN

Many factors may influence the toxicity of mercury. Studies on animals have indicated that the length of exposure to methylmercury plays an important part in determining the outcome of adverse effects. Berglund *et al.* (1971), in a review of the literature, point out that most studies on the toxicity of methylmercury on animals have not been carried out long enough to determine the lowest toxic dose. Chronic daily exposures lasting for weeks or months followed by an extensive latent period are necessary in most species before the first signs of poisoning appear. The stage of the life cycle at which exposure occurs may also be a decisive factor in determining the lowest toxic dose. Animal studies reviewed by Clegg (1971) suggest that the prenatal stage of life may be most sensitive to insult from methylmercury. The administration of mercury-binding compounds can result in a reduction in the toxicity of mercury. In the case of methylmercury, the administration must take place before irreversible damage has occurred to the nervous system. In effect, these mercury-binding agents are modifying the toxicity of mercury by effectively reducing the dose. However, more recent work, reviewed below, indicate that other types of interactions with chemicals are possible, resulting in a modification of the toxicity of mercury.

In recent years, some information has become available on factors modifying the toxicity of metallic mercury vapor and methylmercury in man. This information is rather sparse, and conclusion drawn from it must be regarded as somewhat tentative.

A. Importance of Length of Exposure

The period of exposure to methylmercury in the outbreak in Iraq was approximately 2–3 months (Bakir *et al.*, 1973). Assuming a 70 day clearance half-time from the body, the body burden would remain elevated for a period of approximately 1 year after the end of exposure (Fig. 3). Thus, the victims of mercury poisoning in Iraq experienced an exposure period of not more than 15–18 months. An opportunity presented itself to study a group of Korean contract fishermen working off American Samoa who had unusually high intakes of methylmercury from fish. The period of exposure was for at least 6 months. Their average exposure time was 6.5 years. Therefore, from the point of view of lengths of exposure to methylmercury, it was of interest to compare this population with the one reported in Iraq.

Marsh and co-workers (1974) and Clarkson *et al.* (1974) reported blood levels of mercury in fishermen and shoreworkers in American Samoa employed in a fish canning factory. Excellent agreement was noted between organic mercury measured in blood by selective atomic absorption and methylmercury determined by gas chromatography (Fig. 4). The slope of the line relating the two types of determinations of mercury had a gradient of 0.95, insignificantly different than unity, and the square of the correlation coefficient was 0.94. A histogram describing the blood levels of methylmercury in units of nanograms of mercury per milliliter of whole blood is reported in Fig. 5. Most of the fishermen had blood levels less than 100 ng/ml, but some had blood levels in

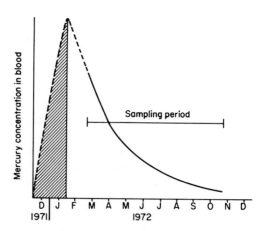

FIG. 3. A diagrammatic representation of the levels of mercury in blood during and after consumption of contaminated bread. The shaded area is the period of consumption.

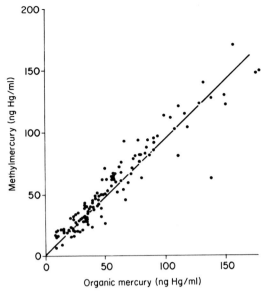

FIG. 4. The relationship between organic mercury determined by atomic absorption and methylmercury determined by gas chromatography in blood samples from Korean contract fishermen based in American Samoa. The equation of the line calculated by linear regression analysis is $y = 0.95x + 0.79$, and the correlation coefficient is $r = 0.97$. Reproduced from Clarkson et al. (1974).

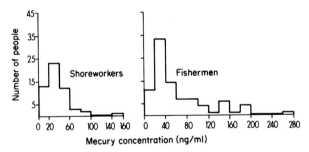

FIG. 5. A histogram describing the distribution of mercury concentrations in samples of whole blood collected from Korean contract fishermen and from shoreworkers based in American Samoa. Reproduced from Marsh et al. (1974).

the range of 100–200, and one fisherman was found with a blood level of 218 ng Hg/ml. The shoreworkers had substantially lower blood levels, though still considerably higher than the normal level found on the North American continent. The shoreworkers had a medium blood level in the range of 20–40 ng/ml, with most of the workers being substantially below 100 ng/ml. The highest recorded blood level was 140 ng/ml.

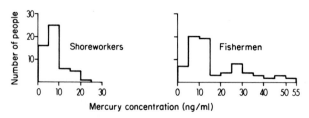

FIG. 6. A histogram describing the distribution of mercury concentrations in samples of hair collected from Korean contract fishermen and from shoreworkers based in American Samoa. Reproduced from Marsh *et al.* (1974).

A histogram describing the distribution of organic mercury determined by selective atomic absorption in hair is reported in Fig. 6 from the paper by Marsh and co-workers (1974). The distribution in hair generally followed that seen in blood, except that the absolute level in hair is about 300 times higher. Most of the fishermen had hair levels below 30 μg/gm, but some had hair levels as high as 55 μg/gm. The shoreworkers had levels substantially lower than those seen in the fishermen, with most falling below 10 μg/gm and all of them below 25 μg/gm.

In order to compare the blood levels in the Korean fishermen with the body burdens reported in the Iraq study, one may make use of the metabolic parameters published by Miettinen (1973). In studies of volunteers taking methylmercury, Miettinen reported that approximately 1% of the body burden was contained in 1 liter of whole blood. The average body weight in the adults studied in Iraq was 51 kg. Therefore, the threshold dose at which effects became detectable, i.e., 0.5–0.8 mg Hg/kg body weight, is equivalent to a blood level of 250–400 ng/ml. Thus, the highest blood level recorded in the Korean fishermen just overlaps the threshold range reported from Iraq. If time of exposure is important in determining man's response to insult from methylmercury, we might expect to see a substantial number of cases of poisoning in these Korean contract fishermen, since their exposure on the average was five times longer than that seen in Iraq. The clinical data in Table II, taken from Marsh *et al.* (1974), indicate that no signs or symptoms attributable to methylmercury exposure could be found in the population. Marsh *et al.* (1974) pointed out that one of the fishermen complained of a mild aching in his limbs, but this was attributed to a brainstem lesion of an undetermined type. They noted that he did not have the full clinical syndrome of methylmercury poisoning.

These results suggest that length of exposure is not an important factor in determining response to methylmercury in man. However, it must also be admitted that these data on the Samoan fishermen suffer

TABLE II   **Correlation of Symptoms and Signs with Those of Early Methylmercury Poisoning**[a]

| Signs and symptoms | Number with sign and symptom | | Occurs in methyl-mercury poisoning |
	Fishermen[b]	Shore-workers[c]	
Symptoms			
Paresthesias of limbs distally	0	0	Yes
Paresthesias, perioral, tongue	0	0	Yes
Ataxia of gait	0	0	Yes
Ataxia of limbs	0	0	Yes
Slurred speech	0	0	Yes
Impaired peripheral vision	0	0	Yes
Deafness	0	2	Yes
Abdominal discomfort	8	0	No
"Tired after work"	0	7	No
Lumbar or leg pain	5	1	No
Hemoptysis	2	0	No
Signs			
Symmetrical hypesthesia of fingers, toes	0	0	Yes
Astereognosis of hands	0	0	Yes
Impaired sensation of lips	0	0	Yes
Ataxia of gait	0	0	Yes
Ataxia of limbs	0	0	Yes
Dysarthria	0	0	Yes
Concentric constriction of visual fields	0	0	Yes
Hearing deficit	3	5	Yes
Of focal brain stem lesion (medulla)	1	0	No

[a] From Marsh et al. (1974).
[b] Total population, 88.
[c] Total population, 45.

from the weakness that only a few fishermen have blood levels in the range of those associated with signs and symptoms in the Iraq study. The majority of the fishermen and all the shoreworkers, except one, have blood levels lower than 100 ng/ml. This is more than a factor of 2 below the minimum threshold effect noted in Iraq.

Nothing is known of the relationship between length of exposure and toxicity of elemental mercury vapor. Occupational exposures may vary from days or weeks to periods of 10–20 years or more. Information is also lacking on the kinetics of elimination of mecury from man following exposure to metallic mercury vapor. The rate of elimination may not be the same immediately following a single dose as that seen after long-term chronic exposure. We do not know the length of exposure necessary to bring an individual into a steady state of balance with respect to his body burden of mercury.

B. Prenatal and Early Postnatal Exposure to Methylmercury

The outbreak of methylmercury poisoning in Iraq provided an opportunity to observe the effects of prenatal exposure to methylmercury and early postnatal exposure to ingestion of methylmercury by breast-fed infants. Iraqi infants are normally breast-fed for the first 2 years of life. They usually begin to consume some solid foods about the age of 1 year. Thus, infants born in the 6 months just prior to the consumption of the contaminated bread by the mother had exposure only to methylmercury in breast milk. Infants older than this would receive mercury not only from breast milk but possibly also by eating some contaminated bread. Figure 7 shows the levels of mercury in infant blood and in the blood and milk of the mother in a case where exposure had occurred only from breast milk. The first samples were collected in July of 1972, approximately 6 months after the end of the consumption of the con-

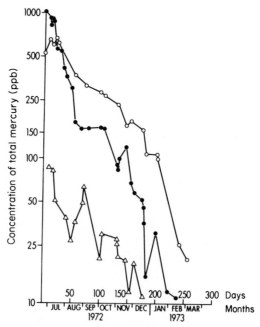

FIG 7. Concentration of total mercury in blood of infants (○) and mothers (●) and milk (△). The date of birth was June 1971. Reproduced from Amin-Zaki et al. (1974a).

taminated bread by the mother. The concentration of mercury in infant blood was observed to decline at a slower rate than that of the mother. Thus, in July, the infant's blood was lower than that of the mother, but after August, infant blood mercury levels were generally higher than those seen in the mother. The main reason for this lower rate of decline in infant blood level is the continued ingestion of methylmercury from mother's milk. Although the milk levels are significantly lower than the blood level, the daily intake of methylmercury from milk could make a substantial difference in the overall methylmercury balance in the infant. Methylmercury is only slowly excreted from the body (in adults 1% of the body burden is excreted per day), so a small intake could significantly affect blood levels of methylmercury.

Unfortunately, it was not possible to follow a large number of infant–mother pairs for the period of time reported in Fig. 7. However, it was possible to collect occasional samples from infant–mother pairs, and the results of these studies are presented in Fig. 8. In this figure, taken from the publication by Amin-Zaki *et al.* (1974a), the ratio of the concentration of methylmercury in infant blood to the concentration in mothers' blood is plotted against the date of collection. It may be seen that the ratio is less than unity in July of 1972, indicating that

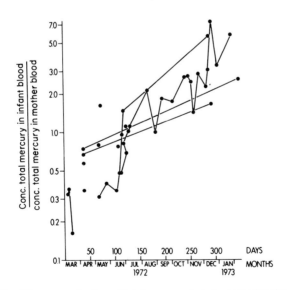

FIG. 8. Ratio of the concentration of total mercury in infant blood to the concentration in mothers' blood in infant–mother pairs sampled over the period March 1972 to January 1973. Data points for each pair are connected by straight lines. The broken line represents equivalence of mothers' and infant's blood concentrations. Reproduced from Amin-Zaki *et al.* (1974a).

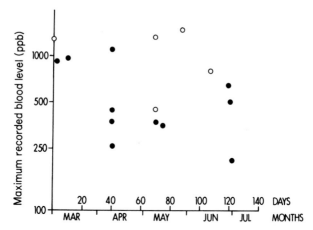

FIG. 9. The maximum recorded concentrations of total mercury in each infant's blood plotted according to the date on which the sample was collected. These data points do not necessarily indicate the true maximum level in the infant's blood. Key: ● = exposure only from milk, ○ = exposure from milk and possibly from contaminated bread. Reproduced from Amin-Zaki *et al.* (1974a).

the infant's blood is less than the mother's blood. The ratio becomes unity in about August of 1972 and thereafterwards becomes in excess of unity, thus confirming the relationship reported in Fig. 7, namely that the infant blood mercury levels decline more slowly than those seen in the mother.

Despite the slower decline in infant methylmercury levels than those seen in the mother, no signs of methylmercury poisoning were seen in infants studied in the months of March to July of 1972 who had received only postnatal exposure to methylmercury. Figure 9 indicates the maximum recorded blood levels of infants having postnatal exposure to methylmercury. Most infants received methylmercury only from milk, but some infants may have received some directly from contaminated bread. Despite blood levels as high as 1000 ng/ml, no signs of poisoning were evident at this early stage after exposure. These and other infants having postnatal exposure are the subject of an extensive follow-up study, and it is possible that signs of methylmercury poisoning may manifest themselves as the infants get older. However, as these preliminary data stand at present, they offer no reason to suppose that the infant is unusually sensitive to methylmercury as compared to the adult.

A group of fifteen infant–mother pairs in which prenatal exposure had occurred were the subject of a report by Amin-Zaki *et al.* (1974b). Clinical evidence of methylmercury poisoning was evident in six of the fifteen mothers and in at least six of the fifteen infants. Five of the infants were severely affected, suffering from gross impairment of motor and mental development. The relationship between evidence of poisoning and the maternal blood levels is reported in Table III, taken from Amin-Zaki et al. (1974b). It may be seen that the fraction of those poisoned for a given range of blood levels in the mother is not significantly different in the infant versus the mother. In only one case was it found that the infant had signs of methylmercury poisoning and the mother was free of signs and symptoms herself. This is in marked contrast to the report from Minamata (Harada, 1966) in which evidence was presented that twenty-one infants were born suffering from severe cerebral palsy, whereas the mothers were free from or exhibited only minimal signs and symptoms of methylmercury poisoning. The reason for this difference is not known, but the Japanese infants were examined several years after birth, whereas the preliminary report on Iraq was based

TABLE III   Comparison of Frequency of Cases having Signs and Symptoms of Methylmercury Poisoning in Mothers and Their Infants[a]

Mercury level in maternal blood (ng Hg/ml)	Poisoned cases/ total cases	
	Mother	Infant
1–100	0/2	0/2
101–500	1/2	0/2
501–1000	0/4	0/4
1001–2000	3/4	3/4
>2000	3/3	2/3

[a] The mother–infant pairs were grouped according to the estimated blood level in the mother. The data are taken from Amin-Zaki et al. (1974b). The first blood sample from each mother was collected at different dates. In order to categorize the infant–mother pairs in the table, the mercury concentrations reported in the first blood samples were corrected to a common date (March 1, 1972) assuming a clearance half-time from blood of 65 days (Bakir et al., 1973).

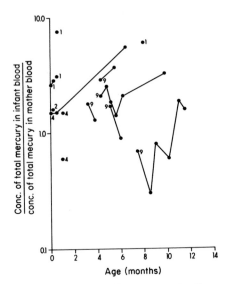

FIG. 10. The ratio of the total mercury in infants' blood to the concentration in maternal blood in infant–mother pairs according to the age of the infant. Points from the same infant–mother pairs are connected by straight lines. The numbers adjacent to the points indicate the estimated month in gestation when the mother ceased consuming the contaminated bread. Reproduced from Amin-Zaki et al. (1974b).

on studies within approximately 6 months of the outbreak. Mercury levels in blood of infants and mothers were not reported in the cases of prenatal poisoning in Japan.

In general, blood levels in the infants following prenatal exposure are always higher than the simultaneous blood level in the mother. The data in Fig. 10, taken from Amin-Zaki et al. (1974b), indicate that the blood levels at birth may be substantially higher in the infant than those seen in the mother, and this difference persists after birth up to a period of 12 months. One reason for infant blood levels higher than the mother's after birth is probably the ingestion of methylmercury from breast milk.

The ultimate question on the relative sensitivity of prenatal versus adult life has not been settled by the Iraq data. The reports of Amin-Zaki et al. (1974a,b) are only preliminary, based on clinical examinations in the first few months after the epidemic. At this time, the possibility cannot be excluded that the infants prenatally exposed and those postnatally exposed from milk may develop problems in mental and physical development at a later stage in life. There is a clear need for careful long-term follow-up studies on the infants exposed to methylmercury in Iraq.

There are no reports in literature of prenatal poisoning due to exposure to elemental mercury vapor. Substantial numbers of females of childbearing age have been and still are employed in industries where occupational exposure occurs. The absence of reports of prenatal poisoning therefore suggests that elemental mercury vapor may not present a significant hazard to prenatal life. Nevertheless, we do not know how carefully such effects have been looked for in exposed populations. The effects of elemental mercury vapor on prenatal life, if they were to occur at all, may not manifest themselves in the developing infant in the same way as they do in the mature adult. It would be reassuring to see the negative results of a carefully planned follow-up study of infants whose mothers have been exposed to elemental mercury vapor during pregnancy.

Studies on animals reported by Clarkson et al. (1972) indicate that elemental mercury vapor can cross into the fetus much more rapidly than ionic mercury. Data from the report is presented in Table IV, where it may be seen that the mercury content of the fetus is ten times higher after exposure to elemental mercury than following a similar dose of mercuric chloride. In contrast, the accumulation of ionic mercury in the placenta is much higher after $HgCl_2$ than that after exposure to elemental mercury vapor. When the mercury level in the fetus is compared to that in maternal blood, the distinction between the two forms of mercury is even more dramatic. The fetal tissue to maternal blood ratio is almost sixty times higher after exposure to metallic vapor than after an equivalent dose of mercury chloride.

The preferential transport of elemental vapor versus ionic mercury across the placenta parallels the same type of selectivity in the case of the blood–brain barrier. Elemental mercury vapor produces adverse effects primarily on the central nervous system, in distinction to ionic

TABLE IV   Maternal–Fetal Transport of Inorganic Mercury[a]

Form of mercury[b]	Mercury content (ng)		1 ml fetal blood
	Placenta	Fetus	
$HgCl_2$	0.8	0.01	0.003
Hg^0	0.2	0.11	0.2

[a] Data from Clarkson et al. (1972).
[b] Dose 0.1 μg Hg/rat.

inorganic mercury, which affects primarily the kidneys and gastrointestinal tract. The preferential transport of elemental vapor into the fetus warrants further studies on possible fetotoxic effects.

C. Interaction of Mercury with Other Chemicals

Except for reports of patients given mercury complexing agents, no information is available in man on interaction of other chemicals with mercury compounds. Studies by Ganther et al. (1972) on rats and Japanese quail suggest that the presence of selenium in the diet may diminish or at least delay the toxic effects of methylmercury compounds. The mechanism of this interaction is not known. If it could be shown that selenium were protective in man, the significance would be considerable. Certain species of oceanic fish, such as tuna, which are a source of methylmercury in the diet, also contain quantities of selenium, which could diminish the hazard from methylmercury. Unfortunately the dose–response relationships reported on the outbreaks in Japan and in Iraq do not report on the selenium levels in the populations in the study.

Elemental mercury vapor on contact with blood and tissues is oxidized to ionic mercury (for review, see Clarkson, 1972). The process of absorption, oxidation, and distribution to the brain is depicted diagrammatically in Fig. 11. Elemental mercury vapor, on entering the alveolar spaces of the lung, rapidly crosses the pulmonary membranes and dissolves in blood. The dissolved vapor rapidly crosses into the red cell where it is oxidized to ionic mercury. The process of oxidation is believed to be enzyme mediated, and Kudsk (1973) speculated that catalase may be the enzyme involved. Despite transport into and oxidation within the red blood cells, sufficient elemental mercury remains dissolved within the blood stream so that appreciable amounts are present when the blood passes by the blood–brain barrier, allowing diffusion of elemental vapor into the brain. In this tissue, it is believed to be oxidized to

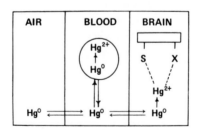

FIG. 11. A diagrammatic representation of the pulmonary absorption, transport, and oxidation of elemental mercury vapor. The structure of the binding site of ionic mercury in brain is hypothetical and is taken from the ideas of Weiner et al. (1962).

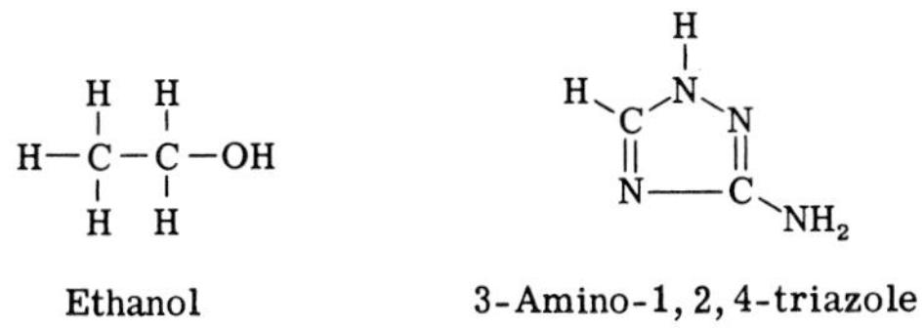

H H
| |
H—C—C—OH
| |
H H

Ethanol

3-Amino-1, 2, 4-triazole

FIG. 12. The chemical structure of ethanol and aminotriazole, two chemicals that inhibit the biotransformation of elemental mercury vapor.

ionic mercury. Once transformed into the ionic form, mercury rapidly reacts with protein sulfhydryl groups and is retained in the tissue.

The retention and deposition of elemental mercury vapor can be influenced by other chemicals, probably through inhibition of the oxidation process. Ethanol and the herbicide 3-amino-1,2,4-triazole, chemicals having no obvious structural similarities (Fig. 12), both produce similar and dramatic effects on the retention and distribution of mercury after exposure to elemental mercury vapor. Kudsk (1965) observed that the retention of mercury was dramatically diminished in workers ingesting moderate amounts of alcohol under conditions of occupational exposure to elemental mercury vapor. The data in Table V, taken from Magos et al. (1973), illustrate the effects of alcohol on the deposition of inhaled elemental mercury in rats. For example, the lung content in control animals was 17% of the inhaled dose as compared to only 1.5% in animals given alcohol. The reverse relationship was observed in liver tissue, where the content in controls was 2.7% versus 19% in the alcohol-treated animal. Brain and blood levels of mercury were also affected but to a less dramatic extent. Nevertheless, the ratio of blood to brain content of mercury was changed by alcohol, the brain content being approxi-

TABLE V   Effect of Alcohol on Deposition of Inhaled Metallic Mercury in Rats[a]

Tissue	Mercury content (% dose)	
	Control	Experimental
Blood	0.3	0.1
Brain	1.1	0.6
Lung	17.0	1.5
Liver	2.7	19.0

[a] Data from Magos et al. (1973).

mately three times the blood content in control animals versus six times the content in those given alcohol. The blood level of mercury is used as an indication of the level of mercury in the central nervous system. Mercury blood levels may give misleading information in people who have ingested alcohol.

Aminotriazole produces effects essentially similar to alcohol except that the levels in blood are not influenced to the same extent. This herbicide is an inhibitor of the enzyme catalase, and it may be that both alcohol and aminotriazole are inhibiting this enzyme, which may be responsible for the oxidation of elemental mercury vapor. These changes in the retention and deposition of mercury following exposure to alcohol or aminotriazole indicate the potential for modifying the toxic effects of this form of mercury. However, no studies have been reported to date measuring the effects of these chemicals on the toxicity of inhaled vapor.

IV. RESEARCH NEEDS

An improvement in our knowledge of the quantitative toxicity of mercury in man will always be an important research theme. Obtaining such information depends upon the availability of populations occupationally or accidentally exposed to unusually high amounts of mercury. From the public health point of view, elemental mercury vapor and alkyl mercury compounds are the two forms of mercury in most need of study. Studies should concentrate in that range of doses where adverse effects first manifest themselves. In the case of elemental mercury vapor, this dosage range would correspond to atmospheric levels of 10–100 μg Hg/m^3 and for methylmercury in range of dietary intake between 280–420 μg per day. Of special importance is the study of pre- and early postnatal exposures to both forms of mercury. These studies should include long-term follow-up observations on infants such as those recently exposed to methylmercury in the Iraq outbreak. The study of interactions between mercury and other chemicals is still in its infancy. Further research is needed on the effects of selenium on the toxicity of methylmercury and on the influence of alcohol and aminotriazole on the toxicity of elemental mercury vapor. Whereas the pharmacokinetics of uptake, distribution, and excretion of methylmercury in man are well described, little is known of the metabolic state of inhaled mercury vapor in human subjects. This lack of knowledge makes it particularly difficult to formulate accurate dose–response relationships for inhaled metallic mercury vapor.

V. SUMMARY

The dose–response relationship is the usual way of expressing quantitatively the toxicity of chemicals. This amounts to establishing a relationship between the estimated dose and the observed frequency of signs and symptoms of poisoning. Such relationships have been reported on human populations either accidentally or occupationally exposed to mercury compounds. This paper reports on the human toxicity of methylmercury compounds and elemental mercury vapor as these two forms of mercury are the most likely to be involved in human exposures.

The dose–response relationships for both mercury vapor and methylmercury share certain featues in common. The type of effect seen depends upon the dose. Symptomatic complaints (symptoms) appear at the lowest doses, whereas objective signs of poisoning are seen at higher doses. The first symptoms are not necessarily characteristic of mercury poisoning, and the key problem in interpreting dose–response relationships is to distinguish these symptoms from background symptoms due to causes other than mercury poisoning. Adverse health effects become manifest in occupational exposures to air concentrations of elemental mercury vapor above 100 $\mu g/m^3$. Effects due to elemental mercury vapor have been claimed at air levels in the range of 10–100 $\mu g/m^3$. The first detectable adverse effects of methylmercury in adults is paresthesia exhibited by a loss of sensation in the extremities and around the mouth. These effects become manifest at a body content of methylmercury in the range of 0.5–0.8 mg/Hg/kg body weight.

Factors influencing the toxicity of mercury in man have not been widely studied. Comparison of populations briefly exposed (Iraq) to populations undergoing long-term exposure (Samoa) to methylmercury suggest that the maximum body burden is more important in determining frequency of signs and symptoms than is length of exposure. Sensitivity to methylmercury depends upon age. A more generalized damage to the nerve system (cerebral palsy) appears to result from prenatal exposure. Evidence in laboratory animals indicates that various chemicals may modify the toxicity of mercury. Dietary selenium may reduce the toxicity of methylmercury. Alcohol and the herbicide aminotriazole dramatically influence the absorption and distribution of elemental mercury vapor. No information is yet available on the effects of these chemicals on the toxicity of elemental vapor.

ACKNOWLEDGMENT

This article is a review of some of the collaborative studies conducted by the faculties of the University of Baghdad (Iraq) and Rochester, New York. We are indebted to Dean Muallah of the Medical College, University of Baghdad and to Dean Orbison, University of Rochester School of Medicine for helping to arrange the interuniversity collaboration and to Professor F. Bakir, chairman of a scientific committee appointed to coordinate all studies of the methylmercury outbreak in Iraq. The University of Rochester acknowledges support from NSF (RANN) GI-300978 and NIGMS (GM 15190 and GM 01781).

REFERENCES

Amin-Zaki, L., Elhassani, S., Majeed, M. A., Clarkson, T. W., Doherty, R. A., and Greenwood, M. R. (1974a). Studies of infants postnatally exposed to methylmercury. *J. Pediat.* **85**, 81–84.

Amin-Zaki, L., Elhassani, S., Majeed, M. A., Clarkson, T. W., Doherty, R. A., and Greenwood, M. R. (1974b). Intrauterine methylmercury poisoning in Iraq. *Pediatrics* **54**, 587–595.

Armstrong. R. D., Leach, L. J., Belluscio, P. R., Maynard, E. A., Hodge, H. C., and Scott, J. K. (1963). Behavioral changes in the pigeon following inhalation of mercury vapor. *Amer. Ind. Hyg. Ass., J.* **24**, 366–375.

Bakir, F., Damluji, S. F., Amin-Zaki, L., Murtadha, M., Khalidi, A., Al-Rawi, N. Y., Tikriti, S., Dhahir, H. I., Clarkson, T. W., Smith, J. C., and Doherty, R. A. (1973). Methylmercury poisoning in Iraq. *Science* **181**, 230–241.

Berglund, F. *et al.* (1971). Methylmercury in fish. *Nordisk Hygienisk Tidskrift.* Suppl. 4.

Clarkson, T. W. (1972). Recent advances in the toxicology of mercury with emphasis on the alkylmercurials. *CRC Crit. Rev. Toxicol.* **1**, 203–234.

Clarkson, T. W., Magos, L., and Greenwood, M. R. (1972). Transport of elemental mercury into fetal tissues. *Biol. Neonate* **21**, 239–244.

Clarkson, T. W., Smith, J. C., Marsh, D. O., and Turner, M. D. (1974). A review of dose response relationships resulting from human exposure to methyl mercury compounds. *Proc. Conf. Heavy Metals Aquatic Environ., 1973* (in press).

Clegg, D. J. (1971). Embryotoxicity of mercury compounds. *In* "Mercury in Man's Environment" (Royal Society of Canada, ed.), pp. 141–148. Roy. Soc. Can., Ottawa.

Friberg, L., and Nordberg, G. (1973). Inorganic mercury—a toxicological and epidemiological appraisal. *In* "Mercury, Mercurials, and Mercaptans" (M. W. Miller and T. W. Clarkson, eds.), pp. 5–23. Thomas, Springfield, Illinois.

Ganther, H. E., Goudie, C., Sunde, M. L., Kopecky, M. J., Wagner, P., Oh, S. H., and Hoekstra, W. G. (1972). Selenium: Relation to decreased toxicity of methylmercury added to diets containing tuna. *Science* **175**, 1122–1124.

Harada, Y. (1966). Study on Minamata Disease. *In* "Minamata Disease" (M. Katsuma, ed.), pp. 93–117. Kumamoto University, Japan.

Kudsk, F. N. (1965). Absorption of mercury vapor in the respiratory tract in man. *Acta Pharmacol. Toxicol.* **23**, 250–262.

Kudsk, F. N. (1973). Biological Oxidation of Elemental Mercury. *In* "Mercury, Mercurials, and Mercaptans" (M. W. Miller and T. W. Clarkson, eds.) pp. 355–372. Thomas, Springfield, Illinois.

Magos, L., Clarkson, T. W., and Greenwood, M. R. (1973). The depression of pulmonary retention of mercury vapor by ethanol. Identification of the site of action. *Toxicol. Appl. Pharmacol.* **26**, 180–183.

Marsh, D. O., Turner, M. D., Smith, J. C., Choi, J. W., and Clarkson, T. W. (1974). *Proc. Int. Congr. Mercury, 1st, 1974* (in press).

MAC Committee. (1969). Maximum allowable concentration of mercury compounds (MAC). Report of an International Committee. *Arch. Environ. Health* **19**, 891–905.

Methyl Mercury in Fish. (1971). *Nord, Hyg. Tidskr., Suppl.* **4**.

Miettinen, J. K. (1973). Absorption and elimination of dietary mercury (Hg^{++}) and methylmercury in man. *In* "Mercury, Mercurials, and Mercaptans" (M. W. Miller and T. W. Clarkson, eds.), pp. 233–247. Thomas, Springfield, Illinois.

Smith, R. G., Vorwald, A. J., Patil, C. S., and Mooney, T. F., Jr. (1970). Effects of exposure to mercury in the manufacture of chlorine. *Amer. Ind. Hyg. Ass., J.* **31**, 687–701.

Weiner, I. M., Levy, R. I., and Mudge, G. H. (1962). Studies on mercurial diuresis: Renal excretion, acid stability, and structure—activity relationships of organic mercurials. *J. Pharmacol. Exp. Ther.* **138**, 96–112.

Author Index

Numbers in italics refer to the pages on which the complete references are listed.

Chesters, J. K., 307, *313*
Chetty, K. N., 282, 289, *299*
Chida, N., 192, 194, 208, 215, *228*
Chiemchaisri, Y., 29, *44*
Chisholm, J. J., Jr., 447, 449, *451*
Chitharanjan, D., 148, *159,* 169, 175, 176, *223*
Cho, G. J., 110, *130,* 142, *160*
Chodos, R. B., 83, 86, 92, *102*
Choi, J. W., 460, 461, 462, 463, *474*
Chow, C. K., 182, 184, 185, 188, 199, 200, 203, *221, 231*
Christophersen, B. O., 166, 171, *221*
Chutkow, J. G., 6, 13, *16,* 62, *74*
Ciambellotti, V., 209, *220*
Cibis, P. A., 206, *221*
Claffey, W. J., 250, *267*
Clarke, P. C. N., 8, *16*
Clarkson, T. W., 363, *369,* 454, 457, 458, 459, 460, 461, 462, 463, 464, 465, 466, 467, 468, 469, 470, 471, *474*
Clawson, A. J., 236, *246,* 282, 288, *300*
Clegg, D. J., 459, *474*
Clement, R. M., 53, *74*
Clements, F. W., 301, 305, *311*
Cline, M. J., 214, *226*
Clostre, F., 70, *76*
Coble, Y., 347, *366*
Coburn, J. W., 29, 34, 36, 37, 39, *45, 46,* 65, *76*
Coch, E. H., 139, *158*
Coffin, D. E., 406, *415*
Cohen, G., 166, 192, 205, *221*
Cohen, G. H., 447, *452*
Cohen, G. N., 139, *158*
Cohen, M. I., 8, *16*
Cohlan, S. Q., 310, *311*
Cohn, D. V., 31, *44*
Colby, R. W., 3, *16*
Cole, B., 363, *367*
Coleman, J. E., 241, *247*
Collier, H. B., 186, *222*
Collins, E. M., 207, *233*
Colucci, A. V., 435, 437, *440*
Combs, G. F., 306, *310, 311*
Comporti, M., 204, *221*
Conen, P. E., 9, *20,* 37, 39, *45*
Conner, T. B., 37, 38, 39, 40, 42, *44*
Conrad, M. E., 209, 211, *223*

Consolazio, C. F., 57, *74*
Constant, M., 206, *221*
Cooper, C. W., 33, *44,* 66, *73*
Cooper, M. R., 194, *221*
Cooper, W. C., 106, *129*
Cooperberg, A. A., 196, 197, *231*
Cope, O., 57, 63, 68, *73*
Corcoran, C., 147, *158,* 176, *223*
Cornatzer, W. E., 405, *414*
Cornblath, M., 209, *221*
Corneliussen, P. E., 406, *414, 415*
Cosens, G., 308, 309, 310, *312, 313*
Cotlove, E., 2, *21*
Cotta-Ramusino, F., 401, 406, *414*
Cotzias, G. C., 236, 237, 238, 240, 244, 245, 246
Couch, J. R., 206, *222*
Coughlin, L. L., 407, *415*
Court, J., 238, *246*
Cousins, R. J., 403, *414,* 436, *440*
Coussons, H., 55, *74*
Cowie, D. B., 139, *158*
Cowlishaw, B., 29, *44*
Cox, A. J., Jr., 403, *416*
Craig, J., 108, *131*
Craigie, J. S., 271, *278*
Creek, R. D., 239, *246*
Criddle, R. S., 136, 138, 139, 144, 146, 159
Crocker, W. C., 407, *415*
Csima, A., 29, 34, 35, 42 *46*
Cuevas, M. A., 108, 116, 121, *130*
Cummins, L. M., 107, 123, *129,* 144, *158*
Cuppett, S. L., 108, *131*
Curnutte, J. T., 193, *219, 221*
Curran, G. L., 94, *102,* 389, *397*
Curtis, P. B., 207, *221*
Cuthbert, J. E., 178, 209, 210, 211, *222*
Czerniejewski, C. P., 80, *102*

D

Dahl, L. K., 59, 60, *77*
Dalakos, T. G., 87, 88, *102*
Dale, E., 336, 337, 338, *342*
Dalgarno, A. C., 307, *313*
Dam, H., 198, *221*
Damluji, S. F., 457, 458, 459, 460, 467, *474*

Trashjian, A. H., Jr., 65, 77
Troughton, V. A., 31, 45, 65, 76
Trout, J. R., 403, 414, 436, 440
Truesdale, A. W., 205, 232
Truhaut, R., 401, 406, 414
Trump, B. F., 202, 219
Tsai, H. C. C., 239, 247, 302, 305, 311, 314
Tsang, R. C., 8, 9, 21
Tsay, D. T., 150, 162
Tsibris, J. C. M., 151, 161, 162
Tsubaki, T., 401, 406, 414
Tsuchiya, K., 401, 403, 413, 415, 435, 441
Tucker, S. G., 5, 16, 37, 38, 39, 44
Tudhope, G. R., 190, 192, 210, 216, 225, 233
Tupikova, N., 5, 19, 71, 76
Turk, D. E., 306, 313, 314
Turner, B., 118, 129
Turner, D. C., 106, 133, 141, 162
Turner, M. D., 460, 461, 462, 463, 474
Tuve, T., 138, 162
Tytko, S. A., 116, 132

U

Ugazio, G., 204, 233
Ulbrcy, D. E., 29, 45
Ullberg, S., 389, 399
Ullmann, W., 363, 367
Ulmer, D. D., 12, 21, 67, 68, 77, 401, 405, 416
Underwood, E. J., 240, 247, 250, 268, 274, 275, 278, 279, 302, 303, 314, 317, 345, 353, 354, 357, 369, 389, 393, 394, 399
Unge, G., 124, 130
Ury, H., 336, 342
Utley, H., 178, 201, 224
Utter, M. F., 242, 246

V

Valassi, K. V., 352, 353, 369
Valberg, L. S., 235, 247, 282, 300
Valentine, W. N., 167, 178, 179, 190, 209, 210, 226, 229, 233

Vallee, B. L., 12, 21, 63, 67, 68, 77, 80, 104, 241, 247, 272, 279, 385, 399, 401, 404, 405, 415, 416
VanBergen, F. H., 14, 15
Vance, P. G., 242, 247
Vander, A. J., 428, 430
Vanderhoff, G. A., 156, 159
Vane, J., 198, 229
van Heyningen, R., 204, 205, 206, 233
Van Itallie, T., 209, 224
VanWormer, D. E., 215, 219
Vargaftig, B. B., 197, 233
Vassallo, C. L., 194, 233
Vaughan, G., 204, 231
Vecchione, L., 206, 232
Veen, M. J., 328, 333, 345
Venkateswarlu, P., 250, 267
Vergin, H., 171, 224
Vernie, L. N., 120, 133, 156, 157, 162
Vessey, M. P., 335, 343
Vesterberg, O., 404, 415
Vetrella, M., 193, 209, 210, 233
Victor, M., 5, 19, 70, 71, 76, 78
Victor, N., 11, 21
Vigdahl, R. L., 197, 227
Vigliani, E. C., 436, 441
Vinton, W. H., Jr., 94, 104, 418, 419, 423, 430
Vinyard, E., 395, 398
Vitale, J. J., 29, 46
Viteri, F., 116, 118, 119, 125, 126, 128
Vivian, S., 385, 397
Vlasáková, V., 148, 162
Voelter, W., 168, 169, 174, 175, 176, 223
Vogt, M. T., 194, 233
Vohra, P., 386, 399
Vo-Khactu, K. P., 428, 429
von Sallman, L., 207, 233
Vorbeck, M. L., 52, 73
Vorob'eva, A. I., 352, 354, 358, 362, 363, 369
Vorwald, A. J., 455, 456, 475
Vostal, J. J., 363, 369, 401, 413

W

Wabnitz, C. H., 144, 160
Wachs, B., 251, 266
Wachsman, J. T., 139, 163

Cumulative Subject Index

Entries that refer to volume I are indicated by italic page numbers.